SECOND EDITION

Introduction
to
Clinical Pediatrics

Edited by

DAVID W. SMITH, M.D.
Professor of Pediatrics
University of Washington School of Medicine

W. B. SAUNDERS COMPANY
Philadelphia, London, Toronto

W. B. Saunders Company: West Washington Square
                           Philadelphia, PA   19105

                           1 St. Anne's Road
                           Eastbourne, East Sussex BN21 3UN, England

                           1 Goldthorne Avenue
                           Toronto, Ontario, M8Z 5T9, Canada

Library of Congress Cataloging in Publication Data

Main entry under title:

Introduction to clinical pediatrics.

    Includes bibliographies and index.

    1. Pediatrics.   I. Smith, David W., [DNLM: 1. Pediatrics.
WS100 1625]

RJ45.I58 1977   618.9'2   76–50157

ISBN 0–7216–8396–7

Introduction to Clinical Pediatrics   ISBN   0-7216-8396-7

Last digit is the print number: 9   8   7   6   5   4   3   2

To students

CONTRIBUTORS

E. RUSSELL ALEXANDER, M.D., Professor, School of Public Health, University of Washington School of Medicine

Immunization

MARVIN EARL AMENT, M.D., Associate Professor of Pediatrics, Chief, Division of Pediatric Gastroenterology, University of California, Los Angeles, School of Medicine Center for Health Sciences

Pediatric Gastroenterology

IRWIN D. BERNSTEIN, M.D., Associate Professor of Pediatrics, University of Washington School of Medicine

Malignant Diseases

C. WARREN BIERMAN, M.D., Clinical Professor of Pediatrics, University of Washington School of Medicine

Allergy Disorders

W. ARCHIE BLEYER, M.D., Assistant Professor of Pediatrics, Adjunct Assistant Professor of Medicine, University of Washington School of Medicine

Principles of Drug Therapy in Infants and Children, Hematology

RONALD L. CHARD, JR., M.D., Clinical Professor of Pediatrics, University of Washington School of Medicine

Malignant Diseases

RUSSELL W. CHESNEY, M.D., Assistant Professor of Pediatrics, University of Wisconsin School of Medicine

Parenteral Fluid Therapy in Children

M. MICHAEL COHEN, JR., D.M.D., Ph.D., Professor of Oral and Maxillofacial Surgery and Pediatrics, University of Washington Schools of Dentistry and Medicine

Oral Disorders

NORA E. A. DAVIS, M.D., F.A.A.P., Clinical Associate Professor of Pediatrics, University of Washington School of Medicine

Sudden Infant Death Syndrome

JACK M. DOCTER, M.D., Clinical Professor of Pediatrics, University of Washington School of Medicine

Cystic Fibrosis

PETER M. DUNN, M.A., M.D., M.R.C.P., D.C.H., D. Obstet. R.C.O.G., Consultant Senior Lecturer in Child Health, University of Bristol, United Kingdom

Congenital Postural Deformities

NANCY B. ESTERLY, M.D., Associate Professor of Pediatrics, Pritzker School of Medicine, University of Chicago

Skin Disorders

JAMES H. FEUSNER, M.D., Hematology-Oncology Fellow, Children's Orthopedic Hospital, Seattle, Washington

Hematology

MARC A. FORMAN, M.D., Professor of Psychiatry and Professor in Pediatrics, Temple University Health Sciences Center

Developmental Issues and Psychosocial Problems in Childhood: I. Normal Development and Minor Behavioral Problems, II. More Serious Behavioral and Performance Disorders

FRANK J. GAREIS, M.D., Clinical Instructor in Pediatrics, University of California, San Francisco, School of Medicine; Assistant Chief of Pediatrics, Department of Pediatrics and Adolescent Medicine, Naval Regional Medical Center, Oakland, California

Endocrine Disorders, Including Diabetes Mellitus

ROBERT D. GUTHRIE, M.D., Assistant Professor of Pediatrics, University of Washington School of Medicine

The Newborn

JUDITH G. HALL, M.D., Associate Professor of Medicine and Pediatrics, University of Washington School of Medicine

The Genetic Approach to Childhood Disorders

SHERREL L. HAMMAR, M.D., Professor and Chairman, Department of Pediatrics, University of Hawaii School of Medicine

Adolescence

ROBERT H. A. HASLAM, M.D., F.R.C.P.(C), Professor and Chairman, Division of Pediatrics, University of Calgary School of Medicine

Neurological Disorders

WILLIAM H. HETZNECKER, M.D., Professor of Psychiatry and Associate Professor in Pediatrics, Temple University Health Sciences Center

Developmental Issues and Psychosocial Problems in Childhood: I. Normal Development and Minor Behavioral Problems, II. More Serious Behavioral and Performance Disorders

HARRY R. HILL, M.D., Associate Professor of Pediatrics and Pathology, University of Utah College of Medicine

Prenatal Infectious Diseases

WILLIAM ALAN HODSON, M.D., Professor of Pediatrics, Head, Division of Neonatal Biology, University of Washington School of Medicine

The Newborn

JAMES R. HOOLEY, D.D.S., Professor and Chairman, Department of Oral and Maxillofacial Surgery, University of Washington School of Dentistry

Oral Disorders

ROBERT E. KALINA, M.D., Professor and Chairman, Department of Ophthalmology, University of Washington School of Medicine

Ocular Disorders

ISAMU KAWABORI, M.D., Assistant Professor of Pediatrics, University of Washington School of Medicine

Cardiovascular Disorders

C. HENRY KEMPE, M.D., Professor of Pediatrics, Director, National Center for the Prevention and Treatment of Child Abuse and Neglect, University of Colorado Medical Center

Child Abuse and Neglect

LuVERN H. KUNZE, Ph.D., Professor of Speech and Hearing Disorders, Duke University Medical Center

Hearing, Language and Speech Disorders

RICHARD E. MARSHALL, M.D., Associate Professor of Pediatrics, Washington University School of Medicine

History and Physical Evaluation

BEVERLY C. MORGAN, M.D., Professor and Chairman, Department of Pediatrics, University of Washington School of Medicine

Cardiovascular Disorders

JANET H. MURPHY, B.Sc., M.B., Ch.B., Instructor of Pediatrics, University of Washington School of Medicine

The Newborn

JAMES WYCHEMANIER OWENS, M.D., M.P.H., Clinical Associate Professor of Pediatrics, University of Washington School of Medicine

Infancy and Childhood

WILLIAM E. PIERSON, M.D., Associate Clinical Professor of Pediatrics, University of Washington School of Medicine

Allergy Disorders

JOHN L. PRUEITT, JR., M.D., Assistant Professor of Pediatrics, University of Washington School of Medicine

The Newborn

C. GEORGE RAY, M.D., Professor of Pathology and Pediatrics, University of Arizona College of Medicine

Common Infectious Diseases, Severe Life-Threatening Diseases

WILLIAM O. ROBERTSON, M.D., Professor of Pediatrics, University of Washington School of Medicine

Accidents and Poisonings

NANCY M. ROBINSON, Ph.D., Associate Professor of Psychiatry and Behavioral Sciences, University of Washington School of Medicine; Adjunct Professor of Psychology, University of Washington

Educational Intervention for the Mentally Retarded Child

MICHAEL BRUCE ROTHENBERG, M.D., Professor of Psychiatry and Pediatrics, University of Washington School of Medicine

Reactions of Children to Illness and Hospitalization

JANE GREEN SCHALLER, M.D., Professor of Pediatrics, University of Washington School of Medicine

Rheumatic Diseases (Inflammatory Diseases of Connective Tissues, Collagen Diseases)

BARTON D. SCHMITT, M.D., Associate Professor of Pediatrics, University of Colorado Medical Center

Child Abuse and Neglect

BILL S. SCHNALL, M.D., Clinical Instructor of Pediatrics, University of Washington School of Medicine
Common Pediatric Procedures

C. RONALD SCOTT, M.D., Professor of Pediatrics, University of Washington School of Medicine
Inborn Enzymatic Errors

WILLIAM E. SEGAR, M.D., Professor and Chairman, Department of Pediatrics, University of Wisconsin School of Medicine
Parenteral Fluid Therapy in Children

THOMAS H. SHEPARD, M.D., Professor of Pediatrics, University of Washington School of Medicine
History and Physical Evaluation, Common Pediatric Procedures, Prenatal Life

DAVID W. SMITH, M.D., Professor of Pediatrics, University of Washington School of Medicine
History and Physical Evaluation, Prenatal Life, Infancy and Childhood, Malformation, Growth Disorders, Mental Deficiency

FRED G. SMITH, JR., M.D., Professor and Chairman, Department of Pediatrics, University of Iowa College of Medicine
Renal Disorders in Childhood

NATHAN J. SMITH, M.D., Professor of Pediatrics, University of Washington School of Medicine
Nutrition in Infancy and Childhood, Including Obesity

LYNN T. STAHELI, M.D., Associate Professor of Orthopedics, Head, Division of Pediatric Orthopedics, University of Washington School of Medicine
Orthopedics

E. RICHARD STIEHM, M.D., Professor of Pediatrics, University of California, Los Angeles, School of Medicine
Immune Disorders

GARY THOMPSON, Ph.D., Associate Professor of Speech and Hearing Sciences, University of Washington
Hearing, Language and Speech Disorders

RALPH J. WEDGWOOD, M.D., Professor of Pediatrics, University of Washington School of Medicine
Historical Perspective, Common Infectious Diseases

RICHARD P. WENNBERG, M.D., Professor of Pediatrics, University of California, Davis, School of Medicine
The Newborn

DAVID E. WOODRUM, M.D., Associate Professor of Pediatrics, University of Washington School of Medicine
The Newborn

PREFACE

The purpose of this book is to provide a reasonably concise core of basic information about pediatrics that will allow the reader to rapidly achieve a basic plateau of knowledge about life and its disorders from conception until adulthood. This introduction should assist you in your pediatric clinical experience and allow you to move more rapidly toward higher level discussions with your teachers and in-depth knowledge about your patients and their problems. Thus it is hoped that this book will assist you in becoming more able in the task of improving the health and welfare of infants and children.

This book evolved from a University of Washington, Department of Pediatrics, student teaching synopsis, initially developed purely to assist our own students. Its popularity led to the publication of the first edition of *Introduction to Clinical Pediatrics* in 1972, with the co-editorship of Richard E. Marshall, M.D., who is now Associate Professor of Pediatrics at the Washington University School of Medicine in St. Louis. Though the second edition is still predominantly from the University of Washington Medical School, there are now a number of contributors from other medical schools in the United States, Canada and England as well.

We invite your participation in recommending future changes in this text. A questionnaire for this purpose has been set at the beginning of the text.

DAVID W. SMITH, M.D.

ACKNOWLEDGMENTS

Richard E. Marshall, M.D., now Associate Professor of Pediatrics at Washington University School of Medicine in St. Louis, was the co-editor and of great assistance in the development of the first edition of this text while he was at the University of Washington. Ralph J. Wedgwood, M.D., Professor of Pediatrics at the University of Washington, provided a great deal of support and many recommendations for the first edition while he was chairman of Pediatrics.

The editor wishes to acknowledge the assistance of the following individuals and departments in the development of the second edition of this text:

Mary Ann Sedgwick Harvey, M.A.: Ms. Harvey provided invaluable editorial assistance.

Christine A. Hansen: Ms. Hansen provided most valuable secretarial assistance.

Phyllis J. Wood: Ms. Wood and others in the University of Washington Department of Medical Illustration developed and prepared most of the illustrations in this book.

The Department of Medical Photography at the University of Washington.

The support of Beverly C. Morgan, M.D., Professor and Chairman of the Department of Pediatrics at the University of Washington, for the expanded second edition of this text is greatly appreciated, as were the recommendations of Waldo E. Nelson, M.D., the editor of editors, toward the reorganization of this second edition.

CONTENTS

QUESTIONNAIRE

This book is to be revised every three to five years, and we invite your comments toward its improvement.

NAME (*optional*):_____ Age:_____

Training status and location:_____

_____

Overall comments about the book:_____

_____

_____

_____

_____

Sections which should be revised, and comments:_____

_____

_____

_____

_____

Sections which should be added or omitted, and comments:_____

_____

_____

_____

_____

David W. Smith, M.D.
Department of Pediatrics, RD-20
University of Washington
School of Medicine
Seattle, Washington 98195

PART 1

BACKGROUND

1 Historical Perspective

Ralph J. Wedgwood

Children are the basic resource for all human endeavor. Mankind is dependent upon children, not only for the perpetuation of the species, but also for continued social evolution. As children thrive, so mankind may thrive. To the extent that any generation fails to fulfill this potential, mankind suffers. Children in a very direct sense represent man's only access to the future. Health of children has been of vital importance to all societies.

Modern pediatrics is concerned with the health of children and with the illnesses which affect their growth and development. The emphasis is upon optimal development, and upon disease as it affects development. Within the field are joined a historic concern for child health and special attention to children's diseases of more recent origin.

ANTIQUITY

In European civilization the separation of children's diseases and child health from other fields of medicine goes back to the beginning of recorded history. Hippocrates (460–370 B.C.) repeatedly refers to the special features of diseases in childhood; one of his treatises is devoted solely to the period of dentition. Aristotle (384–322 B.C.) continued the tradition, placing particular emphasis on generation, teratology, birth processes and early infancy. Celsus (before A.D. 5) stated that "children require to be treated entirely differently from adults" and described many childhood diseases and procedures, including infantile diphtheria, tonsillectomy and herniorrhaphy. Pliny the Elder (A.D. 23–79) recorded the first pediatric predictor of height—as good

today as it was 2000 years ago: at three years the length of the body is half that which it will eventually attain. Soranus (98–117) established the precedent for the joint consideration of maternal and child health. Galen (130–200), the authority in medicine for 50 generations of physicians, emphasized the need for special consideration of the nurture (and diseases) of children. Rhazes (850–932), who represents perhaps a more direct line to modern medicine, devoted an entire treatise to children's diseases—probably the first "pediatric text." Avicenna (980–1037) devoted large sections of his works to carefully organized, age-related discussions of child rearing and children's illnesses.

THE RENAISSANCE

The revival of learning in medicine after the Middle Ages came about with the invention of printing, and the first known medical treatise on any subject to appear in print was devoted solely to child rearing and diseases of children (Bagellardus, *Libellus de Egritudinibus Infantium*, Padua, 1472). It was followed within only a decade by two others (Metlinger, 1473; Roelans, 1483). Similarly, medical poems devoted to children, based on the *Regimen Sanitatis Salernitanum* (Arnald of Villanova, 1233–1312), appeared with increasing frequency. One of the earliest, written and printed in English, was Thomas Phayre's *The Boke of Chyldren* (London, 1553), although other popular maternal and child health texts in the "vulgar" had appeared before in other languages (e.g., E. Roesslin, *Rosegarten*, Strassburg, 1512).

The birth of modern medicine with the

encyclopedists and systematizers of the sixteenth century established a new trend, which has continued to modern times. Perusal of the compendia of such greats as Paré, Gesner and Mercurialis provides fascinating documentation for the recognition in the medical renaissance of the unique attributes and importance of maternal and child health, and child development.

THE AGE OF REASON

Entry into the era of modern science maintained tradition. The curious tracts of Nicholas Culpeper (1651) contain special pediatric sections, and Mauriceau's famous obstetric text (1668) contained 18 chapters devoted to children's diseases (which were included in the translation into English by Chamberlen, the "inventor" of the obstetric forceps). Sylvius, an anatomist, published a separate medical text on children in 1674. His student, Gower, included a treatise on rickets in his English translation (1682). These two texts introduce clinical detail (Sylvius was one of the first teachers to use the hospital for bedside teaching) and attempt to relate symptoms to pathology in a logical manner. Thomas Sydenham (1624–1689) brought his extraordinary skill in observation to bear on children, giving the first accurate, modern clinical descriptions of diseases such as scarlet fever, chorea and measles. The anatomist Willis (1621–1675) similarly portrayed epilepsy and whooping cough.

Thereafter many books solely on childhood diseases appeared, resembling the pediatric texts of today. The overpublished (18 editions in 50 years) book of Walter Harris in 1689 is probably the most famous. A rash of books on child upbringing—particularly on schooling—appeared in England and on the Continent in the mid-seventeenth century, extending the concept of child rearing beyond infancy (by authors such as William Petty and John Locke). In the beginning of the eighteenth century, attention was turned again to congenital malformations ("the influence of maternal impressions on the unborn"); in 1743 Andry's text, "Orthopedia," or "the art of correcting or preventing deformities in children," extended the field further, coined a new word in medicine and gave rise to the modern specialty of orthopedics.

THE AGE OF SCIENCE

It was still many years, however, before the treatises on child health ceased to depend on the authority of tradition and became based upon observation, deduction and experiment. In 1741 the Foundling Hospital was established in London. William Cadogan, appointed physician to the hospital, questioned many existing traditional practices. Suggesting that the hospital be used to introduce and study more rational methods of child care, he laid the cornerstone for modern infant hygiene as, 100 years later, Semmelweis laid the basis for obstetric antisepsis.

Over the next 25 years no one man is clearly identified with major general advances, although many great names appear with unique contributions: Desessartz's comparison of various milks for infant feeding; the founding by Armstrong of a dispensary for the infant poor, which led (after techniques had been developed to allow safe, artificial feeding of infants) to the establishment of children's hospitals; Home's descriptions of croup and his successful experiments with measles inoculation (similar to Lady Montague's variolation) are typical.

In 1765 a text came forth that established the author as one of the two founders of modern pediatrics. The book, "The Diseases of Children and Their Remedies," by Rosen von Rosenstein, Professor of Medicine at Upsala, discards quotation of ancient authority and refers systematically to the latest writers and contributions of scientific societies. The other work of equivalent impact was that of Michael Underwood, published in 1784. With Underwood, as Still comments in his history of pediatrics, the dawn of modern pediatrics and the proper study of child disease appeared.

THE BIRTH OF MODERN PEDIATRICS

The explosion of science and medicine in the nineteenth century makes it difficult to identify the parentage of modern pediatrics accurately thereafter. Certainly Jenner set a new basis for prevention of infectious disease through vaccination in 1796. Pasteur, Koch and their pupils provided the basis for immunization and serum therapy. Von Pirquet and Schick initiated the study of allergy; Ehrlich developed the basis for chemotherapy; Mendel outlined the basis for genetics; Darwin defined the basis of selection and mutation (and also described early child motor and personality development); and Freud founded psychiatry and delineated the impact of child rearing on psychologic development.

PEDIATRICIANS IN THE UNITED STATES

In no sense can child health be considered the domain of a single professional group. The field of pediatrics reflects the contributions and continued activity of many professions. Nevertheless, during the past century in the United States there has been an extraordinary development of the medical specialty "pediatrics," and the "pediatrician." Similar specialization has occurred in other health professions, e.g., in dentistry, nursing and public health. The emergence of the pediatrician in the United States is not unique; it exemplifies a general process.

As with much of American medicine, the development of the medical specialty of pediatrics was strongly influenced by German medical tradition. The first professor of pediatrics in the United States was Abraham Jacobi (1830–1919). Born and trained in Germany, he was one of many German physicians forced to emigrate because of political convictions. His initial official position (1861) was Professor of Infantile Pathology and Therapeutics at New York Medical College. In 1870 he was appointed Professor of Diseases of Children at the College of Physicians and Surgeons (Columbia University). In 1888 Harvard followed suit by the appointment of Thomas Morgan Rotch (1849–1914), who also was trained in Germany. L. Emmett Holt (1855–1924), through his efforts to establish the Babies' and Children's Hospital in New York, made it clear that in American medicine a new specialty had emerged. In 1888 the American Pediatric Society was founded, four papers being presented (one of them by Holt, and two by Jacobi, the first president). One year later there were 43 members. At the turn of the century, von Pirquet came to Johns Hopkins, and later Béla Schick came to Mt. Sinai Medical School in New York.

Pediatricians participated also in two other great changes in medicine. The first successful, truly full-time university clinical department was created at Johns Hopkins in pediatrics by John Howland (1873–1926), a student of L. Emmett Holt, who succeeded von Pirquet in 1911. Under Howland a group of American-trained pediatricians was developed, allowing the specialty to spread, both in practice and in medical schools throughout the United States. In 1929, at a meeting of the American Medical Association in Portland, Oregon, J. B. Bilderback and three pediatricians, feeling that the American Medical Association did not sufficiently represent the needs of child health or the practicing pediatrician, founded the American Academy of Pediatrics. In 1932 the Society for Pediatric Research was established through the efforts of J. L. Gamble (one of Howland's students). In 1933 the pediatric societies joined together to found the American Board of Pediatrics for certification of pediatricians.

Today in the United States, pediatrics flourishes as a medical specialty. The 43 members of the American Pediatric Society in 1889 have grown to 15,000 pediatricians. They have a justifiable pride in their origins and, with other health professions, have contributed significantly to the conquest of many childhood diseases.

The evolving emphasis on child health was not solely reflected by the activities of pediatricians, however. For example, in the late 1800's and early 1900's the state of children in the developing industrial and rural slums became of increasing concern to a variety of persons and agencies. In 1911, by legislative act, the Children's Bureau was established as a federal agency for the protection of the health and welfare of children. For many years the Bureau was ably directed by a student of Howland's, Martha Eliot. Through the Bureau a complex series of interlocking state and federal service and training programs for children were developed that continue to this day. These programs are characterized by their multidisciplinary nature and involve many health professions, of which pediatrics is one. Through this process and other similar programs (such as Head Start), the established medical specialty of pediatrics has become increasingly interrelated to the many other professions that provide child health services. Their combined efforts have achieved far greater contributions for the improvement of child health than would have been possible by any one of the professional groups alone.

PEDIATRICS TODAY

Recent history is difficult to condense. The generations from 1930 to the present have seen greater change than any other similar era. Child health in the United States has evolved from a private interest of the privileged few, to become a matter of public policy for all, as indicated by the establishment of the National Institute of Child Health and Human Development in 1963, and the Child Health Acts of 1967 and 1968. Both in the science and the public policy of health, change has occurred at an ever increasing rate. It is difficult under the circumstances to attribute change to individuals or specific innovations. The following is a biased view of recent progress; the historical validity requires time for proper perspective.

In 1930 the principal causes of mortality and morbidity in childhood were infections and nutrition. The main changes in the past three decades have undoubtedly resulted from improved standards of living and public health procedures — clean water, sanitation, housing and better food production and distribution techniques. In nutrition, milestones include the definition of nutritional requirements for growth — calories, protein and amino acids, vitamins and trace elements. Inexpensive artificial formulae for infants were developed that could be made readily available in a sanitary form. The identification, isolation and synthesis of vitamins gave these essential nutrients wide distribution. In the United States, although malnutrition still exists, rickets, scurvy, beriberi and goiter have virtually disappeared.

Better food also had impact on the scourge of infants — diarrhea and dehydration. Each summer in the 1920's and 1930's, epidemic diarrhea would crowd the hospitals, with its attendant death from dehydration. Understanding of fluid and electrolyte balance, along with nutrition, became the *sine qua non* of pediatrics. The classic studies of Gamble, Darrow, Butler, Cooke and Wallace provided the essential information to develop proper fluid replacement techniques for correction of dehydration and acidosis. The technical innovations of flame photometry and microchemical methods in the post-World War II years made this knowledge generally applicable so that while public health measures were eradicating the disease, the lives of those infants who did become afflicted could be saved. Today the knowledge gained on body fluids, renal physiology and homeostasis is applied to other diseases, e.g., diabetic acidosis and renal insufficiency.

In infectious diseases the impact of immunization and antibiotics has been equally extraordinary. Diphtheria immunization (Schick, von Pirquet) and pertussis vaccine (Sauer) have made these once common diseases rarities. Poliomyelitis has been virtually eradicated by isolation of the virus (Enders, Robbins and Weller), preparation and trial of killed vaccine (Salk and Francis) and live vaccine (Sabin). Similarly, measles has become a preventable disease; German measles, mumps and infectious hepatitis will probably follow suit shortly. The introduction of chemotherapy with sulfonamides (Domagk, 1935), following the developments by Ehrlich and the introduction of antibiotics (Fleming, Florey, Waksman), made possible the effective treatment of fatal infections such as pneumonia and meningitis. Understanding the epidemiology and pathogenesis of streptococcal infections and rheumatic fever has resulted in the virtual disappearance of rheumatic heart disease. Similarly, tuberculosis and congenital syphilis have become uncommon.

As these causes of morbidity and mortality disappeared, other causes of death and disability have become more apparent. Perinatal mortality has gained in public concern, for in spite of other advances the United States remains sadly behind many other civilized nations in infant death rates. Prematurity was given emphasis (C. A. Smith, Ethel Dunham, Levine, Gordon) in the 1940's, and a new specialty concerned with the perinatal period has arisen. Concomitantly, congenital and heritable defects have become an increasingly important area of interest. The classification of such disorders and the techniques for genetic analysis, such as biochemical screening and chromosome studies, have made identification and family counseling an important segment of health care. Advances in diagnosis and surgery have allowed repair of heart defects once considered fatal (Cournand, Gross, Blalock, Taussig), and even children with serious multiple defects such as meningomyelocele and hydrocephalus are no longer ignored and allowed to vegetate or die.

The residual mortality in childhood now bears little resemblance to that of a few years ago. After the neonatal period, the sudden death syndrome, cancer and accidents have replaced pneumonia, diarrhea and infections as the principal causes of death. Increasing emphasis has been given recently to attempts to reduce death by accident, including poisoning, through anticipatory guidance in the home, and with public health measures accompanied by new legislation. Some of the most effective mass screening studies for cancer chemotherapy have been carried out on children. In the past few years, attention to the sudden death syndrome has at least defined more clearly the epidemiology and provided facts for parental support.

It is a striking fact that when von Rosenstein and Underwood wrote their pediatric texts 200 years ago, three out of every four infants surviving the neonatal period died before the age of five years. Today, better than 99 out of every 100 infants will live to become adults. The issue is no longer survival of the individual child, but rather the quality of life for the future adult. The nature of society may be profoundly affected by the attention given to child health. Thus as the organic causes of death and disability have been diminished, pediatrics has become appropriately more concerned with optimal development than with disease. The provision of services so that all children grow up to participate happily, effectively and productively in our complex technologic society has become a primary concern. Such interests, reflecting those of antiquity, were marked in this generation by increased attention to child rearing and child development (Aldrich, Gesell, Spock). As a result, today there is greater awareness of those factors which contribute to perceptual, intellectual, personality and social development. Piaget, Skinner and Brunner have become as much a part of the vocabulary of the 1970's as fluid and electrolytes were 30 years ago.

THE FUTURE

Prediction of any human endeavor requires caution. Nevertheless some trends appear reasonably clear.

First is the immediate need for greater attention to the delivery of health services. A child who becomes ill with a preventable disease represents a failure in the delivery of health care. Inequality in access to and availability of health services for children has become unacceptable, to both the public and the profession. Pediatrics is not alone in this dilemma. The systems for the provision of all health services are under increasing pressure, criticism and analysis. The need for reorganization, redistribution and innovation has become apparent. The development of new ways and new professions to provide health services has emerged as an issue of high priority for the immediate future. Existing knowledge and skills must be made readily available to all children.

Second perhaps is better recognition that some health problems may be solved best by mechanisms unrelated to health care services. Environmental hazards and accidents, now principal causes of childhood morbidity and mortality, are excellent examples. Increasing attention needs to be given to the study of these conditions, in the same manner as was given in the past to the study of infectious diseases, so that the causal factors can be identified and preventive measures can be taken. Although this effort will demand the direct participation of health professionals, the steps required to eradicate this group of presumably preventable entities will depend upon other social, political and economic factors. There are many other health problems whose eventual solution lies beyond the domain of the health professions alone, including fluoride and dental caries, and economics or transportation and access to health services.

Third, we still know very little about many other childhood disorders that cause death and disability. It is axiomatic that prevention is better than treatment, but prevention requires knowledge. Although current emphasis is properly given to health services, equivalent emphasis and support must be given to the research that may provide solutions to these problems.

There are four general fields in which these problem areas can be grouped. One is the field of *developmental biology*. A significant number of the organic handicapping conditions in children today are congenital or heritable disorders. It is not unreasonable to hope that from understanding of the mechanisms by which genetic information is transmitted and translated into the development of the infant, we might be able to prevent or at least reduce the incidence of these often catastrophic occurrences.

Another field is that of *perinatal biology*. The eventual solution to the infant mortality and residual morbidity associated with gestation and birth probably depends upon our acquiring better knowledge of the physiologic processes involved in intrauterine existence, in the factors which result in labor and in the mechanisms necessary for adaptation to independent life after birth. Without such knowledge this critical period of life is left to chance.

The next most critical period of human life is infancy. During these months the most rapid development of intellectual and behavioral function occurs. Failure in development may well result in permanent disability. Prevention of the handicapping conditions attendant upon disordered development might be possible if we had a better understanding of the processes involved. *Developmental psychology* (using the term in its broadest sense) is a vital field of concern for child health; it and the influence of the environment on development should receive increasing emphasis.

The period of puberty and adolescence, the transformation of the child into a mature person, presents another critical time. The striking physical and behavioral changes of this period constitute the final milestone in the attainment of adulthood. Again, failure to achieve orderly development may result in a permanent handicap. Once the proper time for *maturation* has passed, it will never occur again. Equally, the field of maturation requires study so that we may acquire the understanding requisite for proper preventive and curative health services for youth.

These four fields—developmental biology, perinatal adaptation, developmental psychology and maturational development—are perhaps the new "basic sciences" upon which the future of pediatrics will depend. Each constitutes an exciting challenge, not only as a scientific field of its own, but also because any knowledge gained has relevance to the basic resource of all human endeavors—the next generation of children.

SUMMARY

Those involved in health services for children may look to the past with justifiable pride. The tradition for their roles stems from antiquity, and the record clearly notes their contribution to the conquest of disease. They can look forward with equally well based enthusiasm to the future, for they play a vital role in society—the provision of health care for the optimal development of each child, and the rearing of a new generation to become happier, more effective adults in a better world.

REFERENCES

Still, G. F.: *The History of Paediatrics:* The Progress of the Study of Diseases of Children up to the End of the XVIIIth Century. Reprint edition, Dawsons of Pall Mall, London, England, 1965 (originally published by Oxford University Press, 1931).

Major, R. H.: *A History of Medicine.* Springfield, Ill., Charles C Thomas, 1954, Vols. 1 and 2.

Faber, H. K., and McIntosh, R.: *History of the American Pediatric Society.* New York, Blakiston Division, McGraw-Hill Book Co., 1966.

2 History and Physical Evaluation

Richard E. Marshall,
David W. Smith
and Thomas Shepard

The medical evaluation of each patient should be related to his age and problem. The following are general points to consider in obtaining a history and physical examination. First, find a quiet place to talk. The person from whom the history will be taken varies with the age of the patient. For children up to the age of six years the information is usually obtained from the parents. From six years to adolescence it is often possible to obtain additional useful information from the child to supplement that supplied by the parents. Adolescents often do not wish to discuss their concerns in the presence of their family; hence, it is often advisable to talk privately with the patient at this age.

Ideally, it is important to obtain all the pertinent facts from history and physical examination before striving to achieve an overall diagnosis of the patient's disorder. Otherwise there is an insidious risk of making the facts fit a prematurely conceived diagnosis rather than the diagnosis fit the facts. This approach was emphasized by the physician-author Sir Arthur Conan Doyle through his character Sherlock Holmes.

There is no standard form appropriate for all patients. The following outline provides one general approach to the gathering of information. Additional recommendations for history and physical evaluation may be found in Chapter 8 on the newborn infant, Chapter 10 on the adolescent and in most of the chapters dealing with particular types of disorders.

PATIENT HISTORY

Chief Concern

This is basically the same as the chief complaint and constitutes a brief statement concerning the reason the patient is being evaluated.

Present Problem

This is comparable to the present illness and should be a complete story dating from the apparent time or age of onset of the problem.

Patient's Life

This is comparable to the past history and is usually divided into the following subsections. Depending on the age of the patient and nature of the problem, it is not necessary to routinely obtain all this information.

Prenatal. Age of the mother. It may occasionally be important to know whether the pregnancy was planned or not. Were there any maternal illnesses requiring medical attention? Did the mother take any medication other than iron, vitamins or mineral supplementation? What was the intake of alcoholic beverages during pregnancy? When was the onset of fetal activity? What was the duration of gestation and of labor? What was the mode of delivery?

The Genetic Approach to Childhood Disorders

3

Judith G. Hall

Nowhere in medicine are the variations among individuals more apparent than in the growth and development of children. Most of these differences have a genetic basis. All disease processes act upon the genetic constitution of the individual. Some disease processes or malformations occur primarily because of external, exogenous factors; others occur primarily because of internal imbalances or disharmonies in the individual. The internal forces of individual growth and metabolism are regulated by inherited determinants or genes, the chemical basis of which is DNA. Genetic information is expressed through the production and the control of the production of enzymatic and structural proteins in the cell. In genetic disorders, we postulate that at some time during development an abnormal amount or type of protein allowed abnormal function or structure to occur.

The genetic approach to pediatrics consists of asking the question, "Could this disorder, disease, malformation or condition have a genetic basis?" This question is particularly important for the better understanding of treatment and prevention. Individual genetic conditions may be quite rare, but the principles of clinical genetics are broadly applicable. Genetic disorders are usually experiments in nature in which a normal function or process is disrupted. Often, only because of its disruption, do we learn that the process even exists. Thus, through the study of rare genetic abnormalities we can learn more about the normal way in which our bodies function.

Definitions

Congenital means present at birth. It is not synonymous with genetic. Genetic factors may or may not be primarily responsible for producing congenital abnormalities and malformations. Conversely, hereditary conditions may be present at birth or may not appear until old age. *Inherited, hereditary* and *genetic* are used interchangeably, and they imply conditions that are dependent on genes for their expression. *Familial* is used in connection with disorders that occur in aggregation within families but may not have been proved to have a genetic basis. There are three main categories of genetic problems: chromosomal, single gene and multifactorial.

CHROMOSOMAL DISORDERS

Human beings normally have 46 chromosomes in each cell, present as 23 pairs that can be recognized according to size and shape. Each pair has been assigned a number. When the chromosomes of a cell are analyzed and arranged, it is called a *karyotype* (Fig. 3-1). Normally, one chromosome of each pair comes from the father and one from the mother, so an individual is truly genetically half his mother and half his father. Twenty-two of the pairs of chromosomes are normally identical. These are called the autosomes. The other pair is called the sex chromosomes. The sex chromosomes can be either X or Y chromosomes.

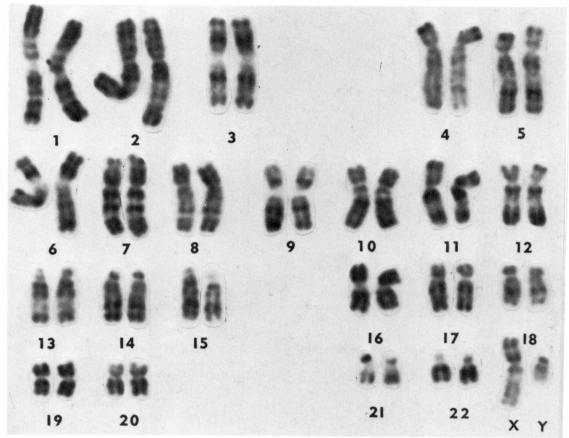

Figure 3–1   Karyotype of chromosomes from a normal male. Note X and Y chromosomes. Giemsa staining brings out the banding pattern on the chromosomes. (Courtesy of Dr. Holger Hoehn.)

Females have two X chromosomes, and males have an X and a Y. The presence of the Y chromosome normally leads to maleness.

Chromosomal disorders are present when there are abnormal numbers of chromosomes or an abnormal position of part of the chromosomal material; e.g., whole chromosomes can be missing, extra chromosomes can be present, small parts of chromosomes can be missing or in extra amount, parts of chromosomes can be in an abnormal position such as being stuck together (translocated) or broken up in abnormal ways. Occasionally, individuals have some cells with normal chromosomes and some cells with a chromosomal abnormality; these individuals are called *mosaics*. Abnormalities in any chromosome can occur, but only some are viable. As many as 50 per cent of early first trimester spontaneous abortions have chromosomal anoma-

lies. Children are more likely to be born with chromosomal abnormalities when there is advanced maternal age or when chromosomal abnormalities have occurred previously in the family.

If there is an abnormality of a chromosome, multiple systems of the body are usually affected. When a large part of a specific chromosome is missing or an extra chromosome is present, a characteristic pattern of abnormalities is usually seen. For example, trisomy 21 (an extra 21 chromosome) leads to Down syndrome, and 45 XO (a missing chromosome) leads to Turner syndrome. Each condition involving abnormal chromosomes is relatively rare (see Table 3–1), but 0.5 per cent of all viable newborns have a chromosomal anomaly. Recently, new techniques for staining chromosomes have allowed identification of small pieces that are missing or extra. The associated clinical features of such small

TABLE 3–1 FREQUENCY OF SOME
COMMON CHROMOSOMAL
ABNORMALITIES

	Frequency/Live Births
Trisomy 21	1:660
Trisomy 18	1:3500
Trisomy 13	1:7000
Turner, 45 XO	1:5000 (1:3500 females)
Klinefelter, 47 XXY	1:1000 (1:500 males)
47 XXX	1:1000 (1:500 females)
47 XYY	1:1500 (1:750 males)

chromosomal abnormalities are just beginning to be recognized.

When and how should chromosome studies be done? Usually, chromosomes are studied in the peripheral white blood cells after drawing sterile heparinized blood and culturing the cells for three to five days. However, skin fibroblasts can also be studied by growing cells from a specimen taken at surgery, skin biopsy or from an autopsy. In general, children with unknown patterns of malformation including short stature, mental retardation and multiple system abnormalities should have chromosomal analysis with banding. A family history of children with different patterns of malformation, multiple stillbirths or abortions should alert the physician to study the chromosome of the parents. Chromsome studies should be done when a chromosomal abnormality syndrome is suspected in order to establish the expected chromosome constitution of the child and to rule out translocation or mosaicism. If translocation is found, it may run in the family, and studies of the parents would be needed. If mosaicism is present, the degree of abnormality in the child may be less severe depending on the relative percentage of abnormal cells.

GENE DISORDERS

The second major category of genetic disorders is that of conditions caused by abnormal genes. Individually, these conditions are quite rare, but together they account for about 5 per cent of hospital admissions. They are the disorders usually thought of as genetic. On a biochemical level, a gene is thought to be a small piece of DNA that codes or controls the production of single polypeptide or protein. An abnormal gene is recognized when it produces an abnormal trait or disorder. Traditionally, the traits and disorders are said to be either dominant or recessive. A condition is dominant when only one abnormal gene is necessary to produce it. A condition is recessive when a double dose of an abnormal gene (e.g., two abnormal genes, one on each of a pair of chromosomes) must be present to produce it. The genes that produce dominant and recessive conditions can be carried on any of the autosomes or on the X chromosome. The specific position of the genes producing most known genetic conditions is unknown, but it is assumed that the position of a specific gene is always the same on a specific chromosome. Because genes are much too small to see on the chromosomes, chromosomal analysis is not indicated in disorders produced by abnormal genes.

Autosomal Dominant Disorders

In autosomal dominant disorders, there will usually be vertical transmission from one generation to another (Fig. 3–2). An affected individual has a 50 per cent chance of passing on the gene that causes the condition to each of his children. There is often a difference in the severity of the condition in affected individuals, even within the same family. We call this difference among affected individuals *variability in the expression of the gene.* In dominant disorders, there is usually some sign of the condition in a person who carries the abnormal gene. An autosomal dominant disorder, however, can be seen in an individual whose parents are not affected. Such affected individuals represent a mutation. The occurrence of new mutations in autosomal dominant disorders is associated with advanced paternal age. Autosomal dominant disorders include achondroplasia, neurofibromatosis, Huntington's chorea and the Marfan syndrome.

Autosomal Recessive Disorders

In families with autosomal recessive conditions, parents and grandparents are usually normal. There can be several affected children of both sexes in one gener-

DOMINANT
INHERITANCE

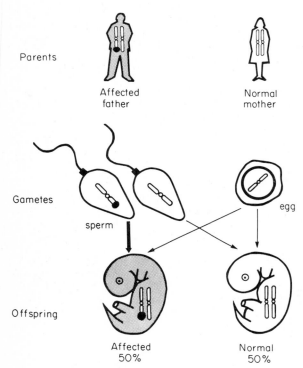

Parents

Affected
father

Normal
mother

Gametes

sperm

egg

Offspring

Affected
50%

Normal
50%

Figure 3–2   Diagram of inheritance of an autosomal dominant trait caused by a mutant gene.

ation. Often, in such a situation, a family says, "there has never been anyone affected in our family previously, so how can this condition be genetic?" In fact, this is exactly what we expect in autosomal recessive conditions. The parents are the carriers of the abnormal gene (in other words, have only one abnormal gene), and since the condition is recessive (and it takes two abnormal genes to produce it), they are not affected. In most recessive conditions the carrier state is perfectly normal, but a carrier can be recognized in some autosomal recessive conditions by specific biochemical tests. When two carriers have children, there is a 25 per cent chance of having an affected child each time they have a child, boy or girl (See Fig. 3–3). In addition, two thirds of their normal children will be carriers just as they are. Autosomal recessive conditions are much more likely to occur if relatives marry (consanguinity) since relatives are more likely to have the same

genes. It has been estimated that all of us carry five to eight genes that would cause serious defects or death in a child if we happened to marry someone else who carried the same gene. Well-known autosomal recessive conditions include cystic fibrosis, phenylketonuria and sickle cell anemia. Most inborn errors of metabolism have autosomal recessive inheritance.

X-Linked Disorders

Traits and disorders produced by genes carried on the X chromosome are said to be X-linked. They can be recognized by the pattern of inheritance within families. Since women have two X chromosomes, they are usually protected from having X-linked disorders by the normal gene on their other X chromosome. Since males have only one X chromosome, if they carry an abnormal gene on their X chromosome, they will manifest the abnormal condition. Most X-linked disorders are recessive and thus affect only males. X-linked inheritance is characterized by the presence of several affected males in a family with the condition being transmitted through apparently normal carrier females. Carrier females of X-linked conditions have a 25 per cent chance of having affected sons, a 25 per cent chance of having normal sons, a 25 per cent chance of having carrier daughters and a 25 per cent chance of having normal daughters (see Fig. 3–4). In some X-linked recessive disorders, such as hemophilia and color-blindness, when affected men have children all of the daughters will be carriers, since they receive their father's X chromosome carrying the abnormal gene (this is what makes them female), and all of the male children will be normal, since they receive his Y chromosome (see Fig. 3–4). Thus, one of the characteristics of X-linked conditions is that male-to-male transmission never occurs. When no previous family history of affected males is present, a new mutation in the affected boy or in his mother (making her a carrier) must be considered.

MULTIFACTORIAL INHERITANCE

The third type of genetic problem is called multifactorial or polygenic. Most of

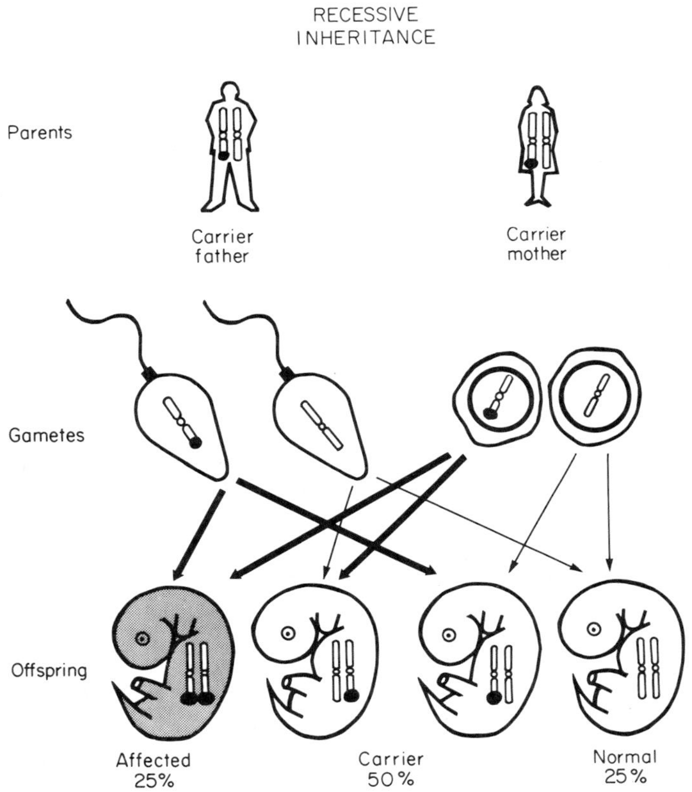

RECESSIVE
INHERITANCE

Parents

Carrier
father

Carrier
mother

Figure 3–3 Diagram of inheritance of
an autosomal recessive trait caused by a
mutant gene.

Gametes

Offspring

Affected
25%

Carrier
50%

Normal
25%

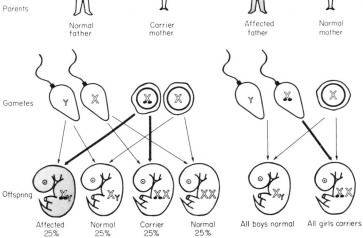

X-LINKED RECESSIVE
INHERITANCE

X-LINKED RECESSIVE
INHERITANCE

Parents

Normal
father

Carrier
mother

Affected
father

Normal
mother

Figure 3–4 Diagram of inheritance
of an X-linked recessive trait in a carrier female and an affected male.

Gametes

Offspring

Affected
25%

Normal
25%

Carrier
25%

Normal
25%

All boys normal

All girls carriers

TABLE 3–2   RISKS FOR SOME MULTIFACTORIAL CONDITIONS

	Incidence for General Population (Per Cent)	For First Degree Relative When One Individual Affected (Per Cent)	For First Degree Relative When Two First Degree Relatives Affected (Per Cent)
Common Congenital Defects			
Cleft lip and/or palate	0.1	2–5	9
Club foot	0.1	2–5	10–25
Congenital heart disease	0.5	2–5	10–15
Mental retardation (IQ <70)	2	6	10–20
Neural tube defect (anencephaly, spina bifida, meningomyelocele)	0.2	2–6	10
Common Diseases of Postnatal Life			
Allergies	18	40	—
Cancer	5	5–15× increased	—
Diabetes	1–5	5–15	10–40
Hypertension	4–20	8× increased	—
Schizophrenia	1	7–15	40
Seizures	0.5	3.5	10–15

these conditions are relatively common. They include many of the common malformations and many of the common diseases of adulthood (Table 3–2). The genetic mechanism involved in these conditions is poorly understood. It is felt that multiple genes (polygenic) as well as environmental factors play some role in producing this type of condition. Therefore, the term *multifactorial* is utilized. These conditions have been observed empirically to have an increased recurrence risk in families.

When discussing the recurrence risk in multifactorial disorders, we talk about the degree of relation: first degree relatives are parents, siblings or offspring; second degree relatives are grandparents, aunts and uncles, nieces and nephews, grandchildren and half-siblings. In general, in conditions that are multifactorial, if a first degree relative (that is, a parent or sibling) is affected with the condition, there is an increased risk that the next child born to the couple will have or develop the defect, while other relatives have relatively less risk of having affected children. The exact risks have been empirically determined and can be obtained for each condition by consulting appropriate references. Risk is usually influenced by race, sex, degree of severity in the affected person, age of onset and environmental factors that can sometimes be identified. If another affected child is born (making two first degree relatives), the risk becomes further increased in subsequent

pregnancies. Polygenic-multifactorial defects or conditions do not have fixed recurrence risks like single gene disorders but increase with the number of relatives affected (see Table 3–2).

When a specific disorder is diagnosed, implicit in that diagnosis is that it will occur in the family in a specific way. It is possible to identify the way in which conditions occur in families either by making a specific diagnosis or by analyzing the family tree.

FAMILY HISTORY

A very useful shorthand method for taking family histories is a pedigree. This involves drawing a diagram of the family tree by the use of certain symbols (Fig. 3–5). Circles are used for females, squares for males, blackened-in areas for affected individuals and an arrow to indicate the person who brought the family to attention. Lines are drawn between married individuals. Siblings are connected by lines drawn up and over. Parents and children are connected by lines from the marriage line to the sibship line. Information concerning a specific individual can be written under his symbol, i.e., name, age, illnesses, symptoms, age at death and cause of death. When taking a family history, it is common practice to ask about familial disorders and conditions that are known to occur fre-

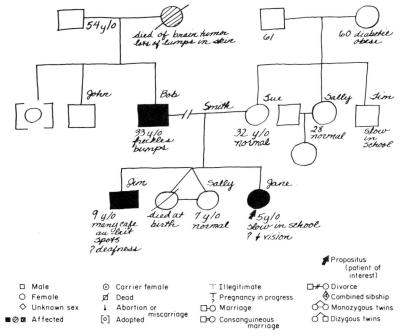

Figure 3-5 Sample pedigree and pedigree symbols.

quently in families, such as diabetes, hypertension, cancer and mental disorders. In addition, questions should be asked about any congenital malformations, stillborn children, intermarriage of relatives, the national background of the family, the age of parents at the time of birth of children, whether or not there are any other individuals with a problem like that of the individual in question and, if indicated, whom he looks like in the family.

Once a family history has been taken, it can be analyzed to make a determination of whether or not the condition is familial and specifically how it is occurring in the family.

ACCURATE DIAGNOSIS

A correct diagnosis is important in genetics since it implies a specific inheritance pattern and a specific natural history, no matter whether there has been a previous family history or not. Thus, if the diagnosis is not properly made, the wrong inheritance pattern and natural history will be expected by the family and patient. One of the problems in reaching a correct diagnosis is *genetic heterogeneity*. This concept implies that more than one condition can

have very similar clinical characteristics, but each has a different genetic basis. The problem of reaching an accurate diagnosis is further complicated by *pleotropism,* the concept that a single gene may cause multiple effects in different parts of the body. The abnormalities are not inherited as independent disorders but rather altogether since they are caused by one gene. Thus, in order to make a correct diagnosis, we must know what problems and complications can occur in a specific condition and the variability that is known to occur within a family. Finally, accurate diagnosis is dependent upon knowing the age of onset of the specific complications of the disorder. Some conditions, such as Huntington's chorea, do not usually have onset until middle or late middle age. Others are present at birth or prenatally. Genetic disorders are known that have onset during every age period in life. Generally, a specific condition has a fairly characteristic age of onset, and this may help in arriving at an accurate diagnosis.

MUTATIONS

Changes in the genetic information of an individual can occur, and these are called

MUTATION
IN GAMETE

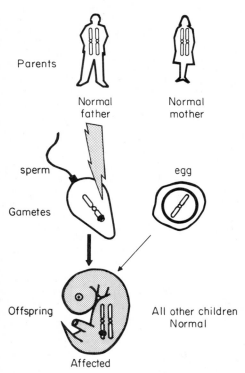

Figure 3–6 Diagram of a new dominant mutation.

PRENATAL DIAGNOSIS

Prenatal diagnosis is the process of diagnosing whether or not a fetus has a particular abnormality prior to birth. Many parents would not have children if they felt there was a significant risk of having a child with a serious abnormality. Prenatal diagnosis is performed when the family is known to be at risk for an abnormality, but it is not yet available as a screening technique. The implication is that if an abnormal fetus is found by prenatal diagnosis, most families would choose to have an abortion, but this is left up to the individual family. Most often, the prenatal test is normal, and the family can be reassured that the fetus does not have the abnormality. They can never be told that they will have a perfectly normal child since there is no way of testing for that.

Several techniques for prenatal diagnosis are available. They include amniocentesis, ultrasound, roentgenography, fetoscopy, electroencephalogram and electrocardiogram. The most common test used at this time is amniocentesis, which is the process of taking some of the amniotic fluid to examine the fetal cells or the chemical content of the fluid. When used for prenatal diagnosis, the procedure is done between 14 and 18 weeks of gestation and would appear to have only minimal risk to mother or fetus (less than 0.5 per cent complication rate). Most often, the fetal cells are cultured so biochemical or chromosomal studies can be performed, but the amniotic fluid may be analyzed directly as well.

The most frequent indication for amniocentesis is advanced maternal age, since with advancing age the mother has an increased risk of having a child with a chromosomal anomaly. It is now generally advocated that all pregnant women over 35 years of age have amniocentesis. However, if there has been a chromosomally abnormal child previously in the family, the risk of having another chromosomally abnormal child is increased, and such a mother should have access to amniocentesis at any age. If either parent is a carrier of a chromosomal translocation, amniocentesis should be done. In X-linked disorders in which the diagnosis of the condition cannot be made prenatally but the sex of the fetus can be determined, amniocentesis can de-

mutations. The concept implies that usually genetic information is passed on unaltered from parent to child. Mutations are recognized when they produce an autosomal dominant disorder, in an individual whose parents are unaffected (Fig. 3–6). When an individual has a dominant condition and neither of his parents had it, we recognize that a "mutation" or change in the genetic information of the affected individual has occurred. We do not usually recognize mutations in genes for recessive or X-linked conditions. Once a mutation has occurred, the individual carrying the mutant gene can pass on the abnormal gene to his children. Mutations are known to be caused by a number of environmental factors, such as drugs, chemicals, illnesses and irradiation (this is the reason for gonadal shields when taking x-rays), and they increase in frequency with older paternal age.

termine whether the fetus is the sex at risk for having the disorder. And finally, amniocentesis should be available to all families with a history of a child with a neural tube defect (anencephaly, multiple vertebral defects, meningomyelocele, hydrocephalus), since most cases of neural tube defects can be diagnosed prenatally. Other indications for amniocentesis or any of the other techniques of prenatal diagnosis are extremely varied. Some inborn errors of metabolism can be diagnosed prenatally. When there is a family with an increased risk of having a child with an abnormality, one should ask the question: Could this condition be diagnosed prenatally and how? It is the responsibility of the physician to suggest that this kind of procedure should be available in a future pregnancy.

GENETIC COUNSELING

Genetic counseling is the process of educating a family about their situation so parents can make an informed decision for themselves about whether or not to have more children and how to best manage an affected individual. Because genetic counseling is a process of education, it is important to do background reading in order to be familiar with the condition so that one can educate the family properly.

The process of genetic counseling involves five specific areas. The first is diagnosis: how the diagnosis was arrived at and what the diagnosis is. Second is the natural history of the disorder: the extent of the disorder, how severe it can be, how mild, what complications can be expected. The third is the recurrence risk: for parents, for a normal child, for affected individuals and for other relatives. The fourth is prevention: of complications and of future affected children. This may include prenatal diagnosis and contraceptive information. The fifth is therapy: specific symptomatic therapy and other kinds of preventative therapy, such as physical therapy, psychological help, social services and community facilities.

REFERENCES

McKusick, V. A.: *Mendelian Inheritance in Man. Catalog of Autosomal Dominant, Autosomal Recessive, and X-Linked Phenotypes.* Baltimore, Johns Hopkins University Press, 1975.

Nora, J. J., and Fraser, F. C.: *Medical Genetics.* Philadelphia, Lea & Febiger, 1974.

Stevenson, A. C., Davison, B. C. C., and Oakes, M. W.: *Genetic Counselling.* Philadelphia, J. B. Lippincott Co., 1970.

Thompson, J. S., and Thompson, M. W.: *Genetics in Medicine.* 2nd ed. Philadelphia, W. B. Saunders, 1973.

4 Reactions of Children to Illness and Hospitalization

Michael B. Rothenberg

The "FAGS syndrome" represents a mnemonic device created to focus on four critical reactions of children to illness or hospitalization. These reactions—fear, anger, guilt and sadness—are shared by the child, his family and the professional. Although they are most prominent in relation to serious illness or hospitalization, they exist to some extent every time a child becomes ill. The degree to which these reactions can affect everyone's response to the child's illness, and even the course of the illness itself, warrants a closer examination.

THE "FAGS SYNDROME"

In the following diagrammatic representation it becomes clear that each of the four critical reactions may manifest itself in one of two behavior patterns, and that, depending on which of the two patterns is manifested by the patient, he may be labeled as "good" or "bad." Which of the two patterns appears in a given patient will be determined by a combination of factors derived from his premorbid personality and from the total milieu in which he currently has become ill.

		"Bad" Patient	"Good" Patient
FEAR	Panic and agitation	+	
	Anxious withdrawal		+
ANGER	Disruptive behavior	+	
	Depression and immobilization (anger withheld because of fear or guilt)		+
GUILT	Anger at being made to feel guilty, with disruptive behavior	+	
	Withdrawal, out of shame or fear of punishment		+
SADNESS	Agitation, with crying or clinging	+	
	Quiet withdrawal, e.g., to thumbsucking, stuffed animal		+

It can be seen that the patient who is least able to express his feelings openly and directly, and who in this sense requires the most help, will often have the least attention paid to his emotional reactions and needs. If we substitute the parent for the patient in our diagrammatic representation, it becomes obvious how the parent–health professional relationship can be affected by each of the reactions, espe-

22

cially if the professional is unaware of the emotion beneath each behavior pattern. Finally, the health professional may experience each of these reactions, and the less he is aware of them, the more likely it is that they may deleteriously affect his functioning to help the patient.

An added note is necessary about sadness. This is the reaction least often recognized, partly because it is confused with depression. Sadness is a reaction to loss. In the frame of reference of this discussion, loss may be represented by: (1) a child's loss of his family (due to his hospitalization) and of his normal routines altogether, (2) the family's similar loss or (3) the health professional's loss of competence (when the patient has a chronic disease) or of his patient altogether (when his patient has a fatal disease). Although depression may involve loss, its distinguishing characteristic is that it always involves withheld anger and therefore demands a different therapeutic response.

"THE 3-D REACTION"

This is another mnemonic device, created to remind us of the normal child's triphasic reaction to separation from his family. This reaction is seen primarily in children between the ages of approximately nine months and four years, and is especially important when the separation results from illness and hospitalization.

For mnemonic purposes, I have called the first phase, lasting approximately from 24 to 72 hours after separation, the phase of *dismay.* Here we see the agitated child crying loudly, calling for his parents, utterly inconsolable — and more than likely labeled a "bad" patient! Phase one gives way to the phase called *despair,* which may last several days or more. Now we are presented with a "good" patient, one who lies quietly in his crib or bed, or sits impassively in a chair in front of the ward television, heavily "sedated" with a compound of sadness and depression. The third phase is that of *denial,* and is the one most likely to be overlooked altogether. The child, with his normal great capacity to simply deny the existence of what is distasteful to him, appears cooperative and uncomplaining and

indeed may carry on his daily routines as if he were not even in a hospital. Needless to say, he will be seen by one and all as a "good" patient.

The importance of recognizing this triphasic reaction is that the recognition makes it possible for the health professional to respond to each phase appropriately. The phase of dismay will require support and reassurance, to allow the child's grief to be vented. Although younger children, particularly, may be distracted, an attitude of "Now, now, don't you cry — you're a big boy, aren't you?!" is clearly contraindicated. The therapeutic response to despair will entail giving the child the opportunity to express his sadness or anger verbally. The "third person technique," described later, is most useful in this regard. The response to denial requires the longest clinical experience for the development of real expertise. Here, again leaning heavily on the third person technique, the health professional must find the sometimes hazy line between permitting the child sufficient ventilation to reduce underlying conflicts and fostering so much ventilation of underlying material that the vital and normal defense mechanism of denial cannot be used at all by the patient.

SOME COMMON PSYCHOLOGICAL DEFENSE MECHANISMS

Emotionally normal children may use many psychological defense mechanisms to handle the stress of physical illness. It is not the intent of this chapter to cover such a subject in detail. A working knowledge of some of the most common of these mechanisms can be very helpful to the pediatrician on a day-to-day basis, however.

Perhaps the most common, and certainly the most easily detected defense mechanism is *regression.* This represents a situation in which a child, in the face of stress and without any conscious intent, moves backwards in his psychosocial growth and development to a point at which he received, in times past, more protection from his total environment. For example, we may find a child returning to thumb-sucking, to soiling or wetting, to having difficulty feeding himself, or to infantile speech patterns.

Denial, the capacity to simply deny the existence of that which is distasteful to him, is a defense mechanism used constantly by the normal child in sickness and in health. If we were to plot the amount of denial against chronological age on a simple graph, we would find that the normal limits of denial decrease as age increases, until the two lines cross as the child reaches adolescence. Thus, the pediatrician may accept a fairly massive amount of denial of illness as within normal limits in the young child. A similar amount of denial in the adolescent, however, would raise the doctor's suspicion concerning the patient's capacity to utilize normal psychological defense mechanisms.

Reaction formation is the mechanism by which the child will form a reaction against what he is feeling by manifesting exactly the opposite behavior. This is most often seen in excessive compliance with the orders of all personnel, total cooperation during all procedures and perhaps even "falling in love" with the doctor or nurse. The functional importance of recognizing such a reaction is that it is invariably covering up a great deal of anger and resentment.

Identification with the aggressor is most commonly seen in children who have undergone many procedures, especially plastic surgery. This is somewhat similar to the reaction formation just described in the sense that we are presented with a child who informs everyone that he has decided to become a doctor, usually a doctor just like the one who is most involved in subjecting him to painful procedures. This mechanism has been given the subtitle, "turning passive into active." This simply means that, by identifying with his doctor, the child may psychologically turn away from his passive position as the helpless recipient of painful procedures and see himself instead as the active party who controls the situation and inflicts these procedures.

Displacement refers to the mechanism by which an emotion initially directed at one person by the child creates too much anxiety in him because of his relationship with that person, leading the child to displace the same emotion onto a less anxiety-provoking person. Thus, the child's anger at his parents for failing to visit him at the hospital, for example, may be displaced onto his doctors and nurses.

Projection is a defense mechanism whereby one's own emotion, too anxiety-producing to be accepted as one's own, is projected instead onto someone else who is then seen as having the emotion in question. The angry child, for example, may perceive his doctor as being angry at him, unaware that this is his (the child's) own anger.

Finally, we may find *isolation of affect* in children from about the age of five onward. Here the physician is confronted with the child who talks about his feelings in an intellectualized manner as a substitute for making contact with and directly manifesting these feelings.

The functional importance of the health professional recognizing these psychological defense mechanisms lies in the consequent ability to penetrate the defenses sufficiently to be able to give the child the opportunity for therapeutic ventilation, with support and reassurance concerning anxieties about his illness. We elaborate on this in the last section of this chapter.

SPECIAL PROBLEMS OF THE INJURED CHILD

The injured child may view his accident and subsequent injury as "punishment" for real or imagined errors of omission or commission. This is particularly true if the child was engaged in some forbidden activity at the time of his injury.

If others are injured in the same accident, especially if they are more seriously injured or killed, the child may feel inordinately guilty about his being "spared." Such guilt may also arise because his preaccident fantasies or wishes for injury to or death of his parents or siblings apparently have come true. Young children normally have many omnipotent feelings and fantasies and can become quite terrified when it appears that their fantasies have become fact.

It must also be remembered that the parents and siblings of the injured child may feel inordinate guilt about the patient because of their own past destructive wishes or fantasies about the child. The guilt of siblings following the sudden infant death syndrome ("crib death") is a striking example of this situation. Clearly, the person attempting to provide comprehensive care will view the exploration of such feelings with the family as his responsibility.

The guilty patient will often feel that he does not deserve the care he is receiving, and may even resist therapeutic procedures on this basis. Guilt is an uncomfortable feeling and normally leads the person to feel angry at those who cause guilt feelings. Thus it is not uncommon to find a vicious circle of guilt, anger and more guilt (at being angry at those who are trying to help) building up rapidly. The health professional may therefore find himself with an angry child resistive to treatment. This can lead to his becoming frustrated, angry and guilty himself if he fails to recognize and then explore this reaction in the child.

WHAT CAN THE HEALTH PROFESSIONAL DO?

This welter of reactions and defense mechanisms requires only one response. The professional must *talk to the child,* and in so doing provide the answers for the following six questions, always present, but seldom explicitly stated:

1. What do I have?
2. How did I get it?
3. Why did I get it?
4. Will I get well?
5. When will I get well?
6. Why did my parents leave me in the hospital?

The question, "Will I get well?" includes all the questions that are concerned with the specific procedures and medications involved in the child's treatment. The sixth question is usually encountered with the younger child who is experiencing "the 3-D reaction" already described. It is important to note that the fifth question, *"When* will I get well?" is the most frequently asked, and that is often the *only·* question asked. This is because the other questions frequently are so anxiety provoking that the only one the child or his parents are able to verbalize is, "When will I go home?" The repetition of this question in the face of specific answers should alert the health professional to the probable inability of the patient to articulate the other questions.

All these questions have to be answered for the parents and, through them, the siblings as well. Remember also that answering these questions only once will rarely suffice to provide the comprehensive care to which we are addressing ourselves here. The first answers will inevitably undergo some distortion as they are filtered through the patient's defense mechanisms, and at least one more session of clarification is critical.

I have found that a three-step process is most productive when talking to children. First, ask the child to tell you whatever he can about his own ideas and feelings in regard to these questions. Second, use the third person technique, again giving the child maximum opportunity to respond with further ideas and feelings. Here you approach the child with something like, "You know, lots of times kids with your kind of sickness find themselves thinking (feeling) . . ." (whatever you suspect is going on); "Does that make sense to you?" This gives the child three options (the "option play"): (1) it does not make sense, (2) it makes sense, but does not apply to him or (3) it makes sense and in fact is just what he has been thinking or feeling. The third step involves providing the child with the necessary factual information, i.e., the truth. When the next chat takes place, start back again at the first step in this process.

This three-step process for talking with children allows one to get at feelings behind defenses. What is important is that the child hear the truth. It is not necessary for him to drop all his defenses in order to have his anxieties allayed, and the professional must not insist that the child reveal all the feelings behind his defenses. It is sufficient for the child to know that his health professional is ready and willing to talk to him and that he is not afraid of the truth.

REFERENCES

Bergman, A. B., and Schulte, C. J. A. (Eds.): Care of the child with cancer. Pediatrics (Supplement), 40:507, 1967.

Kohlberg, I. J., and Rothenberg, M. B.: Comprehensive care following multiple, life-threatening injuries—treatment of an adolescent boy. Am. J. Dis. Child., 119:449, 1970.

Senn, M. J. E., and Solnit, A. J.: *Problems in Child Behavior and Development.* Philadelphia, Lea & Febiger, 1968, pp. 227–230.

Wolf, R. E.: The hospital and the child. *In* A. J. Solnit and S. A. Provence (Eds.): *Modern Perspectives in Child Development.* New York, International Universities Press, Inc., 1963, pp. 409–418.

Wolff, S.: Illness and Going to the Hospital. *In* Wolff, S.: *Children Under Stress.* London, Penguin Press, 1969. (This is the most important of the five references.)

5

Common Pediatric Procedures

Bill Schnall and Thomas Shepard

This chapter illustrates and describes a number of common clinical procedures that are unique to pediatrics. These techniques should be regarded as core skills for the medical student. The student should observe a demonstration and be supervised by an experienced practitioner while learning these procedures.

The *3-times label check* has been in standard use by pharmacists and nurses for many years, but medical students seldom are aware of the technique. It consists of the following:

1. When a medication is removed from the shelf or medical bag, *check the label.*
2. When the syringe or dispenser is loaded, *check the label.*
3. When the medication is returned to storage, *check the label.*

When another person is loading a syringe for your use, ask that person to load it in your line of sight so that you can check the label.

RESTRAINING TECHNIQUES

Clove hitch cloth restraint. For the hospitalized infant and child, restraint of one or more extremities is often necessary. A fairly coarse type of cloth has the advantage that it does not become jammed or create increasing compression with circulatory restriction in the periphery. It is essential that the restraint be attached to the bedside in a way that allows the lowering of the crib siding without injury to the child (see Fig. 5–1).

Mummifying restraint. In the infant and younger child this is used to restrain the whole body in situations in which gastric lavage or external jugular blood drawing are necessary. One arm may be left free for blood drawing. The procedure using a sheet is illustrated in Figure 5–2a to e.

INJECTION TECHNIQUES

Several different routes of administration, as well as many different sites, are available for the injection of numerous medications. Selection of each is based upon the particular situation, while bearing in mind the differences in onset of action,

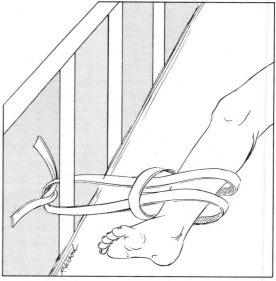

Figure 5–1 Clove hitch restraint. See text for explanation. Figures 5–1 through 5–9 were drawn by Phyllis Wood, A.M.I., Health Sciences Illustration, University of Washington.

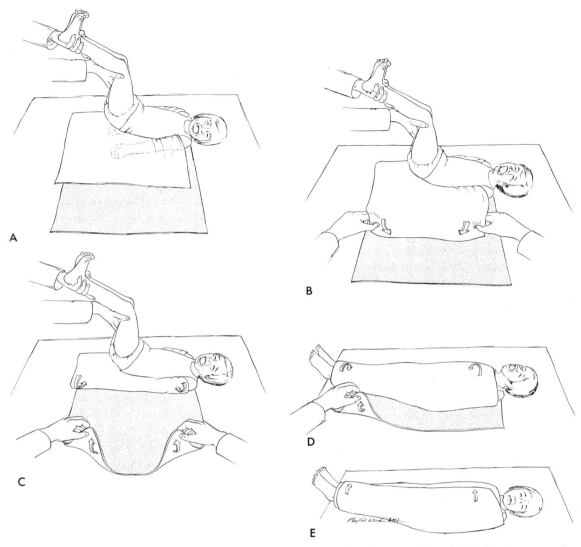

Figure 5–2 Mummifying restraint. The restraining sheet is placed under the child and folded back, pinning the arms down (*A*). Next, the sheet is tucked back under the child's left arm (*B*). The sheet is then wrapped around the entire child (*C, D, E*) and may be fastened with a safety pin.

degree of absorption, trauma to the patient, age and ease of administration, the volume to be injected and whether or not continuous infusion will be necessary (see Chapter 6).

One of the great anxieties among pediatric patients is "the shot." Mention of the word often precipitates fear, crying, acting-out behavior and sometimes even hysteria. Much of this reaction is due to previous negative experiences and is not simply isolated to the pain of the procedure itself but to the atmosphere and attitudes of those adults involved. This must always be kept in mind and a positive approach should be taken. Parents should never threaten a child with a "shot" as punishment for misbehavior in the physician's office; in fact, in most circumstances, the parent should be excused from the room during the procedure so that the child does not associate the experience with the parent. The child should *not* be told that it "won't hurt" because it obviously will. Instead, the procedure should be explained at the child's level of comprehension, and specific information such as "there will be a little stick" should be given at the appropriate time.

Pain from an injection can be decreased by a few simple techniques:

1. Use the smallest gauge needle that still permits easy flow of the injection material.

2. Use alternate sites if recurrent injections are involved.

3. The solution for injection should be at, or near, room temperature.

4. Do not inject more than 2 ml at any site (except for intravenous).

5. The site should be dried of the antiseptic solution before injection. Any alcohol carried in with the needle can be very painful.

6. Apply *dry* cotton or bandage to the site after withdrawal.

Intradermal injection is used for various immunological procedures. Using a tuberculin syringe of 0.5 to 1.0 ml with a 25–27 gauge needle, the injection is usually made on the forearm. After proper skin preparation, the skin is stretched slightly by traction as the left hand partially encircles the forearm (see Fig. 5–3). The tip of the needle is caught in the epidermis and the remainder of the bevel is inserted by aiming parallel or slightly away from the skin surface. This direction helps to keep the needle in the epidermis. After the bevel has disappeared beneath the skin, rotate the needle 180 degrees to prevent the material from being inadvertently squirted into the operator's eye. The injection should raise a wheal if the needle is properly placed. The wheal will clear within seconds in some patients with peripheral edema, but usually it will remain for a few minutes. Record in the patient's chart the place and type of test, and when more than one injection is made, indicate the exact location.

The *subcutaneous route* is most often

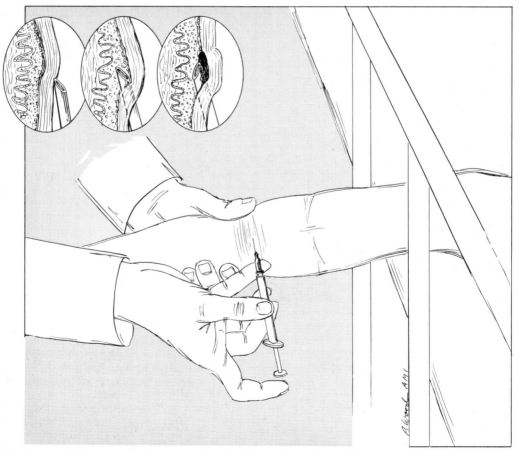

Figure 5–3   Intradermal injection. See text for description.

used for the injection of insulin, allergy medications and epinephrine, but may be employed in a variety of other circumstances. The main advantages are that many sites are available for rotation in cases of long-term administration and there is much less chance of nerve or blood vessel damage because of the relatively superficial depth of penetration. The primary disadvantages include the limited number of medications suitable for injection (no irritants, heavy suspensions or vehicles can be used), the limited volumes (preferably not more than 1.0 ml) that can be injected at one site and the variable absorption from subcutaneous tissues.

The sites most commonly employed for subcutaneous injection are the upper outer third of the deltoid muscle or the mid-thigh area. One may, however, use any site that has loose subcutaneous tissue. A 1 ml tuberculin syringe with a small bore, 25 or 26 gauge, ½ inch needle is used. Cleanse the site selected with alcohol, Betadine or other antiseptic solution and allow to air dry. Prior to injection, pinch a fold of skin between the thumb and forefinger with your opposite hand. Approach and enter the skin at a 45 degree angle. This prevents excessively deep penetration. Aspirate gently to insure that you have not entered a blood vessel, and then inject. Withdraw the syringe and gently massage the area while applying a dry cotton ball.

The *intramuscular route* is usually reserved for injection of larger volumes, which are often suspended in heavy vehicles, and in situations in which rapid onset of action is not deemed critical. The selection of a site is primarily based upon careful consideration of the underlying major blood vessels, nerves and associated anatomy. The "traditional" site remembered from childhood, the buttocks, is *not* recommended any longer for routine use because of the close proximity of the sciatic nerve and the possibility of permanent sciatic palsy. In unusual situations, injections may be made in the *upper outer quadrant* of the gluteal muscles.

The vastus lateralis muscle of the thigh is probably the best, easiest, most readily accessible site for intramuscular injection in the infant and young child. Restraint is simple with the patient in a supine position and the assistant leaning across the abdomen. There are no major vessels or nerves in the area and in cases of adverse or hypersensitivity reactions, a tourniquet may be applied proximal to the site of injection.

The specific site on the anterior surface of the thigh is the area from 3 cm below the greater trochanter to 3 cm above the knee. After the antiseptic is applied and dry, the needle should be inserted perpendicular to the thigh for a distance of 2 to 3 cm. In some thin patients, the tip of the needle may strike periosteum, and partial withdrawal before injection is required. After aspiration, injection should be made slowly. Withdraw and massage the site with a sterile cotton ball for several seconds.

Use of the *deltoid muscle* for intramuscular injection is preferably reserved for the older child in whom restraint is not as much of a problem. The major advantages are those of easy accessibility and tourniquet application in adverse reactions. The disadvantages of smaller muscle mass and major adjacent nerves and blood vessels must be kept in mind. Injection at this site should not exceed 1 ml.

With the arm hanging limp, the site should be cleansed and allowed to dry. The injection should be made perpendicular to the surface, 3 to 4 cm below the acromion process, to a depth of 2 to 3 cm.

The *intravenous route*, unlike the previously described techniques, is used not only for single dose administration, but for continuous fluid or drug therapy as well. Depending upon the type of therapy contemplated and the age of the patient, there are many different sites available. We will be able to discuss only a few, primarily those for continuous therapy. Proper restraint (described earlier) is critical for successful intravenous infusion. Mastery of this technique is as important as the actual intravenous insertion for overall success.

Irrespective of the specific site selected, there are several basic concepts to remember. Distention of the vein is most commonly achieved by application of a tourniquet proximal to the site of infusion. Other helpful additive techniques include application of heat (compresses or submersion in warm water), the use of gravity and exercise (such as repeatedly opening and closing the fist). The "butterfly" needle or cannula to be used should be filled with sterile normal saline to inhibit clotting after

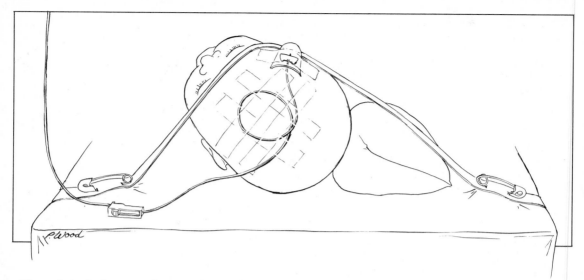

Figure 5–4   Scalp vein infusion and sandbag restraint. Adhesive tape is attached to the head, sandbag and bed sheet. The adhesive on the bed sheets should be reinforced by pins (also see text).

successful entry. This procedure also assures patency of the needle. For insertion of the "butterfly" needle, the vein should be "anchored" with the opposite thumb or index finger and the skin stretched taut to prevent "rolling" of the vein. The needle should be inserted, bevel up, ½ to 1 cm distal to the vein and parallel to it. This will afford increased stability of the needle in the subcutaneous tissue for continuous infusion. The needle should be advanced relatively superficially until blood is seen in the tubing. Appearance of a hematoma usually indicates excessive penetration and perforation of the posterior wall of the vessel and is an indication for withdrawal from that site. After successful entry of the vein, always be sure to release the tourniquet before administration of any fluid.

Single dose "push" intravenous injections are most commonly used to control seizures, give glucose in insulin shock, administer certain antibiotics and give chemotherapeutic agents. In infants, this is usually most easily accomplished via the external jugular vein (see blood drawing technique described later). In older children, the antecubital area is most advantageous.

Only in infants and the very young child are *scalp veins* used for continuous intravenous infusion (Fig. 5–4). Any visible vein on the head is acceptable, with those near the midline being most advantageous for prolonged restraint. The tributaries of the superficial temporal vein or the frontal vein are those most commonly used. The area should be shaved with soap, water and safety razor, in a wide enough radius to permit adhesive taping when the procedure is complete; the immediate area should be cleansed with an antiseptic. The tourniquet applied is usually a rubber band around the circumference of the head.

A 23 or 25 gauge scalp "butterfly" needle, filled with sterile saline, bevel up, is inserted 1 cm distal to the prepared vein while remaining *very superficial*. Watch carefully for a slow blood return and tape the needle to the site, being especially careful to anchor the "wings" of the butterfly with cotton swabs and not to dislodge it at this point.

Numerous branches of the veins on the dorsum of the hand are usually visible even in the very young child. The advantages of using this location are the need to restrain only one extremity (except in the very uncooperative youngster and infant) and the many potential sites in one small area. The major disadvantage is that the veins are not well anchored in the subcutaneous tissue and thus tend to "roll."

The veins in the *antecubital fossa*, while well suited to single injections and blood drawing, are not ideal for continuous therapy. Restraint of the outstretched arm is quite uncomfortable for the patient, and even when attempted, it is difficult to prevent the elbow joint from twisting in the uncooperative youngster. Furthermore, the site easily becomes infiltrated and this is difficult to detect in the early stages.

BLOOD DRAWING

The general approaches and considerations described under Injection Techniques apply equally to blood drawing.

Finger and heel sticks should be initiated after preparing the skin with an antiseptic, using a sterile, pointed blade (usually Bard-Parker). A single "clean" jab should be made so the blood flows without squeezing the site, which may dilute the blood with tissue fluids. Care must be taken to avoid hitting periosteum since osteomyelitis has occasionally been associated with this procedure.

Antecubital veins offer some of the best sources for venous blood (Fig. 5–5). The technique of the person restraining the child is of prime importance. Movement of the body can be prevented by gently but firmly leaning across the thorax. The left hand is placed above the patient's elbow, lifting the antecubital area so the vein is accessible. The other hand is placed on the patient's wrist to prevent rotation of the arm and still not be in the way of the blood drawer. A rubber Penrose drain tubing serves as a good tourniquet and should be

tied with a simple loop to allow easy release. After the vein is visualized or palpated, the needle is inserted through the skin and then into the vein. With experience, the slight give of the needle as it passes into the vein can be detected.

External jugular vein drawing is illustrated in Figure 5–6. The child must be placed in a mummy restraint, crying and have his head down as in the figure. Fingers of the left hand are used to act as a local tourniquet and to prevent rolling of the vein.

Internal jugular, femoral and longitudinal sinus vein drawings are not recommended except in extreme emergencies.

DIAGNOSTIC TECHNIQUES

Nasal instillation. The primary purpose of nasal instillation is to shrink swollen mucous membranes by direct application of medication. Before administration, mucus and other nasal contents should be removed by aspiration with a bulb syringe.

Even in the uncooperative infant, this procedure can be accomplished without assistance and thus taught to the parent for home use. The infant should be placed in the supine position and cradled on the lap with his feet straddling the parent's (or

Figure 5–5 Antecubital vein blood drawing. See text for description.

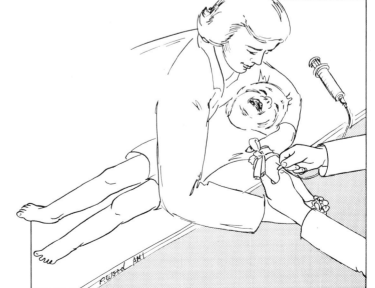

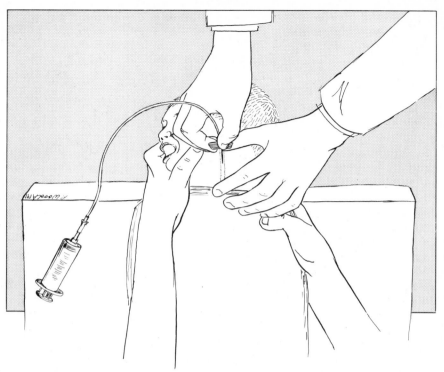

Figure 5–6   External jugular blood drawing. See text for description.

physician's) waist. The head should be slightly hyperextended over the parent's knees and supported with the left hand, leaving the right hand free for administration of the solution. The dropper should be placed just inside the nostril and the solution expelled. The position of the patient should be maintained for 3 to 5 minutes to permit gravitational drainage.

The older, cooperative youngster should lie on the bed, supine, with the head hyperextended over the edge. With the head rotated to the right, the drops are placed in the right nostril; reverse for the left nostril. Maintain each position for at least three minutes. Better dispersion may be attained if the child can be taught to snuff the drops.

Nasopharyngeal cultures. The nasopharyngeal culture is primarily used in infants for isolation of *B. pertussus* and *C. diphtheriae,* avoiding contamination with normal oral flora. The best position for obtaining a specimen and restraint in infants and uncooperative children is with the patient supine with arms extended above the head. The assistant can immobilize the head while also controlling the arms and hands by pressing the patient's arms against the sides of the head.

The culture specimen should be obtained using a thin plug of cotton wrapped on a fine, flexible wire, usually 19 gauge aluminum or copper. Wooden stick applicators are *not* used. Patency of the nasal passage should be assured by aspiration using a bulb syringe. One finger should be used to exert gentle pressure at the inner canthus of the eye, upon the corner of the nose, to prevent the entry of tears into the nasal area, as tears can dilute the specimen.

The sterile cotton swab should be inserted in a posterior direction, with care not to contaminate it by touching the nasal mucosa. It should be advanced until definite resistance is met and then gently rotated and left for several seconds, or at least until the patient coughs. Upon removal from the nasopharynx, the organisms should be transferred *immediately* to the appropriate culture media (usually blood agar, but Bordet-Gengou if pertussis is suspected). The pertussis organism is notoriously difficult to culture.

Nasogastric intubation. Nasogastric intubation is useful in a wide variety of circumstances including lavage of the stomach contents (as in toxic ingestions), short-term gavage of liquid nourishment and suction prior to abdominal surgery. The tubes employed should be transparent but radio-opaque for x-ray visualization. The diameter selected depends, to some degree, on the anticipated use. Lavage would obviously require a larger bore tube than gavage.

Except in the older, cooperative patient, in whom the procedure may be attempted in the sitting position, the patient should be placed supine and be well restrained (see mummifying restraint described earlier). When performing lavage, the patient should be further tilted into Trendelenburg's position but lying on his side. The length of tubing to be passed is approximately equal to the distance from the bridge of the nose to the tip of the xiphoid process. This should be premeasured and marked on the tube before the insertion. The nares should then be inspected to assure patency.

After application of a water soluble lubricant to the tip of the tube, it should be inserted into either naris in the direction of the occiput. When the tube reaches the pharynx, the older patient may be asked to swallow. Continue to advance the tube to the prescribed distance.

Placement of the tube in the proper position may be ascertained by the following checklist:

1. Be sure the tube is not coiled in the mouth or pharynx.

2. The patient should not be having coughing spasms.
3. Aspirate to check for the presence of stomach contents.
4. Place the end of the tube in a glass of water; if bubbles are produced during expiration, placement is in the *respiratory* tree by error.
5. Listen with a stethoscope over the stomach while injecting air through a syringe; this should produce audible sounds over the area.

Extubation is easily accomplished by quick withdrawal while pinching the tube closed.

Lumbar puncture. Lumbar puncture in the infant or child is not unlike that in the adult except that extra special attention must be focused upon adequate restraint to prevent a traumatic tap, and upon the influence of growth, which produces an ever-changing anatomy.

There are several guidelines unique to pediatrics:

1. The distance between the skin and the subarachnoid space varies greatly with age. In infants it is 1.5 to 2.5 cm, increasing to about 5 cm in a five-year-old child.
2. The total volume of cerebrospinal fluid varies from 10 to 20 ml in a newborn to 100 to 150 ml in an adult.
3. The amount of CSF that can be safely removed is roughly 1 ml/kg for infants up to 10 kg.
4. A 22 gauge lumbar puncture needle, 1½ inches in length, is adequate

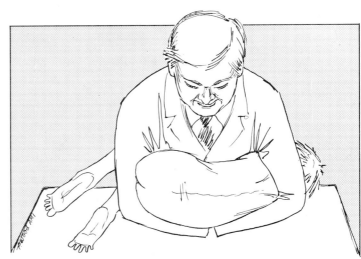

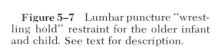

Figure 5–7 Lumbar puncture "wrestling hold" restraint for the older infant and child. See text for description.

for an infant, whereas a 20 or 22 gauge needle, 3 inches or more in length is needed for the older child. A lumbar puncture needle has a short bevel and always a stylet.

5. Restraint is usually best accomplished (as pictured in Fig. 5–7) in the lateral recumbent position, producing maximal spinal flexion. The assistant's one arm is placed around the neck and the other around the flexed knees (the "wrestling hold") each drawing toward the other. The assistant should also hold the child's wrists. The patient's back should be *exactly* parallel to the operating table.

With the patient in the lateral recumbent position, an imaginary line drawn between the superior brim of the iliac crests will bisect the third or fourth lumbar interspace (see Figs. 5–7 and 5–8). With this point as the center, the site should be swabbed with an antiseptic in ever-increasing concentric circles. An area at least 8 to 10 cm in diameter should be prepared. In infants, the inferior end of the spinal cord is usually as low as the third lumbar vertebra (as opposed to adults whose caudal end of the cord is at the first lumbar vertebra). Thus, it is extremely important *not* to mistake landmarks and enter too far craniad. After the site is draped with a sterile towel, an intradermal injection of procaine hydrochloride 1 per cent is made at the L-3 interspace. This skin anesthesia is often omitted in infants.

The needle, with stylet in place, should be introduced at the interspace, directly in the midline, exactly perpendicular to the spine with the bevel of the needle parallel to the axis of the spine. The needle should be advanced in a somewhat cranial direction—essentially "aiming" for the umbilicus. Advance gently and slowly until the characteristic "meningeal pop" is felt. When doubt exists about whether the end point has been reached, remove the stylet and check for cerebrospinal fluid in the needle. This will help prevent excessive penetration or a bloody traumatic tap.

When a successful tap has been made, opening and closing pressures should be recorded (but are invalid in a struggling, crying infant, so wait patiently if necessary)

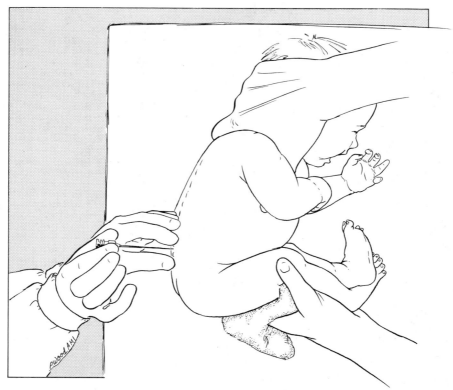

Figure 5–8   Lumbar puncture technique for small infant. See text for description.

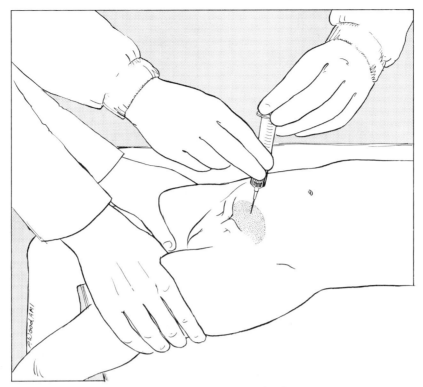

Figure 5–9   Bladder tap. See text for description.

and at least three separate tubes of fluid obtained for cell count, culture and spinal fluid chemistry. The operator should observe for xanthochromia or fresh blood in the fluid. Following a traumatic tap, there will usually be less blood in the tube collected at the end. Remember to obtain a simultaneous venous specimen for blood glucose level when indicated.

Bladder tap (suprapubic aspiration). The suprapubic aspiration of urine in infants and children is one of the more significant recent advances in the diagnostic capabilities of the pediatrician. The procedure enables one to obtain a sterile urine specimen in an infant or young child without the problem of external contamination. We have now reached the point where it is no longer considered acceptable to obtain urine by urethral catheterization except in very unusual circumstances. The collection of urine by bladder tap insures that the initial diagnosis has been made in the most accurate fashion available. Furthermore, in making the diagnosis, it must be remembered that urine obtained in this fashion should *normally be sterile* and thus the

presence of *any* bacteriuria and subsequent growth on culture is significant. For urine obtained suprapubically, the traditional colony counts of greater than 10^5 are not required for significance.

The fluid consumption of the patient should be increased 30 to 60 minutes before the procedure to increase fullness of the bladder. An attempt at aspiration should be postponed if the patient has voided in the previous half hour. In the newborn and infant, the bladder extends above the symphysis pubis even with only a small amount of urine present, but in the older child the bladder needs to be relatively full before becoming as readily accessible. In these children, the procedure should not be attempted unless the bladder is palpable. Remember to have the assistant gently compress the shaft of the penis or exert anterior pressure on rectal examination in the female to prevent untimely urination while the operator palpates the bladder!

With the patient in the supine, frog-leg position, immobilization is accomplished with the assistant's one arm over the trunk and the other over the thighs and hips (see

Fig. 5–9). The operator works from the opposite side of the table. An area in a radius of 5 cm from the symphysis pubis should be cleansed aseptically. No anesthetic is required. A 1½ inch, 22 gauge needle, attached to a sterile 5 cc syringe is used to enter in the midline, 1½ to 2 cm above the symphysis pubis. The needle is directed at a 20 to 30 degree downward (caudad) angle to a depth of approximately 1 inch while exerting a gently negative pressure on the syringe. As with the lumbar pucture, one often feels a "give" on penetration of the bladder. A small amount of urine is aspirated and the needle is quickly withdrawn.

The potential complication of perforation of an abdominal viscera is extremely rare and is greatly minimized if fullness of the bladder is ascertained on palpation. Occasionally, microscopic and even macroscopic hematuria is seen on the subsequently voided urine specimen and, as a single event, is not of great concern.

Principles of Drug Therapy in Infants and Children

6

W. Archie Bleyer

"Doctors pour drugs of which they know little to cure diseases of which they know less into human beings of whom they know nothing."

Voltaire (1694–1778)

Although we may have learned much about humans and their diseases during the 200 years since Voltaire, we still know precious little about drug therapy in children. We are reminded of this gap in our knowledge on the one hand by the occurrence of therapeutic tragedies after the use of the sedative thalidomide and the antibiotic chloramphenicol, and on the other hand by the fact that children are "therapeutic orphans"; that is, many drugs effective in adults are not available to children because they have not been adequately tested in the pediatric age range.[1] In a recent poll of practicing pediatricians the respondents indicated that their greatest need in the clinical practice of medicine was to have more information about drug therapy in children.[2]

This chapter summarizes the principles of pediatric drug therapy and illustrates these concepts with clinical examples and applications. Two specific areas have been singled out: (1) the pharmacological peculiarities of the neonatal period, which help explain why drug therapy in newborn infants must be individualized, and (2) the value of body surface area as a guide to drug dosage determination in children over the age of three months. The important problem of teratogenic or fetal effects of drugs is discussed in Chapter 7.

NEONATAL DRUG THERAPY

Newborn infants have been shown repeatedly to be more susceptible to the action of drugs or chemical agents than the adult organism.[3-7] Perhaps the best known example is the chloramphenicol-induced "gray syndrome" in premature infants, in which administration of the antibiotic to the mother prior to delivery results in cardiovascular collapse and death of the infant. Other examples of therapeutic tragedies are sulfonamide-induced kernicterus in otherwise healthy but jaundiced neonates, brain damage after hexachlorophene baths and blindness caused by high oxygen concentrations. Even feeding practices have had adverse effects—premature infants fed excessive protein have had lower intelligence quotients than those fed normal amounts of protein.

The susceptibility of the newborn infant, especially the premature infant, can be explained by immaturity of those mechanisms that govern the nature, intensity and duration of drug action. These processes include absorption, distribution, metabolism, excretion and protein-binding of the drug. In general, all these factors are incompletely developed in the full-term infant, and even less well developed in the premature infant. In addition, each of these processes undergoes rapid changes during the postnatal period. Clearly, simply adjusting the dosage to the size of the patient is inadequate, and multiple factors must be considered in tailoring drug therapy for infants, as shown in Figure 6–1.[4]

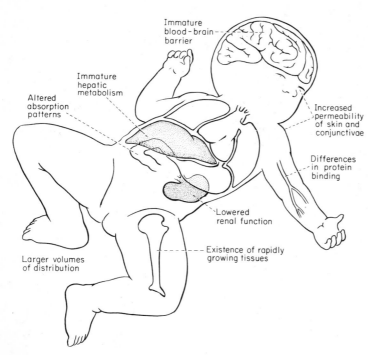

Figure 6–1 Some of the multiple factors that modify drug disposition in the newborn infant (adapted from Hirata, T.: Drug Therapy, p. 29–36, December, 1975).

Absorption. In general, absorption from the intestinal tract is delayed, particularly in premature newborn infants. Vitamin E, riboflavin and several antibiotics are known, for example, to be slowly absorbed from the intestinal tract of newborn infants. In the case of riboflavin, the specialized intestinal active-transport process is incompletely developed, and absorption must take place by passive diffusion over a long segment of the gastrointestinal tract. As a result, absorption in the neonate proceeds for more than 16 hours, whereas in the older infant it is usually complete within 3 to 4 hours. Vitamin E, a lipid-soluble vitamin, is incompletely absorbed in the premature infant, undoubtedly because premature infants produce significantly less bile. These infants are thus susceptible to vitamin E deficiency and the associated hemolytic anemia. Bile salts inactivate certain chemotherapeutic agents, such as polymyxin and nystatin, and their relative absence in newborn infants may enhance absorption of these agents. Triple sulfonamide, erythromycin and tetracycline are poorly absorbed during the first few days of life, although the absorptive processes undergo rapid functional changes and are usually normal within five days after birth. Rarely, the slower intestinal transit time may cause unusually efficient absorption of drugs. The enhanced toxicity of oral chloramphenicol may be such an example.

On the other hand, topically administered drugs are absorbed more readily by the relatively permeable skin and conjunctivae. For example, hypertension can occur in infants who have had their eyes dilated with phenylephrine. Applying a few drops of epinephrine to the skin of a premature infant results in rapid blanching. Hexachlorophene baths may result in progressive encephalopathy. The use of boric acid to treat a diaper rash may result in systemic poisoning. Aniline dyes used to mark laundry have caused methemoglobinemia. Even such innocent-appearing procedures as rinsing infant laundry in antimicrobial agents may cause adverse effects when the chemical is absorbed through the skin of infants.

Distribution. After a drug has entered the circulatory system, its immediate disposition is determined by the volumes of the various body compartments, the rate of transport across biological membranes and the extent of binding to the plasma proteins. The newborn infant has larger volumes of total body water, extracellular fluid and plasma than the adult, and the premature newborn has larger volumes of these body spaces than does the full-term infant. For example, total body water varies from 86 per cent of the body weight in the small premature infant to 70 per cent in the full-term infant. Fat content, on the other hand, is much lower in the premature infant (about 1 per cent) than in the normal full-term infant (16 per cent). With these differences in body composition, differences of distribution are to be expected. It is likely, for example, that marked changes in the amount of fat tissue can affect the distribution of lipophilic drugs such as thiopental, an anesthetic agent, and diazepam, a sedative and anticonvulsant drug. In small babies, the same dosage of gentamicin and ticarcillin (a new penicillin derivative) is distributed in a larger space, and this dilutional effect results in a lower peak concentration of the antibiotic than in term infants.

Protein binding. Distribution of a drug is also affected by differences in binding to plasma proteins. For example, studies with diphenylhydantoin, an anticonvulsant drug, show up to twice as much unbound drug in newborn plasma as in adult plasma. Bilirubin appears to compete for the binding sites, and the jaundiced infant may have three times more unbound drug. This difference in plasma protein binding has been found for other drugs and may be another reason why drugs have much greater effect, and more often cause side effects, in the neonate than in the adult.

On the other hand, drugs with a greater affinity than bilirubin for bilirubin binding sites, will displace bilirubin and result in increased free bilirubin levels. A tragic example of this phenomenon took place several years ago when premature infants were prophylactically treated with sulfonamides in an attempt to prevent neonatal septicemia. A greater number of deaths occurred in the sulfonamide-treated group than in the group that did not receive sulfonamide, and these deaths were related to kernicterus, the toxic effect of indirect hyperbilirubinemia. The mechanism was shown to be displacement of bilirubin from its binding sites by the antibiotic.

Metabolism. Another tragic example of increased toxicity in the newborn is that of the antibiotic chloramphenicol. In premature infants given this drug prophylactically for infections, more than six times as many died as compared to a control group.

The drug-treated group developed the characteristic "gray syndrome": rapid onset of cyanosis accompanied by respiratory distress, hypothermia and flaccidity, followed in 24 hours by death. In this case, the fault was shown to lie in inadequate detoxification of chloramphenicol by glucuronide formation, and hence toxic levels were achieved at a usual dosage.

The encephalopathy of hexachlorophene may also be related to reduced metabolism of the drug in newborn infants. Again, the mechanism appears to be immature glucuronide conjugation of the parent compound.

Excretion. In the newborn infant, renal function has not completely developed; for example, glomerular filtration rate and renal plasma flow are approximately 30 to 40 per cent of adult values. Antibiotics are important drugs for consideration here, since these agents are usually eliminated via renal excretion without prior metabolism. Thus, the limiting factor in the clearance of most antibiotic agents is the rate of renal excretion. The penicillins and the aminoglycoside antibiotics are excellent examples; and their plasma half-lives are markedly prolonged during the immediate postnatal period.

Postnatal changes. Another important feature of developmental pharmacology lies in the rapid changes that take place during the first month after birth. Both hepatic and renal mechanisms mature rapidly, although at different rates for each class of chemical compounds. The development of the process of glucuronidation, for example, may be quite active so that by two or three weeks of age the same dose of a glucuronidated drug that would have been toxic and fatal after a few days' usage in the newborn may be insufficient for safe usage against infection. Ampicillin, ordinarily given every 12 hours during the first days of life, will be inadequate for maintenance of a minimal bactericidal level during the second week of life.

Individualization of therapy. That dosage has to be individualized for newborn infants can be illustrated with the following clinical example. There are three neonates in the nursery whom you wish to treat with ticarcillin. One of these infants is a one-month-old child weighing 2.0 kg, the second is a newly born infant weighing 2.5 kg, and the third is a newly born term infant weighing 3.0 kg. Which infant will clear the antibiotic most rapidly from his plasma? The answer unpredictably is the smallest infant, as determined by the studies of Nelson and his colleagues.[8]

This example illustrates that dosage in neonates cannot be accurately calculated from body weight alone. It is best to consult a neonatologist or the latest publications on recommended drug dosages for newborn infants.[9, 10] In summary, the neonate's physiological functions that relate to handling the drugs are underdeveloped. The neonate cannot, therefore, be considered a miniature adult, and scaling down dosage simply on a weight basis is not a safe or effective method of giving drugs. Particularly in the neonate, dosage must be individualized and a drug's effects closely observed.

DRUG THERAPY IN OLDER CHILDREN

Beyond the neonatal period, the variability in the dose response diminishes. Thus certain dosage guidelines can be applied to most children. An interesting phenomenon occurs as the child matures from the neonatal to the postinfantile period (Fig. 6–2). The ability of the child to metabolize and excrete drugs rapidly increases during the first two to three months so that it actually "overshoots" to a capacity of metabolism

TABLE 6–1

| Drug | Serum half-life (hours) | |
	Children	Adults
Antipyrene	5–9	10–17
Phenylbutazone	24–48	48–96
Phenobarbital	37–73	53–140
Diazoxide	9–24	24–36

and excretion that is greater than that in adults. As a result, the serum half-life for most drugs is significantly shorter in children over the age of three months than in adults (Table 6–1).

What is the best method, then, for calculating dosage in children beyond the neonatal period? Most pediatricians use body weight to determine dosage and they usually calculate a full day's dosage. Thus the total dosage is calculated in milligrams per kilogram per 24 hours and then divided into individual doses. However, the dose-age relationships in Figure 6–2 indicate that several multiples of the adult dose in milligrams per kilogram would have to be administered in order to achieve the same response or plasma concentration in the younger child. This has been the situation for all drugs critically examined in this way, several of which are listed in Table 6–2. One explanation for this observation is that the determinants of drug action do not vary directly with body weight, and one cannot simply scale down dosage according to weight.

There does exist, however, a fairly reliable relationship between the body surface area and many physiologic variables, including extracellular fluid volume, plasma volume, cardiac output, glomerular filtration rate and liver size. Thus body surface area provides a reasonable method for determining the initial dose to use in children over three months of age. Dosage is relatively independent of age when it is based on body surface area, as shown in Figures 6–3 and 6–4. Note that dosage based on body weight varies considerably among different age groups, but that a single dosage generally suffices for infants and children when the body-surface-area method is used. Examples include 1 mg/m² for the digitalizing dose of digoxin, 100 mg/m²/day for gentamicin, and 50 gm/m² for the glucose dose in the oral glucose tolerance test.

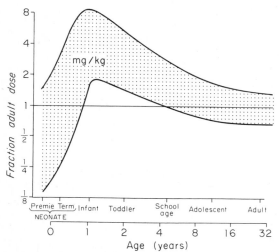

Figure 6–2 Range of recommended dosages based on body weight as a function of age.

TABLE 6–2   COMPARATIVE EFFECTIVE DOSE (mg/kg)

		Multiple of Adult Dose for		
Drug type	Effect	*Infant*	*Toddler*	*School-age*
Barbiturate	Hypnosis	2.8	2.8	1.8
Digoxin	Blood level	5.0	4.0	2.0
Cephalexin	Blood level	2.5	1.6	1.5
Ephedrine	Pressor	3.3	2.8	2.3
Halothane	Anesthesia	1.6	1.4	1.2

Note also that the body-surface-area method can be applied for caloric, electrolyte and fluid therapy.

How does one obtain the body surface area of a patient? This is a simple matter in that one need know only the height and weight of the patient. Body surface area can be readily determined by consulting standard tables or using nomograms relating these body parameters (Fig. 6–5).

The most complete compilation of recommended drug dosages for children is the *Pediatric Dosage Handbook** written by H. C. Shirkey.[11]

ADMINISTRATION OF DRUGS

The route of administration and the prepared form of the drug should be chosen with the age and symptoms of the patient

---

*This handbook can be purchased for a small fee from the American Pharmaceutical Association at 2215 Constitution Ave., N.W., Washington, D.C. 20037.

clearly in mind. The drug must be in a form that the attendant can easily administer. Parenteral injection by either the subcutaneous, intramuscular or intravenous route is the most reliable means of administration. When the child's illness is severe or when vomiting is a factor, parenteral therapy should be utilized. For intramuscular injection, the thigh or the upper lateral quadrant of a buttock should be used. Intramuscular injection into the inferomedial gluteal area is associated with a risk of sciatic palsy, especially in infants. After the needle is inserted, the syringe barrel should always be aspirated to prevent injection of the drug directly into a blood vessel. Objections to the parenteral route include the trauma of administration, a greater risk of drug sensitization and local or systemic reactions.

The oral route can often be utilized unless refusal, vomiting or malabsorption prevents adequate administration. Children under five years of age are frequently unable to swallow tablets or capsules.

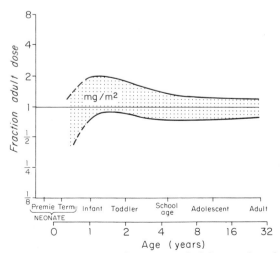

Figure 6–3   Range of recommended dosages based on body surface area as a function of age.

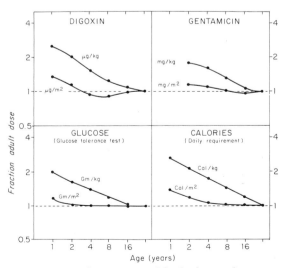

Figure 6–4   Comparison of the body-weight versus body–surface area methods of dosage calculation.

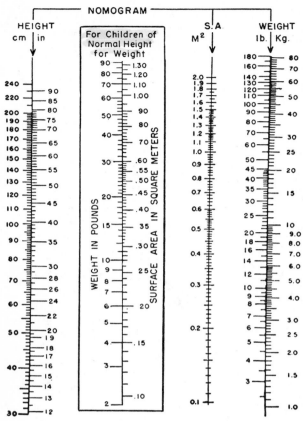

NOMOGRAM

HEIGHT
cm | in

For Children of
Normal Height
for Weight

S. A.
M²

WEIGHT
lb. | Kg.

WEIGHT IN POUNDS

SURFACE AREA IN SQUARE METERS

Figure 6–5 The West nomogram for the estimation of body surface area. The surface area is indicated where a straight line connecting height and weight intersects the surface area column. If the patient is roughly of average size, the surface area can also be estimated from the weight alone (enclosed area). Reproduced here from Shirkey, H. C.: Drug therapy. *In* Vaughan, V. C., III, and McKay, R. J. (Eds.): *Nelson Textbook of Pediatrics.* 10th ed., Philadelphia, W. B. Saunders Co., 1975.

Forced administration to a struggling child may result in aspiration. If liquid preparations are not available, tablets can often be crushed, or the contents of a capsule emptied, and mixed with syrups, jams or honey. Drugs with a bitter taste can be crushed and placed into empty capsules. Unpleasant-tasting drugs should not be put in food served to the child. Some drugs are available as rectal suppositories but because the child's rectum is often filled with stool, rectally-administered drugs are often poorly absorbed. Instillation of drugs into the eyes, ears or nose of a child is often particularly vexing. Solutions are preferred to ointments for this purpose, and plastic droppers should be used rather than glass.

Standardized measuring devices should be used for measuring dosage. The volumes contained by household teaspoons, droppers and plastic medicine cups vary greatly. Calibrated droppers are preferred for the measurement of smaller doses. The volume prescribed should always be large enough to minimize errors in measurement. When prescribing drugs for infants or children, the clinician must keep in mind all possible factors that may interfere with the drug arriving at the desired place in the recommended dose.[11]

REFERENCES

1. Shirkey, H. C.: Editorial comment: Therapeutic orphans. J. Pediatr., 72:119, 1968.
2. Nelson, W. E.: Results of a survey on reader interest and informational needs. J. Pediatr., 77:929, 1970.
3. Giacoia, G. P., and Gorodisher, R.: Pharmacologic principles in neonatal drug therapy. Clin. Perinatol., 2:125, 1975.
4. Hirata, T.: Drug therapy for the premature infant. Drug Therapy, p. 29, December 1975.
5. Chudzik, G. M., and Yaffe, S. J.: Introduction to the special problems of pediatric drug therapy. Drug Therapy, p. 17, July 1973.
6. Yaffe, S. J., and Juchau, M. R.: Perinatal pharmacology. Ann. Dev. Pharmacol., 4:219, 1974.
7. Done, A. K.: Developmental pharmacology. Clin. Pharmacol. Ther., 5:432, 1964.
8. Nelson, J. D., Shelton, S., and Kusmiesz, H.: Clinical pharmacology of ticarcillin in the newborn infant: Relation to age, gestational age, and weight. J. Pediatr., 87:474, 1975.
9. Schaffer, A. J., and Avery, M. E.: *Diseases of the Newborn,* 4th ed. Philadelphia, W. B. Saunders Co., 1971, pp. 871–877.
10. McCracken, G. H.: Pharmacologic basis for antimicrobial therapy in newborn infants. Clin. Perinatol., 2:139, 1975.
11. Shirkey, H. C.: *Pediatric Dosage Handbook.* Washington, D.C., American Pharmaceutical Association, 1973.

PART II

MAJOR PERIODS OF PEDIATRICS

7

Prenatal Life

Thomas H. Shepard and David W. Smith

The intent of this chapter is to stimulate curiosity about the vital biologic prenatal events that shape the ultimate form and function of an individual. This area is still an exciting, untapped frontier of knowledge. We have touched on many aspects of prenatal life, attempting to distill and present some of the more important emerging concepts.

Periods of Development

Three consecutive periods of human prenatal development are the ovum, the embryo, and the fetus. Fertilization may occur within a few hours of ovulation. Implantation begins about seven days later. The period of the ovum lasts from fertilization until establishment of the primitive villi at about 12 to 14 days of gestation. This is followed by the embryonic stage, which encompasses the major events of organogenesis and lasts until a crown-rump length of approximately 32 mm is reached by about 54 to 56 days of gestation. By 22 to 23 days the embryo enters the early somite stages and the heart begins beating. By the end of the embryonic period, organogenesis is essentially complete; consequently, during this period the embryo is more susceptible to the adverse agents that produce major congenital defects such as neural tube defects, limb deficiencies and congenital heart disease. After the embryonic stage, development ensues with relatively less differentiation and a greater amount of growth. The fetal period lasts until the end of pregnancy. In general, a fetus of 600 gm or less is regarded as nonviable and a birth under this weight does not require a birth certificate or burial permission.

44

Maturational Age

Confusion can arise when the age of an embryo or fetus is reported in weeks or months. Often there is no indication whether the dates are from the last menstrual period or are actual weeks of gestation. Accurate dating is especially important. In this text we refer generally to either gestational days or to menstrual weeks. The gestational period is assumed to commence 14 days after the last normal mensis and coincides closely with ovulation, fertilization and copulation ages. Menstrual weeks refers to the time from the onset of the last normal menstrual period.

Methods of Measurement

For the early embryo and fetus the crown-rump length is the best individual measurement. The crown-heel length is generally inaccurate owing to the inability to straighten the fetus. The foot length correlates well with the crown-rump length, and accordingly, it is useful in estimating the length of a disrupted fetus following curettage interruption of pregnancy. The fetal weight is also used in defining growth of the fetus. After 26 menstrual weeks percentile charts of birth weights for premature infants are available (Lubchenco *et al.*). Figure 7–1 is a chart correlating crown-rump length, body weight, foot length and gestational age.

Survival Rate

It has been estimated that 90 per cent of ova become fertilized under ideal condi-

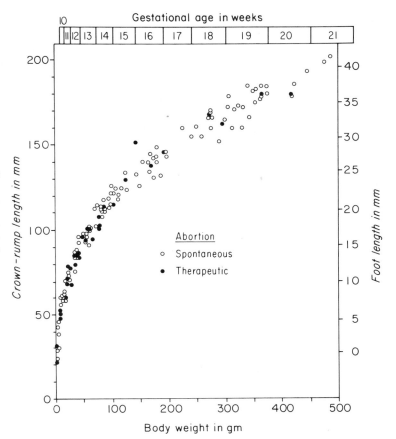

Figure 7–1 The body weight of fetuses, both therapeutic and spontaneous abortion specimens, is shown in relation to crown-rump length on the left, and foot length on the right, with gestational age in weeks (not menstrual weeks) at the top (Tanimura, *et al.*, 1971, Courtesy of Wistar Press).

tions. By interpolation of the findings of Hertig *et al.* (1959), only about 50 per cent of human conceptuses survive through completion of implantation on the fourteenth day of gestation (about the time of the first missed mensis). This 40 per cent loss from the time of fertilization to full implantation is much greater than observed in experimental animals, but the data are limited in number. Can it be that more critical fail-safe systems exist in human gestations? After recognition of pregnancy by the mother, the reported abortion rate is 10 to 25 per cent; the higher figure is probably more correct.

A significant proportion of this early selective mortality is due to genetic errors, which do not allow continued survival. One obvious category is that of genetic imbalance secondary to faults in chromosome distribution. At least 4 per cent of pregnancies start with a chromosomal abnormality, while only 0.5 per cent of babies are born with an aberrant chromosome number; most such fetuses are aborted in

early gestation. Twenty-five to 60 per cent of spontaneous abortions have been shown to have an abnormal chromosome number (Boué, Boué and Lazar). These karyotypes include many XO syndromes, triploid complements and various trisomies (Fig. 7–2).

The lower limits of viability for a premature are between 600 and 700 gm, and the fetal lung begins to be capable of gas exchange at 28 to 30 menstrual weeks. The normal baby is usually born about the fortieth menstrual week (280 days from last menstrual period with a standard deviation of 13 days). As a general rule, the mortality rate in prematures improves by 10 per cent with each week following the twenty-eighth.

Chemical and Physiological Growth

In early gestation, the fetus is approximately 94 per cent water and by full-term is 69 per cent water. He normally loses about 5 per cent of his weight shortly after

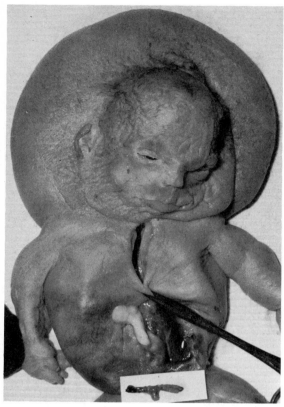

Figure 7–2 Fetus at approximately 23 menstrual weeks with XO Turner syndrome. Peripheral edema is marked, giving a halo effect to the head; the genesis of the associated neck webbing can be envisaged from the finding. A surprising observation is that the ovaries are nearly normal at this stage of fetal development; later, after birth, they degenerate into fibrous streaks.

birth. Weight gain is accelerated during the last eight weeks of fetal life by the accumulation of adipose tissue. The premature infant, deprived of this period, thus appears and is, in fact, very lean.

Fetal blood has a low oxygen tension (30 mm Hg), partly because of the admixture of arterial and venous blood in the intervillous space of the placenta. The fetus does well by virtue of having a high hemoglobin level (18 gm/100 ml), a fetal type of hemoglobin that dissociates oxygen to a greater extent than the adult type and because he is able to utilize anaerobic metabolism better for his energy needs. Thus the fetus and newborn are able to withstand periods of hypoxemia more successfully than the mature individual. The early energy needs are predominantly met by glucose through the entrance of pyruvate into the energy generating cycle (Kreb's cycle and electron

transport system). The early embryo also uses the pentose shunt pathway, which allows production of pentose necessary for RNA and DNA synthesis, to a greater extent than the mature individual. Later in fetal life protein and fat become part of the energy resource with increasing generation of high energy ATP bonds. The availability of glucose seems to be especially important in the presence of hypoxemia.

Three periods of growth may be defined in most organs (Winick): (1) pure hyperplasia increase in cell number with proportionate increase in weight, protein and DNA; (2) hyperplasia and concomitant hypertrophy (increase in DNA but more slowly than the increase in weight and protein); and (3) hypertrophy alone (increase in cell size, weight and protein with no increase in DNA).

TERATOLOGY

A teratogenic agent is one that produces, during embryonic or fetal development, a major or minor deviation from normal morphology or function in the offspring. These agents include chemicals, drugs, physical agents and viruses as well as certain deficiency states. The principles of teratology have been clearly described by Wilson. The period of development when the fetus is exposed to an agent largely controls the conceptus' sensitivity to teratogenesis. Damage during preimplantation and presomite periods (0 to 14 days) produces little altered morphogenesis because generally the ovum either dies or regenerates completely, while during organogenesis (up to about 60 gestational days) the embryo is highly sensitive and exposure may produce major morphological changes. The following fetal period is less sensitive to morphologic alterations, but change in functional capacity such as intellect, reproduction or aging may occur. This time specificity has been found in all cases in which teratogenesis in the human has been proved and studied in detail (see Table 7–1). Another new point of interest learned from experimental animals is that during the later part of the fetal period the conceptus becomes sensitive to transplacental carcinogens, and in some cases, the fetus is much more susceptible than the mother.

A second principle of teratology is that

TABLE 7-1 TIME SPECIFICITY OF ACTION FOR HUMAN TERATOGENS

	Gestational Age (Days)	Malformation
Rubella virus	0–60 0–120+	Cataract or heart disease are more likely Deafness
Thalidomide (removed from the market)	27–40	Reduction defects of extremities
Male hormones to female fetus (Androgens, progestins)	Before 90 After 90	Clitoral hypertrophy and labial fusion Only clitoral hypertrophy
Coumadin, anticoagulants	Before 100	Hypoplasia of nose and stippling of epiphyses
Radioiodine therapy	After 65–70	Fetal thyroidectomy
Goitrogens and iodides	After 180	Fetal goiter
Tetracycline	After 120 After 250	Dental enamel staining of primary teeth Staining of crowns of permanent teeth

some species are much more susceptible to teratogenesis than others. Aspirin, cortisone and several vitamin deficiencies are highly teratogenic in the rodent, but no evidence for their teratogenicity has been produced in humans. The thalidomide epidemic would not have been prevented by tests in pregnant mice and rats, even though the drug is highly teratogenic in rabbits, monkeys and humans. An understanding of the pharmacological, physiological and genetic variations that lead to teratogenesis is critical if we are to be able to protect the embryo and fetus from environmental and drug damage.

Nearly all chemicals and drugs when administered in very large doses to pregnant animals will produce some fetal intoxication, which may be evidenced by fetal growth retardation and immaturity of the skeleton. This does not mean the drugs are

TABLE 7-2 KNOWN HUMAN TERATOGENS (1976)*

Radiation (therapeutic, radioiodine, atomic bomb)

Infections (rubella virus, cytomegalovirus, herpes virus hominis I and II, toxoplasmosis, syphilis and varicella)

Maternal metabolic imbalance (phenylketonuria (untreated), virilizing tumors, alcoholism, diabetes (?) and endemic cretinism)

Drugs and environmental chemicals (androgenic hormones, aminopterin and methylaminopterin, cyclophosphamide, busulfan, thalidomide, organic mercury, chlorobiphenyls, diethylstilbestrol, coumadin anticoagulants and diphenylhydantoin and trimethadione)

*From Wilson and Shepard.

teratogenic or that therapeutic doses in humans will produce damage. More than 700 agents have been shown to alter the offspring of experimental animals, but only about 25 are known to be teratogenic in man (Table 7-2). A summary of studies of 850 animal and human teratogens is available in Shepard's *Catalog of Teratogenic Agents* (1976). The fetal alcohol and dilantin syndromes are described in Chapter 22.

FETUS

The development and nature of certain aspects of the fetus are covered categorically, as are some fetal problems and techniques of assessing the fetus.

Placenta

This organ, largely fetal in origin, serves as liver, lung and kidney for the fetus. In addition, it is responsible for maintenance of the pregnancy and maternal metabolic changes by its production of chorionic gonadotropin, placental prolactin, estrogen and progesterone. Progesterone appears to be a poorly understood factor that may prevent uterine contracture and presumably affects the duration of gestation. Prostaglandins also may be important in maintenance of the uterine homeostasis. If the fetus dies, the first hormonal indication may be decreased estriol levels in the maternal urine. This steroid, produced by the fetal adrenal and modified by the fetal liver, is also often low in the maternal urine when the fetus is anencephalic with a hypotrophic adrenal cortex.

The developing placenta is relatively large in early fetal life; by 15 menstrual weeks the fetus proper has equaled the placenta in weight and thereafter surpasses it in size. New cells are constantly added in the placenta until about 32 menstrual weeks; thereafter the growth rate is less rapid, and degenerative aging changes are sometimes evident by birth. At birth the placenta weighs about 460 gm (14 per cent of fetal weight). If the pregnancy goes beyond about 42 menstrual weeks, the placenta may no longer be an adequate resource; postmature babies may be born showing indications of undernutrition.

The vascular villous bed of the placenta has a surface area of about 160 sq ft. Substances with a molecular weight of less than a few hundred, such as most anesthetic gases and most drugs, pass through by direct or "facilitated" diffusion. Caution must therefore be exercised in terms of both the nature and dosage of agents administered to the pregnant woman. Lipid solubility, protein binding and other factors affect placental transfer. The gradient favors a slightly higher fetal level of many amino acids, water-soluble vitamins, calcium, phosphorus, magnesium, potassium and inorganic iodide. The exchange of iron seems to be unidirectional to the fetus. There is selective transfer of a few large proteins, such as maternal immunoglobulin G (IgG), which increasingly crosses to the fetus after four to five months, providing passive immune protection against certain infections during the first few postnatal months. Immunoglobulin M (IgM) does not cross the placenta, and the presence of IgM in the newborn indicates fetal production of an antibody, which can be a warning sign of fetal infection. No maternal pituitary hormones and relatively little maternal thyroxin cross the placental barrier, and hence the fetus is generally self-reliant in terms of its endocrine function. As an "auxiliary liver," the placenta synthesizes albumin and alpha and beta globulins, degrades certain molecules, stores glycogen and also makes fructose. Minor leaks may occur, allowing a few blood cells to exchange, but the most critical time for the Rh-negative mother to receive a large dose and become sensitized by Rh-positive fetal cells is at

the time of placental separation at birth. It is also around this time that serious fetal blood loss can occur secondary to aberrant position or early separation of part of the placenta. A large resource of blood is available in the placenta at the time of birth and the question still exists about when "the cord should be clamped."

Circulation

(See Chapter 8 on neonatal life.)

Hemostasis in the Fetus

Maturation of the clotting components into an effective hemostatic mechanism continues throughout gestation and in part during early infancy. Extensive hemorrhage occurs in the vast majority of early abortuses in which all hemostatic components are poorly developed. Premature infants have imperfect platelets, fragile vessels and low levels of nearly all clotting factors, and hemorrhage is relatively common. In full-term neonates only platelet function and certain clotting factors (principally the vitamin K factors) are incompletely developed, and bleeding is rare.

Amniotic Cavity

The amniotic fluid space increases from 30 ml at 10 menstrual weeks to 350 ml at 18 weeks. The predominant source of amniotic fluid is fetal urine in later gestation. There is a dynamic fluid exchange with resorption mainly by intestinal uptake of the swallowed fluid. Excessive amniotic fluid (polyhydramnios) may indicate congenital atresia of either esophagus or upper gastrointestinal tract. Lack of amniotic fluid should be a warning of serious defect in the fetal urinary tract. The skin is relatively protected by a layer of material called "vernix caseosa."

Lung

The lung is initially a glandlike organ containing much glycogen and characterized by solid outbuddings, which become canalized into an increasing number of potential air sacs at about 26 to 28 weeks. Capillary networks develop, and the less cuboidal alveolar epithelial cells produce a liquid called "surfactant," which lowers surface tension. By around 28 weeks or later the lung is capable of expansion and gas exchange. By use of ultrasound techniques, the human fetus has been shown to have breathing movements 50 to 90 per cent of the time at a frequency of 30 to 70 per minute. Gasping and fetal apnea have been recorded during asphyxia.

Brain

The flat neural tube appears about the eighteenth gestational day. The neural tube folds begin fusing on the twenty-second day with closure of the anterior neuropore about the twenty-sixth day. There is good evidence that anencephaly results from incomplete fusion of the anterior neuropore and lumbar meningomyelocele from a defect in closure of the posterior neuropore. (Obviously, a search should be made for any environmental teratogen that interferes with neural tube closure.)

Further development of the brain, particularly histogenesis, becomes increasingly complex—a fact that may explain why mental retardation is commonly associated with other clinical signs of abnormal prenatal growth. Cerebellar development is completed relatively late. The 28- to 30-week-old premature is hypotonic with irregular jerking motions, tremulousness and almost no head support, whereas the full-term baby is mildly hypertonic and a bit better coordinated.

Other Organs

In general, the variation in weight of a particular organ relative to body weight correlates with its state of biochemical and physiological function. The brain and the liver weights increase in proportion to body weight, as do the weights of the kidney and heart. Both the spleen and the thymus have a proportional increase in size during the first 120 days of intrauterine life.

Immune System

Early lymphocyte stem cells apparently derive from the thymus. Early in fetal life it appears that the stem cells differentiate into two populations. One type, termed T-cells, are thymus dependent and reside primarily in the bone marrow; they are associated with delayed or cellular immunity. The other line, termed B-cells, populate the lymph nodes and spleen, and differentiate further into the normal antibody-producing (immunoglobulin) cell line including plasma cells. The responsiveness of the immune system to antigenic stimulus is rarely challenged during fetal life. Indeed, one of the unique phenomena surrounding pregnancy is the non-responsiveness of the woman or infant to the foreign antigens unique to the other. The absence of the rejection of what is, to all intents and purposes, a prolonged homograft remains an unsolved mystery. Nevertheless, there is good evidence that while the fetus has perhaps a limited immune capacity, it is capable of response. The humoral response may be partially modified by the transfer of IgG to the fetus from the mother, beginning at 16 weeks.

The embryo and early fetus have a very active macrophage defense system and lack the usual tissue response involving polymorphonuclear cells and fibrosis. This difference helps to explain the absence of fibrous scars at sites damaged in early development; instead, the damaged part may be reduced in size or missing.

FETAL PROBLEMS

Only a few fetal problems are set forth as examples. Malformations and fetal growth deficiency are considered in other sections.

Twinning

The uterus was not designed for more than one fetus. Twins grow at a usual rate until 30 weeks, to a combined weight of about 4000 gm and thereafter tend to grow at a slower rate. They are more likely to be prematurely born. The rate of growth is often unequal, especially for identical twins, who may rarely have a placental vascular communication allowing for unequal blood exchange. Twins are more likely to be relatively undernourished at birth and are more prone to prematurity and problems of neonatal adaptation.

Infection

The early fetus is generally an excellent culture medium for many viral agents. Once a viral agent is acquired via maternal viremia, or (rarely) via the vaginal route, it tends to cause a chronic widespread fetal disease. Serious disease may occur in tissues that are not altered by the same viral agent in the mature individual. A notable example is the rubella agent, which, for unknown reasons, must usually be acquired during the first 12 to 16 weeks to cause fetal disease. Such viral agents may give rise to a fetal IgM antibody response, but it is usually insufficient to rid the fetus of the viral agent at this stage of life. The IgM response can be utilized at birth as a non-specific indicator of prenatal infectious disease, since IgM does not cross in significant amounts from the mother and is only provoked by an antigen stimulus to the fetus.

Opsonic activity, the ability of leucocytes to ingest and kill bacteria, is limited in the premature. Perhaps for this reason, and because of the initial lack of IgM, the newborn baby, especially the premature, is more prone to develop sepsis caused by agents such as *E. coli* or *Pseudomonas*.

Altered Maternal Environment

Maternal hypovolemic shock, acidosis or hypoxemia can seriously affect the fetus. Also, most medications administered to the mother will affect the fetus. Maternal diabetes mellitus is associated with increased rates of abortion, stillbirths, malformation and problems of neonatal adaptation in the liveborn. An increase in maternal serum phenylalanine (PKU), an autosomal recessive disorder, frequently has an adverse effect on fetal brain development, besides being associated with increased incidence of other malformations.

MONITORING OF FETAL DEVELOPMENT AND DISORDERS

Amniocentesis

From 13 to 14 menstrual weeks onward it is possible to insert a needle through the pregnant woman's lower abdominal wall and uterus to obtain 5 to 10 ml of amniotic fluid. This is currently done when there is a known risk of having an offspring with a serious disorder that can be detected in early development. For example, chromosome studies of cultured amnion cells can be done to exclude a fetal chromosomal abnormality, or enzyme studies can be made to exclude a homozygous fetus with Tay-Sachs disease when parents are carriers for this autosomal recessive disorder. More than 25 other inherited metabolic defects can be diagnosed by study of cells from amniotic fluid (Dorfman, 1973). Sex can be determined in the fetus of a woman who is a known carrier for an X-linked recessive disorder such as hemophilia, in which case the male fetus would have a 50 per cent risk of being affected. When anencephaly or meningomyelocele has occurred in a preceding pregnancy, the risk of recurrence of either defect is approximately 5 per cent. Detection of elevated alpha-fetoprotein levels in the amniotic fluid may indicate the presence of anencephaly or meningomyelocele. If the alpha-fetoprotein is not increased, anencephaly can be reliably excluded, but positive results are found in only about 90 per cent of pregnancies with meningomyeloceles. Having obtained the definitive information, the parents can then elect to terminate undesired pregnancies. Since the time limit for therapeutic abortion is 18 menstrual weeks, it is necessary that the laboratory tests on amniotic fluid, especially in which cells must be grown and studied, be performed with expedience and by specialized laboratories.

Fetal Activity

The fetus has movement discernible to the mother at 16 to 20 menstrual weeks. Thereafter he is active every day, and any prolonged periods of inactivity should lead to concern.

Heart Rate

Heart rate can be monitored. During late gestation the rate is about 140 to 160 beats per minute. Bradycardia is a sign of fetal distress, though the rate may normally slow down during uterine labor contractures. Continuous fetal heart monitoring during labor is assuming a more important role in the detection of fetal hypoxia.

Amniotic Fluid

Polyhydramnios or oligohydramnios may be evidence of a fetal problem (see Chapter 22, Malformation). The fetus usually does not pass stool (meconium) until birth unless in distress. Hence, meconium-stained amniotic fluid or "dirty" fingernails in the newborn from meconium lodged there during delivery is a sign of pre-existing fetal distress. Tracheal aspiration should be considered in such babies, since aspirated meconium may impair respiration. If there is any indication of fetal bacterial infectious disease, the amniotic fluid should be examined for evidence of such. Premature rupture of the membranes places the fetus at increased risk of infection.

Scalp Blood

When indicated, fetal blood can be obtained from scalp blood vessels during labor to determine blood gases, hematocrit, bilirubin and so on,

Prelude to Neonatal Adaptations

Finally, the fetus must undergo major adaptations in the transition to an extrauterine environment. Besides the all-important respiration, there are enzyme systems, which have yet to be induced to full activity. The liver cells must now become able to conjugate bilirubin and the infant must now utilize gluconeogenesis to regenerate his glycogen stores and thereby maintain his own blood glucose. Thus he is relatively prone to develop hyperbilirubinemia or hypoglycemia in the first few postnatal days, to mention only two potential problems. If fetal development has been such that he is mature, well-nourished and healthy, there will seldom be any problems in adaptation. He is less likely to adapt readily, however, if he is premature, postmature, underweight for gestational age, has Rh or ABO incompatibility disease, has a prenatally acquired infectious disease or has a serious problem of malformation.

REFERENCES

Boué, J., Boué, A., and Lazar, P.: Retrospective and prospective epidemiological studies of 1500 karyotyped spontaneous abortions. Teratology, 12:11, 1975.

Carr, D. H.: Chromosome studies in spontaneous abortions. Obstet. Gynecol., 26:308, 1965.

Dorfman, A. (Ed.): *Antenatal Diagnosis.* Chicago, University of Chicago Press, 1972.

Hertig, A. T., Rock, J., Adams, E. C., et al.: Thirty-four fertilized human ova, good, bad, and indifferent recovered from 210 women of known fertility. A study of biologic wastage in early human pregnancy. Pediatrics, 23:202, 1959.

Lubchenco, L. O., et al.: Intrauterine growth as estimated from liveborn birth-weight data at 24–42 weeks of gestation. Pediatrics, 32:793, 1963.

Saxén, L., and Rapola, J.: *Congenital Defects.* New York, Holt, Rinehart & Winston, Inc., 1969.

Shepard, T. H.: Normal growth and development of the human embryo and fetus. *In* Gardner, L. I. (Ed.): *Endocrine and Genetic Diseases of Childhood,* 2nd ed. Philadelphia, W. B. Saunders Co., 1975.

Shepard, T. H.: *A Catalog of Teratogenic Agents,* 2nd ed. Baltimore, Johns Hopkins Press, 1976.

Tanimura, T., Nelson, T., Hollingsworth, R. R., and Shepard, T. H.: Weight standards for organs from early human fetuses. Anat. Rec., 171:227, 1971.

Winick, M.: Cellular growth of the fetus and placenta, *In* Waisman, H. A., and Kerr, G. (Eds.): *Fetal Growth and Development,* New York, McGraw-Hill, 1968, p. 19.

Wilson, J. G.: *Environment and Birth Defects,* New York, Academic Press, 1973.

8 The Newborn

Robert D. Guthrie, John L. Prueitt, Janet H. Murphy,
W. Alan Hodson, Richard P. Wennberg and
David E. Woodrum

Of the 3 million infants born in the United States each year, a distressingly large number die during the first year of life (52,000 in 1974), resulting in an infant mortality rate in the United States of 16.5 per 1000 live births. More than 75 per cent of infant deaths occur during the neonatal period (the first 28 days of life), and a major portion of these deaths occurs within the first 24 hours of life. Prematurely born infants account for a large proportion of these neonatal deaths.

A relatively small segment of the population in the United States accounts for an inordinately large proportion of neonatal mortality and morbidity. The infant mortality rate in the low income areas of our larger cities approaches 26 per 1000 live births, a level similar to that in the poorer areas of countries considered to be under-developed.

Perinatal complications can result in life-long mental and physical disabilities. Reduction of mortality and morbidity rates in the neonatal period will require improvement in recognition and treatment of problems in the immediate pre- and postnatal periods, including a better understanding of the causes and prevention of premature parturition, and efforts to improve the social and economic well-being of all pregnant mothers.

The newborn is unique, with rapid growth and major physiological and biochemical changes interacting as at no other time in life. This discussion focuses on perinatal adaptation, management of the infant in the delivery room and the first hours of life, subsequent newborn care, detection of abnormalities and common illnesses of newborns.

MANAGEMENT OF THE INFANT IN THE FIRST HOURS OF LIFE

Several abrupt changes in organ function occur at birth. The first goal of delivery room management is to facilitate adaptation to extrauterine life with particular emphasis on the most vulnerable aspects of adaptation: cardiopulmonary and temperature regulation.

CARDIOPULMONARY ADAPTATION TO EXTRAUTERINE LIFE

Major cardiopulmonary changes are required to allow successful transition from the aquatic fetal state to the air-breathing newborn state. The organ of gas exchange during fetal life is the placenta, which receives one third of the fetal cardiac output. There is a large maternal-fetal gradient across the placenta for oxygen and a small gradient for carbon dioxide (Table 8–1). The fetus compensates for his relatively low PO_2 by having a fetal hemoglobin curve that is shifted to the left (more saturated at a given PO_2) of the adult curve. At an umbilical PO_2 of 32, fetal hemoglobin is 82 per cent saturated.

Fetal blood flow characteristics are illustrated in Figure 8–1. One third of the blood from the inferior vena cava (and umbilical vein) is shunted across the foramen ovale to the left side of the heart to supply the upper portion of the body with relatively well-oxygenated blood—PO_2 of 27 mm Hg. The lower portion of the body receives a mixture of blood from the left ventricle and the right ventricle (via the ductus arteriosus) with a resultant PO_2 of 21 mm Hg. Ninety per cent of the right ventricular out-

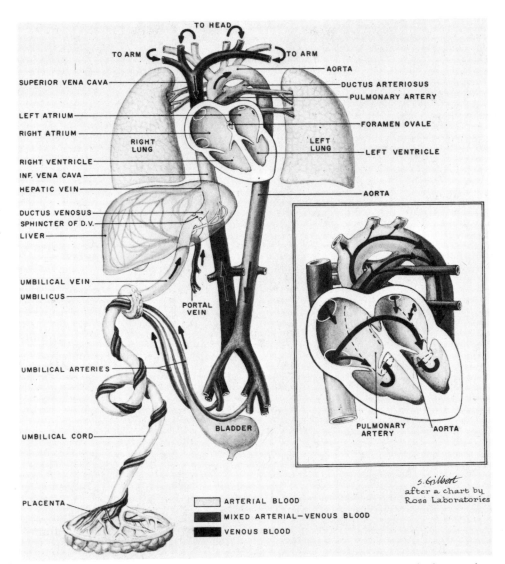

TO HEAD

TO ARM — — TO ARM

SUPERIOR VENA CAVA —————— AORTA

DUCTUS ARTERIOSUS
PULMONARY ARTERY

LEFT ATRIUM ————

RIGHT ATRIUM ————

RIGHT LUNG — LEFT LUNG

FORAMEN OVALE

RIGHT VENTRICLE ———— LEFT VENTRICLE

INF. VENA CAVA ————

HEPATIC VEIN ————

AORTA

DUCTUS VENOSUS ————
SPHINCTER OF D.V. ————
LIVER ————

UMBILICAL VEIN ————
UMBILICUS ————

PORTAL VEIN

UMBILICAL ARTERIES ————

BLADDER

UMBILICAL CORD ————

PLACENTA ————

ARTERIAL BLOOD
MIXED ARTERIAL—VENOUS BLOOD
VENOUS BLOOD

PULMONARY ARTERY   AORTA

S. Gilbert
after a chart by
Ross Laboratories

Figure 8–1 Fetal circulation. Arrows indicate course of blood. Oxygen saturation is highest in the umbilical vein and progressively lower in the vessels to the head and neck, the aorta, and finally the inferior vena cava below the liver, which has the most desaturated blood. The insert illustrates the course and distribution of blood in the fetal heart and large vessels more clearly. Note that the oxygenated placental blood entering the heart via the inferior vena cava flows preferentially to the left ventricle and head. (*From* Bonico, J. H.: Principles and Practice of Obstetric Analgesia and Anesthesiology. Philadelphia, F. A. Davis Co., 1967; adapted from Ross Clinical Aid No. 1, Fetal Circulation, Ross Laboratories, Columbus, Ohio 43216. Reproduced with permission.)

put passes through the ductus arteriosus into the descending aorta and 10 per cent goes through the lungs. This major shunt is due to the high pulmonary vascular resistance and the large caliber of the ductus arteriosus.

The lungs in fetal life contain fluid with a volume equal to the functional residual capacity in the newborn. This fluid origi-nates in the lung and is of a different composition than amniotic fluid. Amniotic fluid does not enter the respiratory tract except under conditions of fetal distress when respiratory efforts are attempted. Passage through the birth canal results in a thoracic squeeze, which expels a portion of the lung fluid. The majority of the fluid is absorbed through the pulmonary capillaries

**TABLE 8–1   ARTERIAL BLOOD
GASES AND pH**

	Maternal	Fetal (Umb. Vein)	Birth	1 Day
PO_2	98	32	15	60
PCO_2	37	42	60	35
pH	7.4	7.37	7.25	7.36

and lymphatics following initiation of respiration.

Chest wall movements associated with phrenic nerve activity occur during rapid eye movement sleep in fetal animals, indicating that the neuromuscular control of breathing is intact and functional prior to delivery. At birth, gas exchange is abruptly switched from the placenta to the lung. Prior to the first breath, the PCO_2 is elevated and the PO_2 and pH are decreased (Table 8–1). The hypoxemia and hypercarbia stimulate central and peripheral chemoreceptors, and along with other sensory stimuli (tactile, proprioceptive and thermal) result in initiation of breathing in the normal infant.

The normal newborn may generate transthoracic pressures as high as 60 to 80 cm H_2O with the first few breaths. Large intrapleural pressures are no longer needed when the fluid has been absorbed and the alveoli are air-filled.

Replacement of alveolar fluid with air increases arterial PO_2, which is a key factor is causing pulmonary vasodilation and constriction of the ductus arteriosus. The increase in pulmonary blood flow elevates left atrial pressure and closes the foramen ovale. The increase in arterial PO_2 causes constriction of the umbilical vessels and ductus arteriosus, and the transition from fetal circulation to neonatal circulation is complete.

TEMPERATURE REGULATION

The infant has a relatively large surface area and relatively little thermal insulation; he is, therefore, easily cooled as he is delivered wet into an air-conditioned delivery room. The environmental temperature at which the metabolism is minimal for the infant is considerably higher than for the adult, i.e., 31 to 33°C for the term infant as compared to 22 to 28°C for the naked adult. The newborn is unique in that he does not shiver, and heat production is primarily by non-shivering thermogenesis. The mechanism of heat production is probably related to norepinephrine release and hydrolysis of fat rich in mitochondria (possibly brown fat) resulting in mobilization of free fatty acids and increased consumption of glucose. Prolonged cooling may result in metabolic acidosis and a reduced PaO_2 and is associated with an increased mortality in premature infants weighing less than 1000 gm at birth.

Delivery Room Management

Patency of the airways is critical for the establishment of respiration. At delivery, the oropharynx should be suctioned to remove mucus, blood or meconium. The baby should be held level to, or slightly below, the perineum to minimize gravitational flow of blood from the infant to the placenta. The blood volume of the infant at the time of delivery is about 70 ml/kg. If cord clamping is delayed or the cord is "milked," the blood volume may be increased up to 100 ml/kg. This may be detrimental to a compromised infant.

The infant should be dried immediately to reduce evaporative heat loss and placed under a radiant heat source. The general condition is recorded at one and five minutes of age by means of the Apgar rating (Table 8–2).

A brief examination should be directed at acute, correctable lesions. If the infant is in respiratory distress or does not become pink with brief inhalation of oxygen, then airway obstruction or a pulmonary lesion should be considered. Cyanosis in the presence of a chest fixed in inspiration along with a shift in the position of the apex beat strongly suggests a pneumothorax, which occurs spontaneously in 2 per cent of births or following vigorous resuscitative efforts. Diaphragmatic hernia (1 in 2200 live births) is suggested by respiratory distress in the presence of a scaphoid abdomen. Meconium aspiration is most likely to occur in the asphyxiated fetus because of intrauterine passage of meconium. Patients with meconium aspiration are particularly prone to develop pneumothorax. Choanal

TABLE 8–2 APGAR SCORE

Sign	Score		
	0	1	2
Heart rate	Absent	Below 100/min.	Over 100/min.
Respiratory effort	Absent	Slow/irregular	Good/crying
Muscle tone	Limp	Some reflexion of extremities	Active
Reflex irritability (slap the foot)	No response.	Some motion	Cry
Color	Blue or pale	Extremities blue; body pink	Pink

Technique of scoring: One minute after the birth of the baby the five signs are evaluated, and each is given a score of 0, 1 or 2. A total score of 10 indicates that the infant is in optimal condition.

atresia, with complete obstruction of the nasal passage, occurs in 1 in 5000 births and is potentially lethal in the newborn infant since he is an obligate nose breather. This defect is easily detected by noting whether the infant can breathe with the mouth closed. Passage of a tube through the nose may cause mucosal trauma and is not recommended as a routine screening procedure for this condition. Idiopathic respiratory distress syndrome is common in prematures, asphyxiated preterm infants and infants of diabetic mothers. Signs of hyaline membrane disease are most often present in the delivery room.

A catheter is passed into the stomach to rule out esophageal atresia (1 in 6000 births). Aspiration of more than 20 ml of fluid from the stomach is indicative of high intestinal obstruction.

Fetal hemorrhage may rarely occur during birth. This is accompanied by pallor, weak peripheral pulses and poor venous filling and capillary refill. The full-term newborn has a hematocrit of 50 to 55 per cent and a blood pressure of 60/40 mm Hg. Changes in the blood pressure or the hematocrit do not necessarily occur with acute blood loss.

Markedly undergrown infants, infants of toxemic or diabetic mothers and erythroblastotic infants are susceptible to hypoglycemia in the first days of life and should be identified as high-risk infants in the delivery room. Infants born to mothers with prolonged rupture of the membranes, particularly in the presence of overt maternal infection, should be identified and closely observed for the signs of sepsis. The gastric

fluid should be examined for polymorphonuclear white cells (indicating the presence of amnionitis if more than 5 per high-power field) if the membranes have been ruptured for more than 24 hours.

Placental size should be 15 per cent of fetal size. A small placenta may be inadequate for the proper nutrition of the fetus. Areas of fibrosis and infarction of the placenta suggest possible fetal compromise. In twin pregnancies, the placenta should be examined to determine whether the twins are fraternal or identical. If the twins are identical and have greatly differing hematocrits, it is likely that anastomosis between fetal vessels allowed one twin to transfuse the other.

Single umbilical arteries occur in 1 per cent of newborns. The presence of a single umbilical artery should call for a closer examination than usual for other congenital abnormalities such as the oligohydramnios tetrad or the VATER* anomalad although the majority of such infants are normal.

Prophylaxis for gonococcal ophthalmia consists of instillation of 1 per cent silver nitrate; this procedure reduces the risk of infection to 2 per cent of exposed neonates.

Resuscitation. Resuscitation of the newborn is directed toward facilitating successful transition from the aquatic fetal state to the air-breathing newborn state. The major factor normally responsible for this transi-

---

*Various combinations of vertebral anomalies, anal atresia, tracheoesophageal atresia, renal defects, radial limb defects, cardiac defects and single umbilical artery.

tion is the elevation of PaO_2 which occurs with the initiation of respiration. Resuscitative efforts, therefore, revolve mainly around establishment of adequate air-blood contact in the lungs by ventilation. In the severely asphyxiated infant, correction of acidosis by the use of bicarbonate aids in increasing cardiac output and perhaps in decreasing pulmonary vascular resistance. Asphyxia can be predicted about 70 per cent of the time if close attention is paid to events during labor and delivery. The presence of "late" or "variable deceleration" patterns in the fetal heart rate and fetal tachycardia or meconium-stained amniotic fluid suggest fetal hypoxia. The risk is increased with juvenile or multigravid mothers, multiple births, abnormal birth presentation, vaginal bleeding and systemic maternal disease.

If respiration is mildly depressed at birth, all that is often required is cutaneous stimulation of the rib cage or slapping of the feet. A few breaths of 100 per cent oxygen may be of benefit. If respiration is gasping in nature or absent and the infant is limp, more active measures must be taken. After suctioning, an oral airway should be placed, and the infant should be ventilated with 100 per cent oxygen by means of a bag and mask. The chest wall is observed for expansion as a clinical indication of the adequacy of ventilation. At times 60 to 80 cm H_2O pressure is required for adequate chest expansion although 30 cm H_2O pressure is sufficient to resuscitate most infants.

If ventilation with a bag is unsuccessful, then an endotracheal tube should be inserted. An endotracheal tube of 3.5 mm internal diameter should be used in the full-term infant and one of 2.5 mm in the infant weighing less than 1000 gm. Due to the frequent presence of areas with low ventilation-perfusion ratios in the lung, it is advisable to use 100 per cent oxygen for resuscitation rather than room air.

An asphyxiated infant develops a metabolic acidosis due to accumulation of non-carbonic acids. If the infant does not respond promptly to ventilation, he is given bicarbonate of soda, $NaHCO_3$ (3 mEq/kg), via an umbilical vessel. This is sufficient to correct approximately one half of the base deficit of moderately asphyxiated infants. This dose may be repeated once or twice at intervals of five minutes if the infant re-

mains non-responsive. Additional buffer therapy should usually follow acid-base and blood gas determinations. As supplied by manufacturers, sodium bicarbonate is in 0.9 M solution. To avoid a hyperosmotic load, it is recommended that the sodium bicarbonate be diluted, with an equal volume of sterile water.

A heart rate of less than 100/min generally indicates asphyxia of at least moderate severity. If the heart rate is less than 50/min or peripheral pulses cannot be felt, closed chest cardiac massage (midsternum) at a rate of 100 to 120/min may be needed until cardiac output is adequate.

The First Six Hours

Since most neonatal problems have their onset in the first four to six hours after birth, the infant should be initially placed in a nursery area where he will receive close observation during a "transitional phase" of his hospital stay. Common problems include excess secretions, airway obstruction, retained pulmonary fluid, cyanosis, respiratory distress (including grunting, flaring of the alae nasi, chest wall retractions), apnea, abnormal posture or movement (jitteriness, seizures).

About 5 per cent of all infants will develop a problem requiring specialized care. Therefore, early identification and triage to (1) an intensive care nursery, (2) another hospital or ward with specialized facilities, (surgery, radiology, laboratory) or (3) to a separate area of the nursery for more intense observation will facilitate management. Nursing observation should include heart rate, respiratory rate, general activity, temperature and ability to handle the first feeding (usually water). Premature infants weighing more than 1.5 kg may require observation for a longer period of time in order to ascertain the level of their special care needs. Since smaller premature infants are at appreciable risk for developing problems in the newborn period, it is advisable to transfer them to an intensive care unit.

The baby should be kept naked under a radiant heater that is servocontrolled to an abdominal skin temperature of 36.5° C. After approximately four hours, if the rectal temperature is above 36.5°C and he is otherwise normal, the infant is given a bath and a feeding of 10 to 15 ml water. He is then dressed, swaddled and placed in a bassinet in the nursery for routine care and feeding.

Nursery Care of the Normal Newborn

During the first 12 hours of life the infant should have a thorough physical examination. The significant events of pregnancy and delivery should be recorded including length of gestation, duration of labor, abnormalities in fetal heart rate, Apgar score, mother's previous pregnancies, blood group incompatibility, premature rupture of membranes and maternal infection.

Physical examination. The physical examination should be of the most thorough nature to rule out underlying congenital malformations, specific neonatal problems and birth injury.

GENERAL APPEARANCE. Note general body proportions, color, activity, distress or growth abnormalities.

HEART. Next, it is preferable to examine the heart and lungs before the infant is disturbed. Note the position of the apex beat, the rate (normal 120 to 160/min) and intensity of sounds. Fifty per cent of newborn infants will have a murmur of a patent ductus arteriosus, which usually disappears by the third day of life. Since there is normally a high pulmonary vascular resistance at birth, shunt murmurs associated with congenital heart disease are frequently not evident until a few weeks.

RESPIRATORY SYSTEM. While the infant is still quiet, observe the respiratory pattern and rate (normal 30 to 40/min). If the infant is having respiratory distress, note retractions, nasal flare, air entry, grunting and whether the A-P diameter is increased or decreased with sternal retractions. Later, note the duration and intensity of his cry as an indication of "pulmonary function."

Subsequent examination involves a head to foot approach.

HEAD AND NECK. The relatively soft calvarium and open suture lines allow considerable molding of the head as it passes through the birth canal. Sometimes there is soft tissue edema (caput succedaneum) and bruising. Subperiosteal bleeding (cephalohematoma) is differentiated from a caput in that the swelling does not extend beyond suture lines. Note the shape of the head and the size and tension of the fontanels. Transillumination of the skull in a dark room should be done to rule out major central nervous system malformations such as hydrocephalus and hydranencephaly. Note the shape and size of the orbital fissures; examine the eyes for hypo or hypertelorism, the conjunctiva for hemorrhage or inflammation, the iris for coloboma and lens for cataracts. Small retinal hemorrhages are seen in about 25 per cent of normal newborns. Retinoblastoma, while rare, can be present in the neonatal period. Low-set, malformed ears may be associated with other congenital anomalies. The amount of ear cartilage is related to gestational age. Examination of the tympanic membrane is rarely helpful. Since the infant is an obligate nose breather, patency or non-patency (unilateral choanal atresia) of the nares can be checked by closing first one nostril, then the other, with the mouth closed, while observing respiration. Occasionally, the tongue may be enlarged (lymphangioma) or protrude slightly from the mouth (Down syndrome, congenital hypothyroidism). The tongue may obstruct the airway if there is a small mandible (Robin anomalad). Clefts of lip or palate or the alveolar ridges should be searched for. While the infant is sucking your finger, feel for a subtle or submucosal bony cleft of the palate and the strength and duration of suck. Seventh nerve palsy may result from birth injury (including injury from forceps) and is characterized by a droop in one corner of the mouth. A thyroglossal duct cyst, branchial cleft cyst, cystic hygroma or hemolymphangioma may present as a neck mass. Loose folds of skin in the posterior part of neck may suggest the possibility of Down syndrome or Turner syndrome. A difficult delivery, especially shoulder dystocia, may cause a fractured clavicle, easily detected by feeling for crepitus.

ABDOMEN. Observe for distention (obstruction or ileus) or flatness (diaphragmatic hernia). The liver is usually palpable 1 to 2 cm below the right costal margin, and the left lobe is frequently quite prominent. The tip of the spleen is often felt. The kidneys can usually be felt by deep lateral abdominal palpation. Lobulated renal enlargement may signify multicystic kidney disease, congenital hydronephrosis, neuroblastoma or, rarely, Wilms' tumor. The umbilicus should be inspected for evidence of bleeding, infection, hernia and number of umbilical arteries.

GENITALIA. Note size and shape of penis, position of meatus, size of scrotum and skin folds of scrotum. The testes should be palpable; hydrocele is very common. Inguinal hernia may result in incarceration in the newborn, and early surgical correction is indicated. Female genitalia are examined for clitoral size and fusion of the labia. A mucoid, creamy vaginal discharge (estrogen effect) is almost always present. Vaginal bleeding, due to withdrawal from estrogen stimulation, is occasionally seen. Digital rectal examination is not recommended since anal fissures commonly result. An imperforate anus will be detected by routine use of a rectal thermometer. The presence of ambiguous genitalia requires additional evaluation.

EXTREMITIES. Asymmetrical arm movement may indicate an Erb's (C5 and C6 nerve roots) or Klumke's palsy (C8 to T2 nerve roots). Extra digits, syndactyly, limited joint motion, skin creases, edema, length of nails or meconium staining should be noted. The right brachial and femoral arterial pulses should be similar in intensity, and coincident. A strong dorsalis pedis pulse suggests a patent ductus arteriosus.

Congenital hip dislocation occurs in 1 per 1000 live births. The recurrence risk among siblings of affected persons is about 40 times as great as the expected frequency. It is five times as common in girls than boys and is rare in blacks. To test for this, the legs and hips are extended, and the feet are brought together in the midline. The knees and hips are then flexed to 90 degrees, with the anterior tibia fitting into the examiner's palm. The femur is held between the thumb medially and the index and middle fingers, which are placed laterally over the greater trochanter. One leg is held stationary, fixing the pelvis, and the other leg is abducted with the index and middle fingers exerting pressure medially and anteriorly. If the hip is dislocated, the femur will be felt to glide over the acetabulum and "thump" into the socket as the hip relocates (Ortolani sign). A normal

hip should abduct 90 degrees. The leg is then adducted to the midline with the thumb pressing laterally and posteriorly. If the hip dislocates, the femoral head will be felt to ride over the acetabular rim and dislocate with a "thump" (Palmen sign). Subluxation of a femoral head does not return to the acetabulum during the above maneuvers, thus the "thump" is absent. Increased mobility of the femoral head in the "telescoping" maneuver detects this condition. Ligamentous hip "clicks" are found in 25 per cent of newborns and should not be confused with the "thump" sensation of the dislocated hip.

SKIN. Note texture, scaling, rashes, milia, edema or meconium. Milia occur in about 40 per cent of newborns. These consist of distended sebaceous glands appearing within the first week of life, most commonly in the cheeks. Erythema toxicum is an erythematous, often blotchy, rash with a whitish-yellow papular center, which occurs in about 50 per cent of all full-term newborns within the first two days of life. It is transient (usually one to two days) and the etiology is unknown. The temperature differential (normally 2.5°C) between the abdominal skin and extremities may be an important clue to illness. An increased temperature gradient indicates cold stress or sepsis. An overheated baby will have warm or flushed extremities. Transient breast enlargement due to hormones can occur in both male and female infants. It usually disappears within several days although it may persist for several months.

NEUROLOGICAL STATUS. Deep tendon reflexes are frequently very brisk in the newborn. When the infant is awake and quiet, examination of other reflexes peculiar to the newborn is helpful in assessing his overall neurological status. These include the Moro (startle), suck, grasp, rooting, snout, crossed extension, tonic neck and stepping reflexes. Motor activity is observed during reflex testing, as is the tone of the extremities, which normally are held in a flexed position and should return to flexion when an extended limb is released by the examiner. The infant should respond to normal cutaneous stimuli such as pain or pressure by crying and withdrawal. The pupils should react to light; the normal infant turns his eyes toward soft light. Hearing is tested by observing the eyes blink in response to a loud noise. A high pitched cry may be indicative of brain injury or meningitis, as may irritability, abnormal posturing or undue jitteriness.

Measurements of weight, length, occipital-frontal head circumference (OFC) and chest circumference should be recorded. The average birth weight for the white American male is 3.4 kg (7.5 lb) and for the female is 3.36 kg (7.4 lb). The non-white birth weight is slightly lower. The average length is 50 cm (20 inches) and OFC 35 cm (16 inches).

STOOLING. The infant swallows amniotic fluid liberally during the last third of gestation. He does not normally stool unless he is asphyxiated *in utero* or born by breech delivery. Epithelial cells, amniotic fluid and bile salts form a thick green-brown mucoid mass called meconium. This material accounts for the nature of the baby's stools for the first few days of life. Initial dark green stools are followed by "transitional" stools, which are yellow or green and often seedy in appearance with relatively large amounts of water. In three to four days the stools are formed, soft and yellow. The first meconium stool usually appears prior to 12 hours. Intestinal obstruction should be suspected if no stools appear by 48 hours. Most infants will have two to eight stools per day.

Nutrition

The normal infant usually loses about 5 to 7 per cent of his body weight in the first three to four days of life and regains his birth weight by 7 to 10 days. There is an obligatory water loss that cannot be prevented by the early administration of fluids. After this, the infant should gain about 200 to 250 gm/week.

The average newborn infant requires 100 to 120 cal/kg/24 hours for optimum growth. This should include 2 to 4 gm protein/kg. Supplemental vitamins should be added at three to four weeks of age for breast-fed infants or infants fed commercial formulae or milk preparations which do not contain adequate quantities of vitamin A (1000 units), vitamin D (400 IU), and vitamin C (40 mg) per day. Breast-fed babies should also receive fluoride drops. The baby can be put to the breast as soon as he has graduated

from the "transitional nursery" at about four to six hours of age. The mother is instructed to begin feedings for about 3 minutes on each breast and gradually increase the time to about 10 minutes at each breast (see Chapter 11).

Talking with Parents

After the infant is examined, the parents should be reassured that the infant is well if this is true. Any concerns about the baby's health should be discussed with the obstetrician and the parents with care not to produce undue anxiety in parents who may have some postpartum emotional lability. Fathers should be included in all discussions whenever possible. An informed father may provide more support for the mother. Early maternal-infant attachment should be encouraged.

Parents commonly ask questions about the feeding and general care of their infants, and discussions in the hospital should include the following topics:

Quantity and frequency of feedings. Formula-fed newborns initially take 2 to 3 oz. every three to four hours round the clock, the quantity taken gradually increasing over the first few days and weeks of life. It is usual for infants to cease awakening for one of the nighttime feedings at about six weeks. Times for feeding at the breast have been outlined earlier.

Formula preparation and care of bottles and nipples. Commercial formulae are all labeled with directions for preparation, and these should be followed exactly. Bottles and nipples should be thoroughly cleaned and scrubbed with soap and water, and rinsed with clean water before sterilization or boiling for 10 minutes. Tap water may be used for formula dilution where the domestic water supply is pure and the prepared formula is to be consumed immediately. Boiled water is used for dilution of formula prepared in advance, which is then refrigerated.

Sleeping. Newborns sleep for the majority of the time between feedings but often have a period during the day when they are more wakeful. Parent-infant interaction should be encouraged during these periods of alertness.

Stooling. Most infants have two to eight stools per day, these being yellow in color.

Laxatives or enemas should not be given to an infant unless a physician so directs.

Bathing and cord care. The cord dries in the first two days of life and is kept dry, being cleaned gently with alcohol swabs once a day. The dry cord usually separates at a week of age. Reddening of the skin around the umbilicus often indicates infection, and a physician's advice should be sought. The infant should be given a sponge bath once a day until the cord separates, but once this has occurred and the exposed base is dry, the infant's trunk may be immersed in water; pure unscented soap is used for bathing and rinsed off well. Usually the use of oils and creams on the skin is not indicated in the first few months of life.

Clothing. This should be fairly loose-fitting and includes a shirt, diaper and overgarment covering arms and legs in a house at 70°, with one or two blankets to cover the sleeping infant. For going outdoors the head, except for the face, should be covered, and in cool weather an extra blanket or layer of warm clothing is necessary.

Visitors. Many visitors may be tiring for mother and infant during the first few weeks of life, and persons with colds or other infectious diseases should be discouraged from visiting the baby during this time, as he is particularly susceptible to infection.

Physician visits. Following discharge from the hospital, the infant should be seen by his physician within several weeks.

THE PHYSIOLOGICAL BASIS OF NORMAL LABORATORY VALUES

The laboratory values for the normal newborn infant represent organ functions that are gradually changing from their fetal to their extrauterine role. In order to differentiate normal from abnormal function, it is important to consider some of the unique physiological aspects of the neonate.

The Hematological System

Because the fetus is in a relatively hypoxic atmosphere, his hemoglobin concentration is high. The average hemoglobin concentration at birth is about 17 gm/100 ml (Hct 53). Marrow hyperactivity is reflected by a reticulocytosis (4 to 8 per cent in term infants) for the first three or four days. The subsequent marrow hypoactivity results in a progressive fall in hemoglobin concentration to 10 to 11 gm/100 ml by six to eight weeks of life. Reticulocytosis then reappears and the hemoglobin concentration tends to stabilize around 10 to 11 gm/100 ml. In the premature infant, the hemoglobin level remains low for a longer period of time because growth is rapid and, despite an increase in hemoglobin mass, there is dilution by the increasing plasma volume. The amount of iron available through red blood cell destruction is adequate to maintain hemoglobin synthesis for four to six months. Beyond this period, exogenous iron is needed. In infants of low birth weight or with perinatal blood loss, the iron stores are lower and supplemental iron (2 mg/kg/day) should be added at two to three months. In addition, prematurely born infants, especially those with birth weight less than 2 kg, have decreased absorption of vitamin E. Supplementation with 25 IU of a water soluble preparation of vitamin E per day is indicated for the first two to three months.

The white blood count at birth is usually between 15,000 and 25,000/mm³ and falls to 8000 to 10,000/mm³ within a day or two. The differential white count is shifted to the left at birth; after several days, lymphocytes begin to predominate and lymphocytosis persists through the first five or six years. The platelet count in the newborn varies between 125,000 and 250,000/mm³ and in the premature infant may be as low as 100,000/mm³.

Until the infant acquires a bacterial flora in his gastrointestinal tract, he is unable to synthesize vitamin K. As a consequence, vitamin K–dependent coagulation factors made in the liver, such as factors II, VII, IX and X, will be decreased during the first few days of life. The premature infant may have a much greater reduction in coagulation factors. One milligram synthetic vitamin K is routinely given to the infant intramuscularly after birth to prevent "hemorrhagic disease of the newborn."

Renal Function

One of the most important handicaps of the newborn is an inability to concentrate his urine as well as the older infant. Under conditions of thirsting, maximum concentration is only about half that of the adult. During the first few days after birth the infant is less able to tolerate a water load and more susceptible to water intoxication. The ability to handle a high osmolar and acid load is also limited. When the infant has a condition that interferes with growth, metabolic acidosis and dehydration quickly supervene. Under normal conditions, the daily fluid requirements for the term infant are approximately 100 ml/kg; however, the needs of the premature infant are 150 ml/kg/day by three to four days. Drug excretion by the kidneys is relatively slow in premature infants during the first few days of life. Hence, blood levels of some drugs such as ampicillin can be maintained by less frequent administration than in the older infant (see Chapter 6).

COMMON PROBLEMS OF THE NEONATE

Prematurity

The incidence of prematurity (37 weeks gestation or less) is 8 per cent, varying from 16 per cent in low socioeconomic areas to about 2 per cent in middle and upper income communities.

The problems of premature infants are related primarily to difficulties in adaptation to extrauterine life. Failure of pulmonary adaptation due to pulmonary immaturity, hyaline membrane disease or apnea is most frequent. Susceptibility to infection, jaundice, cold stress and hypoglycemia is increased. Maintenance of adequate nutrition in the very low birth weight infant is a common and difficult problem.

Idiopathic Respiratory Distress Syndrome (Hyaline Membrane Disease)

Hyaline membrane disease (HMD) is the most common serious disease affecting newborns. Its incidence is inversely related to gestational age. It occurs in 80 per cent of 28 week gestation infants compared to about 0.5 per cent in full-term infants; the average incidence in premature infants is 14 per cent or about 40,000 cases per year in the United States. Respiratory

distress has its onset at birth and progesses in severity over 24 to 72 hours. It is characterized by tachypnea (respiratory rate more than 60 per minute), expiratory grunting, chest wall retractions (xyphoid, suprasternal, subcostal, intercostal) and oxygen dependency. The hypoxemia results from intrapulmonary shunting of blood past atelectatic areas of the lung. Hypercapnia may also occur. Dilated bronchi and bronchioles contrasted against a background of atelectatic alveoli account for the characteristic radiographic appearance of a reticulogranular pattern and an "air bronchogram" (Fig. 8–2).

The etiology of HMD is related to immaturity of the developing surfactant system in the lung of the premature infant. Perinatal factors such as asphyxia also have an additive effect in increasing the incidence in this susceptible group. With alterations in the surfactant system, alveoli are unstable and tend to collapse. This interferes with alveolar gas exchange and accounts for the clinical and pathological features of the disease.

At autopsy there are patchy or focal areas of atelectasis; hyaline membranes, composed largely of fibrin, line alveolar ducts and terminal bronchioles. Hyaline membranes are rarely present before six to eight hours of age; they probably represent the end stage of alveolar or capillary damage with leakage of plasma proteins.

The treatment of HMD is nonspecific and is directed at homeostasis, including correction of pH, respiratory failure and hypoxemia. Supplemental oxygen is provided to maintain arterial PO_2 between 50 and 80 mm Hg. Assisted ventilation is often necessary. Recent studies indicate that continuous positive airway pressure (CPAP) is efficacious in improving blood oxygenation, but an improvement in survival rate has not been shown conclusively. Maintenance of circulation, renal fuction and alimentation and correction of metabolic abnormalities are important aspects of treatment. About 75 to 80 per cent of affected infants survive. The long-term psychomotor prognosis is favorable in about 80 per cent of survivors.

Current emphasis on management of infant respiratory distress syndrome (IRDS) is directed at primary prevention. Lipid components of surfactant are secreted by the lung *in utero* and appear in the amniotic fluid. At 35 to 36 weeks in normal preg-

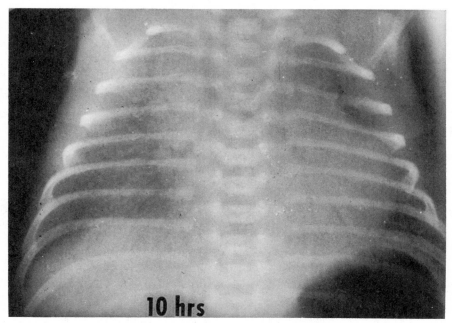

Figure 8–2 Radiograph of hyaline membrane disease at 10 hours of age showing the typical reticulogranular pattern with accentuated air bronchogram.

nancies there is an increase in the ratio of lecithin to sphingomyelin (L/S) which corresponds to a decrease in incidence of HMD after this time. Amniocentesis and measurement of L/S ratios can be useful in timing deliveries in complicated pregnancies. Also of recent interest is evidence that corticosteroids accelerate maturation of the lung; preliminary studies indicate that corticosteroids decrease the incidence of HMD in infants of less than 34 weeks' gestation. Collaborative studies are currently in progress to assess not only the efficacy but also the long-term safety of such agents. This is necessary prior to widespread use of corticosteroids in pregnancies threatened by premature delivery.

Other Causes of Respiratory Distress

Aspiration. Intrauterine stress (hypoxia) may initiate respiratory efforts with resultant aspiration of amniotic fluid or meconium. Aspiration pneumonitis, particularly serious with meconium, has a characteristic "splotchy" radiological appearance, which affects all lobes of the lung.

Aspiration of meconium should be detected in the delivery room. The infant is meconium-stained with depressed function and has irregular gasping respirations. Suction of the oropharynx should be done immediately to remove meconium, which easily obstructs airways. The cords should be visualized; if meconium is present and the baby has not already taken several breaths, tracheal intubation and suction of the meconium is beneficial. Following aspiration, secondary inflammation occurs and hypoxemia or respiratory failure develops. Pneumothorax occurs with increased frequency because of the "ball-valve" effect of partial airway obstruction by meconium. Death rarely occurs.

Pneumothorax and pneumomediastinum. Spontaneous pneumothorax occurs in 1 to 2 per cent of all newborns and is more frequent in infants with respiratory distress due to other causes. The high transpulmonary pressure necessary for the first breaths may cause alveolar rupture and dissection of air along the perivascular sheath to the mediastinum and the pleural space. The use of positive end expiratory pressure in treatment of HMD has been associated with an increased risk of air leak.

Pneumothorax is diagnosed clinically by sudden deterioration in respiratory status associated with a shift in the mediastinum (apex beat). In the newborn with a pneumothorax it is extremely difficult to detect alterations in air entry. As with all forms of respiratory distress in the newborn, a chest radiograph should be obtained immediately. If a pneumothorax is the cause of respiratory distress, a small multiholed polyvinyl tube or trochar catheter (Argyle 8 or 10 French) should be inserted into the intrapleural space and connected to underwater drainage. The tube can be clamped in 12 hours, and then removed in 24 hours if there has been no further accumulation of intrapleural air.

Transient tachypnea of the newborn. Frequently, the newborn infant will have tachypnea (rate of 60 to 120/min) without other signs of respiratory distress. The chest radiograph reveals a hazy appearance of the lung and often a small amount of fluid in the lobar fissures or the pleural space. This condition is thought to represent delayed absorption of lung fluid and usually resolves within 24 to 72 hours without treatment. Supplemental oxygen is necessary to treat hypoxemia.

Apnea of prematurity. Recurrent apneic episodes are common in premature infants of less than 34 weeks' gestation. It is second in incidence to hyaline membrane disease. Periodic breathing (respiratory pauses less than 10 seconds in duration) is very common in prematures. Apnea, however, is defined as a more prolonged respiratory pause (20 to 30 seconds); bradycardia and changes in blood pressure and peripheral blood flow occur in association with the apnea. The frequency of apneic episodes in a given baby may vary from one to two per day to several per hour. The onset is often between 48 to 72 hours of age, and episodes may continue for several weeks. An earlier onset implies apnea from sepsis, severe HMD, a metabolic derangement or CNS damage.

Infants with apnea require intensive care, which includes monitoring of respiration and heart rate with an apnea monitor. Cutaneous stimulation or resuscitation is necessary to re-establish regular respirations. Recently, theophylline or continuous positive airway pressure has been used to decrease the frequency of apnea. Occasionally, artificial ventilation is required.

The etiology remains obscure although sleep state and abnormalities of the chemical and neural control of respiration have been implicated. Long-term prognosis is favorable in the majority of infants.

Congenital heart disease. Congenital heart disease, including hypoplastic left heart syndrome, complex coarctations and obstructed total anomalous pulmonary venous drainage may cause heart failure in the neonatal period. The resultant tachypnea and pulmonary edema may be confused with lung disease. Cardiac catheterization is frequently necessary to establish the diagnosis (see Chapter 31). Cyanotic heart disease such as transposition of the great arteries may also be associated with tachypnea and should be considered in the differential diagnosis of respiratory disease.

Jaundice

Physiological jaundice is common in early infant life and is frequently more pronounced in premature infants. This is primarily due to a delay in the activity of the enzyme glucuronyl transferase. This liver enzyme conjugates bilirubin ("indirect reacting bilirubin") with glucuronic acid to form the water-soluble and excretable bilirubin-diglucuronide ("direct bilirubin"). Maximum indirect bilirubin concentrations are reached on the third or fourth day in term infants and on the fourth to sixth day in premature infants. If the bilirubin concentration rises above a level that can normally be attributed to physiological adaptation (i.e., 7 mg/100 ml on day 1 or 11 mg/100 ml on day 3), the cause of the jaundice should be investigated.

Every infant with unexplained hyperbilirubinemia must be evaluated for possible hemolytic disease. A peripheral blood smear provides a rapid and excellent screening test. Erythroblasts and nucleated red blood cells are seen in erythroblastosis fetalis (Rh incompatibility); 10 to 20 per cent spherocytes are common in hemolysis due to ABO incompatibility; fragmented red blood cells are present in hemolysis due to infection or to red cell metabolic disorders such as glucose-6-phosphate dehydrogenase (G-6-PD) deficiency; pyknocytes are present in infantile pyknocytosis. A hematocrit or hemoglobin level should be obtained, but may be within normal limits in mild hemolytic disease. Isoimmune hemolytic disease should be investigated by blood typing of mother and infant and by performing a Coombs agglutination test on the infant's red cells. Hemolytic disease due to Rh incompatibility will almost always result in a positive direct Coombs test, but this may be only weakly positive or negative in ABO incompatibility. In ABO incompatibility, incubation of the infant's cells with maternal serum with cause hemolysis.

If there is no evidence of hemolytic disease, other causes of jaundice are considered. The mother should be queried about maternal infection, diabetes, hepatitis and family history of jaundice. The infant should be examined for sources of excess bilirubin such as bruising and cephalohematoma. Hepatosplenomegaly, commonly present in hemolytic disease, may also occur in rubella syndrome and in infections caused by a Toxoplasma or cytomegalovirus and in syphilis. Jaundice may occur in hypothyroidism and galactosemia. Jaundice is frequently associated with bacterial and viral infections, and it may be the presenting sign of a potentially lethal infection.

Premature infants have a greater risk for developing kernicterus (toxic damage to the brain) than term infants. This may be due to lower levels of serum (albumin binds bilirubin), hypoxemia, acidemia, infection, hypoglycemia and increased free fatty acids, all of which may potentiate the transfer of bilirubin from plasma and extracellular spaces into tissue. In a healthy premature infant with a normal concentration of serum albumin (3.2 gm/100 ml) exchange transfusion is performed at varying levels of indirect serum bilirubin, depending upon the degree of prematurity and the postnatal age of the infant. These levels for exchange are below the 20 to 24 mg/100 ml values necessitating exchange transfusion in the healthy term infant. In very sick premature infants, it may be necessary to transfuse the infant at 10 to 12 mg/100 ml in order to prevent kernicterus. Exposure to bright light will photo-oxidize bilirubin, and phototherapy can be used to decrease a rise in serum bilirubin concentrations. It must never be used as a substitute for exchange transfusion when the bilirubin concentration reaches hazardous levels.

Hypoglycemia

Hypoglycemia may occur in the neonate in association with a number of conditions. Approximately 5 per cent of infants admitted to a premature or intensive care nursery can be expected to have low blood sugar levels during the first few days of life. Hypoglycemia is defined as a level of true blood glucose below 30 mg/100 ml in the first 48 hours of life and less than 40 to 50 mg/100 ml thereafter. In the premature infant, a blood glucose level below 20 mg/100 ml is considered abnormal. The clinical signs of hypoglycemia in the newborn include jitteriness, limpness, cyanosis, apnea, high-pitched cry, seizures, lethargy and difficulty in feeding. The most common syndrome is transient symptomatic hypoglycemia, which occurs characteristically in an infant who is small for gestational age (SGA), or the smaller member of discordant twins. Hypoglycemia is not uncommon following intracranial injury or neonatal asphyxia.

Infants of diabetic mothers have a high incidence of hypoglycemia. This most commonly occurs between one and four hours of age and is most often asymptomatic. The hypoglycemia is probably due to hyperinsulinism secondary to hyperplasia of the pancreatic islet cells that occurs *in utero* as a consequence of maternal hyperglycemia. Islet cell hyperplasia also occurs in infants with erythroblastosis due to Rh incompatibility. Infants with Rh disease, maternal diabetes or intrauterine growth failure should have routine screening of blood glucose by Dextrostix.

There are a number of other causes of hypoglycemia including inborn errors of metabolism, Beckwith-Wiedemann syndrome, insulinomas, sepsis and iatrogenic causes.

The treatment of both symptomatic and asymptomatic hypoglycemia consists of prompt correction of blood sugar by the rapid intravenous administration of 4 to 5 ml of 25 per cent dextrose/kg body weight, followed by an infusion of 15 per cent dextrose in water at a rate of 75 to 100 ml/kg/day. Once oral feedings are tolerated, the infusion of glucose is slowly decreased and the blood glucose concentration usually becomes stable at levels above 30 mg/100 ml. Hypertonic glucose should never be discontinued abruptly, since reactive hypoglycemia may result. Persistent hypoglycemia is unusual and should be treated with cortisone acetate (25 mg/day IM).

Bacterial Infection

The incidence of sepsis is approximately 1 per 1000 live full term births and 1 per 250 live premature births. Newborns and particularly premature infants are susceptible to serious bacterial infection, especially with enterobacteria and Group B streptococci. This susceptibility is due in part to an impaired ability of leukocytes to phagocytize bacteria (due to decreased opsonins), decreased leukocyte chemotaxis, decreased complement and absence of protective specific maternal antibody. Immune defenses that reside in the gamma G fraction cross the placenta, and if the mother has been sensitized, the newborn will have passive immunity to most viral and some bacterial infections for the first three to nine months of life. Macroglobulins do not cross the placenta. The most common infecting organism is *E. coli* although infections with other gram negative organisms are common. Also, many neonatal care units are currently seeing more infections caused by group B beta hemolytic streptococcus.

Signs of sepsis, especially in the premature, may be very subtle and require careful observation if early diagnosis is to be made. The most common signs are lethargy, poor feeding, residual gastric food, temperature instability (often only a transient 1 degree above or below the normal temperature), unexplained jaundice, abdominal distention and irritability. Hepatosplenomegaly is common in infections due to viruses and in syphilis or toxoplasmosis, but is not seen in bacterial sepsis. The most common forms of infection are septicemia, meningitis, pneumonia and urinary tract infections. Cutaneous infections, often minor, occasionally lead to septicemia. When an infant develops signs of infection, cerebrospinal fluid, blood, urine and cutaneous lesions should be examined and cultured. If the suspicion of infection is strong, the infant should be treated immediately with ampicillin and gentamycin. The treatment can be modified when the infecting organism is isolated. If staphylococcal infection is suspected, methicillin should be used.

The mortality rate from neonatal sepsis is 15 to 35 per cent; 20 to 50 per cent of neonates with meningitis die. It is estimated that more than 50 per cent of survivors of neonatal meningitis will have some neurological damage (see Chapter 14).

REFERENCES

Assali, N. S. (Ed.): *Biology of gestation.* Vol. III. Fetal neonatal disorders. New York, Academic Press, 1972.

Avery, G. B. (Ed.): *Neonatology: Pathophysiology and Management of the Newborn.* Philadelphia, J. B. Lippincott Co., 1975.

Avery, M. E. and Fletcher, B. D.: *The Lung and its Disorders in the Newborn Infant,* 3rd ed. Philadelphia, W. B. Saunders Co., 1974.

Behrman, R. E.: The Newborn. Ped. Clin. N. Am., *174*:759, 1970.

Cornblath, M., and Schwartz, R.: *Disorders of Carbohydrate Metabolism in Infancy,* 2nd ed. Philadelphia, W. B. Saunders Co., 1976.

Dawes, G. S.: *Foetal and Neonatal Physiology.* Chicago, Yearbook Medical Publishers, Inc., 1973.

Oski, F. A., and Naiman, J. L.: *Hematologic Problems in the Newborn,* 2nd ed. Philadelphia, W. B. Saunders Co., 1972.

Schaffer, A. J., and Avery, M. E.: *Diseases of the Newborn,* 4th ed. Philadelphia, W. B. Saunders Co., 1977.

9

Infancy and Childhood

_David W. Smith
and James W. M. Owens_

The slow and orderly process of human development is genetically determined and is dependent on the environment for its full expression. Ideally, we follow parameters of growth and development in the child in order to be alerted to any problems in this dynamic process. The assessment may include measures of actual size or performance as well as *rate* of advancement, as shown for one boy in Figure 9–1. Toward this end, we compare the child's development to that of population standards such as the Stuart growth charts and Denver Developmental Scales (see Appendix). Any individual discrepancy from such general charts should first be interpreted in relation to the immediate genetic background of the child to determine whether this is unusual development for a child of *these* parents. Obviously, this is always important, for we

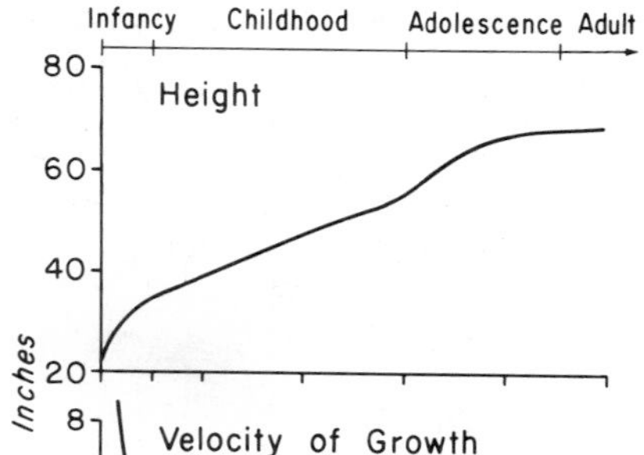

Figure 9–1 Linear growth in one boy showing accelerated growth during infancy and adolescence. (Adapted from Falkner, F.: Pediatrics, 29:448, 1962. Reproduced with permission.)

should not *expect* more of a child than his genetic endowment will allow. If a child's developmental alteration is *not* readily explained as a normal phenomenon for his family, then we should enlarge the search for an explanation of the developmental alteration.

Basically, the physical or performance level of a child should always be viewed in relation to both his chronological age and his biological age. The rate of biological aging, often termed level of maturation, is a variable that need not coincide with chronological age. One of the best indices of biological age, aside from the child's facial bone maturation, is the level of skeletal maturation, or "bone age," which is interpreted from roentgenograms, most commonly of the hand and wrist. Figure 9–2 shows the normal advancement in skeletal morphogenesis in the hand and wrist from four to six years of age. For example, the advent of adolescence correlates better with "bone age" than with chronological age. Thus you can appreciate that the slow maturer, though relatively short and physically immature as a child, reaches adolescence at a later chronological age than usual and eventually achieves normal adult stature. Again, family history provides the best index to whether variance in rate of maturation is a normal feature within that family. In this instance, the family history of interest relates to the age of adolescence in the parents and other close relatives.

The growth pattern of a particular tissue, such as the skeleton or the brain, initially involves increasing cell numbers followed by increasing cell size, in addition to organizational and functional alterations of the cells. The period of greatest vulnerability,

66

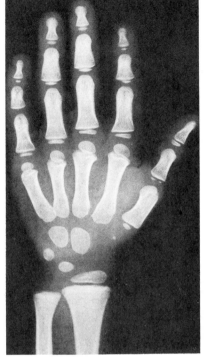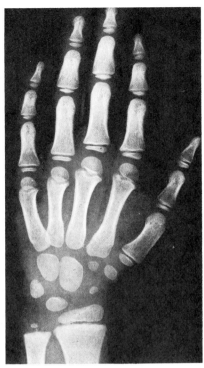

4 years   6 years

Figure 9-2   Roentgenograms of the hand and wrist at the four and six year ages in normal males. The advancement in mineralization of secondary centers of ossification allows for some discrimination of "bone age," crude though it may be. (Adapted from Greulich, W. W., and Pyle, S. I.: *Radiographic Atlas of Skeletal Development of the Hand and Wrist.* 2nd ed., Stanford, California, Stanford University Press, 1959.)

in terms of permanent impairment in growth and development, appears to be the time of increasing cell number. Two critical tissues that are incomplete at birth and hence highly vulnerable to developmental limitation after birth are the skeletal system and the brain. Our standard developmental evaluations are predominantly designed to maintain a surveillance over the adequacy of development of these two systems. Hence they are considered in more detail, followed by discussion of secular changes, sex differences, other changing systems, normal variants in certain aspects of development and anticipatory guidance and the psychology of the child relative to the examiner's approach to him at varying ages.

THE SKELETAL SYSTEM

The most rapid *rate* of skeletal growth is during fetal life with a gradual deceleration during infancy, leveling off to a fairly consistent 2 to 3 inches per year until late childhood. With the advent of adolescence, the final growth spurt takes place prior to epiphyseal ossification, as illustrated in Figure 9-1.

Birth length, averaging 20 inches, relates predominantly to maternal factors and provides little prediction of ultimate stature. With adequate nutrition and lack of chronic disease, the infant shifts into his own genetically determined growth rate. By two to three years of age the child's stature correlates best to the mean height of his parents and the child has usually reached about half of his adult height. Normal expectations for growth throughout childhood as well as for final stature can best be anticipated by envisioning a sex-appropriate mean between the growth patterns and stature of the parents.

Various parts of the skeletal system grow at different rates, thus proportions change with time. For example, the relatively small mandible catches up to the maxilla by two to three years, and the relatively short limbs grow more rapidly than the trunk during childhood.

Throughout its extended period of growth, skeletal development is vulnerable to environmental or disease-related aberrations, especially during early life and during adolescence when the rates are so rapid. The most common environmental limitation is malnutrition, which retards both linear growth rate and maturation of the skeleton. Correction of malnutrition results in accelerated "catch-up" growth toward expectancy for age. However, the more severe and prolonged the growth deficiency, the less is the likelihood of full restoration to the genetic potential for size.

THE BRAIN

Between 15 and 20 weeks of fetal life there is a dramatic increase in the number of neurons, and from 30 weeks of fetal life until about one year of age there is a further increase in the rate of new cell formation, predominantly glial cells. In addition to new cells added after birth, there is modification of existing cells in terms of myelinization and completion of the axonal networks. The brain is growing very rapidly and attains 82 per cent of its adult size by one year of age. Brain volume is readily reflected in head circumference, which increases five times as rapidly during the first year as during the second year (see Appendix).

Because of the incomplete development of the brain a newborn baby has limited function and shows mid-brain controlled reflexes, such as the Moro reflex, which are abolished as cortical centers become functional. Most of the advancing performance of a baby is a direct result of the increasing development of the brain, and only indirectly dependent on environmental stimuli. The progression of neuromotor function is from cephalad to caudad and proximal to distal, as is myelinization of nerve tracts. Most babies smile at about six weeks, sit alone at six to eight months and walk alone around 12 to 15 months of age. Communication progresses from babbling and cooing in the early months to "da-da" and "ma-ma" at 7 to 10 months, to single words and then short sentences by 18 months to two years. The progression is usually similar, but the rate of advancement may vary for particular functions.

Evaluate the status of brain development and function in early life by following head circumference for brain size, and performance for brain function. If indicated, evaluate the overall pattern of developmental performance in terms of motor, language, adaptive and personal-social features by such means as the Denver developmental screening technique (see Appendix). The latter is a crude assessment, but may provide clues about an overall defect in brain development, environmental deprivation or more specific defects in such functions as hearing or vision. We must be cautious not to interpret mild discrepancies too severely, however, since there is poor correlation between mild lag in early performance and eventual intelligence.

Evidence indicates that serious malnutrition during the rapid period of brain formation, especially prior to six months of age, can impair the level of brain development and function. Relatively rare disorders such as hypothyroidism and galactosemia can cause serious brain defect during this formative stage, whereas the same adverse influences have little or no permanent effect on function once the brain is fully developed. Hence you can appreciate the importance of recognizing early developmental lag and alleviating the cause, if possible.

Evaluation for lag in performance can also be indirectly utilized to detect deprivation of stimuli. Certain stimuli are necessary for expression of the developmental potential of the brain. Through neglect or ignorance the parents may not provide the baby with appropriate stimuli for him to utilize his increasing capabilities. This is especially important for language and personal-social advancement. In terms of preventing such problems, it is important to appreciate and nurture early parental attachment for the baby. Initially, the baby is more of a caretaking problem, but by two to three months of age he is usually interacting socially with the parents and comes to be viewed as an increasingly essential person in their lives. Hence the stimuli to utilize full function of the baby's advancing brain potential usually flow forth in a natural manner. If the parents do not develop this personal attachment because the baby was basically unwanted, because he has some defect which has not been accepted, or for other reasons, the baby is more likely to be deprived of appropriate stimuli. Basically, the approach to timing and type of stimuli that should be provided is relatively simple. The baby is the guide, the parents provide the opportunities and stimuli when the baby shows evidence of being ready for them. This applies to language, toys, toilet training and so on.

SECULAR CHANGES IN GROWTH AND MATURATION

During the past 100 years our population has been maturing more rapidly and advancing in height attainment. Thus each generation has entered adolescence about a half year earlier and has been about one inch taller than the previous generation. Since the children of today are more mature and taller at a given age than children of past generations, our old standards for growth comparison are not wholly appropriate for the present generation. The reasons for this dramatic change are poorly understood. "Better" nutrition has been suggested, as has relative lack of serious disease, and the more conjectural possibility of increased outbreeding with "hybrid vigor."

SEX DIFFERENCES IN DEVELOPMENT

The sex chromosomes appear to contain some of the genes that affect growth and maturation. There are preadolescent developmental differences between boys and girls that necessitate separate developmental standards. Girls are more mature at birth and continue to mature more rapidly, reaching adolescence one to two years before boys. Possibly as a corollary to this, girls advance more rapidly in early language development. This is illustrated by the fact that early reading failure in school is three to six times as common in boys. For level of maturation, boys are taller and have better perceptual-motor performance than girls. It is obvious that little boys and girls should not be compared by chronological age, and you may wonder whether they should start school at the same age! See Chapter 10, *Adolescence*, for differences in that age range.

OTHER DEVELOPMENTAL CHANGES OF IMPORTANCE

Each tissue has its own growth characteristics. You should be acquainted with at least these three in addition to the skeleton and brain.

Adipose Tissue

The late fetus develops adipose cells, which increase in number during the first year so that the baby is mildly obese, especially around nine months of age. During the second year there is a gradual decrease in adipose tissue, which may again increase in the preadolescent years. With adolescence, girls maintain the mildly obese state, and boys lose adipose tissue as the increase in muscle mass and strength occurs under the effects of androgen.

Lymphoid Tissue

The amount of lymphoid tissue is relatively great during childhood and decreases at adolescence. Hence during the early childhood years the lymph nodes are more easily palpable, the spleen tip is more likely to be palpable and the tonsils and adenoids appear relatively large.

Dentition

Teeth are developing from five months of fetal age. Deciduous teeth begin erupting at about five to eight months, and all 20 are usually present before two years. The permanent dentition begins erupting at about six to seven years. Dental maturation does not correlate well with bone age and is a poor index of biological age.

NORMAL VARIANTS AND ANTICIPATORY GUIDANCE

It is worthwhile to mention a few functional alterations that are normal features during the developmental process for many children, but may give rise to undue concern from parents or physicians who do not recognize them as variants of normal.

Many of the following common problems

create anxiety on the part of one or both parents about whether they are doing the "right things" for their child. It is important to find out if there are areas of worry, doubt or tension, for these may well be involved in the symptoms the child is showing. It is amazing how even a small infant may be a barometer of tension in the home. It is important to ask more than the traditional "How are things going?" which usually gets the response, "Oh fine!" Ask the mother if she has a chance to get out of the home; watch how the parents handle the baby (fondly, or like a sack of potatoes). This kind of question and these kinds of observations may yield a great deal more understanding about a problem than some of the standard techniques of history taking and physical examination.

The physician should know that certain common features usually appear at various times during the child's life. He should look for signs of problems before they become major disrupters of family life, and prepare with the parents an approach to these problems. The problems are mentioned here at the ages they commonly occur.

Newborns

Hiccupping and sneezing are frequent in the newborn and usually do not indicate disease. Protruding navels represent failure of closure of the rectus muscle around the umbilical opening and almost all of these spontaneously close by 12 to 18 months without *any kind* of treatment such as belly bands or tape. It is not physiologically harmful to support babies under the axillae and let them experience the sensation of bare-footed weight bearing. This will not "bow their legs."

First Three Months

Colic is a condition common in infants up to the age of about three months, in which the infant is extremely fussy, often in the evening. His symptoms suggest "gas cramps," with screaming and drawing the legs up on the abdomen, often with the passage of large amounts of flatus. These symptoms may incorrectly be attributed

to "milk allergy," and parents get on a treadmill of trying different formulae, all of which use cow's milk as their protein source. The etiology of colic is uncertain, but, at least in part, it is due to air swallowing. This may result from improper feeding nipples, in which the holes are too large *or* too small. The formula should slowly drip out of the bottle when it is held upside-down. It is imperative that the feeding situation be as relaxed as possible, as tension and anxiety can be sensed by the baby and can result in increased air swallowing. Frequent burping (after every 1 to 2 oz) and keeping the baby in the semisitting position in an infant seat or with the head of the crib raised for a half hour after feedings may help.

Seven to Nine Months

At the age when the child becomes ambulatory either by crawling or cruising (walking hanging on to objects) safety must be stressed. Room by room checks should be carried out for potential hazards such as poisons, pot handles projecting out from the stove and dangling electric cords.

Eighteen Months to Midchildhood

Strong drives for independence usually appear at this age. Also, children at this age commonly "test" parents to see what their limits *really* are. This testing process often challenges parents at their most vulnerable points. Two of these areas, feeding practices and toilet training, frequently become "hang-ups" for parents and may cause a crisis situation in the family. If you are able to neutralize these situations for a family you often will have helped them immeasurably.

Toilet training. A child is probably physiologically ready to begin toilet training by about 18 months; girls usually achieve this earlier than boys. The only training system that really works consistently is the positive reinforcement method, in which the child is rewarded for successes but nothing is said about failures. Anything that threatens the child's security is likely to cause some regression to more infantile patterns of behavior, and loss of toilet training is one of the most vulnerable.

Feeding. A daily food log for a two-year-old would shock many people unaccustomed to this age group. Breakfast may be fairly good, lunch may be the usual peanut butter sandwich, but often dinner may consist of one diced carrot and a swallow of milk. Parents may react to this by: (1) Telling the child that he is going to sit there until he swallows every bit, even "... if we have to cram it down your throat!" (in the meantime dinner has become a torture for the whole family). (2) Allowing the child who has eaten little to snack frequently on cookies, candies and so on, hoping to maintain his caloric requirements. (3) Insisting firmly that "Mealtime is mealtime." "You may eat what is put on your plate and if you don't want it just leave it there." If you can use this latter approach consistently without emotion and without permitting snacking, most children will respond with a very satisfactory intake over a period of time, even though a particular meal may seem very inadequate.

Discipline. This should be appropriate to the child's age and should be consistent among the family and others who may care for the child. For the nine-month-old, discipline should relate primarily to safety. For instance, slapping his hands when he chews on light cords is perfectly acceptable to make this dangerous practice an unpleasant experience. It is important for both parents to use the same amount and type of discipline since children learn very early to play one parent against the other. Whenever discipline is imposed, especially in the older child, it should be swift and meaningful for that age child. The two-year-old may try the maximum test against limits, a temper tantrum. A good way of handling this is simply to exclude him from the family group by putting him in his room until it is over, and to do this each time his behavior is unacceptable to the family. Breath-holding spells, which are usually seen in the young infant, are simply an earlier response to frustration. Usually occurring when the infant is startled or frustrated, a period of screaming or hyperventilating is followed by a period of apnea and cyanosis, and occasionally a few convulsive movements may be noted at the end of the spell. These are usually brief and self-limited, and the best way of handling them is simply to reassure the parents and to avoid as far as possible the precipitating circumstances.

Physical symptoms such as abdominal pain or headaches may obviously represent symptoms of the child's physical state, his emotional state or both. In the latter instance, the child may be overreacting to a minor ache or pain because of his psychological "set" at the time. It is, of course, important to exclude common physical reasons for these complaints, but keep in mind other factors that may be causing or contributing to the symptoms. Is he afraid of something? Does Daddy always get stomach aches when he is under tension?

Fears. Children at any age may become generally anxious or may develop specific phobias to such things as baths, fire or loud noises. In dealing with these, reassurance and physical demonstration of comfort and love are the most important first steps. Needless to say, some children become so frightened that further help may be required.

THE PSYCHOLOGY OF THE CHILD: THE EXAMINER'S APPROACH

The approach to the pediatric patient by the examiner should be dictated by sensitivity to the usual psychological make-up of a child of that age, and also sensitivity to the feelings, fears and needs of that particular child. What is done in the examination process should also be based on what is really needed. In other words, the very ill child with fever and pallor needs a thorough examination, even if he objects and the whole experience is an unpleasant one for him. On the other hand, consider the 18-month-old who comes in for a well-child evaluation and who is observed without ever touching him to be vigorous and to be developing appropriately in motor, language and social areas. What good will it serve to hold this child down in a violently protesting state while you try to look in his ears? How much better to spend that time with the mother talking about her very real fears and concerns about her child; and how much better the child will feel about coming to your office the next time. You should *always* ask the question, "Is it worth the price?"—for the child, for the family and for your own sense of having accomplished something worthwhile.

Following are a few suggestions concerning different approaches to children of advancing ages. These are by no means always applicable but at least provide you with an initial approach.

Infants (Non-Ambulatory)

Handle the infant gently and firmly while speaking to him in a soft voice. Avoid loud sounds or sudden movements, which may elicit the startle response and vigorous crying, thus limiting your evaluation, for in this age group you are still looking for undetected congenital abnormalities such as heart murmurs, failure to track light or to respond to sound, all of which require a fairly quiet child. Examination just after feeding is preferable, and not at a time that would be interrupting his normal naptime.

Toddlers (Ambulatory)

From the age of six months or so, it is quite common for a child to have a period of wanting to be very close to his mother and being afraid of strangers, especially strangers who are poking at him and doing things he is not accustomed to. If possible, during the examination the mother should have either very close visual contact with the child or the examination may be carried out with the baby on her lap or on her shoulder. Having the infant hugging the mother with his head against hers is often an ideal way to immobilize the head for an ear examination. Children in this age group often respond very well to small gifts such as a tongue blade that they can bite on or throw. This puts them in your camp as a friend. Save the most uncomfortable evaluations such as ear and throat for last, and make sure that these need to be done. Do not bargain with a child for a prolonged period; this simply increases his fear and anticipation of what you are about to do. Discourage parents from using your attentions to the child as threats, such as "If you don't behave I'm going to have the doctor give you a shot."

Older Children

A word about the examination of older children, particularly girls. Depending on a girl's innate sense of modesty plus the attitudes of her parents and peers, it is not unusual for girls to begin to be embarrassed by the usual bare-chested exam even before breast development has begun. For a girl who requires a chest exam and is approaching puberty it is often wise to gown her and examine half the chest at a time. Above all, have either your nurse or the mother in the room at the time. When you note signs of puberty, or preferably before, it is also often wise to determine how well prepared the child is for the changes that are about to occur and whether or not you can be helpful by discussing these with her.

Probably the most important words of advice in examining children of any age is to be sensitive and to be yourself. When you are examining a teenager, use the vocabulary that is your own. Don't try to adopt a different vocabulary or mannerisms in order to achieve rapport with the patient. You usually goof and accomplish the opposite of what you set out to do.

Finally, with older children make sure they understand what you are doing, even the three-year-olds. Make sure that they, especially the teenagers, have a chance to ask questions about procedures, tests, medications and so forth. Do not treat them as though they were passively involved inanimate objects!

REFERENCES

Growth and Performance

Falkner, F. (Ed.): *Human Development.* Philadelphia, W. B. Saunders Co., 1966.

Garn, S. M., and Rohmann, C. G.: Interaction of nutrition and genetics in the timing of growth and development. Pediatr. Clin. N. Am., *13*:353, 1966.

Stuart, H. C., and Prugh, D. G.: *The Healthy Child. His Physical, Psychological, and Social Development.* Cambridge, Mass., Harvard University Press, 1964.

Watson, E. H., and Lowrey, G. H.: *Growth and Development of Children,* 5th ed. Chicago, Year Book Medical Publishers, 1967.

Growth

Bayer, L. M., and Bayley, N.: *Growth Diagnosis.* Chicago, University of Chicago Press, 1959.

Smith, D. W.: *Growth and Its Disorders*. Philadelphia, W. B. Saunders Co., 1977.

Stuart, H. C., and Reed, R. B.: Longitudinal Studies of Child Health and Development. Series II Pediatrics Supplement 24, 875, Nov. 1959.

Tanner, J. M., Goldstein, H., and Whitehouse, R. H.: Standards for children's height at ages 2–9 years alllowing for height of parents. Arch. Dis. Child., *45*:755, 1970.

Winick, M., and Rosso, P.: Head circumference and cellular growth of the brain in normal and marasmic children. J. Pediatr., *74*:774, 1969.

Performance

Erikson, E.: *Childhood and Society*. New York, W. W. Norton & Co., 1959.

Jensen, G. D.: *The Well Child's Problem*. Chicago, Year Book Medical Publishers, 1962.

Robson, K. S., and Moss, H. A.: Patterns and determinants of maternal attachment. J. Pediatr., 77:976, 1970.

Stone, L. J., and Church, J.: *Childhood and Adolescence. A Psychology of the Growing Person*. New York, Random House, 1957.

10

Adolescence

S. L. Hammar

Adolescence is that period in the human life span during which sexual maturity and the ability to reproduce are achieved. This developmental phase is characterized by an increase of growth in body size and by changes in body shape, accompanied by physiological, psychological and psychosocial maturation. Because of the great variations in individual growth patterns and the timing of the growth spurt, defining adolescence on the basis of chronological age is of limited value. On the average, girls begin their pubertal growth spurt around 10 years of age and complete their growth between 16 and 18 years of age. Boys start their pubertal growth spurt approximately two years later than girls, around age 12. Their maximum rate of pubertal growth will be reached at approximately age 14, at which time the average boy will be growing at nearly twice his early childhood growth rate. Most males will complete their pubertal changes around 18 to 19 years of age. Although children have been maturing earlier and getting taller and heavier with each generation since about 1900, the two-year sex difference in the timing of the adolescent growth spurt has remained unchanged.

The average "height-attained" or dis-

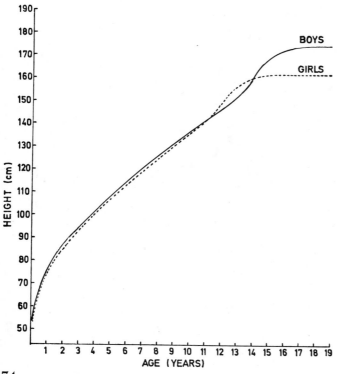

Figure 10–1 Typical individual height distance curves for boys and girls (supine length to age 2). (*From* Tanner, J. M.: Growth at Adolescence. 2nd ed., Oxford, Blackwell Scientific Publications, 1962.)

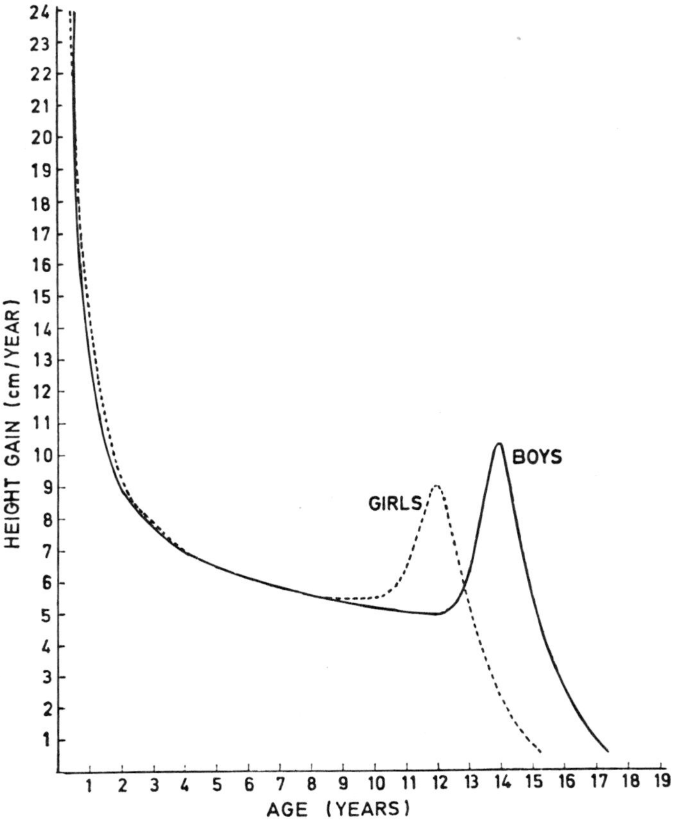

Figure 10–2 Typical individual velocity curves for boys and girls. (*From* Tanner, J. M.: *Growth at Adolescence.* 2nd ed., Oxford, Blackwell Scientific Publications, 1962.)

tance curve for boys and girls is shown in Figure 10–1. Figure 10–2 shows the typical individual velocity pattern for body stature. Velocity is defined as the rate of growth per year (centimeters per year). The male's greater adult height has been attributed to the longer period of preadolescent growth (during which limb growth is most affected) and the greater growth rate during the pubertal growth spurt. The growth pattern for body weight during adolescence is similar.

Although we are most aware of the changes in stature and height during puberty, a similar growth spurt can be seen in other body parameters, i.e., bi-iliac and biacromial diameters, hand and foot length and head circumference.

The precise mechanisms that initiate puberty are still poorly understood. The hypothalamic-pituitary-gonadal axis appears to be intact and functioning in the fetal and prepubertal period of development. Puberty appears to be the result of a changing sensitivity of the hypothalamic receptor sites, which mediate the inhibitory effects of the gonadal sex steroids. With maturation of the central nervous system, increased levels of sex hormones are required to suppress the hypothalamic receptors; consequently, larger amounts of gonadotrophins are secreted that, in turn, stimulate increasing levels of gonadal steroids. The changes of puberty are the results of the increased secretions of sex steroids by the gonads and adrenal cortex.

DEVELOPMENT OF SECONDARY SEXUAL CHARACTERISTICS

The pubertal growth spurt in height and weight is accompanied by rapid maturation of the reproductive organs and development of the secondary sex characteristics. The sequence of events occurring during puberty in the male is shown in Figure 10–3, and the stages are set forth in Table 10–1. The first reliable clinical sign of puberty in boys is a noticeable increase in the size of the testes, with increased pigmentation and stippling of the scrotal sac. A testicular

TABLE 10–1 STAGES OF PUBERTY

BOYS: GENITAL DEVELOPMENT

Stage 1. Preadolescent. Testes, scrotum and penis are of about the same size and proportion as in early childhood.

Stage 2. Enlargement of scrotum and testes. Skin of scrotum reddens and changes in texture. Little or no enlargement of penis at this stage.

Stage 3. Enlargement of penis, which occurs at first mainly in length. Further growth of testes and scrotum.

Stage 4. Increased size of penis with growth in breadth and development of glands. Testes and scrotum larger; scrotal skin darkened.

Stage 5. Genitalia adult in size and shape.

GIRLS: BREAST DEVELOPMENT

Stage 1. Preadolescent: elevation of papilla only.

Stage 2. Breast bud stage: elevation of breast and papilla as small mound. Enlargement of areolar diameter.

Stage 3. Further enlargement and elevation of breast and areola, with no separation of their contours.

Stage 4. Projection of areola and papilla to form a secondary mound above the level of the breast.

Stage 5. Mature stage: projection of papilla only due to recession of the areola to the general contour of the breast.

BOTH SEXES: PUBIC HAIR

Stage 1. Preadolescent. The vellus over the pubes is not further developed than that over the abdominal wall, i.e. no pubic hair.

Stage 2. Sparse growth of long, slightly pigmented downy hair, straight or curled, chiefly at the base of the penis or along the labia.

Stage 3. Considerably darker, coarser and more curled. The hair spreads sparsely over the junction of the pubes.

Stage 4. Hair now adult in type, but area covered is still considerably smaller than in the adult. No spread to the medial surface of thighs.

Stage 5. Adult in quantity and type with distribution of the horizontal (or classically "feminine") pattern. Spread to medial surface of thighs, but not up linear alba or elsewhere above the base of the inverse triangle (spread up linea alba occurs and is rated stage 6).

From the standard illustrations in J. M. Tanner: *Growth at Adolescence*, 2nd ed. Oxford, Blackwell Scientific Publications, 1962.

measurement of 2.5 cm or greater is considered to be indicative of early puberty. Increased testicular sensitivity to pressure and the appearance of axillary sweating are early but less reliable signs of puberty. An increase in growth of the phallus and the appearance of sparse, lightly pigmented pubic hair at the base of the penis follow testicular enlargement. The appearance of axillary hair, facial hair and voice changes are later manifestations of puberty and usually occur after the peak in height growth has passed. Nocturnal emissions usually begin to occur about age 14. Most of the secondary sex characteristics in the male are completed within a span of two to four years after the onset of puberty.

The sequence of pubertal changes in girls is shown in Figure 10–4. The first definite sign of puberty in girls is the appearance of the breast bud at approximately 11 years of age. In a few girls, breast development may be apparent as early as age 8; by age 12, however, breast development is evident in 90 per cent of girls. Pubic hair begins to appear around 11 years of age. Menarche occurs about six to nine months after the peak height spurt has occurred, usually in American girls around 12.6 to 12.8 years of age.

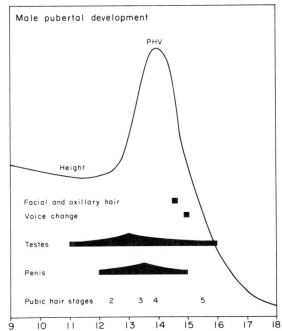

Figure 10–3 Sequence of pubertal events in the male, related to the height velocity curve. (*From* Hammar, S. L.: Adolescence. *In* Kelley, V., Ed.: *Brenneman's Practice of Pediatrics.* Hagerstown, Maryland, Harper & Row Publishers, Inc., Vol. I, Chapter 6, 1970.)

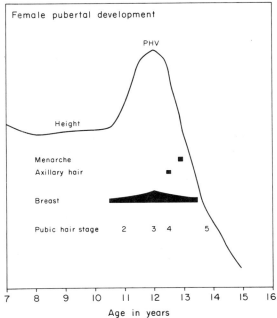

Figure 10–4 Sequence of pubertal events in the female, related to the height velocity curve. (*From* Hammar, S. L.: Adolescence. *In* Kelley, V., ed.: *Brenneman's Practice of Pediatrics.* Hagerstown, Maryland, Harper & Row, Publishers, Inc., Vol. I, Chapter 6, 1970.)

Variations of Pubertal Development

Variations in the sequence of events and in pubertal changes are relatively common. Gynecomastia appears during puberty in approximately 65 to 70 per cent of adolescents, either unilaterally or bilaterally. Though rarely serious, it causes the teenage male much embarrassment and discomfort. Delay in pubertal development is another common variation which affects approximately 2.5 per cent of adolescent males. Breast asymmetry among girls is a common variation, occurring in approximately 8 per cent. Five per cent of girls may achieve menarche while still in their early stages of breast development.

Physiological Changes of Adolescence

Accompanying the physical changes of adolescence are predictable changes in physiological function.

Red cell mass and hemoglobin. Red cell values are relatively high during the neonatal period (5.1 million), but fall by the third month to the average childhood value of 4.5 million. A sex difference becomes apparent during adolescence (5.4 million for boys; 4.8 million for girls).

Hemoglobin values fall from 19.5 to 11.8 gm/100 ml by six months and then gradually rise to 12.9 gm during mid-childhood (6 to 10 years). From 11 to 15 years the average value is 13.4 gm/100 ml with no obvious sex differences. When compared with the stages of pubertal development, however, a sex difference becomes apparent about mid-adolescence, with males attaining a higher mean value (adult male 16.0 ± 2 gm/100 ml, adult female 14.0 ± 2 gm/100 ml). In the adolescent male there appears to be a correlation between hemoglobin levels, increasing muscle mass and 17-ketosteroid excretion, suggesting that testosterone may be responsible for this sex difference, which first appears at adolescence. These are relatively late changes, however.

Girls who have been menstruating for several years tend to have slightly lower hemoglobin levels than those who are prepubertal.

Other hematological changes also occur during puberty. Leukocyte counts tend to decrease slightly in both sexes; platelets increase and the sedimentation rate tends to remain slightly higher in the female. The blood volume increases in both sexes but more in the male than in the female.

Cardiovascular changes. The pulse rate decreases slightly from birth through adolescence. A sexual difference is noted during adolescence, with males having a pulse rate approximately 10 per cent lower than females. The systolic blood pressure rises during the adolescent period in both sexes, with boys exhibiting a greater rise than girls. Accompanying the rise in systolic blood pressure is a rise in the pulse pressure. The diastolic pressures show little change during adolescence and no sex difference. The heart size increases during childhood; from 12 years on boys have larger values for the transverse cardiac diameters. In most girls a sharp increase in cardiac size is closely related to the menarche.

THE APPROACH TO THE ADOLESCENT PATIENT

Adolescents have come to be recognized as a special group of patients. The specific medical conditions or diseases peculiar to this age group are relatively few and are limited primarily to such entities as acne, gynecomastia, Osgood-Schlatter disease or adolescent goiter. Because teenagers are neither children nor adults, they usually have special needs and concerns. They can describe their own feelings and symptoms, ask questions and begin to take responsibility for their own health care. They have usually reached a stage in their development at which they can benefit from a confidential professional relationship.

Generally, it is wise to interview and examine the adolescent without the presence of his parents. When seen together, the examiner naturally tends to direct his questions and explanations to the adult and often forgets that the teenager has and can express his own feelings if given the opportunity. Parents also need the opportunity to express their concerns and to ask questions in private. Initially, it is usually more productive to interview each separately.

Interviewing the Adolescent

Success in working with this age group depends largely upon the interest and comfort of the physician and the amount of time and effort he is willing to invest. Treating the adolescent with respect and conveying interest and a willingness to listen are essential to establishing a good relationship. Although the techniques and approaches used in interviewing and counseling adolescents must be individualized and adapted to fit the particular situation, certain principles apply to working with most adolescent patients.

When dealing with teenage patients, the limits of confidentiality should be established at the outset. The examiner should convey to the adolescent that he will respect his confidences and treat information in a confidential manner, except when the adolescent threatens to harm or injure himself, such as threatening suicide, or divulging plans to run away, or when the patient seems seriously depressed. Since the parents are still legally responsible for the teenager, they must be informed. Such communication should never take place, however, without the knowledge of the adolescent. It is unwise to swear unqualified secrecy or to encourage a teenager to confide and share his feelings with an adult if such a contract cannot be kept. Such an approach usually does not deter the adolescent from confiding his problems, and it keeps the counselor from becoming involved in an untenable situation.

It is easy to overidentify with teenage patients. Their problems, concerns and struggles tend to reawaken the physician's own adolescent experiences. Although a certain degree of empathy and sympathetic understanding is essential, the examiner must assiduously avoid taking sides or making judgments until he has obtained adequate information. Talking with parents, teachers or other involved persons helps the counselor to make a better and more impartial assessment of the adolescent's behavior.

A good observer trains himself to become perceptive and sensitive to non-verbal cues, such as the conduct of the adolescent during an interview, obvious signs of anxiety, flushing, avoidance of particular subject matter, avoidance of eye contact and inappropriateness of dress, affect or appearance. Important also is the effect the patient has upon the examiner. Depressed teenagers often make the physician feel depressed, without verbalizing their feelings. The adolescent who leaves the examiner feeling hostile or angry or who is provocative and manipulative, provides important clues about how he makes other significant adults in his environment feel and reflects his mode of handling situations.

The adolescent patient responds best to an interested counselor who listens and gives him the opportunity to express his opinions. In his attempt to elicit complete information the physician should not be too quick to turn the adolescent off or to redirect questions. Picking up cues from the patient's comments or noting topics that spark interest often provides valuable insights into problems really troubling the teenager. Neither should the counselor be too quick to give advice. To issue advice or directives, the counselor risks becoming involved in a serious power struggle with the adolescent over his right to make decisions. Instead, the patient should be allowed to consider solutions, alternatives and consequences and arrive at decisions without threatening his right to make them.

Providing reassurance too quickly, without an adequate understanding of the teenager's situation, often conveys a lack of appreciation of the patient's feelings.

Medical History

Although some adolescents are seen for routine health checks or for short-term acute medical problems, many tend to be referred because of concerns about behavior, school performance or intrafamily conflicts. It is important with any adolescent to assess more than his physical state. The medical history should reflect the adolescent's progress in completing his developmental tasks and his adjustment to his life situation. It is important to consider three important areas: the teenager's family relationships, his school experiences and his peer group.

The family. The examiner should evaluate how the teenager is getting along with his parents and siblings. Is he showing signs of developing independence? Are the parents allowing him to become more independent? Are the limitations and restrictions placed upon his activities appropriate

to and commensurate with his maturation? Is the adolescent allowed to make an increasing number of decisions for himself? Can he communicate comfortably with his parents? Does he have some responsibility for the operation of the home? Is he showing signs of rebelliousness? Is rivalry among siblings a serious problem? Are the parents' expectations realistic? Problems at home often affect many other areas of the adolescent's functioning.

The school experience. The second area in the adolescent's life situation that should be explored is his school experience. For most adolescents this is their most important and time-consuming job. Is the adolescent taking his school work seriously, or is he failing to perform adequately? In what subjects does he excel; in which subjects is he doing the poorest? What is his attendance record like? Is his schooling relevant to his future vocational or career goals? How does he respond to school authorities and to his teachers? While the adolescent is not expected to have firmly fixed career goals in mind, he should nevertheless give some evidence of having considered future vocational plans. A sign of maturity is the ability to begin to set long-range goals and to delay immediate gratification.

The peer group. As an adolescent begins to emancipate himself from the family unit, his friends and peer group become more important to him. Transferring his attention to friends and peers serves to reduce the intensity of his attachment to his parents and to promote his independence. Is the adolescent showing signs of developing normal heterosexual interests? Is he dating? Is there a special girl or boy with whom the adolescent can communicate comfortably and with whom he likes to spend his time? Does the adolescent have a normal number of friends, or is he isolated or showing a tendency to withdraw?

In reviewing these areas as a part of the medical history the examiner is able to obtain a fairly complete picture of the adolescent patient and how he functions in his total environmental situation.

Physical Examination

Adolescents are usually concerned about their bodies and about their physical changes. A carefully performed physical examination can be not only reassuring, but also an excellent learning experience for the young patient. It is usually preferable to examine the teenage patient without his parents in the room. A nurse or female attendant should always assist in the examination of the adolescent girl; she can provide a great deal of support and reassurance to the patient and help to alleviate much anxiety. The teenager's height and weight should be carefully taken and plotted on an appropriate growth standard. His growth pattern, body type and height and weight percentile should be discussed with him. Unfortunately, peer acceptance depends a great deal on physical appearance, and adolescents are greatly concerned about their physical development. All procedures should be carefully explained to the adolescent. As a part of the physical examination, girls should be instructed how to examine their breasts properly. Performing a pelvic examination as a routine part of the adolescent physical examination has aroused much controversy. The need for this procedure must be individually determined, depending upon the complaints or reasons for the referral, the anxiety level of the girl and, most important, the attitude and comfort of the examiner. The pelvic examination should not be emphasized as a particularly unique part of the normal physical examination, and should never be performed without adequate preparation of the patient. With careful explanation and discussion, most adolescent girls tolerate the procedure without difficulty.

An assessment of sexual age should always be included in the examination of the adolescent. The method developed by Tanner for rating the stage of pubertal development is recommended (Table 10–1). On this scale a rating is given for pubic hair for both boys and girls; in addition, general development in the male and breast development in the female are given separate ratings.

THE PSYCHOLOGICAL CHANGES OF ADOLESCENCE

During the adolescent period, the teenager is expected to accomplish four basic developmental tasks: (1) to establish a stable self-identity, (2) to accept an adult sexual role, (3) to emancipate himself from his family and (4) to make a career or vocational choice.

The self-image or mental picture that an adolescent develops of himself is affected by numerous factors including (a) physical development, physique and appearance, (b) the rate of pubertal maturation compared to peers, (c) the attitudes and esteem that parents have for the teenager and (d) previous sense of success or failure. Adolescent males tend to have less problem with the body image, perhaps because of more acceptable outlets for sexual and aggressive impulses. Adolescent girls, in general, appear to be more conscious of appearance, more oriented toward interpersonal relationships and more concerned about social acceptance.

Adolescents who deviate in their appearance, who are obese, have severe acne or cosmetic defects or who are significantly delayed in their pubertal development tend to have more problems with their self-image or self-identity.

Sexual activity and drives increase markedly during adolescence. Problems associated with teenage sexual behavior have increased during the last decade. Masturbation still causes many teenagers considerable concern. Even though the old wives' tales regarding this practice have been dispelled, many teenagers are concerned about the effects of masturbation on genital size, potency and sexual performance.

Most teenagers still receive the major part of their sexual information, inaccurate and otherwise, from their peers. Heterosexual intercourse and sexual experimentation increase throughout adolescence. More than half of adolescents are non-virginal by 15 to 17 years of age. It appears that attitudes toward adolescent sexuality have relaxed considerably in the past decade, although there is much speculation about whether this is reflected in actual changes in sexual behavior. Incest, sexual abuse, pregnancy in girls less than 14 years of age, abortion, contraception and venereal disease are serious problems related to adolescent sexual behavior that confront the physician.

Establishing independence from the family is often stressful for both parents and teenager. The adolescent often attempts to exert his independence and autonomy through bickering with parents, resisting or testing limits, choosing friends who are unacceptable to parents and questioning family values, political and religious beliefs. Adolescence normally is a time of relaxing limits, assuming increased responsibilities and decision making. By mid-adolescence, most teenagers have begun at least tentatively to consider vocational and career goals.

PROBLEMS OF ADOLESCENTS

The principal cause of death in the adolescent age group is trauma, with motor vehicle accidents, homicides and suicides leading. The leading non-traumatic causes of death during adolescence are malignant neoplasms and cardiovascular disorders.

In special medical facilities for adolescents and in established adolescent clinics the most common problems seen are school underachievement, obesity, behavior disorders, growth deviations, seizures, venereal disease and drug abuse. Obviously, patients referred to these clinics represent a selected population and reflect the kinds of problems that the practitioner finds the most difficult to handle.

School Underachievement

Adolescents who present with school underachievement generally fall into three groups: (1) those with mental subnormality who have decreased intellectual functioning, (2) those with specific learning disorders but with normal intelligence and (3) those whose school failure has a psychogenic basis.

Adolescents with mental subnormality. Most adolescents who present as school underachievers fall into the mild disorder area or borderline range of intelligence. The peak age for diagnosing mental retardation is during the early adolescent period, when maturation and increased educational demands make defects more obvious to educators. Problems about future vocational training, anxiety about potential sexual behavior and concern about future disposition, supervision and care require

professional attention. Psychological and vocational testing to better define the students' strengths and weaknesses, referrals to special educational facilities, appropriate sex educational help with pregnancy prevention and family counseling are often indicated.

Specific learning problems. Adolescents with specific learning disabilities most commonly have severe reading handicaps. A few may be reading at their appropriate grade level, but exhibit specific defects related to spelling, mathematics and handwriting. Although they may be of normal intelligence, evidence of visual-perceptual problems, soft neurological signs or other findings suggestive of mild central nervous system impairment may be present. Poor memory retention, short attention span, distractibility and impulsive behavior are frequent complaints of the teacher. Behavior problems resulting from years of frustration, repeated school failures and inadequate educational programming are common. Special academic programming utilizing channels of communication other than reading, such as student readers, tape recorders, reading tutors using multiple modality techniques and oral examinations are frequently necessary. The prognosis for remediation of specific reading disorders during adolescence is poor. These teenagers often require intensive vocational counseling and programming to help them function adequately and achieve in spite of their disability. The counselor must utilize the special resources of psychology, education and psychiatry in order to determine the type of treatment and training program that is necessary.

Psychogenic underachievers. In the group of psychogenic underachievers the academic problems are secondary to primary emotional problems and environmental factors. Preoccupation with and reaction to family stresses may interfere with scholastic efficiency and school progress. School refusal or inconsistent school attendance in an adolescent who is bright, sensitive, overanxious and unable to cope with the school situation represents a more serious school problem that usually requires immediate psychiatric intervention. Parents are often ineffective and unable to set limits on the teenager's behavior without professional assistance. In some adolescents, school underachievement appears to be related to intense parental demands for scholastic achievement. School failure is often an effective passive-aggressive method of retaliation. In others, cultural expectations, peer group values and familial patterns of underachievement may be largely responsible for school failure.

Since the physician is usually the first professional to be consulted in such cases, he must be able to define the school problem, communicate effectively with the school personnel and make the appropriate referrals for evaluation and treatment.

Obesity

It is estimated that about 15 per cent of the adolescent population is obese. Generally, an adolescent's obesity is not of recent onset, but has been present since mid-childhood. Girls are affected more frequently than boys; in 65 to 70 per cent of cases one or both parents are also obese, indicating perhaps a strong genetic tendency to the development of obesity. More than 95 per cent of this population appear to have exogenous obesity; rarely can endocrinopathies be diagnosed as a causal factor. There is increasing evidence that cellular differences are present in obese and non-obese juveniles. Not only is cell size in adipose tissue enlarged in the grossly obese, but the number of adipose cells is also increased, possibly because of long-standing chronic hypernutrition during critical periods of growth (see also Chapter 11).

Exogenous obesity in the young adolescent is frequently characterized by advanced height age and slightly accelerated skeletal age, and early onset of pubertal changes. The age of menarche, particularly in girls with long-standing obesity, is frequently advanced. The total daily caloric intake of obese adolescents may not seem excessive to maintain their body weight, but these patients are often physically inactive. In addition, they are usually socially isolated and ostracized from the peer group, a fact that contributes to their inactivity. One of the main problems in treating the obese adolescent is lack of motivation. Often the parents or a school nurse are more concerned about treatment than the adolescent. Most teenagers cannot be threatened, coerced or bribed into adhering to a weight reduction regimen. Since many social and emotional problems are often associated with obesity in the adolescent, it is important to evaluate his psychological status carefully before placing him under the additional stress of a weight reduction program. Depression is frequent. Severe environmental stress and family conflicts often potentiate the weight problem, since many obese patients tend to react to anxiety and stress by eating compulsively. If weight loss is to be achieved and maintained, careful attention must be given to the emotional adjustment, self-image, sexual feelings, social adaptation and activity patterns, in addition to providing nutritional education. The goals in treating obese adolescents should be to modify eating patterns, encourage exercise, improve hygiene and appearance and encourage social activities. Having the teenager record a three- to five-day food diary can be a motivational test, and can provide useful information on which to build a well-balanced, calorically reduced diet. Frequent contacts with the physician are essential to provide psychological support. Crash diets, starvation periods, pills and fad diets are of limited value and should be discouraged.

Seizure Disorders

The actual incidence of seizure disorders in adolescent and young adult populations is difficult to establish because of the reluctance of the patient and his family to reveal this affliction. It has been estimated that one in 100 persons in the United States suffers from some type of seizure disorder.

Seizures often become difficult to control at the time of puberty. Frequently, adolescent girls experience seizures just before the onset of their menstrual period. This may be related to the complex hormonal changes that occur during the menstrual cycle or to the increased fluid retention, which may irritate the central nervous system and lower the seizure threshold. Hyperventilation, water loading, sudden environmental changes, stressful and highly charged emotional situations or family disruptions have been known to increase seizure activity.

Adolescents with convulsive disorders often have many unnecessary restrictions placed upon them. Many school personnel have overemphasized the need for rest for the epileptic and prohibit participation in physical education or competitive activities. It is important for these patients to be stimulated mentally and physically, and the benefits from normal participation in peer group activities usually far outweigh the small risks that may be involved.

In many cases, the epileptic adolescent must learn to conduct his social activities without the use of a car. This is usually upsetting to the adolescent male, unless he is well prepared in advance. Many epileptic adolescents are concerned about the advisability of marriage. In most cases there is no contraindication to marriage provided the patients are otherwise able to assume the responsibilities that marriage involves. Girls are often concerned about the possible adverse effects of pregnancy. In some instances, seizures occur more frequently during pregnancy, particularly when complicated by fluid retention, excessive weight gain or toxemia. Pregnancy may require a modification of the anticonvulsant medication in order to obtain the best possible seizure control. Recently, concerns have been raised about the possible teratogenic effects of some anticonvulsants.

Epileptic adolescents require occupational counseling in order to steer them into appropriate vocations. Successful management of the adolescent with a handicap requires patience, an appreciation of the adolescent's feelings about his disease and tolerance of his anger, frustration and rebellion.

Sexual Problems

Venereal disease has increased dramatically and has reached pandemic proportions throughout the world. At best, the reported cases represent only a small portion of the actual number, since many patients are treated either purposefully or inadvertently by their private physicians and are not reported. More than half the cases reported in this country and in Western Europe involve the 15- to 24-year age group. The increased incidence appears to be directly related to changing sexual mores and behavior among young adults and is not peculiar to any particular social class or stratum. The apparent increase in male homosexual activity is also a significant factor in the spread of venereal disease among older adolescents and young adults. The active adult homosexual poses the greatest public health threat because of his mobility and transient encounters, often with a multiplicity of unknown partners, that make an epidemiological approach to case identification difficult.

Acute gonorrhea in the male generally appears as a urethritis or urethral discharge and is diagnosed by culture or smear of the exudate. In adolescent girls the diagnosis can be easily missed since symptoms may be few until the infection spreads to the uterus and fallopian tubes and pelvic inflammation develops. Since the organisms do not usually attack the urethra in the female, dysuria is not a presenting complaint.

Every non-virginal and sexually active adolescent girl should have a pelvic examination with smears and cultures for gonorrhea without exception. Recommended treatment for both sexes consists of 4.8 million units of procaine penicillin with 1 gm probenecid (orally). For adolescents unable to take penicillin, tetracycline (2 gm daily for five days) or spectinomycin injections of 2 gm for males and 4 gm for females may be substituted.

Contraceptive information should be made available to all adolescents. In general, acceptance and effective use of contraceptive methods have been unsuccessful among adolescents, since premeditation, preparation and planning are involved. Many physicians are reluctant to prescribe contraceptive pills to sexually active minors because of potential medical-legal problems. The adolescent should be made aware, however, of the community resources available to provide counseling, contraceptive materials and medical care.

Approximately 10 per cent of girls become pregnant before completing adolescence, and the incidence of pregnancies in girls less than 15 years of age appears to be rising. These adolescents are at risk of producing low birth weight infants, and infant mortality rates are twice as high as in the 20- to 34-year age group. Toxemia, anemia, prolonged labor, cephalopelvic disproportions and hemorrhage appear to be increased in young pregnant teenagers. Pregnancy accounts for two thirds of female high school dropouts, of whom a significant number never complete their secondary education. In recent years, a number of communities have offered specialized programs for pregnant teenage women, designed to meet the needs for prenatal care, education and postnatal family planning and to reduce recidivism. The dynamics of teenage pregnancy are complex and best handled by a multidisciplinary team approach.

Acne

Acne is one of the most common skin problems encountered during adolescence. Often the psychological scars resulting from the skin lesions are more serious and permanent than the physical scars. Two types of acne are seen: non-inflammatory acne, characterized by closed and open comedones, and inflammatory acne, characterized by papules, pustules and nodulocystic lesions, which produce residual scarring.

Acne must be viewed as a chronic problem in which control rather than cure is a more realistic goal. Although incorrect, many adolescents relate acne to masturbation, sexual intercourse, venereal disease and uncleanliness.

Treatment includes general measures of careful face washing, good general hygiene, avoidance of greasy, occlusive cosmetics and other oily substances or coal tar distillates and self-manipulation of lesions. Dietary restrictions are ineffective. Specific measures for non-inflammatory acne include the sparing use of mild peeling agents, such as topical vitamin A (acid-retin A), acne creams and gels, astringents and natural ultraviolet light. Comedo extractors may be useful. Chemotherapeutic agents, such as low doses of tetracycline (250 mg qd or qod) or a combination of topical retin A and oral tetracycline, have been effective in controlling inflammatory acne.

Behavioral Disorders

Emotional problems are common in adolescence. Most emotional reactions and adjustment difficulties have a good prognosis. Severe obsessive-compulsive behavior, acute psychotic episodes, suicide attempts and severe behavioral derangements are more commonly seen in teenagers who have established a pattern of maladjustment prior to adolescence. Antisocial behavior in teenagers appears to be increasing, however. Referrals to the juvenile courts indicate that the antisocial boy is more frequently involved in car theft, drug abuse, running away and stealing, while girls are usually referred for sexual acting out, drug abuse and running away.

Teenage depression is not uncommon. Although mood swings are characteristic of this period of life, some teenagers will exhibit severe depressive reactions and, unfortunately, some will carry them to their ultimate extreme by attempting or committing suicide. The incidence of teenage suicides has increased markedly and ranks fourth as a cause of death in the 15- to 19-year age group. Adolescent girls tend to make more suicidal gestures than boys, but the adolescent male is at greater risk for committing suicide and less likely to give warnings or seek help. Problems with parents, loss of a loved one, broken romances and pregnancy are common reasons for suicide attempts among adolescents. All suicide attempts should be taken seriously, and hospitalization even for a brief period is strongly recommended. Social isolation appears to be an important prognostic factor in recidivism among those males who attempt suicides. Psychiatric crisis intervention and counseling is essential in managing teenage suicidal behavior. Depression often goes unrecognized because the busy physician has little time or avoids discussing such feelings with the teenager. The symptoms of depression in the adolescent may be disguised or present as depressive equivalents, chronic fatigue, hyperactivity and aggressiveness. Early recognition of depressive reactions and referral to appropriate treatment resources are an essential part of effective suicide prevention.

Drug use among teenagers and young adults has become a serious contemporary problem. Many adolescents who use drugs are not necessarily alienated, rebellious or even emotionally disturbed, although they may be. Many are "experience seekers"; some take drugs to prove their courage by indulging in risk-taking experiences, to relieve loneliness, because of peer social pressure or in an attempt to find meaning in life. The manner in which drugs are used is important. Some adolescents are simply experimenters; others use drugs as a means of escaping home situations; still others use them in a malignant and self-destructive way. Investigation often reveals a serious disintegration of the family unit, an absent or detached father, a mother preoccupied with her own problems, alcoholism, marital discord and family turmoil. The use of drugs is a presenting symptom. Therapeutic efforts should be directed at improving the total life situation of the teenager, rather than focusing on drug use alone.

In many communities drug abuse has become a recognized and accepted hazard of modern day teenage life and appears to be decreasing. In contrast, excessive alcohol use and alcoholism among young teenagers are rapidly increasing. This insidious problem is appearing more frequently in hospital emergency rooms. Teenage alcohol abuse must be recognized as another potentially maladaptive behavior and a serious public health problem requiring professional intervention.

CONCLUSIONS

Adolescence is a period of dynamic personal change and immense variation. In evaluating and treating the adolescent patient, the examiner must approach each as a unique person with his own particular pattern of growth, behavior, emotional responses, problems and concerns. Each teenager must be examined in the context of his environment, his family and his peer group, and management of his medical illness and developmental problems must be highly individualized.

REFERENCES

General

Gallagher, J. R., Heald, F. P., and Garell, D. C.: *Medical Care of the Adolescent.* New York, Appleton-Century-Crofts, 1976.

Hammar, S. L., and Holterman, V.: Interviewing and counseling adolescent patients. Clin. Pediatr., 9:47, 1970.

Marshall, W. A., and Tanner, J. M.: Variations in pattern in pubertal changes in girls. Arch. Dis. Child., 44:291, 1969.

Marshall, W. A., and Tanner, J. M.: Variations in the pattern of pubertal changes in boys. Arch. Dis. Child., 45:13, 1970.

Tanner, J. M.: *Growth at Adolescence,* 2nd ed. Oxford, Blackwell Scientific Publications, 1962.

Usdin, G. L.: *Adolescence, Care and Counseling.* Philadelphia, J. B. Lippincott Company, 1967.

Weiner, I. B.: *Psychological Disturbances in Adolescence.* New York, John Wiley & Sons, 1970.

Adolescent Obesity

Collipp, P. J. (Ed.): *Childhood Obesity.* Acton, Mass., Publishing Sciences Group, Inc., 1975.

Hammar, S. L., Campbell, M. M., Campbell, V. A., *et al.:* An interdisciplinary study of adolescent obesity. J. Pediatr., 80:373, 1972.

Wilson, N. L. (Ed.): *Obesity.* Philadelphia, F. A. Davis Company, 1969.

Adolescent Sexuality

Sorensen, R. C.: *Adolescent Sexuality in Contemporary America.* New York, World Publishing, 1973.

Acne

Reisner, R. M.: Acne vulgaris. Pediatr. Clin. N. Am., 20:851, 1973.

Venereal Disease

Blount, J. H., Darrow, W. W., and Johnson, R. E.: Venereal disease in adolescents. Pediatr. Clin. N. Am., 20:1021, 1973.

Drug Use

Koumans, A. J. R.: Treatment of acute drug intoxication. Newsletter Supplement, Mass. Med. Society, 10: No. 5, October, 1970.

Litt, I. F., and Cohen, M. I.: The drug-using adolescent as a pediatric patient. J. Pediatr., 77:195, 1970.

PART III

WELL-CHILD CARE

11

Nutrition in Infancy and Childhood, Including Obesity

Nathan J. Smith

Nutritional demands and requirements are directly influenced by growth. Food provides the essential building blocks and energy to satisfy the needs of growth. Thus, the rapidly growing fetus, infant, older child and adolescent have relatively large nutrient requirements, and along with pregnant women are at greatest risk of developing deficiency diseases and growth retardation.

In the past, the child's physician concentrated his efforts in nutrition counseling of young families toward prevention of deficiency states, such as rickets, scurvy and severe anemia, and assuring an average growth experience. There is still need for such effort in the vast developing populations of the world. An unlimited supply of nutritious, clean food is available in the United States, however. Hence even among the poorest in this country, deficiency states such as rickets and scurvy are rarely seen. In addition, American parents are better informed regarding the food and nutrient needs than ever before. However, recent surveys have identified some nutrition-related health problems that still exist in this informed society.

As many as 15 per cent of families in the United States have inadequate financial resources to provide sufficient food to meet their needs. Children in these families are smaller than children in upper-income families and have a greater prevalence of iron deficiency anemia. Occasional instances of hypoproteinemia and folate deficiency are found among children in poor urban populations. There are no significant differences in food purchasing practices of the well-to-do and the poor—the low-income family buys essentially the same food as the high-income family, only less of it. Nutrition-related health problems are not limited to low-income families but are also common in those with middle and high incomes. Obesity is widespread in both men and women of all income levels. Between 10 and 20 per cent of middle and upper income American women from 12 to 45 years of age are biochemically assessed as iron depleted. Thus, in the presence of abundant food and a well-educated, literate population, the quality and possibly the duration of life is often compromised by less than optimal nutrition. Solutions must be found to the national economic problems that find large numbers of poor children without access to an adequate amount of food. Energy expenditure through physical activity must be recognized as an essential component of good nutritional health in prevention of obesity and in prompting a food intake that will provide an adequate intake of essential nutrients.

An appropriate goal for the child's physician can be optimal nutrition for every child. Optimal nutrition is provided by a diet that is sufficient to support full genetic potential for growth and to provide optimal body composition, and that satisfies the need for all essential nutrients. In addition, the eating experience should enhance the communication, security and self-image of the individual. These latter are needs that man has traditionally met in large part through his eating experience.

In contrast to the abundant food supplies available to most children in the industrialized communities of the world, those living in the so-called developing countries may receive very limited amounts of highly contaminated food. Most of the world's children do not have access to an adequate diet. Depending upon the location and season of the year, any one or a combination of known essential nutrients may be lacking in the diet. Limited growth, compromised development, severe nutritional anemia and chronic enteric infections are the norm for much of the world's child population. This "third world" is not ready for a goal of optimal nutrition for every child. Nutrition for survival must be the goal until more food is provided and sanitation increases the efficiency of food utilization.

INFANT FEEDING

The specific goals of infant feeding may be the following:

1. To meet the nutritional needs of infants as they relate to requirements of growth, energy expenditure, maintenance of homeostatic mechanisms and various functions involved in resisting disease.

2. To experience by healthy feeding the gratification, affection and communication that can be associated with eating.

The nutritional requirements of infants are unique. The infant is completely dependent on being fed during the first several months of life. His nutritional demands are great owing to growth, a high metabolic rate, large insensible water loss and the kidney's limited ability to conserve water. Requirements for calories and particularly water are very high (see Table 11–1). In the absence of an adequate supply of these essentials, growth deficiency and dehydration may readily develop.

The adequacy of an infant's feeding experience is carefully monitored. At each physician visit, gains in length and weight are assessed. In some instances skin fatfolds are measured to estimate the level of body fatness. At 6, 9 or 12 months of age iron nutrition status may be assessed through measurement of hemoglobin concentration, or more precisely, by using some biochemical parameter such as erythrocyte protoporphyrin.

Breast Feeding

Human milk from a well-nourished mother can optimally meet the nutritional needs of an infant during the first two to four months of life, and in some instances, even longer. It is necessary to supplement breast milk with vitamin D and fluoride. This food provides 67 Kcal/100 ml (20 Kcal/oz), with 7 per cent of the calories derived from protein, 42 per cent from carbohydrate, and 51 per cent from fat. An infant weighing 3.2 kg at 10 days of age and receiving 500 ml of breast milk daily will meet his caloric requirements for 350 Kcal, his daily water requirement of 480 ml and his protein requirement of 6.4 gm.

Considerable latitude may be given in initiating breast feeding. In a traditional hospital setting, healthy infants are offered the breast for the first time at 6 to 12 hours of age after a trial feeding of water has been offered in the nursery. The breast is subsequently offered on a four-hour schedule during the remainder of the hospital stay. In a practice that may be more conducive to successful breast feeding the infant is put to the breast soon after being born while the mother is still in the delivery area. Then, under rooming-in conditions, the infant is offered the breast for brief periods of time at much shorter intervals than the traditional four-hour schedule. Most infants will establish an approximate three- to four-hour schedule only after several days. The milk supply will be limited during these early days, and a normal weight loss of approximately 5 to 7 per

TABLE 11–1 RECOMMENDED ALLOWANCES FOR CALORIES, WATER AND PROTEIN PER 24 HOURS

	Calories/kg	Water ml/kg	Proteins gm/kg
Infants	117	150	2.0–3.5
Children (7–9 yr)	80	75	1.2
Adults	40	50	0.8

cent of birth weight will be experienced by the infant.

To satisfy the infant and for the security of the mother, it may be advisable to offer an occasional supplemental feeding of water or cow's milk formula. During the first few days of breast feeding, an atmosphere of confident tranquility is of greater concern than meeting specific nutritional requirements.

It is important that initial periods of breast feeding be limited to no more than three to five minutes on each breast. The normal tenderness and breast discomfort associated with initiation of breast feeding may become accentuated if nursing is prolonged. After several days, the infant will be nursing at one breast for approximately 15 minutes at each feeding and nursing at the other for 5 minutes. In general, the infant should not be nursed more frequently than every three hours and no longer than 20 minutes at a feeding. The adequacy of the feeding experience is monitored by following weight gain and, later, levels of fatness.

The indications and contraindications for breast feeding are greatly influenced in the United States by the fact that there has been no demonstrable biological advantage for the breast-fed infant when compared to a formula-fed infant who has received a sanitary and nutritious formula. The psychological advantages of breast feeding for those mothers who wish to do so are not to be minimized. The mother who is disinterested or ambivalent about breast feeding her infant will, however, probably not be successful, and most important, should have no concerns that she will necessarily be compromising her infant's nutritional health. Valid contraindications to breast feeding are essentially confined to serious health problems of the mother. The advantages of breast feeding that can be most readily documented exist under those conditions in which an infant is born into an environment where sanitary milk supply and facilities for sterilization and sanitation are not available. Here, the health of the infant will be positively influenced by breast feeding, which may be continued advantageously well into the second year and longer.

Nearly all drugs and related products ingested by the mother can be expected to be excreted into the milk. Most antibiotics, aspirin, antihistamines and other commonly used drug preparations, however, are clinically insignificant to the infant in the concentrations found in breast milk. Thus, drug administration to the mother is generally not an indication for discontinuing breast feeding. Specific information should be sought about new and unusual drugs.

Formula Feeding

Infants not fed human milk are most commonly fed infant formula mixtures prepared from cow's milk. These are, most often, commercially prepared infant formulae and only rarely, formulations prepared in the home from evaporated milk.

Cow's milk differs in many respects from human milk (see Table 11–2), and it is modified to meet more adequately the nutritional needs of human infants. Addition of water to the cow's milk reduces the protein and mineral concentration. This conserves water by lessening renal solute load. Carbohydrate is added to maintain the same caloric concentration as human breast milk: 20 Kcal/oz or 67 Kcal/100 ml. In the manufacture of commercial formulae, the butterfat of milk is replaced by vegetable oils, and lactose or sucrose are the carbohydrates added. The protein concentration is reduced to levels similar to human milk. Vitamins are added and iron is usually supplemented. The milk protein used in these formulae is subjected to heat in order to reduce the curd tension to that of breast milk.

The formulation of cow's milk mixtures in the home from either homogenized or evaporated cow's milk is being practiced less commonly than in the past. Less than 5 per cent of infants are fed home-prepared infant formulae. Though somewhat less costly, using such milk mixtures affords no significant economic advantage and compromises the quality of the feeding. A formula that provides 20 Kcal/oz is made with one can of evaporated milk (13 oz) to which is added 19 oz water and 1 oz (2 tbs) of sugar. The sugar may be sucrose, corn syrup (Karo) or a dextrose-maltose mixture (Dextri-Maltose). Large intake of non-heat–treated cow's milk (homogenized or simple

TABLE 11–2 COMPARISON OF HUMAN
AND COW'S MILK

	Human	Cow
Total protein, gm/100 ml whole milk	1.1	3.3
Casein	0.4	2.8
Lactalbumin	0.4	0.4
Lactoglobulin	0.2	0.2
Lactose, gm/100 ml whole milk	7.0	4.8
Fat, gm/100 ml whole milk	3.8	3.7
Energy, Kcal/100 ml whole milk	67	67
Per cent from protein	7	20
Per cent from lactose	42	30
Per cent from fat	51	50
Water, gm/120 ml whole milk	87.6	87.3
Total solids, gm/100 ml whole milk	12.4	12.7
Ash, gm/100 ml whole milk	0.21	0.72

pasteurized milk) may induce a blood losing enteropathy, and can create a high renal solute load. Half the calories are contributed by saturated butterfat. For these reasons, unmodified homogenized and pasteurized milks are not recommended as infant food in the first year of life.

Required Supplements

A healthy infant receiving an adequate caloric intake of human milk from a well-nourished mother receives all necessary nutrients for the first several weeks of life with the exception of vitamin D, iron and fluoride. Fluoride is not present in prophylactic concentrations in breast milk, and thus a supplement providing 0.5 mg of fluoride each day should be given. This is often administered as a vitamin, iron and fluoride mixture. The vitamin D supplement recommended for the breast-fed infant is 400 IU daily. It is common to assure an adequate intake of vitamin C with a supplement of 25 mg daily. Iron supplementation is given as 10 mg/day of elemental iron. The vitamin, iron and fluoride supplement for the breast-fed baby is usually started after the first physician visit, at two weeks of age.

Evaporated milk is fortified with vitamin D (400 IU/13-oz can). The infant taking an evaporated milk formula should receive supplemental vitamin C, iron and fluoride, if fluoride is not added to community water supplies.

Commercially prepared formulae are most commonly purchased as liquid concentrates in 13-oz cans. Powdered and ready-to-feed products are also available. The liquid concentrates are diluted with an equal volume of water for feeding. These infant formulae have supplements of vitamins added in the process of manufacturing. Formulae to be recommended contain 8 to 15 mg of elemental iron per can. As long as the infant takes a commercially prepared infant formula with iron added, the only additional supplement needed is fluoride (0.5 mg/day). In communities in which fluoride is added to the municipal water supply, approximately this amount of fluoride will be provided through water added to the formula concentrate. In other situations, a medicinal supplement of fluoride should be provided.

In December 1970 the Nutrition Committee of the American Academy of Pediatrics recommended that *all infants who were not being breast-fed human milk be fed a commercial formula supplemented with iron (8 to 15 mg/13-oz can) until one year of age.* This recommendation was made in light of the prevalence of iron deficiency in the United States and the adverse effect of drinking large quantities of homogenized milk during the first year of life. In the past, formula feeding has been used only until five to six months of age. The advantages of formula feeding throughout the entire first year are now being recognized, and pediatricians are more commonly implementing the Academy's recommendation in the interest of optimal nutrition. The extended use of such formulae will provide dependable vitamin supplementation and softer curd, as well as much-needed iron, and will reduce butterfat consumption. Milk, usually as 2 per cent milk, should be started only at the beginning of the second year and limited to approximately one pint a day.

Because of rapid growth, the infant's requirement for energy (calories) by 2 to 4 months of age may exceed that which can usually be provided by human milk or a reasonable quantity of infant formula. At about this age, the infant is able to accept spoon feeding of semisolid foods. The caloric needs of the infant can now be met by gradually adding cereals and other pureed foods to the diet. Many mothers may begin to feed these foods at a much earlier age. The ready availability of infant foods, the mother's enthusiasm for "feeding" her infant and the "competitive maturation complex" ("My friend fed cereal at four weeks; I'll do it at three weeks") all contribute to this practice. The very early feeding of solids may be harmless and provide some real pleasure for the mother and infant. Excessive feeding of strained foods and cereals, however, can affect the caloric and nutrient intake. Prepared soups, some "dinners" and certain vegetables have less caloric content per unit volume than formulae. Feeding these lower caloric foods in large amounts can decrease the infant's appetite and reduce nutrient intake to less than desirable levels. Eggs, meat, cereals and desserts, on the other hand, have caloric densities per unit volume that are 1.5 to 3 times that of milk formula. When fed indiscriminately, these foods compromise nutritional quality of the diet and can make a significant contribution to caloric overfeeding and obesity. An appropriate schedule for introducing solid foods can vary greatly. With proper support and guidance, the early feeding of various new foods provides an appropriate opportunity for reinforcing pleasurable and satisfying parent-child relationships. The following is a suggested schedule for the introduction of solid foods:

2 to 4 months	Cereals
3 to 5 months	Vegetables and fruits
4 to 5 months	Meats
6 to 8 months	Zwieback, teething biscuits
6 to 12 months	Normal table foods, and start weaning

The following guidelines are observed in introducing new foods in the infant's diet:

1. Introduce new foods singly, in small amounts (1 to 2 teaspoonfuls) and when the infant is hungry.

2. Foods in each group least likely to be associated with allergic reactions should be introduced first, e.g., rice rather than wheat cereals, vegetables rather than citrus fruits, and lamb rather than beef.

3. Feed solids at the same time as milk in order to reduce the risk of excessive caloric intake.

4. Utilize appropriate family table foods whenever possible, but avoid excessive in-

take of bland carbohydrates such as breads, pastas and rice.

5. A feeding schedule of three meals a day is appropriate by the end of the first year, at which time all liquids taken during the day can be taken from a cup.

An almost limitless number of pureed food mixtures and combinations for feeding infants are available in the market. The majority have no place in a desirable diet for an infant. Mixed dinners, breakfasts, high meat dinners, puddings and a variety of desserts all have excessive caloric density because of high carbohydrate content. They may have a changing and often unknown composition. In addition to satisfying caloric needs beyond those met by a reasonable amount of milk, the second important reason for introducing solid foods into the infant diet is the educational function of introducing the infant to new tastes and textures. Too many pureed mixtures available in the market bear little resemblance to either taste or texture that the infant will encounter in later life. There is the obvious advantage in introducing food items from the family table prepared to a suitable consistency, and the increasingly popular practice of preparing infant foods in the home is to be encouraged.

Avoiding the Use of Skim Milk

Parents concerned about over-fatness during the first year of life may attempt to control caloric and fat intake by replacing formula feeding with skim or half skim milk. This practice is contraindicated for the following reasons:

1. Non-heat–treated milk (homogenized or skimmed) is not a desirable food in the first year of life, as noted earlier.

2. Infant diets using skim milks are deficient in essential fatty acids.

3. Providing adequate caloric intake using skim milk requires an inappropriate protein intake and results in a high renal solute load.

4. Commercial infant formulae with the advantage of fats of vegetable origin and adequate vitamin and iron supplements are recommended as superior nutrition for the first year of life.

5. Weight gain will be most effectively controlled by avoiding various infant foods

of high caloric density, controlling the volume of formula intake and providing non-food–related stimulation to promote increased physical activity.

SOME COMMON NUTRITION–RELATED PROBLEMS IN INFANCY

Growth Deficiency

The most practical method of evaluating the adequacy of dietary intake is the regular measuring of length and weight. This allows one to calculate *daily gains* and compare them to known standards.

Weight gains of breast-fed infants and those fed formulae are expected to be similar. If an infant's growth rate is below the tenth percentile expected for his age, a careful review of his feeding experience is indicated. If the weight gain is more than two standard deviations below the mean over a period of 45 to 60 days in infancy, a more intensive search for the cause should be pursued. Such growth deficiency may be due to one or more of the following causes:

1. Inadequate food intake
2. Recurrent vomiting
3. Abnormally great fecal losses, i.e., malabsorption

By far the most common factor involved in growth deficiency is inadequate food intake due to an inadequate volume of human milk, a poorly devised formula, compromised feeding techniques or parental neglect.

Overfeeding and Diarrheal Stools

The stool of the breast-fed infant is softer than that of the infant fed a cow's milk formula. From about the third to seventh day of life the so-called "transitional" stools are greenish-yellow, contain mucus and may actually appear watery. After this, the stool will be the typical "milk-stool"—soft, yellow and not offensive. True diarrhea in the breast-fed infant is unusual, but may be encountered following the ingestion of particular foods by the mother or subsequent to her use of laxatives.

In the formula-fed infant, loose stools may result from overfeeding, particularly in the first 2 to 3 weeks of life. On occasion, true diarrheal disturbances may be encountered in the formula-fed infant, and these are most commonly caused by contamination of food or may be secondary to some infection such as otitis media.

Regurgitation

A significant number of healthy, thriving babies spit up gastric contents with disturbing frequency, usually in small amounts with no relation to the type of feeding, and accompanied by good growth performance. Infants fed human milk and infant formulae may participate equally in this phenomenon. The infant formulae containing vegetable fats cause regurgitation of milk that is essentially odorless and more tolerable as opposed to babies fed homogenized milk, in which the butterfat produces the offensive, rancid odor of butyric acid. This harmless but unpleasant practice of spitting up may, on occasion, persist until the end of the first year.

Overfeeding and Obesity

Various attempts at permanent weight reduction of the chronically obese child, adolescent or adult have resulted in almost complete lack of success. Therefore, prevention of obesity is of prime importance.

Two indicators of infants at risk are the obesity in one or both parents and a rate of weight gain that significantly exceeds the rate of height gain.

Obesity in infancy is diagnosed by the evaluation of body weight in relation to body length, as shown in Table 11–3, which provides a rough guide for diagnosing obesity. A more precise definition of obesity is obtained by estimating the level of body fatness by measuring skin fat-fold thickness. The mean skin fat-folds and standard for infants are listed in the Appendix. Values that exceed two standard deviations for the triceps and subscapular skin fat-fold thickness are considered evidence of obesity.

Genetic factors significantly affect body composition; those influencing obesity are multiple and complex, and have not been clearly defined. By identifying obese

TABLE 11-3   TENTATIVE DEFINITION OF OBESITY

Age (months)	Males		Females	
	Length (cm) less than	Weight (kg) more than	Length (cm) less than	Weight (kg) more than
Birth	48.1	3.4	47.8	3.4
	48.9	3.8	48.4	3.6
	50.3	4.1	50.2	3.9
	51.7	4.3	50.9	4.1
1	52.0	4.3	50.4	4.0
	53.4	4.6	52.3	4.3
	54.6	4.9	54.0	4.5
	55.9	5.4	55.1	5.0
3	58.4	6.1	56.4	5.6
	59.6	6.6	58.2	6.0
	60.9	7.1	59.7	6.3
	62.7	7.5	61.3	6.8
6	64.8	8.1	63.3	7.5
	66.2	8.7	64.5	8.0
	67.6	9.1	66.0	8.3
	69.4	9.9	67.6	9.1
9	69.2	9.3	67.5	8.7
	70.8	10.0	68.4	9.2
	72.3	10.7	70.0	9.6
	73.4	11.3	71.9	10.5
12	72.8	10.5	71.2	9.7
	74.7	11.3	72.8	10.4
	76.3	11.5	74.4	10.7
	77.8	12.8	76.1	11.9

The table is based on combined data for white infants from the studies of Kasius et al. (1957) and Garn and Rohmann (1966). At each age the values for length for each sex are the tenth, twenty-fifth, fiftieth and seventy-fifth percentiles, while the values for weight are the fiftieth, seventy-fifth and ninetieth percentiles and the mean plus two standard deviations. (Courtesy of S. J. Fomon: *Infant Nutrition.* Philadelphia, W. B. Saunders Company, 1967.)

parents or endomorphic parents who tend to be obese, one can be alert to the risk of obesity in an infant as indicated in the following experience:

GENETIC OBSERVATIONS

Parents	Children
Slender × Slender	Slender (rarely obese)
Obese × Slender	Obesity likely (few slender)
Obese × Obese	Obese

Identifying the infant at risk should prompt the professional to initiate the following preventive program early in infancy:

1. Inform the parents of the genetic, kinetic and sociological aspects of obesity.

2. Supervise feeding practices to maintain weight gain parallel with gain in length, limiting high-caloric infant foods, desserts and bland carbohydrates.

3. Initiate long-range planning to provide for energy-expending activities involving not only the infant but the entire family at risk.

4. Orient family dietary practices to nutritious diets with limitation of snacking, unnecessary fats, and bland carbohydrates.

Note: Whether such measures will have lasting value for the child with familial obesity remains to be determined. For the moment the effort appears meritorious.

Milk Intolerance — When to Change the Formula

Almost all infants do well with commercially available milk and milk substitute formulae. On occasion, parents may become displeased with some aspect of behavior of their young infant, e.g., the normal daily fussy period, or an inconvenient number or nature of stools. There is then a temptation to conclude that it will do no harm and may do some good to change the formula. This practice is to be discouraged, and more will be gained by appropriate counseling and guidance of the parents.

In certain unusual situations, true intolerance to milk may be encountered. True allergy to cow's milk occurs in less than 1 per cent of infants. It is manifested by diarrhea, vomiting, respiratory or cutaneous symptoms, which disappear when all milk and milk products are removed from the diet. After significant episodes of infectious diarrhea, intestinal lactase may be temporarily absent and ingestion of lactose-containing milk formula poorly tolerated for a time. Genetically controlled lactase deficiency occurs among a majority of blacks, Orientals and American Indians, but is not manifest in the first year of life. Congenital absence of disaccharidases is very rare.

Infants with true intolerance to milk should receive feedings free of milk protein or milk sugar. Most commonly used are formulae based on soy protein. Several soy-based formulae are commercially available, none of which contain lactose. These formulae are supplemented to meet recommended vitamin and mineral requirements, and are distributed as concentrates in 13-oz cans. They are commonly fed after mixing with an equal volume of water.

Malnutrition and Brain Development

The clinical consequences of specific nutritional deficiencies are not described here. Rickets, scurvy, xerophthalmia and nutritional hypoproteinemia are adequately described in reference texts and are not expected to be encountered in American infants. The relation of nutrition to development of central nervous system function, however, has received considerable attention in recent years and warrants comment.

Relatively rapid brain growth continues until two to three years of age, by which time the brain has achieved approximately 80 per cent of its adult weight. Measurements of head size, brain cell number and a variety of intellectual and behavioral tests have been made which indicate that permanent deficits can occur in children who have suffered severe and prolonged malnutrition in the first 18 to 24 months of life. The older child who is severely undernourished will be apathetic and unable to learn. These handicaps associated with severe malnutrition with onset after the third year are thought to be reversible and should disappear after adequate nutritional rehabilitation.

Chase and Martin have studied a unique population of severely malnourished infants in the United States. When neglect and malnutrition, as evidenced by severe failure to gain, existed for more than four months in the first year, permanent impairment of central nervous system function occurred. Thus, there is a certain degree of urgency in dealing with the complex social and psychological problems that are responsible for neglect and inadequate nutrition in early infancy. The time required to implement effective psychotherapy, social manipulation or foster care should not be so long as to result in permanent damage.

NUTRITION IN CHILDHOOD

By the end of the first year, the infant will be eating three meals a day with an occasional snack, increasing his self-feeding activities and at times sharing mealtime with other members of the family. The infant participates in family meals, which often prompts parents to express concern about the essentials of a well-balanced diet for the family.

The physician may give a practical answer to this question if he understands how national recommendations for nutrient intakes are established and how they are translated into menu planning.

Fifty of the country's leading nutrition experts were called together in 1940 because large numbers of men were found unfit for military service at the beginning of World War II owing to nutrition-related health problems. The nation's leaders asked this group to define nutrient requirements for the American people. Known as the Food and Nutrition Board of the National Research Council of the National Academy of Sciences, a non-governmental scientific body, the group published a report, "Recommended Dietary Allowances," commonly referred to as the RDA. Recommended allowances were developed for both males and females and were categorized by age groups. Special allowances were defined for pregnancy and lactation.

The word "allowance" was chosen very advisedly. The recommended allowances are indeed *allowances* and not nutrient requirements; nor are they recommended intakes for any given person. As *allowances* they merely provide an informed guideline for planning and evaluating food intake and define the nutrient level that will provide the nutritional needs of essentially *all* normal healthy people in the United States. It was implicit from the first that the RDA would be reviewed periodically and would be revised to keep up with advances in nutrition knowledge and changing American life styles. The allowances have been revised seven times, most recently in 1974. (A summary of the current RDA is provided in the Appendix.)

The RDA tables obviously do not answer the question posed by the parents about what foods should be included in a desired daily diet. Home economists and nutritionists have devised a program that can be most practically implemented via the Four Food Group Plan. The Four Food Group Plan can be readily used to advantage by interested parents and children, particularly adolescents as they experience increasing independence in their food choice. It has almost limitless flexibility, is particularly well suited to the American food supply and is easy to communicate to parents and older children. It is the basis of nutrition education in primary and secondary schools as well as in most public programs of nutrition education. Each of the four food groups are composed of common food items that have been grouped together because of the similar nutrient contribution they make to the diet:

1. Milk and milk products
2. Meat and high protein foods
3. Fruits and vegetables
4. Cereal and grain products

The Four Food Groups

Milk and milk products. After the first year, all children should receive the equivalent of a pint of milk or two servings of food from the milk group each day, either directly as a beverage or included in the preparation of other foods or as an alternate milk product such as cheese or ice cream.

Milk products provide a good source of protein, calcium and riboflavin. Yet, despite all of its virtues, milk is frequently drunk to excess. Older infants, preschool children and particularly young American males are prone to excessive milk-drinking habits. This consumption of large quantities of milk often tends to displace other important foods and may add excess animal fat, protein, salt and electrolytes to the diet. Young children and adolescents who desire more than two glasses of milk a day would be well-advised to drink skim milk. Unmodified milk products, particularly cheeses made from whole milk, are high in animal fat and salt and have a high caloric density.

In addition to contributing other nutrients, milk, particularly fortified powdered milk, can be a low-cost source of high-quality protein.

Meat and high protein foods. This group includes meats, fish, poultry, eggs and such alternate vegetable items as dried beans, peas and nuts. In addition to their protein contribution, these foods are a major source of B group vitamins and iron. Many of the animal protein foods are rich in readily adsorbed heme iron. Their presence increases the absorption of iron from vegetable foods that may be eaten with them.

Two or more servings from this group should be eaten each day (the basic serving of meat is 3.5 ounces of edible portion).

Because of concern over the saturated fat content of many meats and meat products, a prudent diet for Americans as defined by the American Heart Association would limit the intake of red meat to three servings a week and eggs to three per week. The remainder of the week's servings from this group would come from fish, chicken and the high protein vegetable alternates such as beans, peas and nuts.

Fruits and vegetables. Fruits and vegetables, including the potato, have a high nutrient to calorie ratio. Vegetables are particularly important sources of minerals and vitamins. Leafy vegetables such as spinach, lettuce and cabbage provide desired bulk in the form of undigestible cellulose. Citrus fruits, canteloupes, strawberries, tomatoes, leafy vegetables and vegetables that are commonly eaten raw are significant sources of vitamin C and folic acid.

Four or more servings of fruits and vegetables should be included in the daily diet. When not served with butter or high calorie salad dressings, their caloric density is relatively low so they can be eaten in large amounts by people restricting caloric intake.

If there is no fresh fruit or raw vegetable included in the daily diet, an adequate intake of vitamin C and folic acid will probably not be provided.

Cereal and grain products. Bread, cereals, flour and baked goods can be relatively inexpensive carbohydrate sources of energy. In addition, they contribute protein, minerals and a number of vitamins. Most people have little difficulty getting the recommended four daily servings from this group. The active and growing adolescent with high energy needs will find his most economical source of energy in this group.

A Basic Diet Plan

The recommended daily servings from the four food groups are: two servings from the milk group and from the meat and protein-rich foods groups and four servings each from the cereal group and the fruit and vegetable group. These 12 servings in themselves will supply all necessary nutrients no matter how large the individual or how rigorous his growth experience. Such a basic diet will *not*, however, meet the energy (caloric) needs of moderately active, growing children.

The energy contribution of this basic diet will depend on the selection of foods and the size of servings. It will usually not exceed 1200–1500 Kcal per day, however. As a result, it can be used as an effective reducing diet, and it will assure an adequate intake of all essential nutrients for children of all ages, sizes and degrees of activity. (The exception to this is the increased iron requirement for girls after the menarche.)

Obviously, all children beyond the age of three to four years will need additional foods to satisfy their energy needs. Once the need for essential nutrients has been satisfied there is ample room in food selection for individual choices. An old axiom holds true: "First eat what you need (the four food groups) and then eat what you want."

Most young people will respond to their increasing energy needs by making servings from the four food groups much larger than the so-called "normal serving." They will also eat extra helpings and will add high-calorie density foods such as desserts and snacks. One should be sure that these high preference foods are added to, and not substituted for, essential items in the basic diet. Caution should be practiced in avoiding high intake of animal fat by the alternate use of vegetable shortenings, sherbets and milk drinks such as shakes and malts made with non-fat dairy products.

Using the Four Food Group Plan, the physician can readily evaluate the diet of a patient and the dietary practices of the family. After a brief consultation, parents can evaluate food utilization practices within the family to be reassured that adequate amounts of essential nutrients are being provided.

A patient's diet may be evaluated using the so-called "24-hour recall." The patient is asked to record or to recall all the food and drink ingested during the past 24 hours, recalling specific intake hour by hour. One can readily discover whether an appropriate number of servings from each of the four food groups has been included within the 24-hour period.

In circumstances associated with growth deficiency or suspected inadequate nutrient intake a more detailed evaluation of the diet may be needed. Under these circumstances, the patient or parent is asked to keep a detailed record of all food and beverages taken during a five to seven day period. When available, the services of a nutritionist can be called upon for analysis of this record.

NUTRITION PROBLEMS IN CHILDHOOD AND ADOLESCENCE

Caloric Deprivation

The physician will encounter inadequate food intake most commonly in poverty populations. As many as 15 per cent of American families cannot afford to provide adequate food to meet their needs. This results in suboptimal growth, easy fatigue and an increased prevalence of iron deficiency. Less well-documented are altered behavioral patterns such as poor learning and food stealing that may be associated with inadequate diet, particularly in the older child and adolescent living in poverty. Individuals in poor families who have the largest food needs are those who suffer most. The rapidly growing adolescent male with his high food demand is particularly vulnerable. Pregnant women who have increased caloric needs are also at high risk. When both adolescence and pregnancy occur simultaneously, nutritional status may often be severely compromised. Under these circumstances, even the best of diets may fail to meet the combined nutritional demands of pregnancy and adolescent growth.

Voluntary restriction of caloric intake by teenage girls is common in middle- and upper-income populations. Social pressures to maintain a sylphlike figure associated with an inactive urban life style demand a severe caloric restriction. Daily caloric intake of less than 1200 to 1400 calories a day is not uncommon among teenage girls. A significant part of this diet may be contributed by snack foods of low nutrient content. Increased physical activity permitting more healthy eating habits, while maintaining an attractive figure is a proper answer to this problem, though difficult to implement at times.

"Johnny Won't Eat"

Appetite and spontaneous food intake are directly related to the energy demands of the child and reflect the needs of growth and activity. Thus, appetite varies greatly with the age.

The large caloric demands of the rapidly growing infant have been mentioned previously. As the rapid growth rate of infancy declines in the preschool period, caloric demands and appetite decrease proportionately. The three- to five-year-old child will normally have less appetite and less interest in food than a younger child. This normal, small appetite may be a source of considerable anxiety and result in unhealthy stressful encounters at mealtime. The conflict that can arise between parents and child over the parents' unrealistic demand for food intake can put stress on the entire family relationship. Mealtime conversations limited to Johnny "cleaning his plate," "eating the good food which could save the starving Indians" or never "growing up to be a major league player" or "no television for a week unless you eat your vegetables" all change table time from a period of pleasant family interaction to a battle ground. Invariably, the parents' most intense offensive will fail to dent the impenetrable defense of Johnny's petite appetite. Defeat of the combined parental forces by a five-year-old cannot be tolerated and the battle intensifies.

Brief anticipatory guidance that makes the parent aware of the decreasing food needs of the preschool child will avoid these unpleasantries. An active life style, limiting milk to no more than 8 to 16 oz/day and avoiding bland carbohydrate and snack foods will all combine to assure good nutrition for children of this age group. The five-year-old with a normal small appetite should elicit congratulations on avoiding obesity, and parents should be reassured of the adequacy of the child's food intake. Vitamin supplementation is to be avoided, as are between meal snacks. Offering between meal snacks under the excuse that "I must get something into him" will only perpetuate the problem.

New Life Style Diets

Eating and meeting nutritional needs is a dominant determinant of behavior and life style. As the adolescent and older teenager experience increasing independence and begin to develop individual patterns of living, it is expected that they will explore a variety of differing dietary practices. They will enjoy the adventures of eating a variety of new foods. Many young people choose to experience meat-free diets, meeting nutritional needs with fruits, vegetables and dairy products. Such a diet can optimally meet nutritional needs if their life style includes a reasonable energy expenditure and their selection of foods includes a wide variety. Individuals who participate in extremely restricted diets such as prolonged fasting, or macrobiotic diets will develop a variety of forms of malnutrition. Likewise, restricted weight reduction diets such as Dr. Atkin's Diet, the grapefruit diet or the fried chicken diet not only are ineffective but if used for a significant period of time can only lead to symptomatic undernutrition.

The use of "organic foods" has become an interesting part of the present-day nutrition experience among young people. In a chemical sense, all foods are organic. But in the context of modern usage, organic foods are those grown without the use of chemical fertilizers or pesticides and contain no preservatives or additives. Taste, nutrition and ecologic advantage are claimed as advantages of so-called organic foods. Plants use only isolated elements such as nitrogen, carbon, magnesium and calcium in growing and do not use complex chemical compounds. Whether these elements come from a compost pile, the barnyard or a chemical manufacturer does not have any impact on the nutrient composition or flavor of the seeds or fruits.

One is more apt to encounter unclean food in the organic food market inasmuch as many products are grown locally and may not be controlled by the regulations of interstate commerce. A significant consideration for many is the cost differential of so-called organic foods. Recently, it was found that a basket of vegetables, cereals and breads was purchased for $17.43 in a supermarket conventional food section but cost $26.00 in the health food section and $33.74 in a local health food store. Individuals with a necessary concern about unit pricing will do well to avoid this cost differential.

Iron Deficiency

Nutritional deficiency of iron is the only specific nutritional deficiency recognized as being widespread in industrialized nations. Several reasons explain this continuing occurrence of iron deficiency in affluent, food-excess societies: Total food intake is decreasing as individuals expend less energy. Iron concentration of clean, mass produced food is reduced as soil contami-

nation of the diet is eliminated and iron cooking utensils are no longer used. Iron requirements are increased as children grow more rapidly to larger sizes and the menstrual experience is initiated at a younger age. Lastly, man's ability to absorb iron is distinctly limited. These factors combine to place affluent industrial populations at risk for deficiency.

The very rapid growth rate of infants and the low iron content of the infant's milk diet result in a high prevalence of iron deficiency in the first two years of life. Appropriate introduction of a varied diet and the recommendation of routine supplementation with iron through either iron supplemented formulas or medicinal iron for the breast-fed infant can essentially eliminate this problem.

The high risk of iron deficiency in the older child has recently been demonstrated with the ability to assess the status of iron storage in growing children of differing ages. Levels of plasma ferritin in a population of well-nourished children are compared to the ferritin values in adult males and females in Figure 11–1. Ferritin is the body's iron storage compound, and the level of plasma ferritin reflects the level of iron stores. Females with essentially no

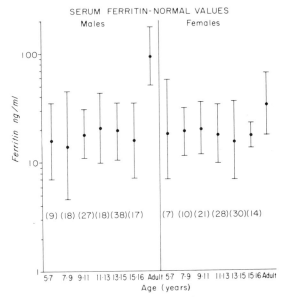

Figure 11–1 Serum ferritin concentrations in populations of males and females of various ages. All had normal hemoglobin, hematocrit and transferrin saturation values. The absence of significant iron stores, as reflected by this measure, extends throughout the entire growth experience of childhood and adolescence.

iron reserves will have only 20 per cent of the mean level of plasma ferritin of adult males. All through childhood, it will be noted that ferritin levels remain even lower than those encountered in the adult female, reflecting an essential absence of significant storage iron in growing children. Iron stores accumulate only in males when growth stops and fail to accumulate to a significant level in present-day American women during their reproductive years. When a child without significant storage iron experiences a compromised intake of dietary iron, unusually rapid growth or blood loss, iron deficiency with or without frank anemia will develop.

Compromised dietary intake of iron is the most common cause of iron deficiency in the young child; excessive milk and bland carbohydrates are the primary dietary factors responsible. Inadequate diet explains the high prevalence of iron deficiency in teenage boys in low-income families. Menstrual losses are the determining factor in iron deficiency that is encountered in approximately 20 per cent of girls in all income levels. This prevalence of iron deficiency in these girls continues through their childbearing years, increasing with age in low-income women.

The effect of iron deficiency on work performance and learning behavior has been documented in recent years. Children with mild anemia, hemoglobin deficits of only 1 to 2 gm/100 ml, have been found to have limited learning ability. Older individuals with similar degrees of anemia have been found to have limited work ability. Recently, iron-deficient rats with normal hemoglobin and hematocrit levels have been shown to have limited work abilities and specific abnormalities in intracellular energy metabolism. Thus the large numbers of individuals suffering from mild degrees of iron deficiency with or without anemia may have learning and work disabilities. Therefore, early detection of iron deficiency assumes importance. Hemoglobin and hematocrit levels are influenced by age, sex and a variety of environmental factors, and therefore do not provide a precise index of iron nutrition. Biochemical assessment of iron status by measuring erythrocyte protoporphyrin or plasma ferritin concentrations will become increasingly important as indices of iron deficiency.

The physician should identify those individuals at risk for iron deficiency: the rapidly growing young child, the teenager living in poverty, and the girl with greater than average menstrual iron losses. Many will need diet and activity counseling, and many adolescent girls particularly may need a daily medicinal iron supplement.

OBESITY

The Prevalence of Obesity

Obesity is widely recognized as a major public health problem in the United States. Obesity is more common among males than females, it increases with age and there is an increasing prevalence of obesity in males with increasing family income. In females, the opposite is true. The prevalence of obesity is lowest among women in the highest income families. Obesity is more prevalent in eastern and southern United States than it is in the north and west. There are also distinct genetic influences, with obesity occurring in family groups.

Recognized Causes of Obesity

Obesity, or over-fatness, represents a positive imbalance in energy intake and energy expenditure. Fat represents storage of excess energy in fat cells with differing distribution in males and females after adolescence.

Creating a positive energy balance that will result in over-fatness may result from an excessively large intake of calories or from the expenditure of minimal energy in an unduly sedentary existence. Inactivity and sedentary living are more commonly the major contributor to obesity in present-day American populations than is uncontrolled, excessive eating. Most commonly, the obese individual will be found to have a caloric intake that is less than the caloric intake of non-obese persons.

Rarely, endocrine disturbances may be associated with disturbed energy balance and resultant obesity. Abnormalities in thyroid function and insulin action and a response to growth hormone frequently identified in the chronically obese individual are almost always secondary to the obesity rather than a primary causative factor.

In the presence of chronic obesity, important contributing factors are accentuated. Over-fatness reduces the facility of physical activity, insulating layers of adipose tissue conserve body heat and thus, basic caloric expenditures and requirements decrease.

In recent years, considerable attention has been directed at the characteristics of fat cells in obesity. Studies of fat tissue have demonstrated that enlargement of fat depots in the extremely obese are due primarily to an increase in the number of fat cells with varying increases in adipose cell size. Subjects with a childhood history of obesity tend to display the most marked degree of increase in cell numbers. Obesity occurring after puberty has a greater contribution of adipose cell enlargement. In both situations, weight reduction is accompanied only by reduction in fat cell size without any appreciable effect on fat cell number. The number of fat cells cannot be reduced, and a permanently increased population of fat cells places an individual at chronic risk of obesity. The first two years of life and early adolescence are periods in which positive caloric balance are most particularly apt to result in an increase in fat cell numbers. Obese children have greater numbers of adipose cells than do non-obese children, and in all instances the fat cells of obese children are larger in size than are those of non-obese children.

The Diagnosis of Obesity

Gross obesity can obviously be diagnosed by inspection; however, the subjective evaluation of over-fatness makes diagnosis by inspection imprecise. Weight-height relationships have been traditionally used to identify overweight persons. Overweight is not synonymous with over-fatness, however, and a large bony structure and large muscle mass may result in weight that is in excess of height in the absence of over-fatness.

A more critical definition of obesity can be made by clinically estimating body fatness with a skin-fat-fold caliper. Values for skin fat-fold as measured over the tri-

ceps area at different ages in boys and girls are given in the Appendix. Measurements of skin fat-fold in early infancy are less reliable than at a later age. A general rule in infancy is if weight exceeds height by more than 20 to 25 percentile points at a given age, a diagnosis of obesity is appropriate and corrective measures should be implemented.

Management of Obesity

Inability to successfully reverse obesity which had its onset in early life indicates that attention be directed to prevention (see Infant Feeding). Failures in correcting chronic obesity may be due to the inability to reduce fat cell numbers once large populations of adipocytes have been established, as well as the parental harassment and devastation of self-image that is associated with chronic obesity in childhood. The first essential of a program in obesity management is the establishment of realistic goals. This will often be merely the reduction in rate of weight gain or weight maintenance rather than any striking reduction in over-fatness. The obese individual must be prompted to establish an active life style and must have a clear understanding of the caloric densities of various foods. He must receive psychological support at home and at the hands of professional counselors. Whether sophisticated counseling in behavior modification can be successful in weight control has not been demonstrated, but at the present time, it is probably the most promising avenue of management available.

DIET AND THE PREVENTION OF CORONARY ARTERY HEART DISEASE

Evidence of coronary artery atherosclerosis has been reported in at least 45 per cent of American young men under 30 years of age killed in war time. Although coronary artery disease does not manifest itself clinically until later in adulthood, its origins must be in earlier life. The Committee on Nutrition of the American Academy of Pediatrics (1972) has summarized the evidence relating cholesterol intake to coronary artery disease as follows:

1. Some inborn and acquired diseases with hypercholesterolemia are associated with premature atherosclerosis.

2. Serum concentrations of cholesterol are frequently relatively high in persons with coronary heart disease.

3. In prospective studies, persons with high serum concentrations of cholesterol are more prone to develop heart disease than are those with lower serum concentrations.

4. The mortality rate from coronary heart disease in different countries varies in relation to the average serum concentrations of cholesterol.

5. Experimentally induced hypercholesterolemia in animals is associated with the development of atherosclerotic deposits.

6. Atherosclerotic plaques contain lipids similar to those in blood.

In addition, one might add that serum concentrations of cholesterol are unequivocally related to diet, especially to cholesterol content.

Although it would appear that coronary atherosclerosis has its onset in childhood, there is no evidence to suggest that dietary intervention early in life will exert a preventive influence on its development. In the present state of uncertainty regarding the advantages or complications from dietary intervention in early life, it seems unreasonable to recommend a major departure from the model of breast feeding in infancy. It is possible that limitation of dietary intake of cholesterol during this period may be harmful. With respect to diet after infancy, circumstantial evidence would suggest that there is indeed harm from high intake of cholesterol, and thus it is appropriate to recommend limitation. A moderate restriction of cholesterol intake seems reasonable. Dietary patterns to follow are well described in the material available from the American Heart Association, which defines a "Prudent Diet" for American males. The recommended diet would reduce the caloric contribution of fat to the diet to less than 35 per cent, with half of that coming from unsaturated vegetable sources. Children in families in which there is a history of coronary disease of early onset and in those with serum cholesterol concentrations of greater than 200 mg/100 ml may well have inborn errors in cholesterol metabolism requiring specific consultation and intervention.

REFERENCES

Anderson, T. A., and Fomon, S. J.: Commercially prepared strained and junior foods for infants. J. Am. Diet. Assoc., 58:520, 1971.

Chase, H. P., and Martin, H. P.: Undernutrition and child development. N. Engl. J. Med., 282:933, 1970.

Fomon, S. J.: *Infant Nutrition*, 2nd ed. Philadelphia, W. B. Saunders Co., 1975.

Smith, N. J., and Rios, E.: Iron metabolism and iron deficiency in infancy and childhood. *In* Schulman, J. (Ed.): *Advances in Pediatrics*, Vol. 21. Chicago, Year Book Medical Publishers, 1974.

Smith, N. J.: *Food in Sport.* Palo Alto, Bull Publishing Co., 1976.

Winnick, M. (Ed.): *Childhood Obesity.* New York, Wiley-Interscience Publication, 1975.

Developmental Issues and Psychosocial Problems In Childhood

I. Normal Development and Minor Behavioral Problems

William Hetznecker and Marc A. Forman

This first behavioral chapter deals predominantly with normal development and minor behavioral problems. Chapter 28 relates to the more serious behavioral disorders.

GENERAL CONSIDERATIONS

All of us were once children. This is not a surprising notion, but we occasionally need to be reminded that squealing infants and negativistic toddlers change, grow up and develop into adults. Some even become physicians.

Our dealings with children are influenced by our concepts about childhood and by our own experiences as children. We may mistakenly view children as either innocent little flowers or as savage animals. We may unwittingly make them passive recipients of our frustrated ambitions and dreams—or unknowingly encourage them to adopt those aspects of our own personalities that we least desire. We can also, of course, provide them with those elements of love, nurturance, consistency and guidance that will allow them to become independent, caring and responsible adults who will carry our culture forward.

There is little question that what happens during childhood is crucial in shaping the personality of the adult. Children, however, are not merely blank screens upon which parents project their values and conflicts. Children come into the world with their own genetic heritage and temperamental individuality. Motor activity levels, sleep and feeding rhythms, responsiveness to stressful stimuli and frustration tolerances vary from one infant to another. The infant's "style" of behavior is, in part, a reflection of his constitution. Each child is unique from the moment of conception, and his ultimate personality is the result of a constant interplay between endowment and environment. It is not a matter of nature *or* nurture, but rather how the two *interact* to create the total child. The child is an active participant and contributor to this interchange, affecting his parents as they, in turn, influence him. Any medical or psychological intervention occurs within this context of reciprocal relationships among all family members.

The development of children can be viewed as a progressive attempt to master intersecting biological, cognitive and emotional tasks. Major developmental issues are illustrated in the following table:

	Biological Tasks	Emotional	Cognitive
Infant	Sleep and feeding rhythms; increasing postural control; prehension; eye-hand coordination	Sense of trust; attachment behavior and affectional ties to parents	Progression from "reflex" behavior to reciprocal inter-action with environment; social smile; rudiments of speech
Toddler	Locomotion; bladder and bowel control	Increasing autonomy from parents; exploration; need for limits	Language; capacity for social-ization
School-age Child	Continuing physical maturation	Appropriate "student" role; relations to peer group; sense of competence and industry	Reading and math skills; mental operations of classify-ing, ordering, numbering; progression to abstract thinking

It should be noted that as a child de-velops, physical and biological factors be-come less important — unless illness inter-venes — and social-emotional and cognitive challenges are more critical. Very young children react to stressful situations via their physiologic apparatus, as exemplified by sleep and feeding disturbances, or by relatively global expressions of anger or fear, as evidenced in such responses as temper tantrums, avoidance and withdraw-al. Older children tend to show their prob-lems in troubled relationships with peers and family, through impairment of school performance, by the development of spe-cific psychological symptoms such as de-pression and phobias, as well as by "re-gressing" to earlier modes of functioning. Each child's response to stress is depend-ent on his developmental level, the nature and duration of the stress and the coping and adaptive capabilities of his family. Ac-cordingly, responses to stress will vary from child to child and family to family. Often the advice, support and anticipatory guidance given by pediatricians during periods of difficulty may have a significant effect in altering the outcome.

Whether a particular behavior is a devel-opmental variation or evidence of a more serious psychosocial disturbance depends upon such factors as the age of the child; the frequency, intensity and resistance of symptoms; their association to a more gen-eralized disturbance, and the degree of functional impairment.

Various "symptomatic" actions and reac-tions have been shown to be part of normal development throughout infancy and child-hood (Lapouse and Monk). Loss of temper can be part of the negativism of two- to three-year-old toddlers. The same behavior at age six or occurring in response to the slightest frustration or disappointment can be a sign of psychosocial disturbance. The decision to seek help is determined by the characteristics of the behavior, its duration and intensity and the degree of distress to the child or others. Requests for interven-tion are determined by parental anxiety and past experience in seeking help, as well as pressure from other sources such as grandparents, school, neighbors and friends. Parents tend to compare their chil-dren's behavior and development with other children and with journalistic ac-counts about childhood. The results of such comparisons can either relieve or enhance the parents' anxiety.

The responsibility is not solely that of the parents. The physician must have ade-quate knowledge of child development and family dynamics to initiate the proper in-quiry and judge whether parents are un-duly concerned, falsely secure or accurate in their assessment of the child.

The Clinical Interview

The clinical interview is the most ubiq-uitous of all procedures in medicine. It requires great skill and continuous atten-tive practice throughout one's professional life. It is also the skill most likely over-looked or taken for granted in the formal education of medical students.

The clinical interview is often portrayed erroneously; it is not history-taking or an obsessive completion of the form provided for physical diagnosis. It is not a cross ex-amination. It is an alliance between two persons—one who is seeking to be helpful and the other who possesses the knowledge, skill and social sanction to offer help. In a formal sense, it is one example of a particular social contract. From the physician's perspective, the clinical interview is the major means of engaging the patient in the active process of caring for himself.

In addition to collecting historical medical data and the signs and symptoms of present illness, there are several other aspects of the patient's life that require careful attention. These include the patient's present emotional state and his reaction to stress and conflict, his self-concept, his value system, the nature of his personal relationships, his coping mechanisms and his strengths and liabilities.

Several factors should be considered in order to make the best possible conditions for a clinical interview.

Time. An adequate interview that explores these dimensions can not be done in 10 minutes. At least 30 to 40 minutes should be set aside for any significant clinical interchange that is more than the perfunctory medical exchange. After one knows a patient well it is possible to conduct a satisfactory clinical interview in 10 minutes but such shortening depends upon the nature and duration of the physician-patient relationship and the purpose of the particular interview.

Setting. Privacy should be sought. It is very difficult to conduct an interview with a child at a bedside with curtains drawn to shield off the other beds in the room, or in an outpatient cubicle with no door. To attempt such a venture is to load the dice against the physician and inadvertently to show inadequate respect and sensitivity to the situation of the patient. This dictum is more likely to be overlooked with children, who are usually regarded with less respect and sensitivity than is accorded adults in these matters.

Hospitals are often set up to preclude adequate privacy. Nevertheless one should try to use a treatment room, an empty conference room or even an unoccupied patient room to promote the greatest possible privacy. A basic question to consider in this, and many other similar clinical situations, is: How would I wish to be treated if I were a patient being interviewed in this fashion?

Goals. One of the basic failures of interviewing is that the clinician has not clearly defined and delineated the goals of that particular interview. A single interview of 20 to 30 minutes or even an hour seldom accomplishes everything. Therefore, it is critical that the clinician define his priorities. Judging from his own style and experience he can gauge what can be accomplished in one interview and how much should be delayed until the next. If the first interview is designed to establish a working alliance with a child and family and identify the primary problems or concerns, then it is a mistake to be led into attempting a total developmental or family survey at this time.

Communication. The major goal of the clinical interview is communication, which we define as an exchange of information between two or more people. In the clinical interview this exchange is between patient and physician. When dealing with children, this exchange is between parent (usually mother) and physician, between child and physician and between child and parent.

There are two major aspects of any interpersonal exchange to be considered in the context of the clinical interview—the *content* or *message* and the *process* or *relationship*. The content refers to the literal meaning of the words exchanged. This meaning can be denotative, the dictionary definition, or connotative, the suggested meaning or allusion of a word.

The process or relationship aspect refers to the non-verbal part of the communication. This includes tone of voice, rate of speech, inflection, facial expression, head movement, hand gestures and body posture and movements. All these aspects of communication are monitored, moment to moment, by each sender and receiver. The non-verbal aspects of communication express the state of the sender and indicate how the content is to be received.

A child learns to interpret non-verbal communication before he or she understands the meaning of words. He communicates basic feelings and emotions with sound, gesture and expression long before he can identify his feelings or know what words are or how to use them as expressions of feelings. A physician must be aware of how his facial expressions, tone of

voice or gestures can influence a child's reaction and thus indicate how a given message is to be "taken" or received.

A physician must be able to correctly
recognize and interpret a child's emotional
state by careful observation of facial expression, body posture and response. A
child who says little in response to a question may be upset by the loudness of the
physician's voice or the suddenness of the
initiation of the examination. The child
may have a temperament that is made anxious quite easily by new and unfamiliar situations. Though the physician may not be
responsible for a child's fear or anxiety, he
may be responsible for not recognizing the
signs of anxiety in a child. He may also be
responsible for frightening a child by lack
of attention or sensitivity to the child's non-
verbal communication of his or her emotional state.

Parental Attitudes and Expectations

A child lives in the minds of its parents
before it is born or even conceived. Attitudes of prospective or actual parents can
be determined by questions such as:

How did you and your spouse make the decision to have a baby now? (or when you had
Sally?)
What had you hoped or expected Sally to be
like before she was born?
How is she similar or different from what you
expected?
What are your hopes or expectations for her
future?

It is normal and healthy for the parent to
harbor certain wishes for a child and to expect some gratification from the child in
exchange for parental concern, sacrifice
and hard work. This promotes the affec-
tionate social ties between parents and
child.

When listening to parents talk about a
child, extreme reactions or expressions
should be noted, whether overly negative
or positive. A parent may make subtle comparisons of the child to family members
whom he dislikes, fears or envies. Parents
may speak of a child as if he were an object
designed to fulfill their needs and wishes,
to compensate for a lost child, to bolster a
failing marriage, to substitute for an indifferent spouse, to provide the vehicle for an

unfilled dream or to give them a chance to
relive their own childhood.

A clinician needs to be sophisticated—but not cynical—about human behavior. Parent-child feelings and attitudes
are highly emotional issues, and the physician is not exempt. Therefore, the physician needs to be clear about his or her own
sensitivities, distortions and expectations
as these relate to parent attitudes. The
physician must develop the knowledge
base to evaluate the wide range of normal
variation in parent attitudes. He must also
be scrupulous in not imposing into clinical
practice the idiosyncratic values or attitudes
that he may hold.

Parents of children who are physically
handicapped, mentally retarded, emotionally disturbed or socially inept and who may
provide little gratification to the parents are
at particular risk of developing unhealthy
and destructive attitudes toward those children, toward society or toward themselves.
The last thing such parents need is a similar
negative or condemning attitude from their
physician.

HEALTHY RESPONSES, DEVELOPMENTAL DEVIATIONS AND PSYCHOSOCIAL DISTURBANCES

ATTACHMENT

Attachment is a specific enduring relationship between two people that is mutually established and maintained. Klaus and
Kennell indicate that the "operational behavior of attachment includes fondling,
cuddling, and prolonged gazing which
serves to maintain contact and show affection between individuals." Attachment of
infant to mother and mother to infant com-
prises the social bond. This is the primor-
dial social experience and provides a foundation for future and more differential
social bonding with father, siblings,
friends, lovers, spouses and children.

Studies of mothers of premature babies
who first had contact with their infants
some hours or days after birth have been
supplemented by observations and films of
mothers of normal infants who had immediate postnatal contact with the newborn.
Both groups of mothers tended to follow a
certain ritualized behavior. Because they

occurred over a longer period of time these actions were more discrete and easily observed in mothers of premature infants. The same actions were carried out by mothers of normal newborns, but the behavior was telescoped into a short period of time immediately after birth. These include touching the infant's extremities by the mother's fingertips, then moving to the trunk with stroking movements. The mother of the normal newborn would speak to the infant while looking at its face. She was emotionally excited, used a higher-pitched voice than usual, and much of what she said related to the baby opening its eyes. Other studies have shown that in the first day of life the baby attends to and moves in rhythm with adult speech. Thus a major principle of interaction is established in the earliest hours of contact between mother and infant.

Interaction that results in bonding requires mutual, reciprocal and complementary responses. Thus the infant who fails to provide some feedback to the attachment behavior of the mother may diminish those behaviors and induce perplexity, frustration and discouragement in the mother. If such non-responsive behavior continues over time because of illness or physical handicap, the possibility of the mother "rejecting" the baby increases. It is as if she says, "If you won't love me I won't love you." This is clearly not a conscious, explicitly formulated attitude, but it occurs because her overtures do not elicit bonding responses on the part of the child.

In like manner, physical or psychological handicap, or physical absence may prevent a mother from initiating attachment action toward her newborn. The newborn then may have no one who elicits or reinforces his early capacity for attachment. At the two extremes this could result in a withdrawn, apathetic, "depressed" infant or an anxious, irritable, incessantly signaling ("demanding") infant.

A note of caution needs to be injected. Studies of these behaviors are still very early and tentative. The exact notion of how innate temperamental characteristics of an infant relate to the interactional processes of bonding is yet to be determined. One should be cautious in forming judgments about inadequate social bonding or "rejecting" mothers when confronted with complaints about fussy, irritable, lethargic infants or other difficulties in adaptation.

Ineffective or absent attachment behavior can result from psychological deprivation, or more specifically, from maternal deprivation. The infant is not able to establish or maintain intimate contact with a mothering person that is characterized by mutual reciprocal stimulation and gratification. The extreme results of this condition have been described by Spitz and Bowlby. Infants tend to show protest and rage initially, then depression followed by apathetic withdrawal. If the lack of emotional and social stimulation persists long enough the infant may become indifferent or apathetic, and he may stop eating, fail to grow and demonstrate psychosocial and motor regression. He also becomes more susceptible to infection and intercurrent disease, such that death may result. This failure to thrive syndrome exists on a continuum and can be observed in infants who are evaluated in hospital emergency rooms as well as outpatient clinics. Such children are frequently brought to the physician because of intermittent and recurrent respiratory or gastrointestinal disorders or with complaints that the child does not eat, does not behave or is not developing as expected. Frequently, parents of such children are overwhelmed by economic and social stresses. They also tend to be individuals whose own psychological strengths and capacities are limited. The combination of depression, impulsiveness, chronic fatigue, irritability and the possible excess use of alcohol or drugs to relieve the burden of internal or external distress serves to limit their effectiveness and particularly their capacity to be emotionally responsive to the needs of an infant or any of their children.

Sleep Disorders

Transient sleep disorders are common, and their expression can assume a variety of forms. The young child may be afraid to go to sleep at night because he worries about burglars, being kidnapped, strange noises, thunder and lightning, "bogeymen" or bad dreams. Fearful children will either verbalize their concerns or attempt to delay bedtime by such gestures as frequent trips to the bathroom, requests for drinks or claims that they are not tired. Some children unwittingly provoke trouble immediately before bedtime in order to avoid the inevitable trip to the bedroom. Before going to sleep or upon awakening in the middle of the night the child may want to come into the parents' bed.

Anxiety about separation from parents is a significant underlying factor in these disturbances. The child may unconsciously equate sleep with removal from parental love and concern. If marital conflict occurs, or divorce has occurred, the anxiety will be exacerbated. The child's bedtime fears are often related to the normal separation from home that is part of the nursery school or kindergarten experience. As a normal developmental event, a child's increasing awareness of death, though still fraught with distortions, surfaces at night and interferes with sleep. Fears of death will be magnified if a family member has recently died. Ultimately, any conflict situation involving the child, family, peers or school may be expressed as a sleep disturbance.

To alleviate sleep disorders, parents should give emotional and physical support, as well as repeated verbal reassurance. Threats and punishment should be avoided. and a calm, patient parental attitude is essential. A definite and regular time for bed should be established. The child should be discouraged from sleeping with parents, but should sleep in a nearby room with a light on if necessary. Some children feel more secure if temporarily allowed to sleep in the same room as a sibling. The period before bedtime should be a quiet one—a warm bath and a light snack are helpful—and overstimulating television programs should be avoided. As with other childhood disturbances, contributing environmental factors should be elucidated and ameliorated, if possible. Most children respond well to a supportive approach. If problems persist, referral to an appropriate mental health professional is indicated.

Tension-Discharge Phenomena

Included in this category are such habits as head banging, rolling, body rocking and other rhythmic actions involving large muscle groups. Thumb sucking, nail biting, hair pulling and grinding of teeth are considered habit disturbances that probably have the same function. Involuntary tics such as facial grimaces, eye blinking, finger snapping, throat clearing and various clicking noises can occur as somewhat more serious and fixed reactions to internal distress or external stress.

Rhythmic movements such as head banging and rocking often begin in infancy and can persist into late childhood. They frequently occur before the child falls asleep. Seen by themselves, they are *not* signs of disturbance. They are best appreciated as ways in which the infant stimulates himself in order to promote sleep or relieve internal tension. They can also occur during waking hours under stressful conditions. As the child becomes older he learns to inhibit these habits in social situations. Usually parental reaction to this behavior is important in determining its outcome. Children usually relinquish them as they enter elementary school and feel the pressure of peers and non-familial adults. Children who continue to rock or bang their heads regularly during daytime activities with or without apparent provocation are probably seriously disturbed emotionally. The persistence of these habits in social situations can also be noted in mentally retarded children and children who suffer from maternal or emotional deprivation.

Teeth grinding usually occurs in sleep and possibly can have adverse effects on dental occlusion. Usually this behavior is associated with a fair amount of anger and resentment that the child does not otherwise discharge. Making bedtime an enjoyable, relaxing experience in which the child and parent can spend 15 minutes together reading, talking and reviewing the day's events may be helpful. The parent should find ways to reassure, praise or comfort the child for the hurts, disappointments or accomplishments of the day. For these and all children, bedtime is not a time to engage in lectures, moralizing or sermonizing a catalogue of faults and failures.

Thumb sucking that is persistent, intense and prolonged is alleged to interfere with normal alignment of the teeth. For children who persistently suck their thumb day and night a system of rewards and deprivations based on learning and conditioning can be used. Generally the best strategy for dealing with mild to moderately persistent habit behaviors is to ignore them when they are occurring. When the child is *not* doing them the parents should recognize and praise him. If the child is able to restrain the behavior for a longer period than usual, this should be noted, and the parents should provide social as well as small material reward. (For a more detailed discussion of these techniques, see Becker, 1971.)

When a tension-release behavior or habit becomes more intense or persistent or if it recurs after disappearing, it may be a signal of increased subjective distress. This increase in internal tension may result from difficulty in mastery of a developmental or social stage. Occasionally, these behaviors are among the many signs of more significant psychosocial disturbance. To establish whether this is the situation the physician needs to conduct a careful inquiry into various areas of the child's life such as relationship with parents, siblings and peers, adjustment to new home or school, academic difficulties or the stress of a physical illness.

Tics

Tics are non-functional, repetitive movements of voluntary muscle groups. Although involving voluntary muscles, tic activity is characterized by automatic non-intentional movement, only partially under conscious awareness. Tics usually cannot be inhibited or initiated at will. They often involve muscles of the face, neck shoulder, trunk and hands. Examples are repetitive blinking, lip smacking, grimacing and throat clearing. Tics can occur as an isolated symptom, in conjunction with a variety of psychiatric disturbances or as postencephalitic sequelae. Tics are distinguished from seizure phenomena in that there is no disturbance of consciousness or attention. There is a variety of theoretical explanations for the occurrence of tics. The simplest is that the tic represents a means of discharging tension and anxiety that can be related to persistent intrapsychic conflicts or social and environmental situations. Tics can be short-lived, representing merely a transient response to stress that may disappear spontaneously.

If tics persist, a thorough psychiatric evaluation is indicated. Treatment can involve behavior modification approaches, or individual psychotherapy directed at ameliorating underlying intrapsychic or interpersonal conflicts and stresses. Frequently, helping these children to be more confident, assertive and comfortable in socially demanding situations such as school or peer groups will reduce their tendency to react with anxiety, which in turn decreases the resultant tic phenomena. Occasionally, a mild tranquilizer or diphenhydramine (Benadryl) can be helpful in modulating the anxiety.

One severe disorder, characterized by tics accompanied by barking, guttural phonation and coprolalia is the Gilles de la Tourette syndrome. Although a relatively rare condition, it is seen in children with severe psychopathology. Some may be borderline psychotic or have severe personality disorders. In addition to psychotherapy for the child and counseling and guidance of parents, medication has been found helpful. Haloperidol (Haldol) has been used with good effect in these children to lessen the frequency and intensity of the tics and to reduce the underlying anxiety.

Disturbances in Motor Behavior

There is wide variability in motor behavior in the normal infant and preschool child. The physician needs to be cautious about labeling a child "hyperkinetic" on the basis of activity and intrusiveness, which may be upsetting to distorted parental expectations for self-control or may be in marked contrast to the sedate behavior of the older sibling. Differences in activity level are one dimension of temperamental variation. A small four-room apartment located on the floor above an elderly couple provides the environmental conditions for almost any degree of activity to be mislabeled "hyperactive." Similarly, a slow to activate, placid child in a family of energetic, active children and adults can be viewed as alarmingly "hypoactive." By false inference, physical slowness or low activity level may be construed as a sign of mental slowness, leading the parents to become anxious unnecessarily.

During infancy the clinician should be

alert to evidence of asymmetry in the degree or range of movements of extremities. The child with a minimal hemiplegia may show only slight variability in the use of the affected extremities. Premature lateralization—or handedness—in the toddler period may be a sign of minimal hemiplegia. Examination of the infant should include observation of type and spontaneity of activity and whether developmental landmarks are passed within normal age range. In addition, listening carefully to the mother's observations and concerns and recording these can be the best source of early identification of motor, as well as other disturbances or deviations. The physician who labels a mother as "overanxious" or a "chronic worrier" and then disregards or minimizes her observations of her child is discarding his most important source of data and his most reliable colleague in the diagnosis and treatment of children.

A reduction in the normal level of behavior can occur as an early sign of illness, especially febrile illness. Diminished motor activity may ensue after a separation from parents or a significant change in the environment, such as a family move or a vacation trip to strange surroundings. An infant or preschool child who is sad as a result of a loss or upset at even a brief interpersonal conflict, may react with reduced motor activity, social withdrawal, emotional blunting, irritability and tearfulness. After a severe fright or shock a young child may limit his mobility and become more dependent and clinging.

Behavior Relative to Safety

One of the most basic parental concerns is that of physical safety. From the time he is able to walk, climb and run, the child is confronted with environmental hazards. His physical ability matures more rapidly than his recognition of and judgment about hazardous situations. Temperamentally, the child who is a highly active, intense reactor and who intrudes upon the environment to satisfy his interest and curiosity is more likely to have falls, to run into the street, to taste dangerous substances or to touch dangerous objects such as hot stoves or unfamiliar dogs.

Children who are experiencing various emotional and behavioral difficulties often engage in hazardous risk-taking and careless behavior without sufficient cognitive awareness of the serious, even fatal, consequences.

Hyperactive children are the most obvious ones in this group. It is important, however, to know that emotionally deprived children, depressed and sad children, children who have inadequate control of their anger for whatever reason, mentally retarded children and children with organic impairment of the brain are all at higher risk for accidents, ingestions and injuries. Children with unsatisfied emotional needs, the overly friendly child and the retarded child can often be the victims of the predatory aggressive or sexual activity of other children, adolescents and adults.

When a child has a history of such problems as "accident proneness," impulsivity, ingestion or willingness to go off with strangers, the physician needs to do several things. First, he must make a complete assessment of the physical, psychological and developmental status of the child. Second, a careful evaluation of the family, especially the parental situation, is indicated. Parental strife and discord, especially maternal withdrawal and depression, alcoholism or addiction may be found. Parents' preoccupation with their own needs and interests can exclude or markedly reduce parenting activities. Unresolved, and often unrecognized, parental anger, resentment and ambivalence directed toward a child in the family can result in neglect of his safety. As a child gets older, his risky, careless behavior may be an intended or unintended way of getting the parent involved, or the behavior may reflect the child's own perception that he is not wanted. He thus internalizes a negative view of himself and acts as if he did not care about his safety and health. Third, the physician must assess the environmental influences of housing and neighborhood.

If the physician judges that the primary difficulty does not lie in parental or marital disturbance, he can rely on careful instruction to the parent to protect the child and decrease hazards and risks to health and safety. If the accident proneness or careless, risky behavior is seen as a sign of childhood disturbance or reflective of parental or familial disturbance, then the physician should refer the family and child to a child mental health facility or practitioner or to a family social service agency.

As in all work with parents, the physician should be careful not to imply that the parent is intentionally guilty of not protecting his child or of being negligent of the safety issue. Some very impulsive, active children require careful and almost constant monitoring until they have developed the controls and judgment to be appropriately cautious. The parent should recognize and reward small improvements in control and judgment on the part of the child.

Anger and Control

A major issue in the socialization of children is the expression and control of feelings of displeasure or dissatisfaction. The infant is biologically equipped to express his subjective displeasure by a cry of protest. The quality of this cry can be identified readily by parents, and they respond by attempting to relieve such causes of distress as hunger, wetness or cold. This expression of feeling is labeled by adults as anger. Throughout childhood, the variation in the manifestation and control of anger is a central task of the child and his parents.

Common developmental manifestations of anger are crying and screaming, breath holding spells, temper tantrums and physical aggression against objects or people. When crying and screaming are deemed solely the expression of anger, they are best managed by ignoring them.

Breath holding is fairly common in the first two years of life. It is best handled by advising parents to ignore it. If the infant is not reinforced for this behavior he will usually give it up. A small percentage of children lose consciousness as a result of breath holding. Their faces become florid, and occasionally they will show some twitching of face and extremities. The episode lasts a few seconds and recovery is complete. These children are not at higher risk for developing various seizure disorders. Occasionally those who have repeated and frequent loss of consciousness as a result of intentional breath holding can be treated with small doses of mephobarbital.

When the child is able to walk and handle his body more competently, he expresses his anger by using his muscles, throwing his body around and kicking, stomping and using a newly discovered tool, language in the form of the word "No!" or "I won't!"

Temper outbursts can have infinite variations, but the basic issue is essentially the same. The child is faced with (1) the refusal on the part of parent or others to grant his wish or fulfill his need or (2) the expectation of the parent for the child to carry out a desired action ("go to bed") or to stop a disapproved action ("don't make that noise"). The child usually refuses to comply by persisting in what he is doing. The parent then may repeat the request several times. Finally, lack of compliance on part of the child leads the parent to intervene physically to carry out the desired action or punish the lack of compliance. It is then that the child responds with the expression of anger in the form of an outburst or tantrum. In another instance, the child may persist in his unfilled request, and the parents' refusal to comply will result in the child's loss of temper.

It is very important to note whether the child has adult models for his loss of temper. Adults are loath to label their own loss of control as a tantrum, but what else can one call the loud, angry voice, contorted facial expression, the slamming of doors or the breaking of objects? Often, infliction of pain accompanies parental anger at the child. Frequently, the original etiology as well as the concurrent cause of a child's temper outbursts is the model provided by parents or older siblings.

When temper tantrums become full blown, they are best handled by ignoring or, if necessary, firmly but calmly removing the child to his room or some other place of social isolation. Attempts to divert, cajole, wheedle, intimidate, bribe or placate the child usually are ineffective, and only serve to reinforce the future, instrumental use of such outbursts. Angry loss of control and physical punitive action communicates to the child: this is what you do to others when you are angry and want to control them.

Demeaning statements, teasing or attempts to "kid" the child out of his anger are fraught with potential danger. These adult approaches are power-oriented and tend to disrespect the right of the child to be angry. Equally wrong is the parent who is entertained by toddler or preschool tantrums. Adult laughter at the child's anger either can provoke more intense rage or can give the message that Dad or Mom approves of his anger—why else would they smile and seem so pleased? Whether intended or not, such parental behavior can reinforce the temper outbursts.

Prevention is the best method of handling temper tantrums. This requires that the parent carefully observe the early warning signals of temper outbursts and intervene before the child and the parent each loses control. By knowing the early warning signals, the parent is in a better position to divert the child, institute calm gentle tones and defuse the emotional intensity. If necessary, the parent can help the child voluntarily isolate himself to gain control before a full-scale tantrum has occurred. The normal development phase for temper outbursts of a global diffuse type is between two and four years. After that, the child has learned more limited and less disorganized and destructive ways to express his anger.

Learning how to appropriately express negative feelings is a long-term process similar to learning effective and appropriate use of language, or competent mastery of the neuromuscular apparatus to walk, run and climb. Patience and firmness are essential. A cardinal principle to use in guiding parents is that the child has the right to any feeling but not to any means of expressing those feelings. Children are often frightened by the strength and intensity of their negative feelings as well as by the intensity of negative feelings they provoke in loved adults. The child wants to learn to control himself, and he should be rewarded whenever he can express his anger or dissatisfaction in ways that stop short of tantrums and outbursts. The child should also be praised for controlling himself in situations in which he previously lost control or was tempted to lose control.

Aggressive behavior is assertive, intrusive behavior directed at the environment, be it human or non-human. The aims of aggressive behavior are achievement of mastery, control and protection against real or imagined threats. Verbal and physical aggressiveness are common in preschool and school-age children. When combined with affects of anger or hostility, aggressiveness can be termed violence.

The preschool child learns to modulate and control his aggressive behavior by means of verbal instruction, models and teaching. Rewarding cooperative behavior, such as taking turns and sharing, helps the child learn control. Learning social control is a process that extends throughout childhood and adolescence. The sometimes painful give and take learned from peers who are just as assertive help a child learn the limits of reasonable aggressive behavior.

Sexuality

A child's sexual self-identification, as boy or girl, is fairly well established by age three. Sexual standards and behavior of parents are important determining factors in molding a child's gender role identification, as well as the child's conscious and unconscious identification with the same-sex parent. The formation of gender role is more dependent on the sexual roles and expectations assigned to a child and how he is raised than it is on biologic drives or constitutional variables. Sexual standards are clearly culturally influenced. In our society, boys are traditionally supposed to be more aggressive, more sports-minded and more mechanically facile. Girls are typified as more emotionally expressive, passive and nurturant. Parents may become worried when their children deviate from these cultural expectations, e.g., when a boy pursues a "feminine" interest in cooking, or a girl wishes to play football. The pediatrician should not view such behavior as pathological, but rather look at the totality of the child's life. He should also be aware that such parental concern may reflect sexual conflicts between or within parents. Traditional sexual role stereotypes are quite legitimately being challenged by the women's liberation movement, and we can anticipate that in the future, boys and girls will have less restricted and more diverse options for their interests and activities.

Parents may occasionally be concerned about the sexual behavior of their children during the preschool and early school age period. Masturbation, sexual exploration and undressing during play (doctor games), mutual handling of genitals and homo- and heterosexual play are all quite common.

These activities are probably innocuous and, if transient, do not have any implications for sexual preferences and habits during adulthood.

In situations involving alleged or actual sexual molestation of a young child, the physician should be cautious not to identify with the anger of the parent at the alleged molester. This reaction is often a manifestation of parental guilt and projection of self-blame for not preventing the event. The child also may be confused, guilty and angry at the molester and at the parent for not protecting him. The physician in such a situation is not the police or district attorney. His job is not to see that justice is done. His role is to help parent and child with the pain, fear, guilt, anger and confusion. One thing he should clearly try to prevent is incessant and repeated parental questioning about the event. Such behavior can only tend to maintain the event in the child's awareness. Consequently, the child may become increasingly anxious, depressed, guilty and ashamed. Some children may unconsciously use the attention generated by the event as a way of initiating or rekindling parental interest.

Enuresis

Enuresis may be defined as involuntary discharge of urine, occurring after the age by which bladder control would usually have been established. According to Lapouse and Monk, nocturnal enuresis occurs in 8 per cent of school-age children once a month or more. Although diurnal enuresis may occasionally happen during periods of excitement at play, it is considerably less common, and generally represents a more serious problem. Many children demonstrate occasional bedwetting after toilet training is completed, especially during periods of fatigue, stress and physical illness. Frequent nocturnal enuresis beyond age five is considered to be a problem or symptom that merits concern and investigation. Bedwetting is more common in boys, shows familial tendencies and gradually diminishes as the child approaches puberty. In the large majority of instances, the causes for bedwetting are developmental and psychological in origin, rather than organic. Physical examination and urinalysis are indicated, but urograms and cystoscopies are rarely warranted.

Bedwetting that has persisted since infancy is often due to inadequate or inappropriate training experiences. Overzealous and exceedingly vigorous attempts at toilet training by parents may create an arena of conflict in which the child unconsciously expresses anger and resistance by the act of bedwetting. Parents who are indifferent about toilet training may undermine a child's attempts at bladder mastery. Chronic psychological stress during the toddler period can also interfere with the child's ability to learn effective bladder control. Bedwetting that occurs as a regressive phenomenon after a child has been dry at night is almost always related to a precipitating environmental event, e.g., birth of a sibling, death in the family or moving to a new house. In these children, prognosis is better and questions of management less troublesome than in those who have never been continent.

Management of a child with enuresis should be based on a specific understanding of presumed etiologic factors, e.g., helping the child deal with feelings about the birth of a sibling or helping parents correct a punitive attitude that has prolonged toilet training. In addition, some general suggestions are in order: (1) The child's cooperation in overcoming the symptom should be enlisted. This often may be accomplished by establishing a simple reward system for being dry at night. (2) Older children should assume responsibility for laundering soiled bedclothes. (3) Fluid ingestion should be kept to a minimum after supper. (4) The child should void before retiring. (5) Parental techniques that employ humiliation, threats and physical punishment should be vigorously discouraged. Conditioning devices have been used with success but are not necessary in most cases. Response to medication (imipramine) is more variable. Referral for psychiatric evaluation should be considered in children whose nocturnal enuresis remains intractable, who have other associated behavioral symptoms or who have frequent diurnal enuresis.

Encopresis

Encopresis refers to the involuntary passage of feces, occurring beyond the age by which bowel control should have been established (usually by three and a half years), and in the absence of any organic defect. It is often associated with enuresis, as both may have their origins in the toilet training period. However, encopresis is much less common than enuresis, rarely occurs during sleep and is viewed as a sign of a more serious and pervasive emotional disturbance. Chronic fecal soiling may persist from infancy or may begin after a precipitating event. Encopresis often alternates with constipation, which can proceed to fecal impaction and psychogenic megacolon. Defecation and constipation are used by the child as expressions of unconscious defiance and anger. The parents may retort with punitive and humiliating measures, as well as the inordinate use of enemas and laxatives. School attendance and performance are affected as encopretic children become the object of peer group derision. While some techniques used in the treatment of enuresis may be useful in encopresis, the symptoms are generally more fixed and disabling. Referral for child psychiatric evaluation is indicated if supportive measures are unavailing.

Problems in Social Behavior

Children, as they develop, move from a self-centered position to a growing realization of the rights, property and feelings of others. Instances of disobedience, fighting, stealing and lying may be frequent as the child struggles with his own wishes and desires and while he accommodates the values of his parents and society. Parents should be firm but reasonable in such situations; a six-year-old who fibs in order to stay home from school to watch an important baseball game on television is not on the road to perdition and should not be treated as a criminal.

Persistent destructiveness, cruelty to animals, violence and rebelliousness, however, are indicative of serious problems within the child and his family. Familial patterns of extreme overpermissiveness will erode a child's ability to learn self-control; extreme punishment often only teaches the child how to inflict physical pain on others. Children can act out their parents' own unconscious angry impulses,

or may act out directly against parents who are inconsistent, neglectful, unloving or excessively seductive. Hostility may also be disguised in more passive forms, such as persistent procrastination, stubbornness or obstructionism. Aggressive behavior directed at siblings often serves as a cloak for the child's angry feelings toward himself or parents. Children who display such behavioral difficulty usually possess poor self-esteem, but may cover it with superficial bravado. Beneath the "tough guy" facade may lie an anxious and sad child who needs help.

Management of children with chronic acting-out behavioral difficulties usually requires psychotherapeutic and educational approaches that lie outside the domain of the pediatrician. The pediatrician can, however, be useful in counseling the parents of children with mild behavior disorders, as well as in ruling out any organic factors that might produce chronic irritability and fatigue. He should be aware that an undiagnosed learning disability can cause the frustrated child to rebel against school and parental authority.

In contrast to those children who act out their impulses, shy and fearful children are overly inhibited in their self-expression. Often these children have been overprotected by their parents, and healthy initiative has been stifled. They tend to cling to their parents, are anxious in social situations, limit their physical activity for fear of injury and display hurt feelings readily. Episodes of physical illness, even if relatively minor, may reinforce the parents' tendency to treat the child as fragile or sickly, and to reduce age-appropriate activities and responsibilities. While some children are naturally more introverted than others, intervention is warranted when the child's functioning at play, home or school is impaired. Successful management depends primarily on the parents' willingness to encourage the child to take normal risks of growing up. The pediatrician's support and reassurance to parents can be very helpful, as the parent helps the child meet new situations in small, calibrated doses. Nursery school for the younger child and organized peer group activities (Boy Scouts, YMCA) for the older child are useful vehicles for helping the child to move psychologically away from total dependence on parents. Small positive changes should be praised and rewarded; expectations should not be raised too high too quickly. Children who display serious obsessions (persistent and repetitive thoughts), compulsions (ritualistic, repetitive actions) and phobias are generally more difficult to help with this supportive approach and frequently require psychiatric referral.

School Problems

School refusal, or school phobia, though not common, may appear in kindergarten, first or second grade children. The condition usually occurs in the beginning of the school year, or after an absence due to illness or holiday. The children involved are usually good students who tend to be obsessive, perfectionistic and anxious in new situations. Frequently, they have demonstrated previous problems in separating from parents or home. Somatic complaints, most often headache or stomachache, usually accompany the refusal to attend school, and while a physical examination is indicated, it is most often non-revealing. The physician should help the parents take a firm stance and insist on the child's early return to school and continued attendance. Otherwise, an early and temporary school refusal may evolve into a chronic and refractory pattern of absence. The teacher must be enlisted to support this approach and tolerate the crying that will occur on return to school.

Academic or behavioral school problems may be the result of chronic physical illness, mental retardation, sensory deficits, emotional difficulties or inadequate teaching. In the early elementary school years, boys lag behind girls in developing the control necessary to sit still, listen attentively and persist at a task. This normal activity may be viewed as a problem by their teachers, most of whom are women. Children who find it difficult to learn may express their frustrations in behavioral symptoms, including restlessness, fighting, withdrawal, passivity and poor peer relations. An underlying educational problem may be missed if attention is directed solely at the more obvious surface disruptive and troublesome behavior. Family conflicts, if present, do not remain isolated in the home, but the child may carry them with him when he comes to school. In similar fashion, an improper educational program may produce failure or underachievement in school and may also interfere with relationships at home. Despite the dangers of mislabeling and inaccurate diagnoses, the early school years provide excellent opportunities for identifying a number of physical, psychological, social and educational problems (including the hyperkinetic syndrome and specific learning disability). Beyond his own skills, the pediatrician aids the diagnostic process by referral to appropriate psychoeducational and mental health services. He must also be aware of the educational resources that exist within the local school district so that he can adequately guide and support the parents' efforts to secure effective remedial intervention.

REFERENCES

Becker, W. C.: *Parents are Teachers.* Champaign, Ill., Research Press, 1971.

Bowlby, J.: *Child Care and the Growth of Love.* Harmondsworth, England, Penguin Books, 1953.

Erikson, H.: *Childhood and Society,* 2nd ed. New York, W. W. Norton, 1963.

Klaus, M. H., and Kennell, J. H.: Parent to infant attachment. *In* Brazelton, B., and Vaughan, V. C. (Eds.): *The Family—Can It Be Saved?* Chicago, Year Book Medical Publishers, Inc., 1976, pp. 115–123.

Lapouse, R., and Monk, M. A.: An epidemiological study of behavioral characteristics in children. Am. J. Public Health, 48:1134, 1958.

Simmons, J. E.: *Psychiatric Examination of Children,* 2nd ed. Philadelphia, Lea and Febiger, 1974.

Spitz, R. A.: *The First Year of Life.* New York, International Universities Press, 1965.

Thomas, A., Chess, S., Birch, H. G., *et al.: Behavioral Individuality in Early Childhood.* New York, New York University Press, 1963.

Vaughan, V. C., III, and McKay, R. J. (Eds.): *Nelson Textbook of Pediatrics,* 10th ed. Philadelphia, W. B. Saunders Co., 1975.

13

Immunization

E. Russell Alexander

Before discussing specific immunization procedures, some review of the principles of active immunization is pertinent. This is particularly relevant to recent advances in the field because great changes are in progress that health professionals will be expected to evaluate in current medical literature. As quickly as summaries of the status of immunization practices are made, new products outdate them. Only by recalling the principles of immunization can one decide whether to accept these new products.

Recommendations are published periodically by the American Academy of Pediatrics, the American Public Health Association and Advisory Committee on Immunization Practices (Morbidity and Mortality Weekly Reports). More specialized recommendations for immunization are designed for the military services, the Peace Corps, for foreign travelers or for a variety of high-risk groups.

PRINCIPLES OF IMMUNIZATION

Antigen. The amount of antigen is critical for immunity of significant duration. For a live (replicating) antigen it is only necessary that a sufficient amount be contained to initiate infection, but for inactivated (nonreplicating) antigen the amount must be sufficient to protect, but not to sensitize. Not only may a primary immune response with a small amount of antigen provide impermanent protection, but in some instances it may also be detrimental; adverse local or systemic responses may follow revaccination or natural infection. Examples of this in recent years followed experimental trials of measles, respiratory syncytial virus, trachoma, *Mycoplasma pneumoniae* and streptococcal vaccines.

Adjuvants. Aluminum salts and endotoxins are among the adjuvants used to augment immune response (such as diphtheria-pertussis-tetanus — DPT). Water-in-oil emulsions are not currently in commercial use in the United States, although extensive field trials of inactivated influenza vaccine have used this adjuvant. Such emulsions, although they do not affect the primary immune response, induce a more prolonged titer of circulating antibody for a smaller amount of antigen. Although potentially of great promise, this method is of no demonstrable value with polysaccharide antigens; experimental use with gram-negative agents such as typhoid or cholera water-in-oil emulsions has resulted in sterile abscesses.

Secondary or booster response. Two or three observations concerning booster response are pertinent to practical consideration of immunizations. First, it appears that a reinforcing dose is more efficient if administered after a particular minimal interval from the initial dose. For example, giving two doses of influenza vaccine one week apart probably provides little reinforcing effect, but is equivalent to splitting the primary antigenic stimulus. Somewhere between one week and one month is the minimal interval for a reinforcing dose response. Second, the secondary response is more sensitive to the type of preparation originally used. For example, it is more critical that the first preparation use an alum adjuvant than the second. Third, the route of inoculation and perhaps the dose are less critical for booster response. Thus intradermal booster reinoculation for typhoid results in reduced side reaction with circulating antibody production equivalent to that of the subcutaneous route.

The duration of protection is relatively short-lived with vaccines such as influenza, cholera or inactivated poliomyelitis (Salk) vaccine, all of which have low antigenic mass. If the primary antigenic stimulus has been above a minimal threshold, however, the immunity may be long-lived. Even though a low level of circulating antibody may be present, the secondary response to booster reinoculation or infection may be maintained for many years. Thus the ability to respond to booster inoculation for tetanus is maintained for at least 20 years after an adequate primary series. For typhoid this interval is 10 years, and it is probably 15 years for yellow fever.

Live versus inactivated vaccines. Active immunization may be by live attenuated strains of disease agents (smallpox, poliomyelitis) or by inactivated components varying from crude suspensions of organisms (typhoid, influenza) to selected antigenic fractions (purified diphtheria toxoid). Inactivated viral vaccines using purified antigenic fractions of viruses have not been developed to date, although there are some hopes for this in the near future. The main advantage of live vaccine is that in multiplication of the agent in the patient a more massive stimulus results with antigen than from the usual inactivated preparation. Furthermore, live antigen may result in permanent local immunity rather than merely stimulating circulating antibody. The advantage of such immunity in reducing virus spread is vital to the aims of disease eradication. The disadvantages of live vaccines are their greater instability when reconstituted, their constant hazard of carrying adventitious agents or contaminants in preparation that cannot be chemically or physically removed as with killed vaccines and the possibilities that vaccine infection may cause disease. This is particularly true of vaccinia, and very rarely, live poliomyelitis vaccine has caused paralytic disease.

Simultaneous vaccination with more than one live attenuated agent is under reevaluation. Because of the theoretic risk of viral interference between the attenuated agents, such practices had been discouraged. Nevertheless, recent experimental studies suggest that simultaneous vaccination is feasible, with no loss of immunity duration. Theoretic and experimental observations suggest that the potential threat of interference can be minimized by simultaneous inoculation or by an interval of one month or more between vaccinations. At lesser intervals interferon production from one attenuated infection may interfere with the viremic phase of a subsequent vaccination. Examples of multiple vaccines currently licensed are measles-smallpox, mumps-rubella, measles-rubella and measles-mumps-rubella.

Acute febrile illness is a contraindication to any active immunization. In the case of inactivated vaccines, the risk of convulsions may be increased. For all vaccines, the intercurrent illness will complicate evaluation of possible adverse reactions. If a severe febrile reaction or convulsions follow DPT administration, any subsequent immunization should proceed cautiously. The pertussis component should be omitted from further schedules following any central nervous system disorder or thrombocytopenia.

Contraindications to all live virus vaccines include the presence of diseases producing disordered cell-mediated immunity (e.g., leukemia, Hodgkin's disease), immunosuppressant therapy (steroids, ionizing radiation, antimetabolites) and pregnancy.

Allergies to components of certain vaccines constitute another caution (e.g., sensitivity to egg protein for vaccines made in eggs, such as influenza). Some theoretic basis for deferring immunization using vaccines prepared in potentially allergic cell culture systems exists with live vaccines, but in practice, few, if any, such effects have been proved (e.g., measles vaccine produced in a chicken cell system).

Age. The significant variation in immune response by age is in the first six months of life. The response to protein antigen differs quantitatively and qualitatively in the first month. The practical significance of this depends upon the efficiency of the antigen, which is the main reason for delaying initial primary immunization of infancy to two months of age. Further delay is not feasible because of the importance of pertussis protection at this age. Pertussis immunization is not necessary after the primary school entrance age, and the risk of encephalitis as a complication increases with age in early childhood. For these reasons it is omitted from combined immunization after the age of five years. For some inactivated antigens or live attenuated agents, the presence of high levels of passive maternal antibody in the first few months of the infant's life impairs initial immune response. Such impaired response may often be overcome completely with a secondary or booster dose.

ACTIVE IMMUNIZATION

Schedules of immunization, dosages and precautions to be considered before immunization for all these agents will not be reviewed. Recommended pediatric immunization doses are summarized in the *Redbook*. Particular attention should be paid to the dosage recommendations for initial immunization for small children (e.g., typhoid) or for persons sensitive to egg protein when vaccines produced in egg, such as influenza vaccine, are used. In all immunization procedures the potentiality for anaphylactic reaction should be borne in mind, and emergency medications (epinephrine) and equipment (for maintenance of airway) should be available. In individual or mass immunization, the child should not leave the premises for 20 to 30 minutes after inoculation.

Table 13-1 lists active immunizing agents in common and limited use, and experimental vaccines that may soon be more widely used. Table 13-2 gives a recommended schedule of the basic immunizing agents most commonly used in the United States. A combination of advantages to the DPT grouping of agents outweighs the one disadvantage—the need for earlier pertussis protection. Attempts to administer *pertussis* vaccine in the first month of life have not been successful. Severe local or systemic reaction to the initial dose of DPT should prompt reduction of the size of the reinforcing dose and subsequent extension of the number of doses to approximately the same total antigenic mass.

Smallpox vaccine has not changed in recent years, although its use has changed dramatically. As a result of the nearly complete eradication of this disease throughout the world, the risk of vaccination is greater than any benefit to be gained. Vaccination is recommended only for persons travelling to a country where endemic smallpox exists (presently only Ethiopia) and for immediate and secondary contacts in the case of an epidemic. For administration of smallpox vaccine, the use of a bifurcated needle dipped in vaccine was probably the single most important contribution in the smallpox eradication effort. In developing countries, where return visits for preventive immunizations are relatively more difficult to assure, simultaneous inoculation of more than one vaccine is often necessary. Examples are yellow fever, smallpox-measles, or smallpox-BCG.

Various modifications of (Sabin) live *poliomyelitis-virus* vaccine continue to occur. Trivalent preparations are most widely used. The extremely rare vaccine-induced poliomyelitislike disease in susceptible adult vaccinees would probably disappear if universal immunization with live vaccine is continued for all infants.

It is of great interest that Sweden and Finland have eradicated poliomye-

TABLE 13-1   ACTIVE IMMUNIZING AGENTS

Widely Used	Limited Use	Future Use (?)
Diphtheria ⎫ Pertussis ⎬ "DPT" (I)* Tetanus ⎭ Poliomyelitis (L)** Measles (L) Rubella (L) Mumps (L) Influenza (I)	BCG (L) Yellow fever (L) Rabies (I) Typhoid (I) Cholera (I) Plague (I) Typhus (I) Smallpox (L) Meningococcus (I)	Adenovirus (L) Parainfluenza (I) M. pneumoniae (I) Jap. enceph. (I) Trachoma (I) Pneumococcus (I) Streptococcus (I) Typhus (L) N. gonorrheae (I) Hepatitis B (I) Cytomegalovirus (I)

*I — Inactivated   **L — Live

TABLE 13-2 RECOMMENDED SCHEDULE FOR MOST COMMONLY USED
IMMUNIZATION AGENTS

2 months, DPT	Trivalent oral poliomyelitis
4 months, DPT	Trivalent oral poliomyelitis
6 months, DPT	Trivalent oral poliomyelitis
15 months, measles — "M-M-R"°	
18 months, DPT	Trivalent oral poliomyelitis
4-6 years, DPT	Trivalent oral poliomyelitis
	(one month or more after above)
14-16 years, TD	Thereafter TD q 10 years

°15 months, measles, mumps, rubella (singly or in combinations)

litis—and poliovirus—by recurrent and widespread vaccination with inactivated vaccines (more potent than the original inactivated vaccines used in the United States). This observation is of interest because it demonstrates that some local (gut) immunity can be produced by repeated use of potent inactivated vaccines and that herd immunity can be achieved. Current recommendations for the United States utilize live vaccines because of the lack of achievement of anywhere near the greater than 90 per cent vaccination rate of the susceptible population that resulted in the Scandinavian success stories, as well as the greater ease of administration of live vaccines.

Widespread use of live attenuated *measles* vaccine has resulted in a large reduction of that disease and initial optimism for regional or national eradication. But recurrence of focal epidemics in communities that have not maintained their initial enthusiasm for vaccination of all susceptible citizens suggests that eradication may be a distant goal, though theoretically feasible. There is no evidence of waning of immunity among the vaccinated, and protective efficacy remains high. Universal immune response is assured by delay of immunization to at least 12, but preferably 15, months of age. Attenuated live virus vaccines have been developed for both *rubella* and *mumps*, which eventually may be reserved for prepubertal administration to girls and boys, respectively, as they are alike in that the serious effects of the diseases they were designed to prevent occur in adults. Combined preparations that are licensed include rubella-mumps. In rubella and mumps vaccines we do not have firm knowledge of the duration of immunity conferred. We also do not know the teratogenic potential of the rubella vaccine. Therefore, the present recommendations

are for widespread use of rubella vaccine in young girls and boys to reduce the prevalence of rubella virus in the community or risk to pregnant women. Mumps vaccine, until the duration of immunity is fully established, should be reserved for susceptible boys shortly before puberty. On the other hand, many prefer to use combined measles-mumps-rubella vaccine at 12 to 15 months of age.

Influenza vaccine is not one of the better immunizing agents. With only moderate potency, and with significant toxicity and poor duration of immunity, it is not as effective as it should be. This is further complicated by the constant change in antigenic pattern, so that current vaccine preparations are usually somewhat behind the antigenic drift. It is included as a widely used vaccine because it is used in the general population, particularly for prevention of death in the aged and the chronically ill. It has limited recommended use in children, being used only in chronically ill children, particularly those with pulmonary, cardiovascular or renal disease.

Those preparations listed as vaccines of limited use in high-risk groups require little additional comment. *Yellow fever, cholera, plague* and *typhus* vaccines are used only for international travel. *Typhoid* vaccine, once widely used in the United States, is now used only for unusual exposure to contaminated water supplies and is rarely indicated. *Bacille Calmette Guérin* (BCG) is usually contraindicated in this country, where the advantage of monitoring the tuberculin skin test response outweighs the protective effect offered. Infants exposed to active tubercular parents who are not to be relied upon for follow-up are an example of this rare use. *Rabies* vaccine is an unusual example. Active immunization with duck embryo vaccine before exposure is applicable only to veterinarians or persons with constant risk of exposure. Prophylaxis of rabies after exposure to an animal bite is a procedure that must be contemplated every time an animal bite or scratch occurs. A number of factors should be considered at that time, including the nature and location of the bite, the species and state of the animal and his whereabouts and the known occurrence of rabies in the community at that time. The recommendations usually given are those of the U.S. Public Health Service, and these are repeated in the *Redbook* and other references cited. It is only necessary to stress that in making these decisions the local health department staff (communicable disease epidemiologist or health officer) should be consulted early for current local data on animal rabies.

Meningococcal polysaccharide vaccines have been developed against serogroups A and C. At present, disease due to A is very rare in the United States. The vaccines are prepared as monovalent and as combined antigens, and are licensed for a limited and unique use—epidemic control. Vaccine will be released for use in the population at risk (to be defined at the time of epidemic occurrence). At that time, its use is restricted to children above age two. Below that age antibody response to vaccine is very poor, and the vaccine appears to be ineffective. In the case of C strain disease, this is less critical because of the relatively small proportion of cases occurring before the second year. For other meningococcal types, the higher proportion of illnesses before two years of age may make effective use of vaccine difficult. These vaccines should be considered an option for travelers visiting countries that are experiencing epidemics of meningococcal disease.

The final list is of preparations in the developmental stages. *Adenovirus* vaccines are of particular interest. The military, which often suffers outbreaks with adenovirus 4 and 7, and less frequently types 3, 11, 14 and 21, no longer uses inactivated preparations because of concern with carcinogenic potential. A live adenovirus vaccine (types 4 and 7) given orally in enteric-coated capsule form has been successfully used experimentally. *Parainfluenza* and *M. pneumoniae* vaccines have not been satisfactory preparations to date, but there is good promise that vaccines will eventually be developed, particularly if antigenic fractions can be used rather than whole organisms. Pneumococcus vaccines in experimental trials appear to be very potent, when polysaccharide antigens are used. In both cases the prime research consideration is what strains to use and whom to vaccinate. Streptococcal vaccines are in a more primitive state of development; to date, the area of most concern is to find the antigenic fraction that will produce immunity without hypersensitivity.

PASSIVE IMMUNIZATION

Immune serum globulin (formerly called gamma globulin) is clearly recommended for only three conditions: measles, hepatitis A (infectious hepatitis) and the hypogammaglobulinemias. Among these, the most common one is hepatitis A, but in most cases immune globulin is recommended for adult household contacts, rather than children, because the disease in children is milder and immunity will result from it. Specific immune globulins used for treatment (and more rarely for exposure) are tetanus immune globulin (human), vaccinial immune globulin (VIG) and human rabies immune globulin (HRIG). Refer to the *Redbook* for specific dosage and precaution in use, and in the case of VIG, for the list of regional consultants from whom it may be obtained. Varicella-zoster immune globulin (VZIG) and hepatitis B immune globulin are under evaluation at this time.

REFERENCES

American Academy of Pediatrics: *Redbook* Report of the committee on the control of infectious diseases. A. A. P., 17th ed., 1974.

American Public Health Association: Control of communicable diseases in man, 12th ed. New York, American Public Health Association, 1975.

Collected recommendations of the U.S. Public Health Service (Advisory Committee on Immunization Practices) Morbidity and Mortality Weekly Reports, Vol. 21, No. 25, 1972.

Coriell, L. L.: Active immunization in the pediatric age group. Med. Clin. N. Amer., *51*:581, 1967.

Edsall, G.: Principles of active immunization. Annu. Rev. Med., *17*:39, 1966.

Inderbitzen, T. M. (ed.): Prophylaxis of infectious and other diseases. *Monographs in Allergy*, Vol. 9. Basel, Karger, 1975.

Plotkin, S. A.: The future of vaccines against viral diseases. Pediatr. Clin. N. Amer. 15:447, 1968.

Smith, D. H., and Peters, G.: Current and future vaccines for the prevention of bacterial diseases. Pediatr. Clin. N. Amer., *19*:387, 1972.

PART IV

INFECTIOUS
DISEASE DISORDERS

14 Prenatal Infectious Diseases

Harry R. Hill

Viral, bacterial and protozoan infections in the pregnant woman may produce adverse effects upon the fetus, leading to death or abnormalities in the newborn infant. Such infections may be clinically apparent or entirely asymptomatic in the mother. Direct infection of fetal tissues may occur via ascending or hematogenous routes and may lead to abortion, stillbirth, prematurity or congenital abnormalities. The outcome may be undesirable even in the absence of actual fetal infection, however, especially when the maternal illness is severe. The exact mechanism by which pneumonia, sepsis or influenza in the mother may lead to complications is not known. The increase in basal metabolic rate and oxygen requirements or the alterations in acid-base status that accompany severe infections may be injurious to the developing fetus.

Almost all known infections have occurred at one time or another in pregnant women. Some are known to affect the fetus adversely (Table 14–1), while others such as adenoviral infections have never been associated with significant complications. A brief description of the more common prenatal infections that affect the fetus is given here.

Rubella

In 1941 Gregg first described the relationship between maternal rubella and congenital anomalies. The overall incidence of malformations following maternal rubella infection during the first trimester is between 10 and 20 per cent. The risk of abnormalities if infection occurs during the first, second or third month is estimated to be 50, 22 and 6 per cent, respectively. Spontaneous abortion occurs in 10 to 15 per cent of cases. Infection after the first trimester may produce fetal loss or neurological sequelae such as deafness, but the incidence is probably low.

The infant with congenital rubella syndrome classically has: (1) cardiac anomalies, (2) cataracts, (3) microcephaly, (4) deafness and (5) mental retardation. The most frequent cardiac lesions are patent ductus arteriosus, pulmonary artery stenosis and septal defects. Eye changes include cataracts, microphthalmia and retinitis (which appears as black pigmentary deposits on the retinae, "salt and pepper retinitis"). Alternating areas of radiolucency and bone density near the meta-

TABLE 14–1 PRENATAL VIRAL, BACTERIAL AND PROTOZOAN INFECTIONS

Common Prenatal Infections Producing Severe Complications

Rubella	Coxsackie virus
Cytomegalovirus	Toxoplasmosis
Herpes simplex	Syphilis

Less Common Prenatal Infections and Infections Causing Less Severe Complications

Hepatitis	Influenza
Variola and vaccinia	Echovirus
Poliomyelitis	Listeriosis
Varicella and herpes zoster	Vibrio fetus
Western equine encephalitis	Group B streptococci
Mumps	Bacteriuria
Rubeola	

physes of the long bones produce a "celery stalk" appearance. Approximately one third of infants with congenital rubella syndrome will excrete live virus in their nasopharynx at six months of age, and 10 per cent will continue to do so at one year. For this reason, such infants should not be allowed to come in contact with pregnant women.

Prevention of congenital rubella syndrome depends upon the detection of susceptible pregnant females exposed during the first trimester of pregnancy. Since 80 to 90 per cent of adult women are already immune, an acute serum specimen taken as soon after exposure as possible will often reveal the presence of protective antibody. If not, increased convalescent antibody titer will confirm infection and indicate the need for considering therapeutic abortion.

Since 1969 an active immunization campaign has been carried out with live attenuated rubella vaccines. The Advisory Committee on Immunization Practices of the Public Health Service and the Committee on Infectious Diseases of the American Academy of Pediatrics recommend immunization of (1) children between 12 months of age and puberty and (2) adolescent and adult women who lack rubella antibody and in whom pregnancy can be prevented for at least two months. A significant decline in reported cases of rubella and congenital rubella has followed the widespread use of this vaccine. In addition, no major epidemics of congenital rubella have occurred. Infection with wild rubella virus may occur in patients with natural or vaccine-induced immunity. In such patients, communicability is probably quite low and viremia does not occur. It is unusual for fetal infection to result in these "immune" patients. Fetal infection with vaccine virus has been reported, however, in instances in which women have been inadvertently inoculated during pregnancy. For this reason, immunization is not recommended for women who may become pregnant during the ensuing two months.

Rubella vaccination has been associated with arthritis and arthralgia in 5 to 10 per cent of vaccinations. These reactions have usually occurred in two to four weeks after inoculation and have lasted one to seven days. A few reports of long lasting joint symptoms have also appeared, as have cases of a transient peripheral neuropathy.

Cytomegalic Inclusion Disease

Approximately 60 per cent of women of childbearing age have serological evidence of past cytomegalovirus infection, and 6 per cent of pregnant women will demonstrate evidence of infection during pregnancy. Fetal wastage, severe neonatal disease or asymptomatic infection in the newborn infant may be produced. In one study, only 1 of 26 infected neonates had clinically apparent infection. In the affected neonate, severe manifestations include thrombocytopenic purpura, hepatitis, pneumonitis and encephalitis. Intracranial calcifications, which are usually periventricular unlike those seen in toxoplasmosis, may appear at several months of age, and microcephaly is common. Chorioretinitis indistinguishable from that seen in toxoplasmosis occurs in 20 per cent of cases, and bone lesions similar to those in rubella may develop.

There is some suggestion in the literature that intrauterine cytomegalovirus infection during the first or second trimester is more likely to produce severe disease than that in the third trimester. Sequelae vary considerably from severe mental retardation with seizures and deafness to no discernible abnormalities. Recently, asymptomatic infection of term neonates delivered to mothers who are carriers of cervical cytomegalovirus has been described. The incidence of viral acquisition by such infants approaches 40 per cent. Fortunately, the majority of these patients have no detectable abnormalities on follow-up examination.

Diagnosis is established by isolating the virus from urine, throat or blood. Typical inclusion-bearing cells are often present in the urine, but this finding is less reliable than that of culture techniques.

Attempts have been made to treat neonates having cytomegalovirus disease with cytosine arabinoside and, more recently, adenine arabinoside. Urinary excretion of the virus has been suppressed, but to date, no long-term beneficial effects of this therapy have been observed.

Prevention of infection is difficult because of the ubiquitous nature of cytomegalovirus. Fetal infection usually occurs only during the initial infection in the mother, and second siblings are only rarely affected.

A live cytomegalovirus vaccine has been developed that, when given to volunteers subcutaneously, results in the development of neutralizing and complement-fixing antibodies. Further studies are necessary to determine the safety and efficacy of this vaccine in preventing maternal or fetal infection.

Herpes Simplex Virus

Herpesvirus hominis can be divided serologically into two distinct types, designated I and II. More than 90 per cent of genital infections are caused by type II, and consequently, the majority of fetal and neonatal infections are also caused by this type (approximately 90 per cent).

Herpesvirus infection of the female genital tract may either be asymptomatic or result in purulent discharge and vesicular lesions. Transplacental infection may occur, or the infant may become infected while passing through the birth canal. The symptoms of neonatal herpesvirus infection, which usually appear three to seven days after birth, are non-specific, resembling those seen in sepsis. These include temperature instability, lethargy, respiratory distress, jaundice and hepatosplenomegaly. In severe cases, disseminated intravascular coagulation, encephalitis and pneumonitis may develop. Chorioretinitis, microcephaly and intracranial calcifications may occur later in the course of the disease. The most characteristic finding in herpesvirus infection is the development of vesicles on the skin or mucous membranes. These usually appear in clusters and may be recurrent. Keratitis is also helpful in establishing a diagnosis. In contrast to Coxsackie virus infection, disseminated herpesvirus infection does not produce cardiac complications.

The virus may be isolated from vesicles, blood or cerebrospinal fluid (CSF) to establish a diagnosis. Morphological examination of infected sites for multinucleated giant cells and intranuclear inclusions may also be of value in establishing the diagnosis of herpesvirus infection.

Available data suggest that approximately 25 per cent of infants delivered to women with genital herpesvirus infection will have severe herpesvirus disease. The risk of colonization or infection of the neonate appears to be dramatically reduced by cesarean section if premature rupture of the fetal membranes has not occurred. This has led a number of authorities to suggest cesarean section of colonized mothers if intrauterine infection can be ruled out (by amniocentesis). Therapy of neonatal herpesvirus disease using 5-iodo-2-deoxyuridine has been attempted with variable results. More recently, adenine arabinoside has been used with initial success.

Coxsackie Virus

Group B Coxsackie viruses, types 1 through 5, produce mild or disseminated infection in neonates. Infection in the mother frequently produces mild upper respiratory symptoms. Transplacental or postnatal infection can occur. The symptoms and signs of disseminated disease are like those produced by herpesvirus except that cardiac involvement occurs in up to 80 per cent of cases. Myocarditis leads to tachycardia, murmurs, electrocardiogram (EKG) changes and congestive heart failure. Central nervous system involvement occurs in fewer than one third of cases.

The virus may be isolated from the throat, stool and occasionally the cerebrospinal fluid. Spread is via the respiratory and fecal-oral routes. Preventive measures other than good sanitation are not available.

Toxoplasmosis

Toxoplasma gondii is a protozoan parasite that infects the mother, crosses the placenta and produces prematurity, severe neonatal disease, and fetal death. Infection in the mother may be asymptomatic or may produce pneumonitis, encephalitis or lymphadenitis. It is more apt to cause disease in the fetus when it occurs during the second trimester. A classic triad of findings (chorioretinitis, cerebral calcifications and hydrocephalus) occurs in 60 per cent of cases of congenital toxoplasmosis. Chorioretinitis is one of the most constant features of the disease, occurring in more than 80 per cent of cases. Both eyes are usually involved. Jaundice, hepatosplenomegaly, rash and purpura also occur. Diffuse cranial calcifications may be present from birth in cases with severe central nervous system disease or may appear several months after birth.

Diagnosis is established by observing the organism in Wright-stained smears of cerebrospinal fluid or by use of the Sabin dye test. Antibody from immune individuals will block the uptake of dye by the organism, which is the basis for this test. Maternal sera taken at acute and convalescent periods and infant sera are necessary. Difficulty exists in determining if the antibody in an infant's serum is being produced in response to infection or if it is maternal antibody that has crossed the placenta. A titer decrease in subsequent infant sera indicates passively acquired antibody. If it rises, this indicates active infection. Recently, a fluorescent antibody test has been developed to detect specific IgM antibody produced by the infant in response to infection.

Syphilis

Treponema pallidum does not cross the placenta and infect the fetus until after the fourth month of pregnancy. Fetal wastage occurs in approximately one fourth of maternal infections. Initially, the neonate with congenital syphilis may appear normal, but in a few weeks typical moist skin and mucous membrane lesions and a rash appear. Severe rhinitis (snuffles) develops, and osteochondritis and periostitis may lead to pseudoparalysis of the limbs. If left untreated, the child may go on to develop the stigmata of congenital syphilitic infection including: (1) cranial frontal bossing, (2) flat nasal bridge (saddle nose), (3) peg-shaped central incisors (Hutchinson's teeth), (4) fine scars at the corner of the mouth (rhagades) and (5) anterior bowing of the tibia (saber shin). Late complications include deafness, keratitis and chorioretinitis.

Prevention of congenital syphilis depends upon the identification and proper treatment of women infected after the fourth month of pregnancy. Since false positive VDRL test results are quite rare in pregnant women, a confirmed positive test at any stage in gestation is an indication for performing an FTA-ABS test. If positive, adequate therapy in the absence of central nervous system involvement consists of the intramuscular injection of 2.4 million units of benzathine penicillin G or procaine penicillin for 10 days. Following adequate therapy, however, a positive VDRL will often persist from 6 to 12 months in the mother. Since the maternal VDRL antibody is contained partially in the gamma G fraction, the cord blood will also be positive. The serological diagnosis of congenital syphilis is complicated. Passively transferred antibody from the mother usually shows a marked decline in titer one to two months after delivery. Waiting for this to occur, however, means that therapy is withheld for an excessive period of time. More recently, a fluorescent antibody test, which demonstrates specific IgM treponemal antibody produced by the fetus, has been developed. This may allow earlier detection of the infected neonate. Congenital syphilis can be treated by the injection of 50,000 units/kg of benzathine penicillin G if central nervous system infection can be ruled out. If there is evidence of central nervous system involvement, then the infant should be treated with 50,000 units/kg/day of procaine penicillin or 100,000 units/kg of aqueous penicillin G per day for 10 to 14 days. This regimen is indicated because the long-acting benzathine penicillin does not result in high enough cerebrospinal fluid levels to kill the treponema.

Hepatitis

Infectious hepatitis (hepatitis A) and serum hepatitis (hepatitis B) occur in the pregnant female, although placental transfer of hepatitis A has not been documented. This may be related to the brief period of maternal viremia. In general, hepatitis A in the neonate does not appear to produce severe illness. In contrast, hepatitis B has been reported to be transferred transplacentally and has caused serious and even fatal infection in neonates. Our understanding of hepatitis B has been greatly advanced by the detection of several antigens of this virus. These include a core antigen, HB_c-Ag, and a surface antigen HB_s-Ag. When the mother develops hepatitis B late in a pregnancy, approximately two thirds of her children will develop antigenemia and biochemical and histological evidence of hepatitis. In contrast, if the mother acquires hepatitis early in pregnancy or is a chronic carrier of HB_s-Ag, then the likelihood of the infant acquiring hepatitis is considerably less. Although evidence suggests that the virus of hepatitis B can cross the placenta and appear in the neonate at birth, this is probably quite rare. Infants also may become infected from maternal-fetal transfusions during delivery. In some of these patients antigenemia is not detected for several weeks or months after birth. Hepatitis B may result in prolonged neonatal jaundice, acute fulminating hepatitis or an asymptomatic carrier state.

Preliminary studies suggest that hyperimmune serum gamma globulin with antibody against the HB_s antigen will significantly modify hepatitis B in adults and even neonates.

Variola and Vaccinia

Smallpox presents no significant problem in the United States at this time. The disease may, however, lead to abortion and stillbirth when it produces a severe toxic reaction in the mother. Transplacental infection also occurs and produces severe neonatal disease.

Vaccinia has caused disseminated neonatal disease and fetal wastage but this is extremely rare. Most large series in which pregnant women were vaccinated have shown no resulting ill effects; however, vaccination is not advised during pregnancy.

Polio

Polio is certainly less of a problem since the introduction of the live virus vaccine. The virus is capable of crossing the placenta and producing abortion, stillbirth and premature delivery. Paralytic disease has occurred in neonates, and congenital defects have been reported, but these are not well documented. There is no evidence to suggest that the live virus vaccine causes any problems in pregnancy.

Varicella and Herpes Zoster

Congenital varicella and herpes zoster have been reported but are quite rare diseases. Varicella is usually quite mild in neonates, but occasionally disseminated disease occurs. Zoster may also occur rarely in newborns, presenting with segmental distribution of vesicular lesions. Congenital malformations have been reported following maternal varicella-zoster infection, but these have not been well documented.

Western Equine Encephalitis

Neonatal central nervous system disease has resulted from transplacental passage of the virus of western equine encephalitis.

Mumps

Mumps virus infection during the first trimester has been associated with fetal death. In one large series, the fetal death rate in pregnancies complicated by mumps was twice that observed in controls. Congenital malformations have also been reported; however, in another large series of 501 pregnancies complicated by mumps no anomalies were found. Congenital mumps parotitis had been reported in the older literature. A live attenuated mumps vaccine is available and appears to offer adequate protection. Inoculation of pregnant women has led, however, to infection of fetal tissues with the vaccine virus.

Rubeola

Rubeola infection during the first 12 weeks of pregnancy has been associated with a slightly increased fetal death rate. The difference was not statistically significant from that observed in a control group of uncomplicated pregnancies, however. Congenital abnormalities have occasionally been reported after measles, but no consistent patterns have emerged.

Influenza

Influenza may have an adverse effect upon the outcome of pregnancy. In general, the number of complications tends to parallel the severity of the maternal reaction to the infection. During the pandemic of 1918, a retrospective study noted, the incidence of abortion, stillbirth or prematurity was 27 per cent in uncomplicated cases and 50 per cent in those with pneumonia. In more recent studies few complications have been noted.

Echovirus Infection

Echoviruses have been shown to cross the placenta and lead to fetal infection. There are no reports that these infections resulted in serious disease or abnormalities. In several prospective studies of Echo type 9 infection, no abortions, stillbirths or congenital malformations were reported.

Listerosis

Infection with *Listeria monocytogenes* may be acquired transplacentally or during passage through the birth canal. The symptoms produced in the mother are similar to those in influenza. Approximately one third of fetal *Listeria* infections have resulted in stillborns. At delivery, the amniotic fluid has a brownish discoloration. Transplacental infection leads to a severe disseminated granulomatous disease with meningitis and pneumonitis. Infection acquired during passage through the birth canal usually does not cause symptoms for seven to nine days after birth and is generally less severe. A gram stain of the meconium will show large numbers of the organisms and can aid in establishing the diagnosis. Ampicillin is the drug of choice.

Vibrio Fetus

Infection with *Vibrio fetus* may lead to abortion, stillbirth and meningoencephalitis. Therapy consists of chloramphenicol or streptomycin.

Group B Streptococcal Infections

Group B streptococci represent one of the two most common types of bacterial pathogens in neonatal sepsis and meningitis. It has been estimated that 2 to 3 per 1000 neonates develop infection with these organisms and 1 per 1000 die. Maternal carriage of group B streptococci has varied from 4 to 26 per 1000, and such carriage has been associated with abortion, stillbirth or premature delivery. Maternal acquisition and carriage of these organisms are usually asymptomatic, but cervicitis, vaginitis or urethritis may be produced. The clinical syndromes in the infected infant are of two main types. An early onset form of infection occurs within the first 24 to 48 hours after birth. These infants often have sepsis, shock or respiratory distress, and roentgenograms are indistinguishable from those showing hyaline membrane disease. The mortality rate in this form of infection ranges from 70 to 90 per cent. A late onset "meningitis" form of infection also occurs. This often has onset 10 days or more after birth and is usually associated with meningitis. The mortality rate is somewhat lower with this form of infection.

Diagnosis of group B streptococcal disease is dependent upon culturing the specific organism or identifying its antigens in infected body fluids by counterimmunoelectrophoresis. Therapy consists of aqueous penicillin G or ampicillin. Efforts are currently underway to determine the significance of antibody to these organisms in preventing disease. Preliminary studies suggest that vaccination or provision of antibody through transfusion may be feasible in this most fulminant of neonatal bacterial infections.

TABLE 14–2 APPROXIMATE PERCENTAGE OF FINDINGS IN NEONATAL RUBELLA, CYTOMEGALIC INCLUSION DISEASE AND TOXOPLASMOSIS

	Rubella	CID	Toxoplasmosis
Hepatosplenomegaly	60	70	40
Petechiae and purpura	55	65	10
Congenital heart disease	80	0	0
Cataracts	50	0	0
Retinopathy	5	20	90
Pneumonia	15	35	10
Cerebral calcifications	0	15	30
Microcephaly	2	40	10
Bone lesions	35	0	0

Asymptomatic Bacteriuria

Asymptomatic bacteriuria was found by Kass *et al.* to be associated with twice the rate of prematurity observed in a group without infection (24 per cent *vs.* 10 per cent). Treatment with antibiotics reduced the incidence to that of a control group. Subsequent studies have yielded differing results. At present, however, it seems wise to detect and treat pregnant women who are bacteriuric.

DIFFERENTIAL DIAGNOSIS OF CONGENITAL INFECTIONS

Tables 14–2 and 14–3 list the approximate frequency of signs and symptoms in the more common congenital infections. Certain characteristics of the diseases are helpful in the differential diagnosis. Thus, heart disease is usually present in rubella (80 per cent) and Coxsackie virus infections (80 per cent). Pneumonia is more common in cytomegalovirus infections, while chorioretinitis is almost always present in toxoplasmosis. Cataracts and bone lesions are almost wholly limited to congenital rubella, although similar bone change has been reported in cytomegalovirus infections. Cerebral calcification may be present at birth in toxoplasmosis and may develop later in cytomegalovirus and herpes simplex virus infections. Microcephaly is most often associated with cytomegalovirus. Coxsackie virus and congenital herpes simplex infections present with signs exactly like those in neonatal sepsis. As mentioned, myocarditis is present in 80 per cent of Coxsackie virus infections. Herpes infection may be indicated by the development of vesicular lesions or keratitis.

These findings may be of value in diagnosing a congenital infection; however, many such infections are not detectable clinically at birth. Screening procedures such as the determination of cord macroglobulin (IgM) concentrations have been advocated to detect occult infections. In one large series from 2 to 4 per cent of cord sera contained elevated concentrations (more than 20 mg/100 ml). After intensive investigation, specific infections were identified in only approximately one third of the patients. In addition, congenital infection has been documented in the face of normal

TABLE 14–3   APPROXIMATE PERCENTAGE OF FINDINGS IN NEONATAL HERPES SIMPLEX AND COXSACKIE VIRUS INFECTIONS

	Herpes Simplex	Coxsackie
Lethargy	80	80
Respiratory distress	60	75
Cyanosis	30	70
Cardiac abnormalities	10	80
Hepatosplenomegaly	50	50
CNS abnormalities	35	30
Vesicular skin lesions	55	0
Keratitis	15	0
Mortality	70	70

cord macroglobulin concentrations. Thus, cord IgM concentrations are at best a nonspecific indicator of infection. If there are clinical or historical findings that suggest congenital infection, a cord IgM level should be obtained. Search for the specific cause should then include: (1) x-rays of the long bones, skull and limbs; (2) urine examinations and culture for viruses and bacteria; (3) blood cultures; (4) cerebrospinal fluid examination; and (5) specific tests for syphilis, rubella, cytomegalovirus and toxoplasmosis, as indicated.

REFERENCES

Alford, C. A.: The immunologic status of the newborn. Hosp. Practice, 88, June, 1970.

Alford, C. A., Schaefer, J., Blankenship, W. J., Straumfjord, J. V., and Cassady, G. A.: Correlative immunologic, microbiologic and clinical approach to the diagnosis of acute and chronic infections in newborn infants. N. Engl. J. Med., 277:437, 1967.

Copps, S. C., and Giddings, L. E.: Transplacental transmission of Western equine encephalitis. Pediatrics, 24:31, 1959.

Eichenwald, H. F., and Shinefield, H. R.: Viral infection of the fetus and of the premature and newborn infant. Adv. Pediatr., 12:249, 1962.

Eickhoff, T. C., Klein, J. O., Daly, A. K., Ingall, D., and Finland, M.: Neonatal sepsis and other infections due to group B beta-hemolytic streptococci. N. Engl. J. Med., 271:1221, 1964.

Emanuel, I., and Kenny, G. E.: Cytomegalic inclusion disease of infancy. Pediatrics, 38:957, 1966.

Feldman, H. A.: Toxoplasmosis. N. Engl. J. Med., 279:1370, 1968.

Hardy, J. B.: Viral infection in pregnancy: A review. Am. J. Obstet. Gynecol., 93:1052, 1965.

Hemming, V. G., McCloskey, D. W., and Hill, H. R.: Neonatal respiratory distress associated with pneumonia due to group B streptococci. Amer. J. Dis. Child., 130:1231, 1976.

Hemming, V. G., Hall, R. T., Rhodes, P. G., Shigeoka,

A. O., and Hill, H. R.: Assessment of group B streptococcal opsonins in human and rabbit serum by neutrophil chemiluminescence. J. Clin. Invest., 58:1379, 1976.

Hood, M., Janney, A., and Dameron, G.: Beta hemolytic streptococcus group B associated with problems in the perinatal period. Am. J. Obstet. Gynecol., 82:809, 1961.

Kass, E. H.: Hormones and host resistance to infection. Bacteriol. Rev., 24:177, 1960.

Krugman, S., and Ward, R.: *Infectious Diseases of Children.* St. Louis, C. V. Mosby Co., 1968.

Modlin, J. F., Brandling-Bennett, D., Witte, J. J., Campbell, C. C., and Meyers, J. D.: A review of five years' experience with rubella vaccine in the United States. Pediatrics, 55:20, 1975.

Overall, J. C., Jr., and Glasgow, L. A.: Virus infections of the fetus and newborn infant. J. Pediatr., 77:315, 1970.

Ray, C. G., and Wedgwood, R. J.: Neonatal listerosis, six case reports and a review of the literature. Pediatrics, 34:378, 1964.

Schweitzer, I. L., and Spears, R. L.: Hepatitis-associated antigen (Australia antigen) in mother and infant. N. Engl. J. Med., 283:570, 1970.

Sever, J., and White, L. R.: Intrauterine viral infections. Annu. Rev. Med., 19:471, 1968.

Siegel, M., Fuerst, H. T., and Peress, N. S.: Comparative fetal mortality in maternal virus diseases. N. Engl. J. Med., 274:768, 1966.

Sparling, P. F.: Diagnosis and treatment of syphilis. N. Engl. J. Med., 284:642, 1971.

Starr, J. G., Bart, R. D., Jr., and Gold, E.: Inapparent congenital cytomegalovirus infection: Clinical and epidemiological characteristics in early infancy. N. Engl. J. Med., 282:1075, 1970.

Stiehm, F. R., Ammann, A. J., and Cherry, J. D.: Elevated cord macroglobulins in the diagnosis of intrauterine infections. N. Engl. J. Med., 275:971, 1966.

Torphy, D. E., Ray, C. G., McAlister, R., and Du, J. N. H.: Herpes simplex virus infection in infants: A spectrum of disease. J. Pediatr., 76:405, 1970.

Wilson, M. G., Hewitt, W. L., and Monzon, O. T.: Effect of bacteriuria on the fetus. N. Engl. J. Med., 274:1115, 1966.

15

Common Infectious Diseases

C. George Ray and Ralph J. Wedgwood

It is difficult to write about infections in childhood without some nostalgia. Thankfully, many of the most striking of these illnesses have become rarities in the United States, and others will surely be eradicated also. Smallpox has been rendered nearly extinct throughout the world, and poliomyelitis, tetanus, measles and others are now only seen occasionally in this country; however, the potential for re-emergence of some of these diseases as major health problems exists, particularly if routine immunization programs are disregarded.

There are some conspicuous absences in this section. We have attempted to include only relatively common diseases that are either peculiar to, or particularly important in childhood—with unique pediatric manifestations. Rare infections, except where they are important to differential diagnosis, have been excluded as have infections that are more common in adults and have few major differences in their manifestations in children (infectious mononucleosis, for instance).

The section is organized, where possible, by the presenting manifestations of the disease as summarized in Table 15–1—not only by the nature of the agents.

Where possible, an outline form is used. Some disease processes do not allow such presentation, and there more general descriptions are provided.

TABLE 15–1 COMMON INFECTIOUS DISEASES

I. Common acute respiratory diseases
   Common cold (excluding streptococcal infections), otitis media, croup, laryngotracheobronchitis, bronchiolitis, bronchopneumonia (viral), mycoplasma pneumonia

II. Acute exanthematous diseases
   Morbilliform or maculopapular: measles, German measles, roseola, erythema infectiosum; other (differential diagnosis)

III. Pox or vesicular diseases
   Chickenpox; other (differential diagnosis)

IV. Acute enanthematous diseases
   Herpangina, herpetic stomatitis, aphthous stomatitis, thrush

V. Other distinctive acute viral infections
   Mumps, viral meningoencephalitis, aseptic meningitis

VI. Distinctive bacterial infections
   Streptococcosis, bacterial pneumonias, pyelonephritis

COMMON ACUTE RESPIRATORY DISEASES (ARD)

The Common Cold

Of all the ills that plague mankind, the common cold is the one most often seen. The best detailed description of this disease is in *Illness in the Home* by Dingle, Badger and Jordan (Western Reserve University Press, 1964), which should be read by all future health professionals. In middle class families, acute respiratory disease accounts for almost two thirds of all illness; the attack rate is five to six illnesses per person per year. Of these illnesses, less than 3 per cent are streptococcal; for all practical purposes there are no other bacterial causes (with the exception of pneumonia). The ARD syndromes are thus more than 97 per cent viral. The use of antibiotics in these non-bacterial diseases is purposeless and potentially dangerous. ARD

130

accounts for the majority of misused antibiotic therapy. The appropriate use in streptococcal disease is described separately.

The problems of ARD in childhood are of special interest. Virtually all known viruses can cause an ARD syndrome, and a large number of viruses have a predilection for the respiratory tract. Without a single agent the epidemiology is difficult to study. An infant is born into a world of seemingly innumerable viruses. As he loses passive immunity he begins to develop disease. Infants have few colds during the first month of life. Half of all infants have had at least one cold, however, by three months of age, and virtually all (95 per cent) have done so by six months. Thereafter the infant, and later the child, is exposed to one virus after another until relative immunity has been acquired, at least to a major portion of the more common agents in the virus pool. Thus at the age of one to two years a child has an average of eight to nine such infections yearly, and frequent infections continue until about age 15 when the attack rate approximates that of adults (four episodes yearly). Since ARD is most common during winter months, the eight yearly episodes in the young child may occur in rapid sequence, often causing parental concern.

The attack rates vary widely among individuals. Certain factors such as crowding, family size, travel and presence of young school children tend to increase the incidence. Single adults living alone have a lower incidence (two to three illnesses per year).

In infants and young children, certain additional special factors influence the manifestation of ARD. Newborn infants and infants who are feeding are obligatory nose breathers. Nasal obstruction is therefore a significant symptom. The lower airway of an infant is smaller, less rigid and surrounded by relatively more lymphoid tissue. From purely geometric considerations, swelling of an infant's airway walls compromises the flow of air more than does equivalent swelling in an adult. The floppiness of the structures further exaggerates the problem. The additional lymphoid tissue increases the amount of swelling. Finally, the infant and young child handle secretions and obstruction poorly.

Similar anatomic considerations apply to the middle ear and sinuses. The eustachian tube of the infant is shorter, straighter and more nearly horizontal than that of the adult. It has relatively more lymphoid tissue. These facts predispose to infection and obstruction. Likewise, the sinuses of the infant are primitive out-pockets of the nasal passage; it is not until facial growth has been almost completed (7 to 10 years) that the necessary maturation and ostia are present to provide functional separation and hygiene.

The symptoms and signs of the common cold are sufficiently well known to make description unnecessary. The incubation period is variable, generally two days (one to six days). Spread is by contact and droplet nuclei. Secondary attack rates are variable, often as high as 40 to 50 per cent in susceptible siblings. There is no worthwhile prophylaxis or prevention. Vaccines are not yet suitable, quarantine is useless and treatment is symptomatic. Antibiotics do *not* prevent secondary infection. Nose drops may relieve nasal obstruction and help infants to suck, but do *not* prevent otitis media. The usual ARD lasts three to four days; however, in younger children nasal discharge and cough may persist for one to two weeks.

Certain age-dependent differences in symptoms exist. Young infants are often afebrile and have only rhinorrhea. In infants and younger children, vomiting and diarrhea are frequent, and otitis media appears early. In older children and adults, soreness and dryness of the throat and hoarseness are more frequent, whereas coryza is less noticeable.

Most common colds leave no sequelae and are thus considered benign. However, otitis media, a frequent complication, can lead to hearing loss. Other bacterial suprainfections often associated with ARD include sinusitis, pneumonia and occasionally bacterial sepsis or meningitis. It is not possible to prevent these by means of antibiotic prophylaxis; indeed, such action seems merely to change the bacterial flora involved in the suprainfection and may be difficult to treat. One must be alert to the possibility of such suprainfection and be prepared to reevaluate the patient with regard to diagnosis and treatment.

Otitis Media

The incidence of otitis media is unknown. It is a common concomitant of ARD in infants and preschool children. Diagnosis is based on pain or pulling at the ear in young infants and the appearance of the ear drum. Health professionals should be aware of two facts: (1) too vigorous manipulation of the external canal will cause at least peripheral reddening of the drum and (2) many ARD's produce some reddening of the ear drums without pyogenic otitis. Purulent otitis media can only be definitely diagnosed when the drum is bulging and the landmarks are no longer visible. Second, not all apparently purulent otitis media is bacterial. Viruses and mycoplasma have been cultured from middle ear exudates, and in about half of younger children and infants with otitis media, cultures of the middle ear are bacteriologically sterile. Of those with bacteria, infants and young children under four years of age generally harbor pneumococci or *H. influenzae;* older children more commonly have pneumococci and rarely group A beta-hemolytic streptococci.

In infants and young children the treatment of choice is penicillin and sulfonamides or ampicillin, whereas penicillin alone will generally suffice for children over four years of age. Neo-Synephrine nose drops are worth trying briefly to relieve obstruction. The acute signs and symptoms generally subside in 24 to 48 hours. Myringotomy is indicated for severe pain. A complication of recurrence is deafness; serous otitis media and chronic otitis media may also occur and may require otolaryngologic consultation regarding surgical and long-term management.

Croup

Acute spasmodic croup (spasmodic laryngitis) is a common condition of children aged two to four years. Generally, in association with an ARD, the child develops paroxysmal nocturnal attacks of laryngeal obstruction. The onset is frequently abrupt, without preceding progressive hoarseness, and there is usually little fever or other systemic symptoms. Croup is a terrifying occurrence for the child and family; the feeling of impending suffocation, labored breathing, cyanosis, hoarseness, brassy cough and stridor are frightening manifestations of a potentially serious, but usually transient, illness from which the child will recover. In most cases the spasms subside over a few hours, to recur less severely on the next and sometimes a third night. This manifestation of ARD tends to be familial, and once a child has had croup, he will probably have it again.

Treatment is symptomatic. High humidity such as running hot water in the bathroom or the shower or cold steam and quiet reassurance generally suffice. Some children become exhausted by the respiratory effort, and some parents cannot handle the apparent emergency. Such children should be hospitalized. Sedation is unwise, as depression of respiration may result. Very rarely, oxygen may be required, but intubation or tracheotomy is rarely necessary. Antibiotics and steroids are not indicated. It is, however, very important to consider in the differential diagnosis the possibilities of foreign body aspiration, epiglottitis or diphtheritic croup. These diseases are discussed in the following chapter.

Laryngotracheobronchitis

The vast majority of cases of this disease group are caused by viruses; the parainfluenza and respiratory syncytial viruses are the most common. The disease presents most commonly at one to four years of age and starts as an upper respiratory infection (URI) followed by hoarseness, brassy cough and stridor. With lower respiratory involvement both inspiratory and expiratory obstruction occur. The onset is not spasmodic, but progressive. As respiratory obstruction increases, the child may become hypoxic, cyanotic, restless and desperately anxious. He struggles for breath, using every possible accessory muscle. On physical examination an extraordinary variety of rales and rhonchi is often heard. Obstruction may produce patchy, or even massive, atelectasis and emphysema. The emphysema is usually not generalized, and the diaphragm is not depressed.

The disease must be differentiated from spasmodic croup, epiglottitis, diphtheria and foreign body aspiration. Most infants should be hospitalized if the symptoms are severe. Intubation or tracheotomy should be performed before the infant is exhausted. The treatment is humidity and quiet reassurance. Antibiotics have not been shown to be effective, and steroids are not helpful. Hydration may be a problem; fluids should be given to replace losses. Sedation is contraindicated. Atropine and similar agents should *not* be used since they cause drying of secretions.

Bronchiolitis

In infants, usually between the ages of 2 and 12 months, a strikingly severe disease occurs as a result of viral infection (most commonly respiratory syncytial virus) of the lower respiratory tract, particularly the terminal bronchioles. The illness starts as a usual ARD, then gets progressively worse over one to three days, to rapid, labored respiration and prominent expiratory obstruction. The chest becomes hyperexpanded, hypoxia and hypercapnia may ensue and may be followed by exhaustion and collapse. The physical findings are those of terminal bronchiolar obstruction with hyperaeration and depressed diaphragm. Radiographically, interstitial infiltrates and patchy atelectasis are also often seen.

The signs and symptoms are very similar to those of severe asthma. True bronchiolitis does not show any significant response to bronchodilator therapy, however. Some infants develop secondary cardiac decompensation, and digitalization may be required. Most infants can be treated with rest, fluids and oxygen as necessary. Antibiotics do not help, steroids are not indicated and sedation should be avoided.

The acute phase of the disease lasts as long as 10 days. The mortality rate is estimated at 2 per cent among hospitalized patients; there are no known sequelae.

Pneumonia

Scarcely any pediatric illness is more frequently over-diagnosed, over-treated and under-studied. Generally the term is applied to any child with ARD whose x-ray shows hilar streaking or patchy interstitial infiltrate ("pneumonitis" or "interstitial pneumonitis"). Sometimes the diagnosis is based merely on auscultation and the finding of rales. Physicians should recognize that most coarse rales in children originate from the bronchi, trachea and upper airway.

Bacterial pneumonias in young children may not localize and can initially present as interstitial pneumonitis; however, alveolar infiltrates will ultimately develop. These are discussed later in this chapter. Viruses are the common causes of pneumonia, and this form of pulmonary infection is not an infrequent concomitant of ARD. The etiological diagnosis of bacterial pneumonia can be difficult. Infants and young children do not produce sputum for examination, and tracheal or transtracheal aspiration is difficult in the very young, with some potential risk to the patient. Generally, the lack of acute systemic signs favors a viral etiology. One should be aware that the patchy atelectasis of laryngotracheobronchitis and bronchiolitis may simulate bacterial pneumonia.

In children who are not severely ill and have no lobular or lobar infiltrates, watchful waiting usually suffices. In children who are severely ill, treatment should be as for bacterial pneumonia, if this cannot be excluded. (See section on bacterial pneumonia.)

Mycoplasma Pneumonia

In patients between the ages of 5 and 19 years, *Mycoplasma pneumoniae* infections are considered the single most common cause of pneumonia. This infection is extremely rare in children under four years of age. In some children the disease may resemble pertussis—there is a gradual onset of malaise, slight cough and fever. The fever becomes variable, and the cough may become severe, lasting 19 to 25 days. The chest radiograph classically shows findings out of proportion to symptoms or signs. Often, "the x-ray looks worse than the child." Serological tests or isolation of *Mycoplasma* confirm the diagnosis. The treatment of choice is erythromycin, which may be effective if begun early, in the first five days of illness.

ACUTE EXANTHEMATOUS DISEASES

Morbilliform or Maculopapular Lesions

MEASLES (RUBEOLA)

Etiological agent—virus.

Incubation period—12 ± 2 days (8 to 16 days).

Prodromata—fever, cough, coryza, conjunctivitis, Koplik's spots (Fig. 15–1).

Epidemiology—irregular epidemics every two to four years; more than 95 per cent in children, highly contagious—airborne and droplet. Secondary attack rate about 66 per cent in susceptibles.

Immunity—transient transplacental immunity; life-long immunity after disease.

Prophylaxis—gamma globulin; quarantine useless.

Prevention—vaccine, live attenuated virus.

Rash—reddish maculopapules (see Fig. 15–2), often becoming confluent, appear first on the face, then trunk and extremities. Branny desquamation, lasting three to seven days.

Other symptoms and signs—high fever, acute respiratory disease (bronchitis, pneumonitis), conjunctivitis, neutropenia.

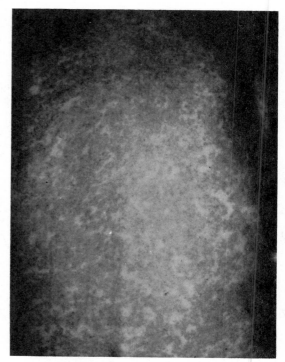

Figure 15–2 Rubeola. Note the confluent nature of the macular rash when fully developed.

Complications—bacterial pneumonia, otitis media, sinusitis, laryngitis, "hemorrhagic" measles and encephalomyelitis (about 1 in 1000 cases).

Treatment—symptomatic.

RUBELLA

Etiological agent—virus.

Incubation period—18 ± 4 days (9 to 25 days).

Prodromata—minimal; retroauricular, postcervical, and post-occipital lymphadenopathy; coryza, exanthem; rarely, rose spots on palate (Forcheimer).

Epidemiology—irregular epidemics, every 6 to 10 years; may be acquired during childhood or early adulthood.

Immunity—transient transplacental immunity; life-long immunity after disease.

Prophylaxis—large doses gamma globulin (efficacy uncertain).

Prevention—vaccine, live attenuated virus.

Rash—very variable; pale rose macules of head, face, spreading to trunk and extremities, may be scarlatiniform on trunk (pinpoint macules); lasts two to three days.

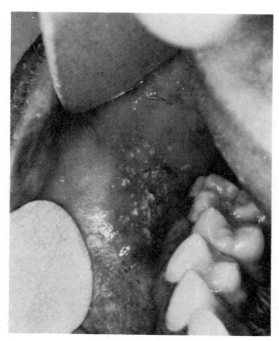

Figure 15–1 Rubeola. Koplik spots on the buccal mucous membrane between teeth and lips.

Other symptoms—low-grade fever, malaise; mild URI; white blood count (WBC) generally normal.

Complications—few in children; arthralgia and arthritis; in pregnant women (first trimester) high incidence of congenital anomalies; encephalitis about 1 in 6000 cases.

Treatment—symptomatic.

EXANTHEM SUBITUM (ROSEOLA INFANTUM)

Etiological agent—? virus (not yet identified).

Incubation period—unknown (? 10 to 15 days).

Prodromata—high fever, 39° to 40°C or higher, often initially of unknown origin.

Epidemiology—unknown; occurs almost entirely in infants between six months and three years; pattern suggests endemic viral infection(s) with high susceptibility in infants.

Immunity—probably transient transplacental, with permanent immunity following disease.

Prophylaxis—none known.

Prevention—none known.

Rash—appears late, after fever declines; maculopapular, rose-colored, evanescent; generally restricted to trunk and head; fades on pressure, fades quickly.

Other symptoms and signs—high unexplained fever for three to four days before rash appears; sometimes very mild upper respiratory infection; neutropenia.

Complications—febrile convulsions at onset.

Treatment—symptomatic.

ERYTHEMA INFECTIOSUM (FIFTH DISEASE)

Etiological agent—probably virus (not yet identified).

Incubation period—10 ± 5 days (probably).

Prodromata—none.

Epidemiology—sporadic, localized, small epidemics in spring and summer.

Immunity—probably life-long from disease.

Prophylaxis—none.

Prevention—none.

Rash—diagnostic; initially (patient often asymptomatic) intensely erythematous, maculopapular, often coalescent rash over malar areas; feels raised, hot, has an "edge" but not tender; one day later on extensor surface of arms, backs of hands, thighs, buttocks; fades to leave a diagnostic, reticular pattern lasting a week or more; rash very variable, often fades and reappears in hours, for two to four weeks, induced by heat, sunlight, trauma.

Other symptoms and signs—generally none (except transient arthritis in adult females).

Complications—none known, no reported deaths.

Treatment—none.

DIFFERENTIAL DIAGNOSIS

Maculopapular or morbilliform eruptions have been associated with various epidemics of both ECHO and Coxsackie viruses. In some epidemics rashes are more prevalent than others; there is no consistent pattern. Rashes are more common in younger patients.

Similarly, morbilliform rashes are seen in some patients with infectious mononucleosis, adenovirus infections, and drug eruptions. Toxic erythema, sunburn and miliaria (heat rash) must also be considered; morbilliform eruptions may herald meningococcemia and rickettsial diseases, including typhus and Rocky Mountain spotted fever. Rat-bite fever (sodoku, *Spirillum minus*) and Haverhill fever (*Streptobacillus moniliformis*) also present fine morbilliform skin lesions.

Scarlet fever is discussed with streptococcal disease.

Pox or Vesicular Lesions

CHICKENPOX (VARICELLA)

Etiological agent—virus (identical with herpes zoster).

Incubation period—15 ± 2 days (11 to 21 days).

Prodromata—fever, malaise for one to two days in older children.

Epidemiology—irregular epidemics in autumn, winter, spring; highly contagious; secondary attack rate of susceptibles greater than 85 per cent with household contact; highest incidence in two- to eight-year-olds; may occur in young infants (even when mother is immune).

Immunity—transplacental immunity not definite; life-long immunity from disease, except that latent virus may persist in host; later reactivation induces herpes zoster.

Prophylaxis—large doses of gamma globulin or zoster immune globulin given within 72 hours after exposure may modify or prevent disease. Quarantine is useless.

Prevention—none.

Rash—appears in "crops" almost from onset, early lesions, erythematous macule with central, thin-walled vesicle ("dew drops on rose petal"); later opacification of vesicular fluid with umbilication and scab; rash primarily on trunk, proximal portion of extremities and mucous membranes. Lesions of all stages may occur in one anatomic area. The rash lasts three to five days.

Other symptoms and signs—high fever, malaise, anorexia.

Complications—hemorrhagic varicella, chiefly in patients using steroids with other disease; varicella pneumonia (usually only in adults); encephalitis (1 in 3000 cases); acute cerebellar ataxia; Reye syndrome.

Treatment—symptomatic.

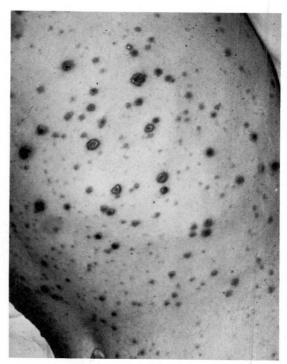

Figure 15–4 Varicella. Fully developed rash shown over lower thorax and upper abdomen. Note the different stages of papules, vesicles and crusts that are present simultaneously.

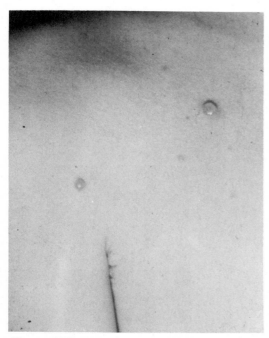

Figure 15–3 Varicella. Early vesicular rash on anterior shoulder and thorax region during first day of the illness.

DIFFERENTIAL DIAGNOSIS

Vesicular (pox) lesions appear in a variety of other diseases, which are all rare. Smallpox (variola) once represented a particularly important differential diagnostic possibility, but now has been nearly eradicated throughout the world.

Rickettsial pox (Rickettsia akari, spread by rodent mites of house mice) has a characteristic primary eschar lesion, followed by a flulike syndrome and then the appearance of very small vesicles on a papular base. The vesicles rarely crust.

Eczema herpeticum (herpes virus) and eczema vaccinatum (vaccinia virus) cause vesicular lesions primarily over involved (eczematous) skin and represent secondary infection of predisposed sites. Dermatitis herpetiformis and molluscum contagiosum can be differentiated by the nature of the skin lesion and the absence of systemic signs. Bullous lesions of the erythema multiforme group, of contact dermatitis, of pemphigus and of certain collagen diseases pose little differential diagnostic problem.

Insect bites, impetigo, urticaria, scabies and papular urticaria also can present with vesicles, but can be differentiated by location, appearance and lack of systemic symptoms.

ACUTE ENANTHEMATOUS DISEASES

HERPANGINA

Etiological agent—Coxsackie group A viruses, occasionally Coxsackie B and ECHO viruses.

Incubation period—two to four days (?).

Prodromata—abrupt onset of fever, anorexia, dysphagia, vomiting, abdominal pain.

Epidemiology—both sporadic and epidemic forms; summer and fall most frequent; highest incidence in one to seven year age groups; contagiousness and secondary attack rates unknown.

Immunity—unknown, probably permanent.

Prophylaxis and prevention—none.

Distinctive features—after two to four days of prodromata, minute vesicles or punched-out ulcers appear on anterior pillars of fauces, tonsils, uvula, edge of soft palate (Fig. 15–5). The pharynx is usually red, the lesions are 1 to 2 mm in diameter, gray-white ulcers on a red areola. These enlarge to 5 mm over a period of four to six days. There are usually less than 20 lesions present. With the ulceration there is often severe dysphagia. The disease subsides in 7 to 10 days.

Other symptoms and signs—genital lesions have been reported.

Complications—usually none.

Treatment—symptomatic.

Differential diagnosis—herpetic stomatitis, aphthous stomatitis (see next section), and erythema multiforme pluriorificialis (Stevens-Johnson syndrome); the latter is distinctive because of conjunctival and rectal involvement, not reported in herpangina, and a tendency to involve the mucocutaneous junction.

HERPETIC STOMATITIS

Etiological agent—herpes simplex virus.

Incubation period—unknown.

Prodromata—abrupt onset high fever, anorexia, irritability, dysphagia.

Epidemiology—herpes simplex is an ubiquitous virus. Most primary infections are inapparent. When they are apparent, however, they are manifest by a group of distinctive vesicular diseases. Following infection, the host apparently becomes a life-long virus carrier. "Secondary" or recurrent manifestations are usually in the form of "cold sores." Most primary infections occur in very young children aged one to four years. Infection is by intimate contact. Contagiousness and secondary attack rates are not known.

Immunity—uncertain and variable. Two types of herpes simplex are now known to exist: type 1 (oral strains) are most commonly involved in childhood infections; type 2 (genital strains) are venereally transmitted, and are responsible

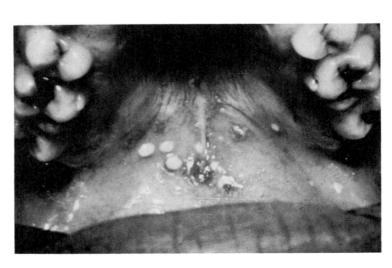

Figure 15–5 Herpangina, due to Coxsackie virus group A infection. This view of the palate shows vesicles and ulcers. The findings may easily be confused with herpes simplex infection. (Courtesy of the Department of Oral Pathology, University of Washington.)

for the majority of genital infections in adults. The type 2 strains are also most frequently associated with intrauterine or perinatally acquired infections of newborns and can cause devastating disease in some.

Prophylaxis and prevention — none.

Distinctive features — shortly after onset of fever and severe constitutional symptoms, striking lesions appear on gums, tongue and anterior portions of oral mucous membranes. Initially there is extreme redness, swelling and friability leading to bleeding. White 2 to 3 mm plaques and shallow ulcers appear in crops over the inflamed base. The anterior cervical lymph nodes become swollen and tender. The disease varies considerably in severity. Most children recover in five to seven days; some with severe infection may continue acutely ill for 10 to 14 days.

Other symptoms and signs — primary herpetic infection may rarely appear as vulvovaginitis. The virus may be "seeded" on an abrasion or wound. One serious primary infection in children with eczema is eczema herpeticum (Kaposi's varicelliform eruption). This potentially fatal disease has the same severe constitutional symptoms. The vesicles occur mainly on the eczematous sites but may appear also on apparently normal skin. Primary herpes infections of the eye are rare, but acute herpetic keratoconjunctivitis does occur and may lead to blindness. This can be treated with topical 5-iodo-2-deoxyuridine (IUDR). Herpes simplex can also cause a meningoencephalitis. There are two forms — one benign and self-limited, the other severe, progressive and sometimes fatal.

Complications — as noted.

Treatment — symptomatic; dehydration is often a serious problem; mouth lesions sometimes preclude ingestion of either fluid or therapeutic agents.

Differential diagnosis — see Herpangina.

APHTHOUS STOMATITIS

Some children have recurrent stomatitis indistinguishable from milder herpetic infections. These are probably not viral but an allergic reaction. One exception is Vincent's angina, which is usually acute herpetic gingivostomatitis complicated by varying degrees of secondary infection by oral bacterial flora.

THRUSH (ORAL MONILIASIS)

Prematures, ill or debilitated infants and severely, chronically ill or undernourished older children may develop a mild infection of the oral mucosa from the normally saprophytic Candida albicans. The pearly white, cordlike lesions are pathognomonic. Diagnostic confirmation can be made from fresh smears. Treatment with local nystatin is helpful.

OTHER DISTINCTIVE ACUTE INFECTIOUS DISEASES

MUMPS (EPIDEMIC PAROTITIS)

Etiological agent — a paramyxovirus.

Incubation period — 13 to 26 days.

Prodromata — fever, anorexia, malaise, headache.

Epidemiology — endemic in urban populations; epidemiology confused by fact that about one third of infections are "subclinical" and inapparent; irregular epidemics; direct contact or droplet transmission; 85 per cent of cases occur in those under 15 years of age; uncommon in infancy, infrequent to age five years; secondary attack rate in childhood susceptibles 30 to 50 per cent.

Immunity — probably transplacental immunity; disease confers life-long immunity.

Prophylaxis — immune (convalescent) gamma globulin not proved to be efficacious; quarantine useless.

Prevention — live vaccine, attenuated virus.

Distinctive features — parotid or other salivary gland swelling, often with pain and tenderness, pain on chewing, and pain on salivary stimulation; salivary gland duct orifices swollen and red; early swelling is associated with much edema, giving a "jellylike" consistency; later the swelling is brawny, with ill-defined borders; with marked involvement there may be presternal edema.

Other symptoms and signs — orchitis, after puberty in 25 per cent of males; 98 per cent unilateral; sterility from bilateral orchitis not proved; aseptic meningitis or meningoencephalitis in about 10 per cent of all cases is usually benign; symptomatic pancreatitis is a severe, uncommon manifestation; oophoritis occurs in women; also sometimes seen are thyroiditis, mastitis, dacryoadenitis, bartholinitis, pneumonitis and myocarditis.

Complications—other than noted already, none; all generally subside uneventfully; rarely neurological sequelae, including deafness, have been described; myocarditis observed in adults; arthritis similar to that in rubella reported.

Treatment—symptomatic.

Differential diagnosis—lymphadenitis of the anterior and preauricular nodes distinguished by anatomic position and defined borders; suppurative parotitis produces redness of overlying skin, and pus may be milked from duct; recurrent parotitis from sialectasis occurs; mumps does not recur. Sialolithiasis generally causes intermittent obstruction; tumors have less rapid onset of swelling; Mikulicz syndrome is rare in children; dryness of mouth and lack of tears are diagnostic; uveoparotid fever (sarcoidosis) may be confused initially with mumps.

VIRAL MENINGITIS AND ENCEPHALITIS

Almost every known virus can produce and has produced central nervous system disease. Certain viruses have a predilection for the central nervous system (Table 15–2). Of special interest in pediatrics are California encephalitis and eastern and western equine encephalitis because of the high attack rates in infants and children. These summer arthropod-borne diseases appear in epidemics in warm weather. There are animal reservoirs; mosquitoes may transmit the virus. Prevention is through mosquito control.

Children have the highest incidence of eastern equine encephalitis infection, with 70 per cent of cases in those under 10 years and 25 per cent under one year of age. St. Louis encephalitis primarily affects patients over 40 years. Western equine encephalitis occurs most frequently in male field workers 20 to 50 years of age and in young infants. California encephalitis is most commonly seen in school-aged children. The onset is generally sudden, but may be gradual, with fever, headache and vomiting, followed by increasing signs of central nervous system involvement. Cerebrospinal fluid (CSF) is usually clear, mononuclear cells are increased, protein is slightly elevated and glucose is normal. Early in the illness the CSF pleocytosis can be predominantly polymorphonuclear. The disease lasts one to two weeks unless fulminating with death in two to four days. Mortality rates vary from 2 to 20 per cent. Recovery in California, eastern and western equine encephalitis is usually complete if the patient survives, except in young infants, for whom residual CNS sequelae are frequent.

Enteroviruses, especially echoviruses, Coxsackie B and some Coxsackie A viruses, are also causes of CNS disease. Most illnesses are believed to be benign, aseptic meningitis syndromes. Severe encephalitis can also result, however, sometimes with neurological sequelae.

Onset may be abrupt or gradual. Presenting features are fever, malaise, vomiting, headache and signs of meningeal irritation.

TABLE 15–2 VIRAL AGENTS MOST COMMONLY ASSOCIATED WITH CENTRAL NERVOUS SYSTEM INFECTIONS AMONG CHILDREN IN THE UNITED STATES

Agent	Age Group Most Frequently Affected	Common Months of Onset	Comments
Mumps	5 to 12 years	November through May	30 per cent of cases may not have associated parotitis
Enteroviruses: (ECHO, Coxsackie)	Birth to 14 years	June through October	Often multiple associated illness in community and family, including febrile exanthematous syndromes
Arboviruses: western equine encephalitis	Birth to 9 years	June through September	Ecological considerations important in suggesting etiology
California encephalitis	5 to 15 years		

Neurological symptoms are variable. Diagnosis is by examination of CSF, with findings similar to those described for arbovirus infections. Specific diagnosis requires virus isolation or significant serum antibody rises.

Treatment is symptomatic.

DISTINCTIVE BACTERIAL INFECTIONS

Streptococcosis

The only significant bacterial infections of the upper respiratory tract are caused by beta hemolytic streptococci, group A and *Corynebacterium diphtheriae*. Streptococcal infections in children are frequent and present a wide range of age-dependent manifestations. For this reason the term streptococcosis is utilized.

Epidemiology. More than half of all streptococcal infections occur in children between the ages of 3 and 13 years. Between the ages of 6 and 12 years, the peak years for infection, the incidence is more than 1 case per 1000 child days; more than 40 per cent of such children have at least one streptococcal infection each year. In adults the incidence is less than 0.2 case per 1000 person days. On the average, by six years of age all children have had one streptococcal infection; by nine years, two infections; by 13 years, three infections. There is great variation among families and socioeconomic groups. In middle class urban families, the average 15-year-old will have experienced 3.5 significant illnesses; some 15-year-olds will have had none, others may have had as many as eight.

There is a marked seasonal variation, as most illness occurs in late winter and early spring months. The disease is spread by contact. In urban areas streptococci are endemic; in isolated communities true epidemics occur.

In most households the disease is introduced by a young school child. The disease spreads most frequently to a preschool sibling first, then to older siblings, rather infrequently to the mother and even less often to the father. Rates in families with young school children are eight times higher than those without. In general, if a clinical case exists in a household, the chances are that 50 to 60 per cent of family contacts will have streptococci in the throat and that 30 to 40 per cent will develop symptomatic illness.

Clinical manifestations. The clinical expression of streptoccal infection is dependent upon the age of the child and prior experience with streptococcal antigens. Generally, a uniform trend can be conceptualized. The young child with no previous experience will present with an insidious non-localized systemic disease; the older child with significant previous antigenic exposure will present with an abrupt, sharply localized syndrome. This concept, in analogy to that of tuberculosis, has been termed streptococcosis. It is thus not sufficient in pediatrics to consider streptococcal infection as a uniform disease with exudative pharyngitis. Similarly, the suppurative and non-suppurative complications are age- and experience-dependent.

INFANTS UNDER SIX MONTHS OF AGE. The disease is characterized in this group by irregular low-grade fever, a watery, mucoserous nasal discharge with crusting around the nares, slight pharyngeal injection, anorexia, vomiting, diarrhea and irritability. The syndrome is often indistinguishable from the common cold. The acute symptoms usually last seven days, but the recovery is prolonged; nasal discharge and irritability may continue for five to six weeks. In the newborn period the disease may be suddenly fatal without any warning signs.

SIX-MONTH TO THREE-YEAR AGE GROUP. The disease has insidious onset, with low-grade fever, mild constitutional symptoms and a mild nasopharyngitis with a purulent discharge. Anterior cervical lymph nodes are generally enlarged and tender. They may suppurate; the peak incidence of abscess formation is in the one- to five-year age group. Sinusitis and otitis media may also occur and can be considered as integral parts of the disease. If untreated, the low-grade fever, with irregular elevation to 38.8°C, continues for as long as one to two months. Convalescence thereafter may take months, with anorexia, weight loss, irritability, pallor and general "lack of pep." In this age group one also sees the pyogenic complications of sepsis, such as pneumonia with empyema and osteomyelitis.

THREE- TO TWELVE-YEAR AGE GROUP. The disease begins to be more similar to that found in adults. This is the period of highest incidence of infection. Scarlet fever occurs most frequently in this age group. The presence or absence of the rash is dependent only upon whether the organism produces the erythrogenic toxin and whether the child has antibody to the toxin.

SCARLET FEVER

Etiological agent—hemolytic streptococcus, group A.

Incubation period—two to five days.

Prodromata—abrupt onset of fever, vomiting, headache, chills, malaise, abdominal pain, sore throat.

Epidemiology—irregular epidemics, predominantly late winter and spring; contact transmission, secondary attack rate approximates 30 per cent.

Immunity—generally transplacental immunity to erythrogenic toxin, prolonged immunity to recurrent toxin form of disease; type-specific immunity to organism lasts probably for life, but many types exist.

Prophylaxis and prevention—penicillin; quarantine useless.

Rash—Enanthem—tonsils enlarged, edematous, reddened and may have patches of exudate. Pharynx, including uvula and soft palate, edematous and beefy red. Can mimic diphtheria in severe cases; appearance may resemble infectious mononucleosis. Tongue initially furred, with white coat posteriorly, tip and edges red; later papillae become red and edematous, producing "white strawberry tongue"; by the fourth or fifth day the white coat peels off and the red glistening tongue is "red-strawberry" appearing.

Exanthem—12 to 48 hours after onset an erythematous, punctiform rash, blanching on pressure and feeling like sandpaper, appears. The entire underlying skin is red. The rash rapidly becomes generalized. On the face, punctiform lesions are absent and the erythema involves primarily the cheeks and lower forehead, giving classically "circumoral pallor." The rash is more intense in skin folds of neck, axilla and groin, and folds may have transverse lines with tiny petechiae (Pastia's sign). If the rash is severe, sweat gland pores become plugged and produce minute vesicles called miliaria crystallina or sudamina. On recovery, the skin desquamates in branny flakes, particularly on hands and feet.

Other symptoms and signs—fever, which usually rises abruptly to 38.5°C or higher, falls in five to seven days without treatment.

Complications—Suppurative: adenitis, otitis, sinusitis; more rarely pneumonia, empyema, septicemia, mastoiditis, osteomyelitis. Non-suppurative: post-streptococcal arthralgia, rheumatic fever, acute glomerulonephritis.

ADULT (MATURE FORM) STREPTOCOCCAL PHARYNGITIS

Sudden onset of sore throat and dysphagia, headache, fever (variable from 38 to 40°C), abdominal pain, nausea and vomiting in children. Signs include beefy-red throat with swollen uvula, generally with exudate on tonsils and tender, swollen lymph nodes at angle of jaw. No single symptom or sign is diagnostic. Clinical diagnostic error in older children and adults exceeds 30 per cent; bacteriological diagnosis is necessary.

DIAGNOSIS AND TREATMENT

The variability in presenting manifestations of streptococcal disease in childhood is so great as to make diagnosis on clinical grounds alone impossible. While it is possible on epidemiological grounds to increase accuracy, this too is haphazard. A throat culture is practical, cheap and effective as an office procedure. A delay of 24 hours in diagnosis does not increase the incidence, severity, morbidity or complications of the disease.

Penicillin is the treatment of choice. Oral penicillin is not always taken faithfully and hence "cure" rates are usually no higher than 85 per cent. On the other hand, intramuscular benzathine penicillin G (600,000 to 1,200,000 units) is cheap, well-tolerated and more than 95 per cent effective. In patients sensitive to penicillin, erythromycin is the drug of choice; sulfonamides and tetracycline, while suppressing infection, *do not* prevent complications and should not be used.

There is disagreement about which patients harboring streptococci require treatment. One important consideration is the prevention of rheumatic fever. In untreated populations with significant infection, the incidence of rheumatic fever following streptococcal disease is 3 per cent. The incidence of rheumatic heart disease in young adults in such populations is about 40 per 1000. Today, with available therapy, rheumatic heart disease rates in college populations in the United States are down to 5.7 per 1000.

It is undoubtedly true that the incidence of rheumatic fever and rheumatic heart disease is far higher in patients who have had significant, symptomatic streptococcal infection. It has been suggested that only such patients require treatment. Such figures may be misleading, however. In most reviews of new cases of rheumatic fever the infection was found to be asymptomatic in at least one third of patients. Usually, an additional one quarter fail to seek medical advice for symptomatic disease. Also, about one quarter see a physician who fails to recognize the streptococcal infection or does not treat it adequately. Thus, attention must be given to less symptomatic infections as well as to classic disease.

Unfortunately, in individual practice, the incidence of rheumatic fever is too low to be meaningful as a method of formulating therapeutic experience. In the age group at greatest risk (7 to 12 years) there will be only one infection per five years, on the average. If *no* therapy is given for the infection, no more than 1 in 25 individuals will develop rheumatic fever, and no more than 1 in 50 to 75 will develop rheumatic heart disease. Rheumatic fever, in contrast to nephritis, is probably dependent upon repeated infection, not isolated disease. If one supposes that 50 per cent of streptococcal infections might be properly treated, rheumatic heart disease will only be rarely visible in a practice containing 500 children between eight and 13 years. Such a practice would have to be very large, with at least 2000 children seen actively, at least once or twice a year. Such practices are unusual, and it is little wonder that individual experience in practice has led to conflicting recommendations.

Thus, we recommend on epidemiological grounds that *all* symptomatic infections should be treated. Patients having such infections usually have a predominant growth of beta-hemolytic streptococci on the culture plate.

PROPHYLAXIS

All children who have had rheumatic fever, most adults with high risk of exposure to streptococcal disease who have had rheumatic fever and all adults with rheumatic heart disease should be given continuous, effective prophylaxis. The studies are quite clear as to the drug of choice: intramuscular benzathine penicillin G once a month is most effective; alternatives include daily oral penicillin or sulfonamide.

Unusual, Often Missed Sites of Streptococcal Infection

Impetigo is generally streptococcal at its onset; there can be a relationship between such skin infections and acute glomerulonephritis. Patients have few systemic symptoms, and most infections occur in summer and fall.

Otitis media in children two years and older is occasionally streptococcal, but the organism is generally also found in the throat.

Suppurative cervical adenitis is frequently streptococcal, usually following a missed or barely symptomatic streptococcal upper respiratory infection.

Vaginitis in young girls is often streptococcal, producing a watery, sometimes serosanguinous discharge without systemic signs of infection.

Pustular insect bites, particularly in summer, may present with acute local pustules and often involve streptococcal infection.

(Rare) Primary peritonitis, osteomyelitis, septicemia, pneumonia.

Epilogue on streptococcosis. We have dealt at length with streptococcal disease in childhood because it presents an excellent model to visualize the age-dependent manifestations of disease from a single infectious agent. It is also the one form of upper respiratory infection seen frequently that can be effectively treated, and such treatment makes a significant difference to the patient.

Bacterial Pneumonias

The most important bacterial pneumonias of childhood are caused by *Streptococcus pneumoniae*, *Staphylococcus aureus*, *Hemophilus influenzae*, *Streptococcus pyogenes* and *Mycobacterium tuberculosis*. Many factors may contribute to the development of pneumonia. Children with cystic fibrosis may develop pneumonia as the first symptom of their disease. Pneumonia may be the only sign of a foreign body in a bronchus. Pneumonia in a newborn infant may be the result of a congenital anomaly, particularly a tracheoesophageal fistula.

PNEUMOCOCCAL PNEUMONIA

This is the most common bacterial pneumonia of infants and children, representing about 90 per cent of all cases. Most infections occur during the colder months of the year. Onset is often abrupt, although symptoms of upper respiratory tract infection may appear several days previously. Signs and symptoms include fever, malaise, rapid shallow respirations, cough and chest pain that is often increased by coughing or deep breathing. Pain may be referred to the abdomen and be confused with appendicitis. Meningismus is common; meningitis may have to be excluded by studies on the cerebrospinal fluid.

Physical findings in the chest may be minimal for the first day or two. The first signs of pneumonia may be only a few rales or diminished breath sounds over the affected area. Later, more characteristic signs of lobular or lobar consolidation will appear. Evidence of pneumonia is often detected in the chest radiograph before physical signs are present.

Pneumococci can be isolated from blood cultures in about 30 per cent of cases and often from pleural fluid, if any is present. Simple throat or nasopharyngeal swabs are of no value in the diagnosis of bacterial pneumonias.

The white blood cell count is usually increased, although severely ill patients may have leukopenia.

Some more common complications include pleural effusion, empyema and abdominal distention.

The treatment of choice is parenteral penicillin and supportive care. Oxygen may be needed for those with cyanosis. The prognosis is excellent with adequate therapy.

STAPHYLOCOCCAL PNEUMONIA

This is the most important bacterial pneumonia of infancy. It is discussed in Chapter 16 on severe life-threatening infections.

STREPTOCOCCAL AND HEMOPHILUS INFLUENZAE PNEUMONIA

Streptococcus pyogenes and *Hemophilus influenzae*, while unusual causes of pneumonia in children, may initially present as an interstitial pneumonia, and lobular patterns may develop later. Compared to pneumococcal pneumonia, these pneumonias are more likely to progress to empyemas. Management is similar to that for pneumococcal pneumonia. Penicillin is the drug of choice for streptococcal pneumonia, and ampicillin or chloramphenicol is preferred for *Hemophilus influenzae* pneumonia.

KLEBSIELLA PNEUMONIA

Klebsiella is an uncommon but devastating pneumonia in infants. Many patients develop abscesses and empyemas. The clinical pattern is similar to that for staphylococcal pneumonias in infants. Diagnosis can only be made by culture, and antibiotic treatment should be based on antibiotic susceptibility testing.

Urinary Tract Infections in Infancy and Childhood

This synopsis will deal primarily with symptomatic infections. Asymptomatic bacteriuria is a common phenomenon, especially in females, with a prevalence of about 1.5 per cent among schoolgirls. The significance of asymptomatic bacteriuria is not yet clear.

The attack rate for symptomatic and asymptomatic urinary tract infections is estimated to be 2 to 4 per cent per year among female infants and children, and 0.1 to 0.5 per cent among males. Because of the frequent subtlety of signs and symptoms, it has been estimated that 60 to 80 per cent of these infections are *not* diagnosed clinically.

It should also be emphasized that use of the term "urinary tract infection" is preferred. Currently, it is not always possible to differentiate between infections involving the upper tract (pyelonephritis) and those primarily affecting the lower tract (cystitis) on clinical grounds alone, particularly when evaluating the infection for the first time.

PREDISPOSING FACTORS

Twenty-five to 40 per cent of cases are associated with neurological deficit such as meningomyelocele and diastematomyelia or urological defects such as urethral valves, ureteral reflux, urethral or ureteral strictures, ureteroceles or duplicated collecting system.

Dictum: Any defect that allows stasis and "puddling" in the urinary tract will predispose to infection. If this condition is allowed to continue without appropriate management, the risk of chronic infection and permanent damage is increased significantly.

CLINICAL SIGNS AND SYMPTOMS

General findings (extremely variable and often subtle): Fever, flank or abdominal pain, dysuria, urinary frequency, enuresis, irritability, anorexia or gastrointestinal complaints with failure to thrive, vomiting, diarrhea and constipation (very common).

Findings pertinent to infants, especially in the neonatal period, which suggest that urinary tract abnormality may exist include abdominal masses, urinary "dribbling" or narrowing of urinary stream. External anomalies such as anomalous genitalia, low-set ears, spine defects, absent abdominal musculature or imperforate anus may be associated with renal anomalies.

LABORATORY DIAGNOSIS

Clean voided urine or urine collected by sterile catheterization or suprapubic bladder aspiration is *essential* in interpretation of the results.

Urinalysis
Albuminuria is infrequent.
Pyuria, i.e., more than 5 white blood cells per $440 \times$ high power microscopic field in centrifuged urine. False positive results are frequent; also, about 25 per cent of urinary tract infection cases do *not* have pyuria at time of examination.
Bacilluria, i.e., bacteria readily visualized in centrifuged urine.

If both pyuria and bacilluria are absent the chance of obtaining a significant result on culture is less than 10 per cent; however, if either or both are present, a culture and colony count are mandatory.

Colony counts of 100,000 or more per milliliter of urine are considered significant; however, colony counts in lower numbers from clean-voided or catheterized urine specimens may also be significant on occasion, particularly if the urine is highly dilute or obstruction is present. Any interpretive dilemmas can usually be resolved by suprapubic aspiration of the bladder.

Urine obtained by suprapubic aspiration should normally be sterile. Any growth should be regarded as potentially significant.

ETIOLOGICAL AGENTS

E. coli is the most common agent in childhood urinary tract infections (70 to 85 per cent); other bacteria, such as *Klebsiella, Proteus sp., Pseudomonas* and enterococcus, occur less commonly but may also be present in mixed infections. Polymicrobial urinary isolates may merely represent contamination but can also suggest a complication of a severely obstructed urinary tract.

MANAGEMENT

ANTIBIOTIC THERAPY. This should be as dictated by sensitivity testing. For infections outside of the neonatal period, sulfisoxazole (Gantrisin) is usually an ideal starting agent in acute, uncomplicated cases. Other agents used include ampicillin and nitrofurantoin. Therapy should be specific and should be maintained for a minimum of two weeks.

FOLLOW-UP CARE. Between 60 and 70 per cent of patients develop a recurrence of infection within the first year after treatment, most of these within the first two months. For this reason, careful follow-up and urine examinations are essential.

Consideration for further work-up. Many cases will need further evaluation, including intravenous pyelography *and* cystourethrography, as well as possible further urological studies depending upon the results of these tests.

The following indications serve as a rough guide in deciding when such procedures may be indicated: any infection in a male; any infection in a patient less than one year of age; more than two infections in a female; failure of clinical response to treatment in 48 hours; persistence of urinary abnormalities for more than two weeks with specific therapy; physical or historic findings suggestive of recurrent infection or urinary tract anomalies.

REFERENCES

Davis, S. D., and Wedgwood, R. J.: Antibiotic prophylaxis in acute viral respiratory diseases. Am. J. Dis. Child., *109*:544, 1965.

Dingle, J. H., Badger, G. F., and Jordan, W. S., Jr.: *Illness in the home. A study of 25,000 illnesses in a group of Cleveland families.* Cleveland, Press of the Western Reserve University, 1964.

DeLuca, F. G., Fisher, J. H., and Swenson, O.: Review of recurrent urinary-tract infections in infancy and early childhood. N. Engl. J. Med., *268*:75, 1963.

Glezen, W. P., and Denny, F. W.: Epidemiology of acute lower respiratory disease in children. N. Engl. J. Med., *288*:498, 1973.

Hill, H. R., and Ray, C. G.: The differential diagnosis of viral exanthems and enanthems. *In Brennemann's Practice of Pediatrics.* New York, Harper and Row, Vol. II, Chap. 30, 1975.

Kaplan, E. L., Top, F. H., Jr., Dudding, B. A., and Wannamaker, L. W.: Diagnosis of streptococcal pharyngitis: Differentiation of active infection from the carrier state in the symptomatic child. J. Infect. Dis., *123*:490, 1971.

Kunin, C. M.: A ten-year study of bacteriuria in schoolgirls: Final report of bacteriologic, urologic, and epidemiologic findings. J. Infect. Dis., *122*:382, 1970.

Kunin, C. M.: Current status of screening children for urinary tract infections. Pediatrics, *54*:619, 1974.

Loda, F. A., *et al.*: Studies on the role of viruses, bacteria, and *M. pneumoniae* as causes of lower respiratory tract infections in children. J. Pediatr., *72*:161, 1968.

Soyka, L. F., Robinson, D. S., Lachant, N., and Monaco, J.: The misuse of antibiotics for treatment of upper respiratory tract infections in children. Pediatrics, *55*:552, 1975.

Wannamaker, L. W.: Perplexity and precision in the diagnosis of streptococcal pharyngitis. Am. J. Dis. Child., *124*:352, 1972.

Severe Life-Threatening Infectious Diseases

C. George Ray, M.D.

This chapter discusses the more common serious infections that should be recognized clinically and for which there is appropriate therapy.

For laboratory diagnosis of these entities the best method is by *direct* demonstration of the infectious agent in the blood or in the site of disease (e.g., cerebrospinal fluid, abscess) utilizing culture and gram stain. Serological and biochemical tests are *not* primary aspects of laboratory diagnosis of the diseases described.

BACTERIAL MENINGITIS (EXCLUDING THE NEONATAL PERIOD)

Etiological Agents

Hemophilus influenzae type b, *Streptococcus pneumoniae* and *Neisseria meningitidis* are most common.

Less common, but to be considered in unusual cases, are tuberculosis, cryptococcosis, staphylococcus, group A beta-hemolytic streptococcus and *Listeria*. In addition, viral meningitis and encephalitis must be considered if a bacterial origin is not identified.

Clinical Manifestations

The manifestations may be variable and sometimes minimal.

Symptoms—fever, nausea and vomiting, headache, irritability, lethargy.
Signs—occasionally may present with convulsions; also stiff neck with positive Brudzinski's or Kernig's signs, and disturbances of sensorium.

Diagnostic Procedures

Lumbar puncture. Examine fluid for cells, protein, glucose (a simultaneously drawn blood glucose specimen is necessary to evaluate this result), gram stain and culture. The usual findings on cerebrospinal (CSF) examination of normal infants and children and in different disease states are summarized in Table 16–1. It should be kept in mind, however, that variations of these findings can occur. For example, bacterial meningitis may be present early with a normal cerebrospinal fluid glucose value, and viral meningitis occasionally begins with predominance of polymorphonuclear cells.

Blood culture. Culture of the blood should always be obtained prior to therapy, to insure an etiologic diagnosis.

Treatment

Antibiotics. The current treatment of choice in acute meningitis when the responsible organism is not immediately known is ampicillin, 75 to 100 mg/kg intravenously as soon as possible, followed

TABLE 16–1 CEREBROSPINAL FLUID FINDINGS (Mean Values in Parentheses)

	Cells/mm³	Percentage of Polymorpho-nuclear Cells	Glucose as Percentage of Blood Glucose	Protein (mg/100 ml)	Other
Normal child	0–1	0	≥60	<30	—
Viral meningitis	2–2000 (80)	≤50	≥60	30–80	—
Bacterial meningitis	5–5000 (800)	≥60	≤45	>60	LDH, GOT, and Lactate ↑, pH ↓
Tuberculous	5–2000 (100)	≤50 (Variable)	≤45	>60	See bacterial meningitis

Neonates

	Cells/mm³	Percentage of Polymorpho-nuclear Cells	Glucose as Percentage of Blood Glucose	Protein (mg/100 ml)	Other
Normal					
Full term	0–32 (8)	≤60	≥60	20–170 (90)	—
Premature	0–29 (9)	≤57	≥60	65–150 (115)	—

by continued therapy with ampicillin, 300 mg/kg/day intravenously, given every four hours. In areas in which ampicillin-resistant *Hemophilus influenzae* are found, it is preferable to begin with intravenous chloramphenicol, 100 mg/kg/day, plus penicillin G, 300,000 units/kg/day until the organism is identified and antimicrobial susceptibility is clarified.

If subsequent testing reveals the cause to be pneumococcus or meningococcus, penicillin G therapy, 300,000 to 400,000 units/kg/day may be substituted. Therapy should be continued *via the intravenous route*, usually for at least 10 days.

Supportive measures. Appropriate fluid and electrolyte therapy with careful monitoring of neurological and metabolic status are necessary. A decreasing serum sodium value is often seen in the acute phase, usually representing inappropriate antidiuretic hormone secretion with resultant excess water retention. This is best corrected by restricting the free water intake.

Other possible measures

1. Mannitol treatment is occasionally employed if cerebral edema develops rapidly. This should accompany careful monitoring of fluid balance and observation of neurological status.

2. Specific treatment of convulsions.

SEPTICEMIA OF THE NEWBORN, WITH OR WITHOUT MENINGITIS

Etiology

The agents noted here are most common in the first 72 hours of life, with decreasing incidence during the next several weeks. After the first month these organisms become infrequent offenders, except in infants with other underlying defects.

Perinatal complications such as prolonged rupture of membranes, prematurity, maternal fever or fetal distress are important predisposing factors in approximately two thirds of cases. Meningitis may coexist with sepsis in about 25 per cent of cases.

The usual agents responsible are, in relative order of frequency: *E. coli*, group B streptococci, *Klebsiella*, *Proteus*, *Pseudomonas*, *Enterococcus* and *Staphylococcus*. Other potential causes are group A streptococcus, pneumococcus, listeria, bacteroides species, *Vibrio fetus* and salmonella.

Clinical Findings

Signs and symptoms may be extremely variable and often subtle at the onset. Signs may include jaundice, refusal to feed, hyperthermia or hypothermia, irritability or lethargy, apneic or cyanotic spells, vomiting, bulging fontanel, convulsions and respiratory distress. Any of these signs should raise a suspicion of sepsis, with or without meningitis.

Diagnostic Procedures

Blood culture, CSF examination and culture and urine culture are the primary procedures prior to initiating therapy.

Age Group	Ampicillin	Kanamycin	Gentamicin
Under 1 week	100 mg/kg/day	15 mg/kg/day (7.5 mg/kg every 12 hr)	5 mg/kg/day (2.5 mg/kg every 12 hr)
1 week to 1 month	150 to 250 mg/kg/day	15 mg/kg/day for low birth weight infants, under 2000 gm; larger infants may require 20 to 30 mg/kg/day for adequate blood levels.	7.5 mg/kg/day (2.5 mg/kg every 8 hr)

Treatment

Antibiotics. Therapy should begin immediately after the suspicion of sepsis has been raised and the appropriate diagnostic procedures completed. Current data indicate that a combination of ampicillin and gentamicin is ideal coverage for the majority of organisms encountered. One organism not well covered by this combination is *Pseudomonas,* for which gentamicin and carbenicillin should be used parenterally. Recommended dosages for the usual antibiotics are seen in the accompanying chart. Remember that the metabolism and excretion of some antibiotics may be markedly delayed in newborn infants.

If meningitis is known or suspected to exist, intravenous therapy is preferable to intramuscular treatment.

FULMINATING MENINGOCOCCEMIA

This entity differs from meningococcal meningitis in that the cerebrospinal fluid may frequently be clear or minimally abnormal, and the clinical course is particularly fulminating, death often occurring within hours unless prompt treatment is instituted. Overall death rates from this syndrome have been variously estimated between 30 and 60 per cent.

Etiological Agent

Neisseria meningitidis.

Clinical Manifestations

Abrupt onset of fever, chills, vomiting, occasionally headache and lethargy, usually followed by an erythematous rash (see Fig. 16–1) that becomes petechial and spreads rapidly to being ecchymotic. Presence of shock, relative *absence* of meningitis, normal or low peripheral white blood cell count and clinical evidence of spreading purpura suggest a poor prognosis.

Diagnostic Procedures

As in bacterial meningitis, drainage of petechial lesions and examination with a gram stain may occasionally be useful in diagnosis. *A normal cerebrospinal fluid does not rule out this diagnosis.* In some endemic areas, one must also consider the possibility of Rocky Mountain spotted fever, which may closely mimic meningococcal sepsis.

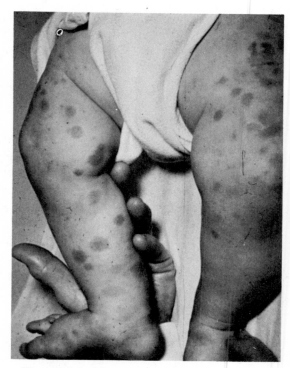

Figure 16–1 Meningococcal rash. The lesions are just beginning to show hemorrhagic change. This can easily be misconstrued as rickettsial disease, or as vasculitis, which may occur with anaphylactoid purpura.

Treatment

Antibiotics. Penicillin G, as for bacterial meningitis, given immediately.

Treatment of shock. The primary goal of treatment for shock is to maintain an adequate circulating blood volume in order to perfuse vital organs. It is mandatory to establish an adequate monitoring system immediately, including frequent observation of blood pressure and other vital signs, hourly urine output and central venous pressure or pulmonary wedge pressure.

Initially, volume expanders, such as saline and salt-poor albumin, are employed. In children, 5 to 10 ml/min for 10 minutes is used at the beginning, followed by an assessment of central venous pressure after a 10-minute "rest" period. The general objective is to increase central venous pressure by about 5 cm of water, and maintain the pressure at 7 to 12 cm of water, if possible. Repeated and continuous infusions are regulated with these goals in mind, paying close attention for possible pulmonary edema, and carefully monitoring urine output.

Pharmacological agents can also be utilized to help maintain cardiac output and arterial pressure. We presently prefer dopamine, used carefully, as a slow intravenous drip, 2 to 5 μg/kg/min. However, dopamine should be used only when the clinician is assured that volume expansion has been appropriate and feels it is necessary to enhance cardiac output. Indiscriminate use can cause ventricular arrhythmias.

Treatment of the disseminated intravascular clotting. Routine heparinization is not recommended in all cases of meningococcemia. If evidence of purpura fulminans or a widespread Shwartzman reaction is present, however, careful heparin therapy, guided by appropriate coagulation studies and monitoring of platelet counts, may be beneficial. This is particularly true in cases with purpura fulminans.

Other treatment. Adrenocortical steroids are variably recommended. Their efficacy is still unproved, but large doses may be useful in modifying the course of an endotoxin-caused myocarditis or shock lung syndrome.

STAPHYLOCOCCAL PNEUMONIA

This is a particularly life-threatening infection that may affect any age group and is especially common in infants. Death may be sudden, often resulting from the abrupt development of a tension pyopneumothorax.

Etiological Agent

Staphylococcus aureus.

Clinical Manifestations

Pneumonia may be preceded by a mild upper respiratory tract infection followed by fever, cough, tachypnea, dyspnea and abdominal distention. The condition may progress to cyanosis and shock.

Physical findings. These may include decreased breath sounds, dullness to percussion and "splinting" on the affected side. Mediastinal shift may be noted on percussion and tracheal palpation. Later on, scoliosis with the concavity toward the affected side may be noted, indicating the presence of an empyema.

Radiological findings. Variable findings include diffuse infiltration, pleural effusion, pneumothorax or abscess or pneumatocele formation.

Diagnostic Procedures

Thoracentesis; blood culture; occasionally, a lung aspirate with culture and smear may be necessary.

Treatment

Antibiotics. Methicillin or nafcillin, 200 to 300 mg/kg/day, given at four- to six-hour intervals intravenously, is the treatment of choice. If subsequent culture and sensitivity data indicate that the agent is sensitive to penicillin, therapy should be changed to penicillin G, as outlined for bacterial meningitis. Treatment should not be less than three weeks in duration, since exacerbations may occur following short-term treatment.

Surgical treatment is an essential part of management. If a significant effusion is present, or if pneumothorax develops, the fluid and air should be evacuated, and continuous closed waterseal drainage insti-

tuted. Close observation is necessary to ensure adequate function of the chest tube as
well as to anticipate the need for change in
tube placement or possible additional
drainage procedures.

Supportive care includes adequate fluids,
oxygen therapy and relief of abdominal distention. There is *no* indication that intrapleural instillation of antibiotics and enzymes or systemic treatment with steroids
is beneficial. In fact, the latter two measures
are contraindicated.

ACUTE EPIGLOTTITIS (BACTERIAL CROUP)

This infection involves primarily the
epiglottis and larynx, with resultant severe
inflammation and edema of the supraglottic
and infraglottic areas. The result is acute
airway obstruction, which may be sudden
and complete. This disease is to be distinguished from "viral croup," which tends to
be accompanied by less inflammation and
is more localized to the subglottic areas.
Viral croup is relatively common and generally more benign among infants and
children. It may occasionally resemble
bacterial epiglottitis clinically, however,
requiring similar treatment.

Etiological Agents

Hemophilus influenzae, type b, in nearly
all cases; occasionally beta-hemolytic streptococci, pneumococci or *Corynebacterium
diphtheriae.*

Clinical Manifestations

There is usually an abrupt onset, with
fever, inspiratory stridor and generalized
toxic conditions, pain on phonation or swallowing and drooling. Physical findings may
reveal aphonia or suppressed phonation
("mashed-potato voice"), cherry-red swollen epiglottis protruding over the base of
the tongue, swollen and tender neck and
prostration.

Diagnostic Procedures

Extreme caution must be taken with
regard to physical examination and obtaining of diagnostic specimens. Acute airway
obstruction may occur if the child is unduly
disturbed by repeated and traumatic procedures. Particularly dangerous maneuvers
include too vigorous or frequent examination of the pharynx, and throat swabs.
Throat swabbing should be postponed
until an adequate airway has been ensured.
A particularly valuable test is a blood culture, which is positive in more than 85 per
cent of cases and serves to firmly establish
the etiological diagnosis.

Treatment

Avoid excessive manipulation of the patient. Place the child in a position of comfort, preferably with the neck extended.
Administer mist, oxygen and antibiotics.
Ampicillin is the current drug of choice,
100 to 150 mg/kg/day intravenously or intramuscularly. Tracheostomy or careful na-
sotracheal intubation should be planned if
any progression occurs. It is preferable to
do this under controlled conditions in the
operating room, and it should be done
early rather than waiting for nearly complete obstruction to occur.

ACUTE HEMATOGENOUS OSTEOMYELITIS

Etiological Agents

Staphylococcus aureus in about 70 to 80
per cent of all cases; streptococcus,
Hemophilus influenzae, salmonella and
gonococcus are infrequently associated
with this disease in young children; tuberculosis may also cause a gradually progressive osteomyelitis. In patients with hemolytic diseases such as sickle cell anemia
salmonellae are frequently found.

Clinical Manifestations

Symptoms—fever, chills, prostration, pain
in affected area. Onset is frequently
abrupt.
Signs—*point tenderness* over the affected
area of bone is the single most important
sign. Swelling, redness and heat of affected extremity may also be present.

Anemia is frequent. Radiographs of the affected bones are usually negative early in the illness; positive radiographs are seen 10 to 14 days later.

Diagnostic Procedures

Blood culture. Aspiration and culture of affected area. Deeper aspiration or specific drainage may be indicated if the early clinical course does not show a satisfactory response.

Treatment

Antibiotics. Treatment is based upon identification of the causative agent. Because of the high frequency of *Staphylococcus*, methicillin is the usual drug of choice, with a course of therapy similar to that recommended for staphylococcal pneumonia.

Surgical management. Depending upon the severity of infection and duration of illness before diagnosis, aspiration or open drainage may be required. If the illness goes beyond three days without adequate treatment, the need for open drainage increases. The chance for subsequent development of chronic osteomyelitis also increases markedly after this time.

Other measures. Bedrest, splinting of the affected extremity for comfort, fluids and correction of anemia.

SEPTIC ARTHRITIS

The comments on osteomyelitis also generally apply to septic arthritis. The signs and symptoms are similar, with tenderness and swelling localized to a joint. Diagnosis may be established quickly by aspiration of the joint in question. Leukocytes may be 15,000 to 200,000/mm³, predominantly polymorphonuclear, and the joint fluid glucose value is usually less than half of the blood glucose value. The distribution of causative agents by age group is as follows:

Birth to one month—any of the agents noted for septicemia of the newborn.

One month to four years—*Hemophilus influenzae* is most common.

Over 4 years—*Staphylococcus aureus* is most common.

This age distribution is useful in selecting initial therapy when the organism is not yet determined. The following agents are suggested for inclusion in initial treatment, while waiting for culture results:

Birth to one month—Ampicillin and gentamicin.

One month to four years—Ampicillin and methicillin or nafcillin.

Over four years—methicillin or nafcillin.

In general, management is similar to that described for staphylococcal pneumonia. Needle aspiration or surgical drainage of the joint is sometimes necessary. Surgical drainage is mandatory for septic arthritis of the hip.

TUBERCULOSIS

Epidemiology

Tuberculosis is spread by airborne infection with droplet nuclei. Infections in patients with tuberculosis are not highly contagious, as are those in diseases such as measles, and close contact is necessary for infection. Since there are no animal carriers, tuberculosis in a child is usually the result of contact with a case of active tuberculosis in the home.

Tuberculosis case rates and death rates have been declining since 1890 (now less than 1 per 1000 per year), and the rate of decline has accelerated since the introduction of streptomycin and isoniazid. It is primarily a disease of adults, most often men over 45 years of age. Case rates are higher in non-whites. In childhood, case rates are relatively higher in the period from birth to three years of age and after 12 years of age.

A recent study showed that less than 5 per cent of naval recruits (males, aged 18 to 22) are tuberculin reactors. Most cases in the future will develop in those persons who have already been infected as the result of reactivation of an old infection. This is the predominant group toward which control measures should be directed.

Clinical Features

Most cases of *primary tuberculosis* in children are discovered by examination of the household contacts of adults with new, active cases of tuberculosis. Most children who are infected simply have a positive tuberculin reaction. A small number of these have active pulmonary lesions, which may be hilar node enlargement with or without pneumonia. A few infected children suffer systemic disease, either miliary, meningeal or osseous.

Most children with active tuberculosis have few symptoms, and only those with systemic infections or pleural effusions are likely to be admitted to a hospital.

Tuberculous cervical adenitis or scrofula in this country is most often the result of infection with atypical myobacteria and not tubercle bacilli.

Progressive primary tuberculosis is rare and occurs when the primary infection does not heal, but progresses to cavity formation. Patients are acutely ill and may require hospitalization for several months.

Tuberculous meningitis is thought to result from rupture of a cortical focus of infection into the cerebrospinal fluid. Initially, patients have only non-specific signs of fever, irritability or apathy. In a few days, untreated patients suffer headache, vomiting, stiff neck and other signs of meningitis. The final stage of the disease is one of deepening coma that without treatment ends in death.

Miliary tuberculosis is the result of an acute hematogenous spread of tubercle bacilli throughout the body. Onset may be insidious or abrupt. Patients have fever and often roentgenographic signs of primary tuberculosis. The characteristic miliary appearance of the chest roentgenogram may not be apparent for several days after the onset of fever. Many patients develop tuberculous meningitis.

Tuberculous pleurisy may be either the result of direct extension of infection from the lung into the pleural space or a manifestation of hypersensitivity to tubercle bacilli. Most often, tubercle bacilli cannot be recovered from the pleural fluid. Onset may be abrupt, with chest pain and fever, or insidious, with only shortness of breath. Patients who have a pleural effusion and a positive tuberculin test result should be treated as if they have tuberculosis.

Tuberculosis may infect virtually any *bone or joint* in the body. Infection of the lower thoracic vertebrae may lead to collapse of the vertebrae and kyphosis. Extension of infection in the bones to surrounding soft tissue produces a cold abscess.

Diagnosis

Isolation of the organism from children with tuberculosis is difficult. Organisms are more often isolated from children with miliary, meningeal or lymph node infections than from those with primary infection. In primary pulmonary infections in children, three early morning gastric aspirates are preferred for culture. In general, the diagnosis of tuberculosis in childhood is most often based on a tuberculin test, a chest radiograph and examination of household contacts.

More than 95 per cent of patients with active tuberculosis react to a tuberculin test. The intermediate strength PPD (purified protein derivative) is the diagnostic agent of choice. The antigen is injected intracutaneously to form a wheal, and the reaction is measured after 48 or 72 hours. Any erythema is disregarded, and the transverse diameter of the induration is measured and recorded in millimeters. More than 80 per cent of patients with tuberculosis have tuberculin reactions of 10 mm or greater. Many small reactions, from 5 to 10 mm, are a result of infections due to atypical mycobacteria. Atypical mycobacterial infections vary widely in prevalence in this country and are most frequent in the southeastern United States. Either for technical reasons or because of serious illness, the tuberculin reaction may occasionally be falsely negative.

Radiographs of children with tuberculosis most often show hilar adenopathy, occasionally associated with pneumonia or pleural adhesions. Calcification is sometimes the result of a tuberculous infection, but more often in the United States, pulmonary calcification is a result of histoplasmosis.

Treatment

Drug treatment is recommended for all children with active tuberculosis, all children with recent conversion of skin tests to positive, all children under the age of five with positive skin test results and all household contacts of a person with an active case of tuberculosis. Isoniazid is the drug of choice in a dose of 5 to 15 mg/kg/day. Patients with systemic tuberculosis often receive a larger dose of isoniazid in combination with other drugs, such as para-aminosalicylic acid (PAS); in severe cases, a third drug is also usually added (ethambutol, rifampin or streptomycin).

Prevention

Isoniazid prophylaxis is highly effective. All persons known to be at high risk of active disease should receive isoniazid prophylactically for one year. These include household contacts of persons with new, active cases, recent tuberculin skin test converters, persons with positive tuberculin reactions and pulmonary abnormalities, diabetics with positive skin test results and tuberculin reactors who are malnourished.

Except for rare cases of progressive primary tuberculosis, children with tuberculosis do not have contagious infection. Thus little will be gained in preventing the spread of tuberculosis by treating only children. On the other hand, the household contacts of children with tuberculosis or with tuberculin reactions often have active tuberculosis.

Health departments commonly have well-organized tuberculosis control programs and will assist in treating patients, giving prophylactic isoniazid and examining contacts.

ACUTE INFECTIOUS DIARRHEA

Although diarrhea is a common problem among infants and young children, a specific bacterial pathogen is isolated from the stool in only 10 to 30 per cent of cases. The commonly recognized viruses, such as enteroviruses and adenoviruses, have *not* proved to be significant causes of diarrhea, although loose stools are sometimes associated with syndromes caused by these agents. The viral agents most commonly associated with diarrhea cannot be isolated in the laboratory with present methods. Their presence can be demonstrated by challenge of human volunteers with stool filtrates, or by immune electron microscopy of diarrheal stools.

The primary aim in treatment of all patients with diarrhea is to provide appropriate fluid and electrolyte replacement until the acute illness has spontaneously subsided. Worldwide, infectious diarrhea remains a major cause of death, particularly among infants.

Bacterial Agents

Shigella. Four basic serogroups of *Shigella* are important to man. Of these, groups B, C and D are most commonly associated with disease in children, and only rarely do they invade beyond the intestinal tract. Group A (Shiga or *dysenteriae*) occasionally causes serious extraintestinal disease, but it is rare in the United States. Shigellosis is characterized by frequent bloody, liquid stools, and polymorphonuclear leukocytes can be seen on a smear of the stool. In addition, fever, generalized convulsions and a predominance of band forms in the peripheral blood smear are often seen.

Antibiotic treatment is recommended *only* if the patient is in the acute phase of illness. Ampicillin, orally or intramuscularly, for four or five days will shorten the duration of the acute illness, if the organisms are sensitive. In ampicillin-resistant shigella infections, absorbable antimicrobials, such as nalidixic acid, chloramphenicol or tetracyclines, may be useful, but the benefits of therapy must be carefully weighed against the potential toxicities of these drugs.

Salmonella. Extraintestinal spread of salmonella can occur, particularly in patients with hemolytic diseases, gastrointestinal tract disease or immunological defects. Nevertheless, salmonella infections are generally localized to the gastrointestinal tract and tend to be self-limited.

Antibiotic treatment of salmonella infections limited to the gastrointestinal tract is *not* generally advised. Such therapy prolongs the duration of the carrier state and also promotes development of multiple drug-resistant strains, without providing symptomatic relief to the patient.

Enteropathogenic E. coli. Ten different serotypes of *E. coli* are recognized that have particular pathogenicity for the gastrointestinal tract in young infants. They are potentially highly contagious, especially in the hospital environment, and strict isolation must be enforced. These enteropathogenic *E. coli* are primarily pathogens for infants under one year of age; after two years of age they appear to cause less significant disease in the host. It is now recognized that many other different strains of *E. coli*, as well as other Enterobacteriaceae, are capable of developing enteropathogenicity similar to those "classical" serotypes. The pathogenicity is primarily due to elaboration of enterotoxins, a trait mediated by extrachromosomal plasmids (R factors). Many such strains are responsible for a large share of cases of "traveler's diarrhea." In proved cases in infants, treatment with either oral neomycin or colistin is recommended, usually for three to four days. The diarrheal disease in infants may be protracted, smoldering over several weeks, and resumption of oral feedings may require exclusion of disaccharide-containing formula during the convalescent phase.

Other causes. Overgrowth of flora, such as *Staphylococcus* or *Candida albicans,* can cause diarrhea on occasion. In general, this is related to broad-spectrum antibiotic use; the best treatment is removal of the antibiotic. Cholera, though not a serious problem in this country, should be considered in the differential diagnosis of patients living in Southeast Asia and the Middle East nations.

causes of malabsorption syndromes, and then examining duodenal contents or duodenal or jejunal biopsy material for presence of the parasite.

Acute gastroenteritis. Acute illness involving the upper and lower gastrointestinal tracts may present primarily with diarrhea, or vomiting may predominate. One of the most common causes of acute gastroenteritis is viral, particularly reovirus-like agents. The incubation period is short, usually less than 48 hours, and explosive outbreaks may be seen, especially during the winter and early spring. The illness is brief, usually lasting two to six days.

The differential diagnosis of acute gastroenteritis includes agents associated with "food poisoning." Staphylococcal food poisoning, with onset usually within one to six hours after ingestion of contaminated food, is one of the most common. *Clostridium perfringens* food poisoning can occur similarly and usually has an onset within 8 to 24 hours after ingestion, salmonella food poisoning occurs within 8 to 48 hours after ingestion and shigella has an incubation period of one to four days. These agents can often be suspected on epidemiological grounds, particularly when there are several or many cases occurring at one time and related to a common food source.

Other agents include various metallic toxins such as cadmium, which can cause acute vomiting and diarrhea within an hour after ingestion of such contaminated liquids as lemonade that have been stored in metallic containers.

Parasitic Diseases

Amebiasis. This disease may resemble acute shigellosis, presenting occasionally with acute bloody diarrhea. One differential point is that a smear of the stool reveals a preponderance of mononuclear cells rather than the polymorphonuclear leukocytes seen in shigellosis. Confirmation of the diagnosis is made by examination of fresh warm feces for trophozoites.

Giardiasis. *Giardia* infection of the duodenum and jejunum has been occasionally associated with diarrhea, abdominal cramps and weight loss. The illness tends to be mild and chronic. Usually the diagnosis is made only after ruling out other

REFERENCES

Ceruti, E., Contreras, J., and Neira, M.: Staphylococcal pneumonia in childhood. Am. J. Dis. Child., *122*:386, 1971.

Davis, S. D., and Ostrow, J. H.: Tuberculosis and diseases due to atypical mycobacteria. *In Brennemann's Practice of Pediatrics*, Vol. II, Chap. 9B, New York, Harper and Row, 1973.

Dick, V. Q., Nelson, J. D., and Haltalin, K. C.: Osteomyelitis in infants and children. Am. J. Dis. Child., *129*:1273, 1975.

Dupont, H. L., and Hornick, R. B.: Clinical approach to infectious diarrhea. Medicine, 52:265, 1973.

Gerard, P., Moriau, M., Bachy, A., Malvaux, P., and DeMeyer, R.: Meningococcal purpura: Report of 19 patients treated with heparin. J. Pediatr., 82:780, 1973.

Goldenberg, D. L., and Cohen, A. S.: Acute infectious arthritis. A review of patients with nongonococcal joint infections. Am. J. Med., *60*:369, 1976.

Gotoff, S. P., and Behrman, R. E.: Neonatal septice-
    mia. J. Pediatr., 76:142, 1970.
Johnson, G. K., Sullivan, J. L., and Bishop, L. A.:
    Acute epiglottitis. Review of 55 cases and
    suggested protocol. Arch. Otolaryngol., 100:333,
    1974.
Lincoln, E. M., and Sewell, E. M.: *Tuberculosis in
    Children.* New York, McGraw-Hill Book Co., Inc.,
    1963.

Mathies, A. W., Jr., and Wehrle, P. F.: Management of
    bacterial meningitis in children. Pediatr. Clin. N.
    Am., 15:185, 1968.
Riley, H. D.: Neonatal meningitis. J. Infect. Dis.,
    125:420, 1972.
Shubin, H., and Weil, M. H.: Bacterial shock.
    J.A.M.A., 235:421, 1976.
Smith, D. H., *et al.*: Bacterial meningitis. A sympo-
    sium. Pediatrics, 52:586, 1973.

PART V

IMMUNOLOGICAL-ALLERGIC DISORDERS

17

Immunological Disorders

E. Richard Stiehm

Introduction

Disorders of the immune system can result from deficient, excess or abnormal immune function. The latter two are discussed in the chapters on allergy and collagen diseases. This chapter considers disorders involving diminished function of the immune system; these are termed the *immunodeficiency disorders* and are characterized by undue susceptibility to infection.

A common and vexing problem is the child with "too many infections." This can mean (1) too frequent infections, (2) too severe infections, (3) too prolonged infections, (4) infections without a symptom-free period, (5) infections with unusual or severe complications and (6) infections with organisms of low pathogenicity. Often the patient has a combination of problems.

Disorders that result in undue susceptibility to infection are noted in Table 17–1.

An important clue to the etiology is the nature of the infection. Infection occurring at one site or involving the same organism is often due to obstruction, poor circulation or skin breakage. By contrast, infections with systemic immunodeficiency occur at multiple sites and with many different organisms. Thus, most of the disorders listed in Table 17–1 can be excluded by a careful history.

The immunodeficiency disorders are divided into primary and secondary immunodeficiencies; the latter are considerably more common. Secondary immunodeficiencies result when there is interference with immune function as a result of some unrelated systemic illness. These are common; indeed nearly every serious illness interferes with the function of the immune system to some degree. Thus, patients with viral disease, leukemia, renal disease and malnutrition, for example, are at increased risk of developing infection. Newborn in-

TABLE 17–1 DISORDERS WITH INCREASED SUSCEPTIBILITY TO INFECTION

Type of Disorder	Conditions
Circulatory disorders	Sickle cell disease, diabetes, nephrosis, varicose veins
Obstructive disorders	Ureteral or urethral stenosis, bronchial asthma, allergic rhinitis, blocked eustachian tubes, lung foreign body, cystic fibrosis
Integument defects	Eczema, burns, skull fracture, midline sinus tracts
Disorders with unusual microbiological factors	Antibiotic overgrowth, chronic infection with resistant organism, continuous reinfection (water supply, infectious contact)
Secondary immunodeficiencies	Malnutrition, prematurity, lymphoma, splenectomy, uremia, immunosuppressive therapy, protein-losing enteropathy
Primary immunodeficiencies	Cellular immunodeficiencies, antibody immunodeficiencies, phagocytic immunodeficiencies, complement immunodeficiencies

fants are particularly affected; infection is liable to be rapid, silent, severe and often fatal. The procedures used to evaluate patients with primary immunodeficiency are also of value in determining the type and extent of secondary immunodeficiency.

CLASSIFICATION OF THE PRIMARY IMMUNODEFICIENCIES

The primary immunodeficiencies are disorders characterized by intrinsic defects in the immune system, leading to increased susceptibility to infection. Most are congenital; many are hereditary. The first recorded case was in 1952, when Colonel Bruton found that an eight-year-old boy with recurrent pneumococcal infections did not have a gamma globulin fraction on electrophoretic analysis of his serum. This patient had X-linked agammaglobulinemia. In 1958 it was noted that some agammaglobulinemic patients had lymphopenia and a more fulminant course; these patients had combined immunodeficiency. In the 1960's, the clinical description of most of the disorders was completed. In 1968, the first bone marrow transplantation for combined immunodeficiency was accomplished.

The primary immunodeficiencies and their relative frequencies are conveniently divided into B cell or antibody defects (50 per cent), T cell or cell-mediated immune defects (15 per cent), combined B and T cell defects (28 per cent), phagocytic defects (5 per cent) and complement or opsonic defects (2 per cent).

The B cell immunodeficiencies are characterized by antibody deficiency without other immunological defects. The onset of problems is usually about six months, when transplacental maternal antibody diminishes. Respiratory infections involving gram-positive organisms are common. Diminished lymphatic tissue throughout the body is noted. There are decreased levels of one or more immunoglobulins and poor or no antibody activity. In some of these disorders, B cells are absent (e.g., X-linked agammaglobulinemia) but in others, B cells are present but do not differentiate into antibody-secreting plasma cells. Others, notably common variable immunodeficiency, have T cells that suppress B cell synthesis of immunoglobulins.

The combined B and T cell immunodeficiencies are the second largest group of immunodeficiencies. These are a heterogeneous group, of which many are hereditary syndromes. Most have thymus abnormalities. They are characterized by onset, within the first few postnatal months, of chronic diarrhea, thrush and chronic respiratory infections.

Patients with isolated T cell defects have normal or near normal immunoglobulin levels and thus are usually not as ill as patients with combined defects. Lymphopenia, cutaneous anergy and decreased lymph nodes and tonsils are characteristic features.

The phagocytic immunodeficiencies include granulocyte and monocyte defects of motility, phagocytosis or intracellular killing of bacteria. These illnesses are characterized by increased susceptibility to infection, intact B and T cell function, hypergammaglobulinemia and lymphadenopathy.

The complement immunodeficiencies are characterized by recurrent bacterial infections, generally of a less severe degree than the others. T cell, B cell and phagocytic functions are intact, but their serum does not support complement-dependent functions such as opsonification and chemotactic factor generation.

CLINICAL MANIFESTATIONS

The primary immunodeficiencies usually are manifested by recurrent upper respiratory infections, severe bacterial infections and failure to thrive (Table 17–2). Remember that normal children often have six to eight colds per year, and this is increased when they are exposed to older school-age siblings or classmates. In the immunologically normal child, however, the respiratory infections are usually mild, lasting only a few days without prolonged fever. Further, the normal child recovers completely between infections. When respiratory infections occur repeatedly as the sole infectious manifestation, allergy should be suspected. Allergic disorders are also characterized by absence of fever, clear non-purulent discharge, prior history of colic, food intolerance, or eczema, a positive family history for allergy, a characteristic seasonal or exposure pattern, a poor

TABLE 17-2 CLINICAL FEATURES IN PRIMARY IMMUNODEFICIENCIES

Usually Present and Highly Suspicious
Recurrent upper respiratory infection
Repeated severe bacterial infections (e.g., pneumonia, meningitis, sepsis)
Failure to thrive

Frequently Present and Moderately Suspicious
Chronic diarrhea
Draining ears
Skin lesions (e.g., rash, pyoderma, alopecia, eczema, telangiectasia)
Thrush
Pneumocystis carinii infection
Malabsorption
Bronchiectasis
Paucity of lymph nodes and tonsils

Occasionally Present and Somewhat Suspicious
Conjunctivitis
Lymphadenopathy
Hepatosplenomegaly
Severe viral disease
Arthritis
Hematological abnormalities (e.g., leukocytosis, leukopenia, thrombocytopenia, hemolytic anemia)

response to antibiotics and a good response to antihistamines or bronchodilators.

Serious bacterial infections such as pneumonia, septicemia, osteomyelitis or meningitis are common with immunodeficiency. While immunologically normal children may have one such episode, repeated episodes should alert the physician to a possible immunodeficiency. Chronic diarrhea is another feature often noted with immunodeficiency. This is often associated with poor weight gain and delayed development. The active, robust child climbing all over the doctor's office is an unlikely candidate for a host defense problem.

A careful history is imperative in all such patients. The birth history should be explored for maternal illness, duration of gestation, birth weight and neonatal illness. The immunization record should be obtained, since a normal response to live virus vaccines generally indicates intact cellular immunity. Family history of consanguinity, early infant deaths and unusual susceptibility to infection, collagen diseases or allergic diseases should be sought. The response of infections to antibiotics, allergy treatment or gamma globulin therapy should be elicited.

Physical examination may yield important clues. Patients having immunodeficiency generally appear chronically ill,

with pallor, irritability, poor subcutaneous fat and a distended abdomen. Skin disorders such as pyoderma, eczema, petechiae, alopecia and macular rashes may be noted. Cervical nodes may be absent despite a history of recurrent throat infections. In certain immunodeficiencies, however, the nodes may be enlarged and suppurative. The tympanic membranes are often scarred or perforated, and purulent ear drainage may be present. Thrush and mouth ulcers are common. The tonsils may be atrophic and appear to have been surgically removed. There is often deep cough, chest rattle, rales or wheezing. The liver and spleen are frequently enlarged. There may be excoriation around the anus as a result of chronic diarrhea. Paronychia may be present.

LABORATORY INVESTIGATIONS

A precise diagnosis of immunodeficiency generally necessitates special laboratory procedures. A recommended initial laboratory screen for suspected immunodeficiency is shown in Table 17-3. A total lymphocyte count of less than 1500/mm³ indicates lymphopenia and is frequently associated with cellular immunodeficiency. Quantitative analysis of immunoglobulins (IgG, IgM and IgA) is recommended as the initial step rather than serum electrophoresis or immunoelectrophoresis, since these must be done eventually in any instance. Levels obtained must be compared with age-matched controls (Table 17-4), since marked variations occur with age, particularly in the first year of life. In general, an IgG level less than 200 mg/100 ml

TABLE 17-3 INITIAL SCREENING TESTS FOR IMMUNODEFICIENCY

Blood Count: Hemoglobin, white blood count, lymphocyte morphology, differential count, platelet estimation or count

Quantitative Immune Globulins: IgG, IgM and IgA

Schick Test or Polio Titers: for IgG function

Isoagglutinin Titer: Anti-A and Anti-B; for IgM function

Infection Evaluation: Erythrocyte sedimentation rate, appropriate cultures, appropriate x-rays

TABLE 17–4   LEVELS OF IMMUNOGLOBULINS IN SERA OF
NORMAL SUBJECTS, BY AGE*

Age	IgG mg./100 ml.	IgG Per Cent of Adult Level	IgM mg./100 ml.	IgM Per Cent of Adult Level	IgA mg./100 ml.	IgA Per Cent of Adult Level	Total Immunoglobulin mg./100 ml.	Total Immunoglobulin Per Cent of Adult Level
Newborn	1031 ± 200†	89 ± 17	11 ± 5	11 ± 5	2 ± 3	1 ± 2	1044 ± 201	67 ± 13
1–3 mo.	430 ± 119	37 ± 10	30 ± 11	30 ± 11	21 ± 13	11 ± 7	481 ± 127	31 ± 9
4–6 mo.	427 ± 186	37 ± 16	43 ± 17	43 ± 17	28 ± 18	14 ± 9	498 ± 204	32 ± 13
7–12 mo.	661 ± 219	58 ± 19	54 ± 23	55 ± 23	37 ± 18	19 ± 9	752 ± 242	48 ± 15
13–24 mo.	762 ± 209	66 ± 18	58 ± 23	59 ± 23	50 ± 24	25 ± 12	870 ± 258	56 ± 16
25–36 mo.	892 ± 183	77 ± 16	61 ± 19	62 ± 19	71 ± 37	36 ± 19	1021 ± 205	65 ± 14
3–5 yr.	929 ± 228	80 ± 20	56 ± 18	57 ± 18	93 ± 27	47 ± 14	1078 ± 245	69 ± 17
6–8 yr.	923 ± 256	80 ± 22	65 ± 25	66 ± 25	124 ± 45	62 ± 23	1112 ± 293	71 ± 20
9–11 yr.	1124 ± 235	97 ± 20	79 ± 33	80 ± 33	131 ± 60	66 ± 30	1334 ± 254	85 ± 17
12–16 yr.	946 ± 124	82 ± 11	59 ± 20	60 ± 20	148 ± 63	74 ± 32	1153 ± 169	71 ± 12
Adults	1158 ± 305	100 ± 26	99 ± 27	100 ± 27	200 ± 61	100 ± 31	1457 ± 353	100 ± 24

*The values were derived from measurements made in 296 normal children and 30 adults. Levels were determined by the radial diffusion technique, using specific rabbit antisera to human immunoglobulins. (From Stiehm, E. R., and Fudenberg, H. H.: Serum levels of immune globulins in health and disease: A survey. Pediatrics, 37:715, 1966 with permission.)
†One standard deviation.

or a total Ig (IgG+IgM+IgA) of less than 400 mg/100 ml indicates clinically significant antibody deficiency. Tests of antibody levels measure the functional capacity of the B-cell system. Isoagglutinin titers, poliomyelitis, antibody titers, Schick test or diphtheria or tetanus antitoxin levels can be used for this purpose. Isoagglutinins (anti A, anti B) primarily measure IgM function, while the others measure IgG function. Finally, the presence of chronic infection can be suspected by an elevated erythrocyte sedimentation rate and documented by cultures or roentgenograms. If

TABLE 17–5   LABORATORY EVALUATION OF B CELL IMMUNODEFICIENCIES

Initial Tests
Ig levels—IgG, IgM, IgA
Isoagglutinin titer
Schick test*
Polio antibody titer

Advanced Tests
B Cell enumeration (by immunofluorescence or EA or EAC rosettes)
IgE, IgD levels
Pre-existing antibody levels (diphtheria, streptolysin O)
Antibody response to injected antigens (e.g., typhoid)
Lymph node or rectal biopsy
Lateral pharyngeal x-ray
Immunoglobulin survival
Immunoglobulin and antibodies in secretions
IgG subclass determinations
Suppressor T Cell activity

*Antigen may not be available.

these screening tests are normal, immunodeficiency is usually excluded. Only if the history is unusually suggestive of immunodeficiency is further laboratory evaluation indicated.

Tests for Antibody Immunodeficiencies

Further evaluation for antibody deficiency is indicated (Table 17–5) if the antibody screening tests are abnormal. B lymphocyte enumeration, either by immunofluorescent study for surface immunoglobulin or by sheep red cell rosette procedures for Fc or C3 membrane receptors, should be done.* Both the percentage and absolute numbers of B cells should be recorded. Very low numbers of B cells are usually indicative of a profound B cell deficit, notably congenital X-linked agammaglobulinemia. Most antibody deficiencies have normal quantities of peripheral B cells, however, despite absence of serum immunoglobulins. IgD and IgE level tests, the latter the reaginic antibody, are next performed. Several syndromes have im-

*B lymphocytes, which make up 10 to 15 per cent of the peripheral lymphocytes, are the precursor cells for the antibody-secreting plasma cells and are characterized by the presence of bound immunoglobulin on their surface membrane. Since B lymphocytes also have surface receptors for the Fc portion of immunoglobulin and C3 complement component, they form rosettes with antibody coated erythrocytes or antibody-complement coated erythrocytes.

munoglobulin imbalance, usually with selective elevations of IgM or IgE. The functional capacity of the antibody system is
next explored, by measuring either pre-existing antibodies or the response to antigenic challenge. The antibody response
to typhoid antigens, typhoid H for IgG and
typhoid O for IgM, are readily available for
this purpose.

A lymph node biopsy is of value, especially when the diagnosis is equivocal or
when there is lymphadenopathy. A biopsy
should be performed after local antigenic
stimulation. A diphtheria-pertussis-tetanus
(DPT) or typhoid shot is given in the anterior thigh, and an inguinal node is obtained from that side five to seven days
later. Structures examined include the
thymic-dependent paracortical area, the
medullary plasma cells and the cortical germinal follicles. B cell defects show decreased plasma cells and follicles, cellular
disorganization, thin cortex and absence of
germinal centers. The rectal mucosa is the
preferred biopsy site of some investigators;
submucosal plasma cells are deficient in
many antibody deficiencies. A lateral
roentgenogram of the pharynx may show a
marked decrease in adenoidal tissue, indicative of poor lymphoid development.

Immunoglobulin survival studies are of
value when there is a suspicion that immunoglobulin is being lost through the gastrointestinal tract. Purified immunoglobulin, usually IgG, is trace-labeled with
iodine-131, injected intravenously, and then
the catabolic rate is determined. A short-
ened half-life (the normal IgG half-life is
25 days) indicates abnormal breakdown or
loss.

Immunoglobulin levels in the secretions
tend to parallel levels in the serum; serum
IgA deficiency is nearly always accompanied by secretory IgA deficiency. Selective
secretory immunoglobulin deficiency is exceedingly rare, but since secretory IgA is
not identical to serum IgA, it can occur.
Measurement of immunoglobulin and antibodies in secretions is hampered by low
levels, variable concentrations and lack of
normal values for each secretion. The nasal
fluid, obtained after saline instillation, is
the most common secretion analyzed, but
tears and saliva are also used.

Selective deficiency of one of the serum
IgG subclasses (IgG1, IgG2, IgG3, IgG4)

may occur in rare instances. Specific antisera for quantitative analysis of subclasses
is available in only a few laboratories.
These studies are indicated in patients
with proven antibody deficiency but normal or near normal IgG levels.

T lymphocytes that inhibit Ig synthesis
of normal B cells have been demonstrated
in common variable immunodeficiency.
Such studies illustrate the interaction of
various cells of the immune system and are
of use in defining the pathogenesis of the
disorder.

Tests for Cellular Immunodeficiencies

Initial studies of cellular (T lymphocyte)
immunodeficiencies include the absolute
lymphocyte count, lymphocyte morphology, thymus size estimation and delayed
hypersensitivity skin tests (Table 17–6). A
chest roentgenogram (posteroanterior and
lateral) for thymus size should be done in
all patients suspected of immunodeficiency, since many syndromes are associated with absent or dysplastic thymus
glands. Normally, the thymus is readily
visualized in the newborn; thus an absent
thymic shadow is particularly significant at
this age. Positive delayed hypersensitivity
skin tests usually exclude cellular immunodeficiency. Since these depend on prior antigenic exposure, several antigens are used
to increase the likelihood of a positive reaction. Positive reactions will occur to strep-
tokinase-streptodornase (SK-SD) and candida without deliberate antigenic exposure, while tuberculin, mumps, and
tetanus toxoid responses will occur only

TABLE 17–6 LABORATORY EVALUATION
OF T CELL IMMUNODEFICIENCIES

Initial Tests
  Lymphocyte count and morphology
  Thymic x-ray
  Skin tests (SK-SD, candida, PPD, mumps, PHA,
    tetanus toxoid)

Advanced Tests
  T Cell enumeration (E rosettes)
  Lymphocyte proliferative responses to PHA, allo-
    geneic cells, or antigens
  Mediator assays (MIF, LT)
  Cytotoxicity assays
  Lymph node biopsy
  Adenosine deaminase, phosphorylase assays

after disease or immunization. In the immunologically normal child who is one year or older, one or more of these skin tests should be positive. Immunologically normal infants less than one year old may have negative skin test results to these antigens because of lack of sensitization. In an immunologically normal infant with a history of thrush, however, the candida skin test should be positive.

The most valuable advanced test for cellular immunodeficiency is T lymphocyte enumeration; this is accomplished by measuring the percentage of isolated peripheral lymphocytes that form rosettes with sheep erythrocytes (E rosettes). Normally 60 to 70 per cent of peripheral lymphocytes will undergo this reaction. In most, but not all, cellular immunodeficiencies, T cells are markedly reduced, both in the percentage and the absolute number.

The proliferative ability of isolated lymphocytes is another valuable test for cellular immunodeficiency. A standard quantity of a mitogen, such as phytohemagglutinin or conconavalin, or an antigen, such as candida or PPD, or mitomycin-treated human lymphocytes is added to a certain number of the patient's isolated lymphocytes and incubated for several days. The culture is pulsed with radioactive thymidine (a DNA precursor) at 48 to 96 hours and the culture continued for 16 more hours. The lymphocyte DNA is separated by filtration or precipitation and its radioactivity determined. The amount of radioactive thymidine incorporated is an estimate of lymphocyte proliferation. Results are generally expressed as a ratio of counts in stimulated cultures to those in unstimulated cultures. Absent or subnormal proliferative responses to mitogens or lymphocytes are regularly seen in severe cellular immunodeficiencies, but this test is often less sensitive than T cell enumeration in detecting subtle or incomplete defects. The absence of a proliferative response to an antigen such as candida in the presence of chronic candida infection indicates a specific cellular immune defect to that antigen.

Another way to study lymphocyte function is to measure the ability of stimulated lymphocytes to synthesize soluble mediators. The two most commonly measured are macrophage migratory inhibitor factor (MIF) and lymphotoxin (LT). In these procedures, supernatants of antigen-stimulated lymphocytes are tested for their ability to inhibit migration of guinea-pig macrophages (MIF) or their ability to kill radiolabeled target cells (LT). Other mediators include chemotactic factor, interferon and transfer factor.

The ability of isolated lymphocytes to kill a target cell (usually a tumor cell line adapted for long-term growth) measures another important cellular immune function, cytotoxicity. If the target cell line is infected with a virus, such assays can be used to measure specific cellular immunity to viruses. Generally the target cell is labeled with ^{51}Cr, and the amount of ^{51}Cr released when the target cells are exposed to test lymphocytes is used as measure of cytotoxicity.

A lymph node biopsy is done in cellular immunodeficiency when the diagnosis is not established or malignancy is suspected. Biopsied nodes show lymphocyte depletion in the deep cortical regions, disorganized structure and histiocytic hypertrophy. Plasma cells may or may not be present.

Tests for Phagocytic Immunodeficiencies

Phagocytic and opsonic deficiencies must be suspected when tests for antibody and cellular immunodeficiency do not provide an adequate explanation for the severity of the child's infections.

Initial tests include the total leukocyte count and the differential and morphological appearance of the granulocytes. White blood cell counts persistently greater than 12,000 or less than 4000 are abnormal. Persistent leukopenia, leukocytosis, unusual vacuolization or the presence of myelocytes in the peripheral blood is an indication for bone marrow aspiration. Another early test is the nitroblue tetrazolium (NBT) dye reduction for chronic granulomatous disease (CGD). Normal leukocytes undergoing phagocytic activity reduce the colorless NBT dye to a deep purple that can be identified visually, microscopically or spectrophotometrically. Deficient dye reduction is characteristic of CGD of childhood.

Advanced tests include the Rebuck skin window, which assesses the morphology and function of inflammatory cells. The skin is superficially abraded with a scalpel, and cover slips are placed over the abrasion sites and changed at intervals over 24 hours. Polymorphs normally appear promptly and are replaced by mononuclear cells within 12 hours.

The most definitive test is quantitative phagocytosis and killing, using isolated leukocytes, opsonin and bacteria. These are incubated at 37° C and agitated for 120 minutes. Aliquots are removed for bacterial counts at the start and every 30 minutes. Leukocytes from a normal subject can phagocytize and kill 95 per cent of the bacteria within 120 minutes. If complete killing has not occurred, the location of the bacteria (within the leukocyte or outside the leukocyte) will determine whether there is a defect in killing or phagocytosis. If a defect exists, leukocyte enzyme determinations will indicate whether or not a specific enzyme deficiency exists.

Leukocyte movement, both directed (chemotaxis) or random, can be assessed, using migration through a millipore filter or agarose gel. Defects in directed and non-directed movement have been identified in several immunodeficiencies, including Job syndrome and the lazy leukocyte syndrome.

Tests for Complement Immunodeficiencies

Initial tests for complement defects include serum levels of C3, C4 and a total hemolytic complement (CH_{50}) titration. CH_{50} will be low or absent in C1, C2, C3, C4 or C6 deficiency. More advanced tests assess individual component levels by hemolytic assays or by immunochemical means. Tests of complement function include the ability of the serum to support phagocytosis of certain organisms (opsonins) or to generate chemotactic factor.

An evaluation of the alternate pathway of complement activation is occasionally indicated. This can be done by a hemolytic assay, using rabbit erythrocytes, or by immunochemical determination of components of this pathway (properdin, Factor B); these are reduced in proportion to the degree of activation.

MANAGEMENT

Prevention of the primary immunodeficiencies can be accomplished only rarely, as the heterozygote state cannot be recognized. Parents of an affected child can be counseled about the likelihood of having another child affected. It is possible to identify an infant who will have severe combined immunodeficiency and adenosine deaminase (ADA) deficiency by enzyme determinations of cultured cells obtained at amniocentesis. Therapeutic abortion could then be performed. Mothers who have had one child with ADA deficiency and are pregnant again should have such a determination done.

General treatment of immunodeficiency disorders includes maintenance of general health and nutrition, prevention and managment of emotional problems and management of their numerous infections. This includes limiting unnecessary exposure to infections, good general diet, maintenance of good dental hygiene and giving appropriate immunizations (as noted later). The complications of chronic infection such as draining ears, sinusitis, chronic bronchitis and bronchiectasis should be managed as in other patients. Special problems such as hearing loss, the need for tutors to make up for school absences and financial help for the family must be anticipated.

Antibiotics are lifesavers in the treatment of patients with immunodeficiency. Because these patients may succumb rapidly to infection, fevers or other signs of infection must be assumed to be secondary to bacterial infection, and antibiotic therapy should best be initiated immediately. Appropriate cultures are obtained prior to therapy. Continuous antibiotic therapy is of value in the management of some patients.

Special precautions must be observed, particularly in patients with cellular immunodeficiency. These patients should not receive live vaccines (nor should their families), because of the risk of vaccine-induced infection. They should not receive unirradiated whole blood or blood products, because of the risk of grafting with non-compatible lymphocytes and a graft-*versus*-host reaction.

Specific therapy for most of the antibody deficiencies is periodic injection of human immune serum globulin (gamma globulin). Gamma globulin must be given at least monthly, by the intramuscular route (severe reactions have resulted from intravenous administration) and in large doses (.7 ml/kg). Plasma and intravenous gamma globulin preparations are alternatives to gamma globulin injections.

Specific therapy for the cellular immunodeficiencies is complex. Bone marrow transplantation from a histocompatible sibling (or rarely another relative) has successfully reconstituted about 30 patients with severe combined immunodeficiency; their profound cellular immunodeficiency permits grafting without immunosuppression.

Fetal thymus transplantation has restored cellular immunity to several patients with DiGeorge syndrome. Thymus transplantation (either fetal or cultured adult thymus) and fetal liver transplantation have also occasionally been successful in severe combined immunodeficiency (SCID) when a donor is unavailable.

Other approaches to restoration of cellular immunity include transfer factor (an extract of immune lymphocytes), thymosin (a hormone from bovine thymus), and ADA-positive human erythrocytes (in a patient with SCID and ADA deficiency). None of these therapies has resulted in the dramatic permanent restoration of immunity such as that associated with bone marrow transplantation.

Specific therapy of phagocytic disorders includes the periodic use of normal granulocyte infusions, particularly to heal an indolent infection. Continuous use of sulfamethoxazole trimethoprim has recently been reported to be of specific benefit in chronic granulomatous disease.

Specific therapy of complement immunodeficiencies consists of the periodic infusion of fresh frozen plasma. Since complement components are relatively short-lived, weekly infusions are necessary.

Complications of the immunodeficiencies are chiefly a result of chronic infection, and include sinusitis, mastoiditis and bronchiectasis. Some of these disorders are associated, however, with an undue susceptibility to malignancy (the cellular immunodeficiencies), autoimmune disease (selective IgA deficiency) or bleeding (Wiskott-Aldrich syndrome).

The prognosis is variable, depending on the specific disorder. In general, however, the immunodeficiencies are life-long, irreversible and associated with a poor prognosis for extended life.

SPECIFIC IMMUNODEFICIENCIES

Some aspects of certain of the more important immunodeficiencies are presented here.

Immunodeficiency of Immaturity

The newborn infant, particularly the premature, has an unusually high incidence of infection. The components of the immune system are present but untested, and because of lack of specific antigenic exposure, there are few if any specific immune responses. The newborn infant makes essentially no immunoglobulin (except small quantities of IgM) but receives IgG transplacentally from the mother. The newborn's cellular immune system has adequate numbers of proliferating T cells, but specific functions of T cells such as delayed hypersensitivity skin reactivity, cytotoxicity and mediator production are deficient. The granulocytes are able to phagocytize and kill, but are labile and may lose this ability with stress. Further, their ability to move to a site of infection (chemotaxis) is limited. Complement levels are about two thirds of adult normal. The monocytes also have a chemotactic defect. All of these abnormalities often combine to make the newborn unable to meet the challenge of an infecting agent, resulting in severe overwhelming infection without the early host responses that aid in early diagnosis (fever, erythema, leukocytosis).

Malnutrition

The most common immunodeficiency on a global scale is that resulting from malnutrition; individuals do not die from chronic malnutrition but from the infections that they inevitably contract. Indeed, measles is a major killer in malnourished African infants. The chief immunological defect in malnutrition is a profound cellular immune defect, associated with skin anergy, thymus, lymph node and tonsil atrophy, diminished number of T cells, decreased *in vitro* reactivity to mitogens and marked susceptibility to viral disease. Serum immunoglobulins are generally normal, although secretory IgA may be impaired. The T cell deficiency is quickly reversed upon initiation of an adequate diet.

Splenectomy

Removal of the spleen may result in increased susceptibility to overwhelming infection, particularly involving pneumococcus and meningococcus. The spleen serves as an important filtering agent to clear the blood of bacteria, particularly in the first five years of life. Accordingly, young children without spleens should receive continuous prophylactic antibiotics, and older children without a spleen should be started on antibiotics at the first sign of infection.

X-linked Infantile Agammaglobulinemia

The first immunodeficiency syndrome described, this is characterized by onset of pyogenic infections at age six to seven months (when transplacental immunity wanes), severe deficiency of B cells, low levels of immunoglobulins (total Ig < 400 mg/dl), paucity of lymphoid tissues and poor or absent antibody response and intact cellular immunity. These patients often develop chronic lung disease, arthritis and malabsorption. Gamma globulin therapy enables many of these patients to live nearly normal lives.

Transient Hypogammaglobulinemia of Infancy

This results from a lag in the onset of the infant's immunoglobulin synthesis after maternal IgG has fallen off. Such infants present at age 6 to 18 months with frequent infections and low levels of all immunoglobulins. The presence of normal numbers of B cells distinguishes it from X-linked agammaglobulinemia. All normal infants (particularly prematures) have physiological hypogammaglobulinemia from age four to six months, and in the absence of symptoms, this requires no treatment; indeed, treatment is contraindicated, since it may turn off the patient's own gamma globulin synthesis.

Selective IgA Deficiency

This is the most common permanent immunodeficiency, occurring as often as 1 in 600 of the general population. It is characterized by serum IgA <10 mg/dl, normal levels of other immunoglobulins and nor-

mal cellular immunity. Some of these patients are symptomatic, but others may have allergies, food intolerance, autoimmune diseases or sinopulmonary infections. These patients lack IgA in their secretions, but may compensate for this by secreting IgM. Gamma globulin therapy is contraindicated, since this may sensitize them to IgA. Antibiotic therapy may be necessary if recurrent infections are severe. These patients have normal numbers of IgA-bearing B cells; occasionally, spontaneous remission of the disease occurs.

Common Variable Immunodeficiency

This illness, also termed acquired agammaglobulinemia, occurs in either sex and usually begins with the onset of pyogenic infection after infancy, usually between ages 15 and 35. Most patients have normal cellular immunity and normal numbers of B cells, but severe antibody deficiency. As the name implies, however, the immunological findings are heterogeneous; further, autoimmune disorders, hematological disorders and partial defects of cellular immunity are not uncommon. Waldmann *et al.* have shown that many of these patients have T lymphocytes (T suppressor cells) that inhibit B cell immunoglobulin synthesis. Treatment with gamma globulin is indicated.

Congenital Thymic Aplasia (DiGeorge Syndrome)

These patients have developmental defects of the third and fourth pharyngeal pouch, resulting in aplasia of the thymus and parathyroid glands and aortic arch abnormalities. These infants may present with seizures in early infancy as a result of hypocalcemia due to hypoparathyroidism. They may have an abnormal appearance, with low-set ears, fish-shaped mouth, hypertelorism, micrognathia and antimongoloid slant of the eyes. Congenital heart disease is common, owing to the aortic arch defects. The immunological defect is a profound cellular immunodeficiency, generally presenting in the newborn period. No thymic shadow is noted on a chest roentgenograph. Treatment with a fetal thymus transplant leads to restoration of T cell immunity, but the hypocalcemia must be treated with calcium, vitamin D or parathyroid hormone. Spontaneous immunological recovery may ensue without transplantation, suggesting that incomplete defects may occur.

Chronic Mucocutaneous Candidiasis

This is a disorder characterized by a cell-mediated immune defect to *Candida albicans* (and a few related fungi), leading to chronic recalcitrant candida infection of the hair, nails, mucous membranes and skin (Fig. 17–1). Most patients have cutaneous anergy to candida antigens, and their lymphocytes do not proliferate in the presence of candida, nor do they make macrophage migratory inhibition factor. Cellular immunity to other antigens is usually normal, however. Endocrine disorders (e.g., hypothyroidism, Addison's disease) may be associated. Treatment with antifungal agents is only of transient benefit; transfer factor has been of benefit in a few patients.

Cellular Immunodeficiency with Abnormal Immunoglobulin Synthesis (Nezelof's Syndrome)

These patients have a cellular immunodeficiency associated with thymic dysplasia and a variable immunoglobulin and antibody deficiency. Patients are generally not as severely ill as patients with combined immunodeficiency, and they may survive beyond the first decade. There are varying patterns of immunoglobulins, including high, normal or low levels of each class, but the antibody response to specific antigens is usually deficient or absent. Unlike the DiGeorge syndrome, they do not have a characteristic appearance, hypoparathyroidism or congenital heart disease. Thymosin has been of benefit in a few of these patients.

Severe Combined Immunodeficiency (Thymic Dysplasia, Swiss-type Agammaglobulinemia)

This is characterized by a profound deficiency of cellular and antibody immunity, thymic dysplasia, early onset of severe infections and a progressive downhill course. Inheritance can be either X-linked or autosomal recessive. One of the autosomal-recessive variants is associated with adenosine deaminase deficiency of erythrocytes, leukocytes with cultured fibroblasts. The latter fact has permitted intrauterine diagnosis of the disorder. Since these patients completely lack T cell immunity, they may develop graft-*versus*-host reactions from maternal cells grafted during pregnancy,

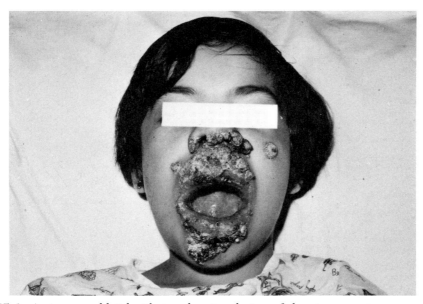

Figure 17–1 A nine-year-old girl with granulomatous lesions of chronic mucocutaneous candidiasis.

from lymphocytes present in blood transfusions or from attempts to reconstitute the patient immunologically. Gamma globulin therapy is of only partial benefit. Bone marrow transplantation from a histocompatible sibling donor is the treatment of choice; approximately 30 patients have been reconstituted since 1968.

Immunodeficiency with Ataxia Telangiectasia

This is an autosomal recessive disorder characterized by progressive ataxia, prominent telangiectasia of the conjunctivae, eyelids and ears (Fig. 17–2), recurrent sinopulmonary disorders, selective IgA deficiency (in two thirds of cases) and defective cellular immunity. Onset is usually by age five, when choreoathetotic movements, disconjugate gaze and extrapyramidal signs develop. Progressive motor and mental impairment occurs. Skin anergy, thymic dysplasia and depressed antibody responses are noted. No satisfactory therapy exists.

Immunodeficiency with Eczema and Thrombocytopenia (Wiskott-Aldrich Syndrome)

This is an X-linked disorder characterized by eczema, thrombocytopenia and re-

current pyogenic infection. Early onset of draining ears or melena occurs (Fig. 17–3). The immunological defects include low levels of IgM, high levels of IgE and IgA, deficient antibody responses, particularly to polysaccharide antigens, partial T cell deficiency with skin anergy, and defective monocyte chemotaxis. Bleeding, infection or malignancy (in 10 per cent of cases) occur, and survival beyond age five is unusual. Transfer factor has been of value in some patients.

Chronic Granulomatous Disease

This is an X-linked disorder characterized by defective intracellular killing of certain organisms, leading to chronic pyogenic infections of the skin, lymph nodes, lungs and bones. Antibody and T cell immunity are normal. Diagnosis is established by inability of leukocytes to reduce NBT dye, which parallels their inability to synthesize hydrogen peroxide for intracellular killing. An autosomal recessive variant with leukocyte glutathione reductase deficiency has been described. Treatment with continuous antibiotic therapy (particularly sulfamethoxazole trimethoprim) has been of considerable benefit. Leukocyte transfusions may also be used.

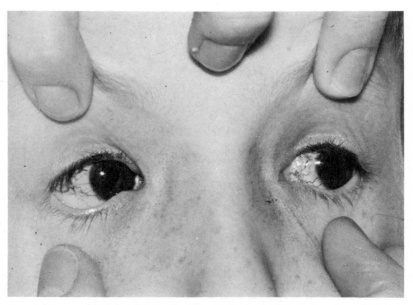

Figure 17–2 An eight-year-old girl with ataxia telangiectasia demonstrating the characteristic conjunctival telangiectasia. She also had bronchiectasis and sinusitis.

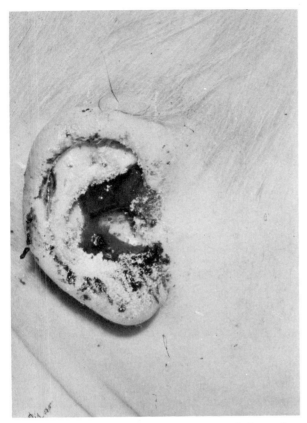

Figure 17–3 *Pseudomonas* infection of the middle ear of a four-year-old boy with the Wiskott-Aldrich syndrome. He lost the ossicles of the ear and developed a partial facial paralysis.

Job Syndrome

This is a disorder of granulocyte chemotaxis, characterized by staphylococcal abscesses of the skin, lymph nodes and subcutaneous tissues in fair, red-headed girls.

Most of these patients have elevated levels of immunoglobulins, particularly IgE immunoglobulin. Granulocyte phagocytosis and intracellular killing are intact, but chemotaxis is abnormal.

Familial C5 Dysfunction

This is a familial complement defect, with deficient opsonic function and generation of chemotactic factors. C5 levels are normal, but its function is deficient. This leads to a syndrome of failure to thrive, diarrhea, seborrheic dermatitis and susceptibility to bacterial infection. Treatment with plasma to replace the defective complement is indicated.

REFERENCES

Bergsma, D., Good, R. A., and Finsted, J.: *Immunodeficiency in Man and Animals.* National Foundation Original Article Series. New York, Sinauer Assoc., 1975.

Fudenberg, H., Good, R. A., Goodman, H. C., *et al.*: Primary immunodeficiencies: Report of a World Health Organization committee. Pediatrics, 47:927, 1971.

Kersey, J. H., Gajl-Peczalska, K. J., and Nesbit, M. E.: The lymphoid system: Abnormalities in immunodeficiency and malignancy. J. Pediatr., 84:489, 1974.

Meuwissen, H. J., Pollara, B., and Pickering, R. J.: Combined immunodeficiency disease associated with adenosine deaminase deficiency. J. Pediatr., 86:169, 1975.

Stiehm, E. R., and Fulginiti, V. A.: *Immunologic Disorders in Infants and Children.* Philadelphia, W. B. Saunders Company, 1973.

Waldmann, T. A., Burm, M., Broder, S., *et al.*: Role of suppressor T cells in pathogenesis of common variable hypogammaglobulinemia. Lancet, 2:609, 1974.

18

Allergy Disorders

C. Warren Bierman
and William E. Pierson

Definition

Atopic allergy is characterized by hypersensitivity to substances that do not ordinarily cause symptoms in "normal" people. This hypersensitive state is an immunological process, and in childhood it is associated with the increased synthesis of specific immunoglobulin, IgE or skin-sensitizing antibody (reagin).

Clinically, the allergic state is common in the general population. Approximately 15 per cent of pediatric patients have atopic (allergic) symptoms ranging from mild to life-threatening. Allergic disease is usually manifested as hay fever, allergic rhinitis with middle ear effusion, asthma, atopic eczema, urticaria, anaphylaxis, certain drug reactions and gastrointestinal allergy.

Type of Allergic Response

Allergic diseases are an immune paradox. Antibodies (*immunoglobulins*), which play an important role in protecting the child from infectious agents, may also be related to a wide spectrum of diseases in which they are harmful rather than protective. Their adverse effects may occur through one or more of at least four distinct types of immunological responses as noted in Table 18–1.

TABLE 18–1   CLASSIFICATION OF ALLERGIC REACTIONS

	Location of Antigen	Location of Antibody	Result	Examples
Type I	Free	Attached to passively sensitized cell	Release of vasoactive substances	Bronchial asthma
Type II	Cell surface or attached antigen or hapten	Free + complement	Cell damage	Transfusion reactions; Goodpasture's syndrome
Type III	Free	Free	Precipitation of antigen-antibody complexes with secondary cellular or vascular damage	Extrinsic allergic alveolitis; serum sickness
Type IV	Free	No serum antibody; mononuclear cells are specifically sensitized	Cellular infiltration	Tuberculin reaction; graft rejection

After R. R. A. Coombs and P. G. H. Gell.

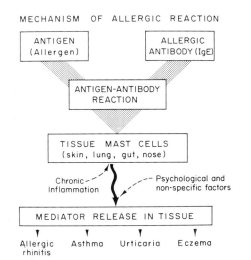

MECHANISM OF ALLERGIC REACTION

Figure 18–1　Pathogenesis of the allergic response.

The isolation and identification of IgE has greatly increased our understanding of immunological hypersensitivity underlying the allergic state. IgE immunoglobulin is synthesized by the plasma cells of the lymphoreticular system in response to exposure to certain "sensitizing" antigens such as house dust, feathers, pollen, mold and animal danders or certain foods. IgE synthesis appears to be under control of suppressor T-cells, which may be decreased in some allergic patients to allow an increase of uninhibited manufacture of IgE. Following sensitization, IgE is produced in sufficient amounts to circulate in the peripheral vascular system and becomes "fixed" or bound to mast cells in the mucous membranes of the nose, skin, lower respiratory and gastrointestinal tracts and on circulating basophils. Subsequent exposure to the sensitizing antigen causes release of inflammatory mediators such as histamine, kinins (kallikrein, bradykinin) and S.R.S.-A (slow reactive substance of anaphylaxis), and E.C.F.-A (eosinophilic chemotactic factor–anaphylaxis) as diagrammed in Figure

TABLE 18–2　INHERITANCE OF ALLERGIC DISEASE

Family History (Asthma, Hay Fever)	Both Parents	One Parent	Neither Parent
Incidence of children with allergy	68%	38%	13%

18–1. These mediators produce dilation of blood vessels, diffusion of fluid from the capillaries, increased mucous gland secretion and viscosity and changes in bronchiolar smooth muscle tone.

Atopic allergic disease (Type I Reaction) is associated with a family history as noted in Table 18–2.

ATOPIC DISEASES

Food Allergy (Gastrointestinal Allergy)

Onset. Food hypersensitivity may begin from the late neonatal period until two years of age. Only rarely does food allergy develop after two years except to certain well-defined allergens such as shellfish or nuts. The peak incidence occurs in the first year of life. Many children have lost their sensitivity to food by five years, and 96 per cent have done so by 12 years.

Pathophysiology. A broad spectrum of manifestations exists, dependent on the antibody and type of reaction involved. In the young infant, symptoms of "colic," pylorospasm, projectile vomiting and chronic diarrhea may be related to food allergy. Food allergy may also present as eczema, allergic rhinitis and asthma in young children.

Major complications. (1) Malabsorption with growth failure; (2) iron deficiency anemia; (3) chronic respiratory disease ("idiopathic pulmonary hemosiderosis") associated with milk precipitins; and (4) iatrogenic disorders from nutritionally inadequate elimination diets.

Diagnosis. Skin tests are of help only in patients with Type I (IgE) allergic disease such as asthma or eczema. Serum precipitins can be identified in children with idiopathic pulmonary hemosiderosis (Heiner syndrome). Antibodies related to allergic gastroenteritis with growth failure have not yet been characterized.

Therapy. Identification of the offending foods and their elimination from the diet.

Atopic Dermatitis (Infantile Eczema)

Onset. The onset of atopic dermatitis occurs in infancy. Fifty per cent of affected patients develop eczema by one year of age, and nearly all cases have occurred by

TABLE 18–3   ALLERGIC MANIFESTATIONS BY AGE GROUP

Age	Allergens		Sex Distribution	Common Allergic Symptoms
Neonatal period to 6 months	Primary Foods		Male > Female 2:1	1. Pylorospasm and "colic" projectile vomiting 2. Chronic diarrhea 3. Atopic eczema 4. Persistent nasal congestion with recurrent respiration infections
6 months to 1 year	Food Environmental Inhalants	66% 34%	Male > Female 2:1	1. Atopic eczema 2. Chronic diarrhea with or without growth failure 3. Chronic nasal congestion 4. Asthma
1 to 5 years	Food Environmental Inhalants Pollens	25% 70% 5%	Male > Female 2:1	1. Atopic eczema (spontaneous improvement in 75% by age 3 years) 2. Chronic respiratory infections 3. Chronic nasal congestion without fever 4. Asthma 5. Persistent middle ear fluid
5 to 12 years	Food Environmental Inhalants Pollens Combined Inhalants (environmental and pollens)	5% 25% 20% 50%	Male > Female 2:1	1. Chronic nasal congestion, eustachian tube dysfunction and hearing loss (serous otitis, secretory otitis) 2. School problems (poor attendance, poor attention span) 3. Hay fever 4. Asthma—Extrinsic > Intrinsic 5. Exercise-induced asthma 6. Urticaria
12 to 21 years	Food Environmental Inhalants and Pollens	<5% 95%	Male = Female 1:1	1. Nasal congestion (perennial) 2. Hay fever (seasonal) 3. Exercise-induced asthma 4. Asthma—Extrinsic > Instrinsic 5. Chronic sinus disease 6. Allergic bronchitis 7. Urticaria
21 to 40 years	Food Environmental Inhalants and Pollens Unknown (intrinsic factors)	<5% 60% 35%	Male = Female 1:1	1. Asthma—Extrinsic < Instrinsic 2. Nasal allergy 3. Nasal polyps and sinus disease 4. Drug reactions 5. Contact dermatitis 6. Occupational lung disease
40+ years	Inhalants Infection Unknown	25% 50% 25%	Male < Female 1:2	1. Asthma—Extrinsic < Intrinsic 2. Nasal allergy 3. Nasal polyps and sinus disease 4. Chronic bronchitis 5. Urticaria 6. Occupational lung disease 7. Drug reaction

six years. Only rarely does it have a later onset. Since more than 75 per cent of children who develop eczema will progress to allergic respiratory disease such as asthma or hay fever, it is important to make an early and accurate diagnosis. This will permit early treatment and allow prevention of subsequent respiratory disease.

Pathophysiology. The pathophysiology of atopic dermatitis is characterized by localized vasodilation in skin subjected to trauma that progresses to spongiosis, or the breakdown of dermal cells and the formation of intradermal vesicles. Scratching produces weeping and secondary infection. Chronic scratching results in lichenification or coarsening of the skin folds. Immunologically, there is a T-cell defect characterized by a decreased Type IV responsiveness (migration inhibiting factor).

Therapy. Therapy consists of the following:

1. *Removal of irritants.* Perfumed soaps, bubble bath and other agents that enhance dryness should be avoided. Wool is a particularly severe contact irritant. Hexachlorophene soaps accentuate dryness and should be used sparingly. The patient's nails should be filed frequently to decrease skin trauma from scratching.

2. *Xerosis.* To counter xerosis, water-miscible ointments (oil in water or water in oil emulsions) should be applied four to six times daily. A variety of hydrophilic ointments is available and should be used successively, letting parents select the most effective agent.

3. *Suppression of inflammation.* Moist compresses decrease pruritus and remove secretions. Acetonated steroid ointments (Synalar, 0.01 per cent or Kenacort, 0.025 per cent) applied three to four times daily most effectively suppress inflammation and promote healing. Occlusive dressings may increase the anti-inflammatory action.

4. *Allergic control* (as noted in the section on Methods and Management).

5. *Systemic steroids* are rarely indicated and should never be used for long-term control.

Allergic Rhinitis, Middle Ear Dysfunction and Hay Fever

Onset. Allergic rhinitis develops early in childhood, with symptoms peaking in the fall and winter months. By age five to six years, seasonal rhinitis may develop during periods of pollination (trees, grasses, weeds).

Pathophysiology. Following cellular release of inflammatory mediators, nasal mucosal edema results from the disaggregation of colloidal ground substance (mucopolysaccharides and mucoproteins), giving the nasal lining the characteristic appearance of gray, wet cardboard. Stimulation of exocrine glands produces a clear serous mucous with a pH greater than 6.5 (normal is 5.0 to 6.5) containing a predominance of eosinophils. The resultant edema impairs epithelial ciliary function and

alters the protective function of nasal mucosa. Vasomotor rhinitis, a non-allergic rhinitis related to reflex mucosal edema, is thought to be due to emotional stress and may be distinguished by the absence of eosinophils and other signs of atopy.

Major complications. (1) Eustachian tube dysfunction leading to middle ear effusions (serous otitis media) and intermittent hearing loss (50 per cent); (2) frequent respiratory infections; (3) paranasal sinus obstruction; and (4) secondary sinobronchitis.

Therapy. Major therapeutic agents are antihistamines or sympathicomimetic amines, alone or in combination. Vasoconstrictive nose sprays should be employed sparingly. Allergic immunotherapy against such allergens as dust, mold and pollens is useful, particularly in the therapy of hay fever.

Asthma (Atopic or Extrinsic)

Onset. Asthma (documented reversible obstructive airway disease) may also begin early in life. Twenty per cent of childhood asthma begins by age one year and 80 per cent by 10 years. In addition to specific allergic exposure, such non-allergic factors as (1) respiratory infections, (2) vagal mediated airway reflexes, (3) cold, (4) vigorous exercise and (5) psychogenic factors may play a role in airway reactivity.

Pathophysiology. The following anatomic changes occur in the lung: (1) Spasm of bronchial and bronchiolar smooth muscle, (2) mucosal edema, (3) hypersecretion and alterations of mucous viscosity, (4) eosinophilic migration into the submucosa, (5) peribronchial inflammation and (6) pulmonary hyperinflation.

Coinciding with these anatomic changes, the following physiological alterations occur: (1) increased airway resistance, (2) decreased forced vital capacity, (3) hypocarbia proceeding to hypercarbia with onset of acute respiratory failure, (4) increased residual volume, and increased functional residual capacity, (5) hypoxemia and (6) abnormal ventilation-perfusion ratio. Effective therapy may reverse these physiological alterations.

Chronic asthma. Chronic asthma is marked by an assortment of all of the anatomical and physiological changes already noted and also has several other unique features. Chronic asthma can result in right ventricular hypertrophy. Also, arterial hypoxemia can result in stunting or linear growth retardation and poor weight gain. Limitation of exercise capacity and excessive school loss and psychological reactions frequently accompany chronic asthma.

Exercise-induced bronchospasm. Exercise-induced bronchospasm is a frequently overlooked handicap of the allergic child. The incidence of asthmatics is 70 to 90 per cent, and in allergic non-asthmatics (hay fever, atopic rhinitis), 40 per cent will have post-exercise bronchoconstriction. Several exercise testing systems are available and clinically useful. Owing to the high incidence of exercise-induced bronchospasm among allergic children, all children over five years of age should be evaluated for this handicap.

Therapy. The therapy of *acute asthma* involves the following considerations: (1) Neutral environment (free of irritants). (2) Increased liquid intake. (3) Adequate oral bronchodilating medications, such as theophylline, on a regular (every six hours) schedule to achieve a serum concentration of 10 to 20 μg/ml. Pressurized hand nebulizers containing isoproterenol are best avoided in children because the hazards of abusive overdose outweigh the advantages. (4) Epinephrine by injection if oral medication is ineffective: .01 ml/kg of 1:1000 aqueous epinephrine injected subcutaneously followed by epinephrine suspension 1:200 (Sus-Phrine) .005 ml/kg. (5) Antibiotics, if indicated for known infection. (6) Short acting steroids for intractable asthma (prednisone, methyprednisolone).

The therapy of *chronic asthma* involves: (1) Neutral environment (as free as possible of allergens and irritants). (2) Adequate oral theophylline to maintain a serum level of 10 to 20 μg/ml (monitored by serum theophylline determinations). The addition of cromolyn sodium may be very useful in patients who do not adequately respond to oral theophylline alone. Finally, several new beta-2 adrenergic agonists may be useful in conjunction with theophylline. These include metaproterenol, turbutaline and salbutamol. (3) Allergic immunotherapy in cases not controlled by (1) and (2). This usually involves desensitization to pollens, mold and house dust. (4) Short-

term or, in rare cases, long-term steroids are indicated if all of these measures fail to control the patient's asthma. Recently, an aerosol form of steroid (beclomethasone) became available that has the advantage of equal clinical effectiveness but markedly reduced side effects when compared with oral steroid therapy.

The treatment of exercise-induced asthma resides primarily with the following agents:

1. Cromolyn sodium: 20 mg by spinhaler, inhalation 10 minutes before exercise.

2. Theophylline (P.O.): 5 mg/kg taken one and a half hours before exercise.

3. Beta-2 adrenergic agonists including metaproterenol, turbutaline or albuterol (under FDA evaluation) taken one to two hours before exercise.

All of these agents have been shown to decrease exercise asthma and to allow patients to more fully engage in recreational or competitive pursuits.

Most childhood asthma is effectively controlled at home by oral medication. Less than 10 per cent of children require epinephrine injections for acute asthma.

Status Asthmaticus

Definition. Status asthmaticus is severe asthma in which the patient has become refractory or non-responsive to catecholamines (epinephrine or metaproterenol) and is at risk of developing acute respiratory failure. It is a medical emergency requiring prompt hospital admission and management.

Initial evaluation. Initial evaluation should include the following: (1) Chest roentgenogram; (2) arterial blood gases (PaCO$_2$, PaO$_2$ and pH); (3) pulmonary function tests: forced vital capacity and forced expiratory volume in 1 second and forced expiratory flow.

Initial therapy. The patient should be admitted to an intensive care unit, for continuous monitoring of vital signs every half hour for at least the first 12 hours. The following therapy is indicated: (1) intravenous fluids for hydration, depletion repair and maintenance with appropriate electrolyte content; (2) intravenous aminophylline 7 mg/kg given in 10 minutes in a volutrol followed by 25 mg/kg/24 hours placed in the intravenous maintenance fluids, and monitored by serum theophylline determinations to insure a level of 10 to 20 μg/ml; (3) intravenous antibiotics, if indicated by presence of bacterial infection; (4) intravenous adrenocorticosteroids; betamethasone 0.3 mg/kg immediately followed by 0.3 mg/kg/24 hours, or hydrocortisone 7 mg/kg immediately followed by 7 mg/kg/24 hours by continuous injection; (5) buffers for metabolic acidosis; (6) ultrasonic nebulization of bronchodilator solution (isotonic saline with phenylephrine, .06 per cent, and isoproterenol, .04 per cent) for 5 minutes every 30 minutes as indicated by patient's condition; (7) humidified oxygen sufficient to keep patient's PaO_2 above 70 mm Hg.

Follow-up therapy. Pulmonary function, blood gas measurements and serum theophylline should be performed initially at one-hour periods and may be spaced out as the patient improves. Generally, the patient can be shifted to oral medications at 24 hours. If, in the course of therapy, the patient's $PaCO_2$ rises above 55 to 60 mm and his PaO_2 falls below 60 mm in spite of appropriate oxygen therapy, he will probably need mechanical ventilation. An anesthesiologist should be consulted early to aid in initiating mechanical ventilation.

Urticaria and Angioneurotic Edema

Onset. Urticaria may occur at any age after birth and is common in childhood. Angioedema is a form of severe urticaria.

Pathophysiology. Histamine or other inflammatory mediators released from tissue mast cells or basophils either immunologically by the reaction of antigen with specific cell-fixed antibodies or non-immunologically by such factors as infectious agents, drugs, trauma, heat or cold. Familial angioedema, a heritable disease of the complement system, may be distinguished by its significant family history, its absence of true urticarial lesions, and chemically by its abnormal complement values, especially C_1 and C_4.

ANAPHYLAXIS

Anaphylaxis is a severe reaction occurring 1 to 20 minutes after bee stings or drug administration and characterized by diffuse "flush" of the skin, hoarseness, dyspnea, urticaria, intense pruritus, hypotension, abdominal cramps and at times fatal upper airway obstruction.

Onset. Anaphylaxis can occur within seconds or up to 30 to 45 minutes after injection or exposure to the etiological agent.

Pathophysiology. The basis of anaphylaxis is a Type I allergic reaction and involves the generalized release of inflammatory mediators that cause a fall in blood pressure, upper airway edema and decreased pulmonary perfusion. Certain agents such as morphine, codeine, curare and contrast dyes induce an anaphylactoid reaction that differs from anaphylaxis only in that an immunological mechanism is not involved.

Therapy. The treatment to be effective must be both *early* and *orderly*. Therapy should be in the following order:

1. *Epinephrine:* 0.2 ml to 0.3 ml (1:1000 aqueous) subcutaneously or intravenously (1:10,000 aqueous) in case of severe hypotension; and the same amount injected directly into and around the site of drug administration or insect sting.

2. *Evaluation and monitoring:* Upper airway patency (laryngeal edema); cardiovascular status (shock).

3. *Oxygen:* Humidified and delivered by mask.

4. *Tourniquet:* Applied to an extremity above the site of injection of offending antigen.

5. *Antihistamine:* Benadryl can be given intravenously (2 mg/kg) or orally (5 mg/kg) every 24 hours.

6. *I.V. Fluids:* If indicated by clinical course.

7. *I.V. Aminophylline:* If indicated due to bronchospasm 7 mg/kg over a 10-minute period followed by 25 mg/kg/24 hours.

8. *Note:* No evidence exists showing a beneficial effect of *steroids* in initial treatment of anaphylaxis, but administration of steroids prior to radiopaque contrast media studies has been beneficial in *preventing* anaphylaxis.

DRUG ALLERGY

Onset. Hypersensitivity reactions to drugs may be encountered at any age after the neonatal period. They may take the form of any of the four classes of allergic reactions. The primary drug reactions in children are to (1) antibiotics and antimicrobials, (2) dermal applications of "caine" and antihistamine drugs and (3) anticonvulsants, especially Dilantin and phenobarbital.

Pathophysiology. The most common drug reaction in childhood is to penicillin. It may present in one of three common forms: (1) immediate explosive reaction (anaphylaxis) occurring within 20 to 30 minutes of administration, (2) accelerated reaction (urticaria) occurring two to 48 hours after administration and (3) late onset reaction (serum sickness, skin eruptions) occurring 48 hours after administration.

Therapy. (1) Treatment of the immediate reaction and (2) identification of the offending drug and withdrawal of it from therapy.

METHODS OF MANAGEMENT

Allergy History

The diagnosis of allergy, as well as identification of specific allergic factors, rests initially on a detailed history of the child, his or her family and physical and social environment. *Seasonal variation* is the hallmark of atopic disease states resulting from airborne allergens, such as house dust, pollen or mold spores. The physician must be familiar with the pattern of such factors in the patient's environment and locale in order to interpret the significance of such seasonal variations.

Symptoms that commonly accompany allergic sensitivity but are not exclusive to it include: "colic," eczema, diarrhea, croup, hives, angioedema, chronic or recurrent "colds" without fever, earaches, hearing loss and behavior problems. The response of symptoms to medication (antihistamine, beta adrenergic or theophylline agents) and temporary changes in environment may also be helpful in documenting an allergic cause.

Environmental history. Especially important is a detailed description of the child's home, noting the following:

1. *Home:* Location, age, type of construction, method of heating, presence of dust filter on furnace, location of clothes dryer and ventilation of dryer

2. *Method of cleaning*

3. *Patient's bedroom:* The bedroom is particularly important. The floor covering, including felt (animal hair) rug pads, as well as the mattress, box springs, bedding and pillows, may contain potential allergens. The closet is often a storage area for the child and, in addition, for the rest of the family. Book shelves, chest of drawers and clutter items may be important.

4. *Pets* (inside and outside)

5. *Number of smokers* in the home

Physical Examination

Significant features of allergic diseases are usually found on physical examination. The *height* and *weight* of the patient indicate the growth pattern, which is affected by both allergic disease and its therapy, and should be recorded on a growth chart. The *ears* should always be examined for tympanic membrane mobility with a pneumatic otoscope, and a 250 Hz tuning fork should be used to perform a Weber and Rinne test to evaluate middle ear function. The *nose* may have pale and edematous mucosa with varying degrees of nasal passage obstruction. Marked adenoidal hypertrophy can result in "adenoidal facies" with flattened maxillary eminences. An atopic pleat of the lower eyelid or *transverse nasal crease* is also seen frequently in allergic rhinitis. *Chest symmetry* and excursion are important to note. Auscultation should be carried out with deep exhalation and after exercise. The skin may be dry and scaly (xerosis), with preferential involvement of the flexor creases of the extremities (especially the antecubital and popliteal fossae).

Laboratory Tests

Nasal secretions. The pH of nasal secretions normally is acidic (pH 5.0 to 6.5) but is nearly always alkaline (pH 7.0) in allergic rhinitis, when measured with pH paper with a narrow band of pH sensitivity (pH 6.5 to 8.0). The collection of the specimen is particularly important. Blowing the nose on plastic wrap or waxed paper yields a far better specimen than that obtained by inserting a swab into the nasopharynx. The specimen should be stained with a special reagent (Hansel's stain) that specifically stains eosinophilic granules. Eosinophils are seen in allergic rhinitis; a predominance of lymphocytes is seen in acute viral infections; and neutrophilic leukocytes and bacteria are noted in acute or chronic bacterial rhinitis. Not infrequently, allergic rhinitis is masked by secondary bacterial rhinitis. Eosinophils may predominate only after the superimposed bacterial infection has been cleared with appropriate therapy.

Blood eosinophilia. Values in excess of 350 cells/mm³ are compatible with allergic disease, although eosinophilia may result from many other conditions (parasitic infection, drug reaction, neoplastic disease, reticuloendotheliosis and during the recovery period of infectious diseases).

Radiographic studies. Edema of the nasal mucous membranes may also involve those of the paranasal sinuses. Roentgenograms may show not only sinus cloudiness but also fluid levels.

Hearing tests. Screening audiometry (250 to 4000 Hz) provides a simple but objective method of evaluating hearing. It is useful for initial evaluation and provides an objective measure of the progress being made by medical therapy. If such therapy does not result in improvement in the patient's audiogram, early referral to an otologist can be made.

In children of early school age, a conductive hearing loss of 25 dB or greater in the range of 250 to 4000 Hz represents a significant hearing or learning handicap. Speech development is significantly delayed with such a conductive hearing loss in young children.

Tympanometry. The use of impedance audiometry (tympanometry) has become a practical and objective indicator of middle ear and eustachian tube function. The various compliance-pressure curves are far more sensitive than any other readily available clinical method of assessing the patency and function of the eustachian tube, detection of middle ear fluid and negative pressure. Allergic patients have a 50 per cent incidence of abnormal tympanograms and thus all should be evaluated by tympanometry. This method is invaluable in determining the results of therapy and need for otological surgery for relief of persistent middle ear effusion (Fig. 18–2).

Exercise testing. Several different systems available for exercise testing are listed here in the order of their capacity to cause exercise-induced bronchospasm.

1. *Free range running:* most asthmogenic, is carried out for five to eight minutes; pulmonary function is monitored for 20 minutes afterward.

2. *Treadmill:* next most asthmogenic system; readily applied to older children and useful in evaluation of drug therapy.

3. *Cycloergometer:* next in order of magnitude; easily applied to even young children.

4. *Others:* (swimming, rowing, ergometer.)

Pulmonary function tests. Assessment of ventilatory function in allergic patients is essential for both diagnosis and evaluation of treatment. The following tests can be performed by even young children (age four to five) and can furnish objective data for proper patient evaluation.

1. Forced Vital Capacity

2. Forced Expiratory Volume in 1 second

3. Forced Expiratory Flow at 25–75 per cent of forced vital capacity

4. Peak Expiratory Flow

These studies (1, 2 and 3) can be performed by use of any one of several readily available spirometers, which allow regular evaluation in most clinical settings. The

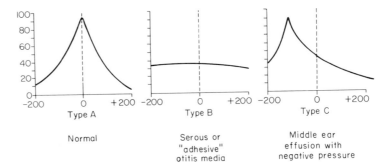

Figure 18–2 Patterns of tympanometry that indicate different states of the middle ear.

peak expiratory flow can be measured by utilizing the Pediatric Wright Peak Flow Meter and offers the advantage of having *no* initial resistance that the small child must overcome to actuate the test device.

Many other more complicated and less readily available pulmonary function tests may be of help in certain patients, but these tests are normally not necessary.

Tests for immune competence. With the recognition that many children with immunodeficiency syndromes may have chronic infections, it has become clinically important to *evaluate* the immune status of those children with recurrent bacterial infections.

Recently, a great wealth of knowledge has been gained and tests have evolved that are useful in measuring the immunological competence of an individual who has recurrent respiratory infections. An overall scheme of immunity in man is diagrammatically displayed in Figure 18–3.

The immediate type of immunity is associated with antibodies that are immunoglobulins synthesized either locally (respiratory tract, gastrointestinal tract, secretions, tears) or by plasma cells of the lymphoid system and circulated in the vascular system. Immunoglobulins (IgM, IgA, IgG, IgD) are easily measured by quantitative radial immunodiffusion, whereas IgE requires a radioimmunoassay. The isohemagglutinin titer (antibodies to blood group antigens A and B) is a functional means of measuring antibody synthesis that can be performed by most blood banks. If a child has been immunized with diphtheria-pertusis-tetanus antigen, a Schick test is a simple method of measuring diphtheria antibody synthesis. Immunization with univalent typhoid antigen with three 0.5 ml injections (0.25 ml in children) intramuscularly one week apart, and subsequent measurement of febrile agglutinins (O and H antibody titers) is another simple, readily available method for measuring antibody response. Humoral immune competence can be viewed as normal if the following tests are in the normal range:

a. Presence of a normal gamma globulin peak on paper or starch block electrophoresis

b. Presence of normal serum levels of IgM, IgA, IgG, IgD, and IgE.

c. Normal anti-A and anti-B titer (isohemagglutin titer)

d. Negative Schick test

Skin tests. IMMEDIATE SKIN TESTS (TYPE I). The immediate skin test is a bioassay for allergic antibodies (IgE, reagins) fixed to mast cells in the skin. A positive response is demonstrated by a wheal and flare reaction that is 5 mm greater in diameter than the control occurring 15 minutes after antigen injection into the skin. The test antigens are aqueous extracts of protein concentrates from foods, animal danders, house dust, molds and airborne pollens of trees, grasses and weeds. The use and interpretation of skin tests can be viewed as corroborative evidence only. *Overemphasis of the importance of positive skin tests that do not correlate with historical, physical or other laboratory findings is the root of great misdiagnosis and mismanagement in allergy.* The following outline delineates the many factors that can alter skin test interpretations.

Factors Affecting Interpretation of Skin Tests

  I. *Skin Factors*
    a. Dermatographism
    b. Vascular supply
    c. Antibody-skin fixing efficiency
    d. Neurological innervation

  II. *Humoral Factors*
    a. Concentration of test antigens
    b. Local skin concentration of allergic antibodies (IgE)
    c. Efficiency of antigen-antibody interaction

  III. *Evaluating Factors*
    a. Positive skin tests help evaluate an immunological reaction — not the presence of a symptomatic allergic condition
    b. Tissue or organ reactivity is markedly variable

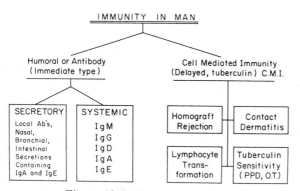

Figure 18–3 Immunity in man.

c. Symptom threshold is also quite variable

DELAYED (TUBERCULIN) SKIN TEST (TYPE IV). Reactions characterized by the tuberculin-type reaction on cell-mediated immunity are determined by this test, in which 0.1 ml of antigen is injected intradermally. A positive test is a skin reaction with 5 mm induration and 10 mm erythema read at 48 hours. It is associated with sensitized lymphocytes and results in a cell-mediated transferrable factor. It has been useful in determining previous exposure to various bacterial, fungal and viral agents. Other tests of cell mediated immunity include mitogen-incuded lymphoblastogenesis, migratory inhibition factor, lymphocyte chemotaxis and lymphokine release.

ARTHUS TYPE SKIN TEST (TYPE III). It is characterized by intense erythema, induration and central necrosis that occurs in four to eight hours after injection of antigen. It has been associated with various diseases that involve precipitin-type antibodies such as many of the organic dust-pneumopathies (allergic extrinsic alveolitis).

Inhalation challenge tests. Confirmation of allergic respiratory sensitivity to pollens or molds may be shown by an increase in airway resistance following aerosol inhalation of these substances under carefully controlled conditions.

Therapy

The cornerstone of allergic management is avoidance of those factors (antigens) to which the child is sensitive.

Dietary avoidance. Foods to which the child is overtly allergic should be eliminated from the diet. Those suspected as being possible offenders can be eliminated on a trial basis. Such avoidance is of greatest advantage in the child who is under five years of age. Elimination diets should be prescribed for only a limited period of time until allergic control is established. But when employed, the physician has an obligation to see that the child had adequate nutrition. On achieving such control, foods that have been eliminated should be reintroduced to determine whether clinical symptoms recur. No child should be placed on a long-term dietary restriction unless the benefits of such therapy can be demon-

strated conclusively. Also, great care must be taken to replace nutritionally comparable foods into the child's diet.

Environmental control. Elimination or avoidance of airborne allergens is of prime importance in the control of allergic rhinitis and other types of respiratory allergy. Effective environmental control not only depends upon a careful history but may also require a home visit by the physician or by a nurse educated in such techniques. These are the points of emphasis:

I. *House Dust Sensitivity*
   a. Careful control of airborne dust particles by frequent (monthly) changes of furnace filters or the use of an electrostatic filter on the furnace
   b. An effective vacuum cleaner equipped with disposable paper bags
   c. A clothes dryer vented to the outside

II. *Mold Control*
   a. A vapor barrier covering all crawl spaces
   b. The cautious use of humidification equipment
   c. The elimination of condensation on windows and resulting mold growth by increased ventilation and adequate insulation

III. *Bedroom*
   a. Removal of bedroom rugs and monthly cleaning of curtains and drapes
   b. Impermeable (e.g., plastic or rubberized fabric) encasings for mattress and box springs, synthetic pillows and non-lint bedspread
   c. Machine washable stuffed toys only
   d. Minimal clutter and storage in closet
   e. Daily bedroom cleaning (damp dusting) with thorough cleaning weekly
   f. Laundering of all bedding at least every two weeks

IV. *Removal of pets from the household.* As a compromise, they may be permitted to remain on an *outside only* basis.

V. *The avoidance of tobacco smoke* and other irritants from the home.

Medications. The basis of appropriate pharmacological (drug) therapy is noted in

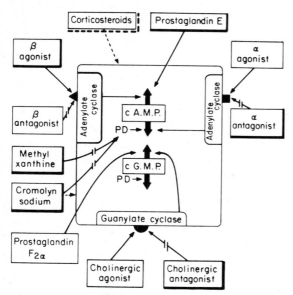

Figure 18-4 Sites of action of various pharmacological agents.

Figure 18-4. Various drugs and their appropriate dosages available for the pharmacological modification of the various allergic diseases are listed in Chapter 6 on pharmacology.

Allergic immunotherapy. Allergic immunotherapy ("desensitization") is used to treat patients who are allergic to unavoidable airborne antigens such as pollens, molds and house dust. Densensitization has no therapeutic effect on food sensitivity or on sensitivity due to animal danders, kapok and wool. In these latter instances, avoidance is the only effective means of treatment.

Allergic immunotherapy appears to act by stimulating production of "blocking antibody" (IgG), which partially protects the individual upon exposure to the airborn antigen. It also decreases cellular sensitivity to antigen-induced mediator release. This therapy has a demonstrated immunological basis and has been evaluated by *in vitro* histamine release techniques showing it to be beneficial to patients.

Use of bacterial vaccines is a source of continuing controversy. Because bacterial hypersensitivity is primarily of the delayed (tuberculin) type, injection therapy for this type of hypersensitivity is not appropriate. Furthermore, no firm immunological or clinical evidence is available that shows that bacterial vaccines have any value. On the basis of available studies, it is our judgment that bacterial vaccines should not be used until better evidence is presented to show their significant benefit.

REFERENCES

Austin, K. F.: Systemic anaphylaxis in man. J.A.MA., *192*:108, 1965.

Beall, G. N.: Urticaria: A review of laboratory and clinical observations. Medicine, *43*:131, 1964.

Bierman, C. W.: Pneumomediastinum and pneumothorax complicating asthma in children. Am. J. Dis. Child., *114*:42, 1967.

Bierman, C. W.: Anaphylaxis. *In* Smith, C. A. (Ed.): The Critically Ill Child. Philadelphia, W. B. Saunders Co., 1972, p. 260–266.

Bierman, C. W., and Pierson, W. E.: The role of the pediatric allergist in the care of patients with eustachian tube dysfunction. Otol. Clin. N. Amer., *3*:79, 1970.

Bierman, C. W., and Pierson, W. E.: The pharmacological modification of atopic disease. *In* Brenneman's Practice of Pediatrics. New York, Harper and Row, Vol. II, Chap. 74, 1970.

Bierman, C. W., and Pierson, W. E.: Hand nebulizers and asthma therapy in children and adolescents. Pediatrics, *54*:6, 1974.

Conference on infantile eczema. J. Pediat., *66*:153, 1965.

Gell, P. G. H., Coombs, R. R. A., and Lachmann, P. J.: *Clinical Aspects of Immunology,* 3rd ed. Philadelphia, J. B. Lippincott Co., 1975.

Ishizaka, T., and Ishizaka, K.: Asthma, physiology, immunopharmacology and treatment. Austen, K. F., Lichtenstein, L. M., Eds. New York, Academic Press, 1973.

McNicol, K. N., and William, H. B.: Spectrum of asthma in children. I. Clinical and physiological components. Brit. Med. J., *4*:7–20, 1973.

Ogra, P. L., and Karzon, D. T.: Role of immunoglobulins in mechanisms of mucosal immunity to infection. Pediatr. Clin. N. Am., *17*:385, 1970.

Pierson, W. E., Bierman, C. W., Stamm, S. J., and Van Arsdel, P. P., Jr.: Double-blind trial of aminophyllin in status asthmaticus. Pediatrics, *48*:642, 1971.

Pierson, W. E., Bierman, C. W., and Kelley, V. C.: A double-blind trial of corticosteroid therapy in status asthmaticus. Pediatrics, *54*:282, 1974.

Rachemann, F. M., and Edwards, M. D.: Asthma in children. A followup study of 685 patients after an interval of twenty years. N. Engl. J. Med., *246*:815, 1952.

Richards, W., and Siegel, S. C.: Status asthmaticus. Pediatr. Clin. N. Am., *16*:9, 1969.

Shapiro, G. G., Bierman, C. W., and Pierson, W. E.: Urticaria: The final common pathway. Cutis, June, pp. 957–962, 1974.

Sheldon, J. M., Lovell, R. G., and Mathews, K. P.: *A Manual of Clinical Allergy,* 2nd ed. Philadelphia, W. B. Saunders Co., 1967.

Stein, M. (Ed.): *New Directions in Asthma.* Park Ridge, Ill., American College of Chest Physicians, 1975.

VanArsdel, P. P., Jr., and Motulsky, A. G.: Frequency and hereditability of asthma and allergic rhinitis in college students. Acta Genet. (Basel), *9*:101, 1959.

Winquist, R. A., and Stamm, S. J.: Arterialized capillary sampling using histamine. J. Pediatr., *74*:455, 1970.

PART VI

ACCIDENT AND NEGLECT DISORDERS

19

Accidents and Poisonings

William O. Robertson

Newspaper headlines, radio broadcasts, public health pronouncements, mass media and professional communications alike combine to stress the mortality and morbidity consequent to "accidents." Skeptics need only recall that in the 1960's accidents accounted for *more* deaths of people between the ages of one and 40 years in the United States than the next eight categories of illness put together, including cancer, heart disease, malformation and infection. This shift in our nation's illness burden is away from the "famine and pestilence" of eons gone by; it reflects more on the relative disappearance of serious infectious disease and nutritional inadequacies than on the emergence of new forms of accidents—save those resulting from the automobile. After corrections for previous inadequate reporting, fatal accidents per 100,000 population—excluding automobile accidents—have actually fallen since the turn of the century. This is partly because of man's better control of his environment and partly because of better patient care programs. Nonetheless, the loss of life continues to be enormous, and the total costs of rehabilitation are high.

STATISTICS

To elaborate, 1974 saw some 13,000 "deaths by accident" occur among the age group from one to 14 years. Automobile accidents, drownings and burns accounted for 70 per cent of those deaths. During the same year, 19 million children sought medical treatment for accident injuries, with more than 3 million of them hospitalized

and more than 12 million school days lost. Figure 19–1 shows the distribution of accidental causes of death for British children.

Automobile accidents lead to almost 55,000 deaths annually, with the 15- to 29-year-old male driver who combines alcohol consumption with an aggressive frame of mind in an inordinate majority. Viewing the overall situation with alarm or predicting next Memorial Day's traffic fatalities fails to alter the impact of accidents on health. Rather, careful study of individual accidents, such as the type done by the Federal Aviation Agency (FAA) of airline catastrophes, or of groups of accidents, such as that done by fire insurance companies after the Hartford (Conn.) Hospital

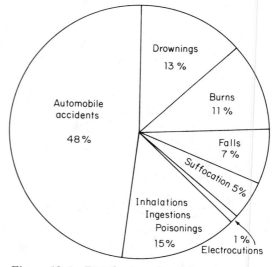

Figure 19–1 Distribution of accidental causes of death in British children under 15 years of age. (Adapted from Jackson, R. H., and Wilkinson, A. W.: Brit. Med. J., *1*:1258, 1976.)

fire, permits pinpointing of contributing agents. Sometimes one or more factors can be modified; witness the effect of automobile seat belts in eliminating extrusion and subsequent crush injuries, of helmets for cyclists, of life guards or of safety patrols at school crossings. The responsible factors have yet to be identified in other instances, or although identified, are not modified for any of a number of reasons. Nevertheless, scientific analysis is uncovering more and more modifiable variables surrounding accidents. The professional, both as an individual and as a member of professional or lay groups, can help bring about the adoption of many of these modifications. More accurate accident statistics have been gathered pinpointing the impact of host factors such as age and sex in relation to particular types of accidents. For example, of children less than five years of age who are killed by automobiles, 35 per cent are pedestrians, while among the five- to nine-year age group, 55 per cent are pedestrians. Among the 15- to 19-year age group, however, only 6 per cent are pedestrians. These data support programs directed at protecting the toddler and child from the street, teaching bicycle safety to the preteen and preparing the young driver through effective driver education programs.

In recent years many attempts have been made to adapt military methods of managing trauma to civilian populations. Community-wide emergency transport systems (ambulance or helicopter), special radio communication networks, specially trained emergency paramedics, elaborately equipped trauma centers and burn centers—these and other programs are springing up across the nation. They are providing services and training and gathering data. Such emergency medical services programs deserve strong physician and community support.

ACCIDENTAL INGESTIONS

One all too prevalent component of accidents in childhood concerns "accidental" poisoning. More than *four million* such episodes occur each year in the United States, and parents of young children can testify to many "near misses" with their own chil-

dren. By actual count, some 560,000 commercially available chemical compounds are "up for grabs" by youngsters; of these, 60,000 change their ingredient composition each year. To cope with this information dilemma—"Johnny just ate something. What's in it?"—a nationwide network of poison information centers, now including more than 540 units, has been developed in the United States since 1950. They inform the professional or the parent of the contents in a given product, its toxicity, approaches to treatment and so forth. An additional resource, The National Center for Poison Control Centers in Washington, D.C., makes available a 5×8 card file information system to all poison control centers. Of great value is the book *The Clinical Toxicology of Commercial Products*, which contains specific ingredient information on more than 25,000 items and general information on many more. The National Clearinghouse has initiated a program to enter the codified information on a computer and is now accessible to nine centers across the country. Microfiche technology has also been applied to solving the problem. Today three microfiche information systems are available for use by the individual poison center; one, Poisindex (Denver), contains ingredient and treatment information on more than 150,000 items and in one study was able to respond to more than 92 per cent of all inquiries. Finally, the National Library of Medicine's Toxicology Program provides complementary information via their quarterly publication, "Toxicity Bibliography," and their online computer program, TOXLINE. About 3000 items still account for 90 per cent of the accidental ingestions. Unfortunately, the remaining 10 per cent still prove to be a difficult information retrieval task.

Identification of Ingestants

For emphasis, the specific composition of the ingestant naturally determines the recommended treatment. Precise identification may be critical. Careful attention to trade name and manufacturer of household products is mandatory; these products account for nearly half the total number of ingestions. Fortunately, the Federal Hazardous Labeling Act requires listing of toxic ingredients on the label for an ever-increasing number of such products. For solid drug forms, the advantages of *imprint codes* are obvious; almost half of ingested items are obtained by the child after they have been transferred from the original container to another. Today, 82 of the 83 manufacturers who illustrate their products in the *Physician's Desk Reference* use imprinting on at least some of their products. Relying on non-imprint characteristics (shape, color, size) results in less than 55 per cent accuracy in identification; relying on imprint codes permits a 97 per cent accuracy in less than 15 seconds. At the same time, host factors also must be considered—age, weight, race, sex—each of these can convert an innocuous ingestion into an accidental poisoning.

Aspirin as an Example

Long the professional's ally, literally tons of aspirin are sold each year. Widespread availability increases the two- to five-year-old's chance to "get into aspirin." A few years ago much propaganda encouraged all parents to put locks on their medicine cabinets as a device to prevent accidental ingestion of aspirin. It made good public relations for many well-motivated interests; unfortunately the fact was overlooked that children get their aspirin from the medicine cabinet *less than 1 per cent of the time.* Careful study of this accident process helped suppress this purported panacea that would have been no more than an expensive placebo. Attractive colors, pleasant tastes, parental claims of "It's only candy" are all said to increase the likelihood of ingestion. Again, current evidence disputes such allegations; immediate environmental circumstances and family situations, as well as personality patterns, appear to be far more contributory to the ingestion process. Obviously, close parental supervision and protection in early life aim to minimize exposure; these gradually give way to the educational process.

Once aspirin has been ingested, if a valid estimate of the amount can be obtained, prediction of its toxicity can be made by consulting any standard pediatric text or calling the nearest poison information center. As a rule of thumb, a single ingestion of 150 to 200 mg/kg necessitates professional intervention; lesser ingestion requires simple observation with a reminder that the child has a 25 per cent chance to repeat the "accident." (The age of the child and his existing state of health—dehydration or fever—may modify the predicted toxic level.) Many times the child will vomit after swallowing aspirin, particularly the adult form; shortly thereafter he usually begins to "look sick." Metabolic acidosis develops within the hour, and hyperpnea becomes evident, sometimes confusing the issue with a primary pulmonary problem. Hypoglycemia may follow. Unchecked, one of the expected 30 annual fatalities in the United States from aspirin poisoning in those under five years may ensue.

Treatment aims. First, treatment aims to rid the child of the ingested aspirin. Two, or possibly three, approaches are currently available. Induction of emesis by syrup of ipecac, *15 to 20 ml with water,* or injection of apomorphine removes more of the ingested material than does gastric lavage. Moreover, while syrup of ipecac can be administered in the home or on the way to hospital, gastric lavage requires hospital equipment, which often accounts for an undue delay in initiation of treatment. As a consequence, a community-wide program has been undertaken in Seattle and other communities to encourage parents of young children to have syrup of ipecac available within the home, and arrangements have been completed with the round-the-clock neighborhood grocery stores to stock this product to limit the delay even at night and on weekends.

Possibly, but not completely substantiated, adsorption of orally ingested toxins by "activated charcoal" may prove even more efficacious. On the other hand, if absorption has already occurred, alkalinization of the urine by intravenous administration of sodium bicarbonate (3 mEq/kg) will increase renal excretion by a factor of as much as 10, if fluid intake is maintained at 4000 ml/m². In children, peritoneal dialysis or hemodialysis is rarely necessary for acute aspirin ingestion. Unfortunately, no specific antidote for aspirin exists, as compared with that of atropine and PAM (pralidoxime) in organic phosphate insecticide ingestion or BAL (dimercaprol) in mercury poisoning. Again, the details of supportive treatment such as fluid therapy and laboratory tests can be gleaned from standard sources. It is better to refresh one's memory about such details at the time rather than try to remember the details of each possibility.

Other Ingestants

Iron preparations, which are frequently prescribed for pregnant housewives, constitute "sleepers." Ferrous sulfate poisoning leads to initial vomiting, which gives way to a period of quiescence. This is followed in two to three hours by vasomotor collapse and death shortly thereafter. Today a new chelating agent, desferrioxamine, is available that binds iron and drastically curtails both morbidity and mortality. It is given orally and by injection; the oral route may preclude absorption, and injection hastens innocuous excretion.

Barbiturate and tranquilizer ingestions continue to burgeon. Both can present confusing clinical pictures, i.e., coma, delirium or extrapyramidal reactions such as with phenothiazines. Best results follow conservative support measures, except for the phenothiazine reactions, which respond dramatically to Benadryl injections. Central nervous system stimulants are universally *contraindicated.*

Hydrocarbons, such as kerosene, gasoline and furniture polish, cause a chemical aspiration pneumonia. *Both* emesis and lavage probably should be avoided. Pulmonary function must be supported. Steroids and antibiotics have not proved effective in controlled studies.

Lye burns of the mouth and esophagus are long-term problems. One must rely on esophagoscopy to establish accurate diagnosis; steroids, antibiotics and dilatations ought only to follow.

Opiates and other narcotics are more of a problem with teenagers and young adults; nonetheless, young children occasionally do gain access to these items or to methadone used for maintenance programs. The specific antidote naloxone (Narcan) is exceedingly effective in such cases.

Tricyclic antidepressants are appearing with increasing frequency and may be associated with central nervous system as well as cardiac symptoms. Since 1975, physostigmine has been introduced as a most specific antidote for the CNS symptoms. The cardiac arrhythmias still tend to be managed by the more conventional arrhythmical drugs such as Lidocaine and Dilantin.

Lead, mercury, arsenic and their inorganic salts and organic compounds produce a wide range of signs and symptoms. Lead constitutes a public health burden among young urban children, who may ingest old lead-containing paint as it chips off window sills.

Pesticides and insecticides pose particular problems, especially the rapidly acting cholinesterase inhibitors used by commercial sprayers. Anyone employing these products ought have the two very specific antidotes, atropine and PAM, on hand for momentary use.

Plants and berries constitute an obvious attraction to inquiring two-year-olds. Their toxic ingredients are legion, and their ability to defy precise identification is infamous. Fortunately, most are relatively nontoxic but a few, varying by region, constitute special hazards. Each community should develop a list of its high-risk items.

COMMENT: Much more could be said on this subject. Suffice it to stress that appropriate intervention may prevent both accidents and accidental poisonings. As a rule of thumb, whenever confronted by any pediatric patient, ask the question, "Could this have been caused by an accident, a foreign body or an accidental ingestion?"

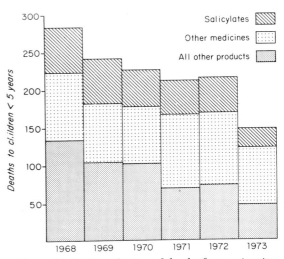

Figure 19–2 Distribution of deaths from poisoning in children under five years of age from 1968 through 1973. Note the decrease in the mortality rate due to salicylates and to non-medications. (Data from Mortality Statistics Division of the National Center for Health Statistics. H.E.W., October, 1976.)

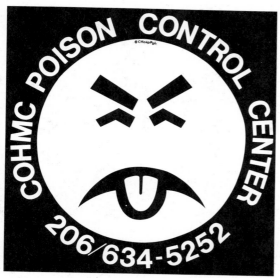

Figure 19-3 The "Mr. Yuk" label for poisonous medication, which contains the telephone number for the regional poison center, in this instance at the Children's Orthopedic Hospital in Seattle.

PREVENTION

Obviously, prevention is better than treatment. Intervention at this stage, as with any accident or illness, represents the ideal. Technological ingenuity—new ideas and modern plastics—make more than 20 varieties of safety caps available to exclude the curious toddler from both solid and liquid products. While obviously not a total solution to the accidental ingestion problem, this innovation has been associated with a dramatic reduction in both morbidity and mortality consequent to accidental ingestions. In the State of Washington, for example, both federal and state laws require the use of safety caps on medicines and on a variety of toxic household products. The use of safety caps for aspirin bottles has decreased the frequency of accidental ingestion of aspirin among study populations from one case for every 190 bottles sold to less than one case for every 5000 bottles sold. In none of the instances was the aspirin actually taken from a closed bottle. Since this innovation, there has been a steady and dramatic decrease in childhood deaths due to aspirin ingestion; i.e., from a mean of more than 100 annual deaths between 1960 and 1970 to less than 30 in 1974. Figure 19-2 shows the decrease in death due to ingestion.

Finally, "regionalization" of Poison Information Programs has evolved, with larger communities serving the needs of smaller ones. Particularly promising has been the "Mr. Yuk" program originated in Pittsburgh. Studies found that the traditional skull and crossbones aimed at deterring children from consuming dangerous products was also being utilized to attract children to watch Saturday morning television and to attend the Pittsburgh Pirates' baseball games. Therefore, the unit went about the scientific development of an alternative label deterrent which, when placed on a dangerous product, not only served to discourage the child from eating it but simultaneously reminded the parents of the emergency phone number to call should an accidental ingestion occur. The "Mr. Yuk" sticker symbol (Fig. 19-3) and prevention program is now being utilized in many parts of the nation, including the Pacific Northwest.

REFERENCES

Arena, J.: Symposium: Advances in the treatment of poisoning. Modern Treatment, 8:459, 1971.

Corby, J., et al.: Clinical comparison of emetics. Pediatrics, 42:361, 1968.

Dreisbach, R.: Handbook of Poisoning: Diagnosis and Treatment, 8th ed. Los Altos, Calif., Lange Medical Publications, 1974.

Gosselin, R. R., Hodge, H. C., Smith, R. R., and Gleason, M. N.: Clinical Toxicology of Commercial Products. Baltimore, The Williams & Wilkins Co., 1976.

Harper, P.: Accidents. In Harper, P. A.: Preventive Pediatrics. New York, Appleton-Century-Crofts, 1962.

Robertson, K. A., Robertson, W. O.: Drug identification by imprint. Clin. Toxicol., 7:83, 1974.

Robertson, W. O., Robertson, K. A., and Peters, J. W.: Poison control: Retrieving stored information. J. Pediatr., 83:461, 1973.

Symonds, J., and Robertson, W.: Drug identification. J.A.M.A., 199:664, 1967.

Child Abuse and Neglect

20

*Barton D. Schmitt
and C. Henry Kempe*

Child abuse and neglect can be broadly defined as maltreatment of children and adolescents by parents, guardians or other caretakers. The physician has two main responsibilities in these cases — detection and reporting. He must be able to diagnose this problem in his own patients as well as to confirm the diagnosis in patients referred by other professionals. Discovery is especially important in the first six months of an infant's life, because the risk of a fatal outcome is high if the diagnosis is missed at this age. In addition, the laws on reporting child abuse are clear. In all 50 states it is mandatory for the physician to report suspected cases of child abuse and neglect to the local protective service agency. The law protects the physician from liability suits if his suspicion should prove to be wrong. Reluctance to report can lead to a recurrence of injuries or even death in the child.

Definition of Child Abuse and Neglect

Physical abuse. Physical abuse or non-accidental trauma can be defined as injuries inflicted by a caretaker. Such injuries include bruises, burns, head injuries and fractures. Severity can range from minor bruises to fatal subdural hematomas. Since physical punishment is acceptable in our society, physicians must have guidelines to when it is excessive and, therefore, represents physical abuse. Corporal punishment that causes bruises or leads to an injury requiring medical treatment is outside the range of normal punishment. Bruising implies hitting without restraint. A few bruises in the name of discipline can easily become a more serious injury the next time. Although discipline is necessary to prevent spoiled children, harsh discipline is not.

Nutritional deprivation. Underfeeding (caloric deprivation) causes more than 50 per cent of cases of failure to thrive (underweight) in infancy. The 3 per cent or more of normal children who are short but well-nourished are not included.

Sexual abuse. Sexual abuse can be defined as any sexual exploitation of a child under age 18 by a family-related adult. This may include incest (sexual intercourse), sodomy (anal intercourse), oral-genital contact or molestation (fondling, masturbation or exposure). Sexual abuse is probably the most underdiagnosed type of child abuse. In most cases the victimized child is a girl. Vulvitis, vaginitis or venereal disease in the prepubertal child must make the physician suspicious of sexual abuse. The initial goal of therapy is first to separate the child from the offending adult, and then to provide the family with intensive psychotherapy.

Intentional drugging or poisoning. This includes drugging children with adult sedatives, sharing narcotics or other dangerous drugs with children and intentionally poisoning children. Parents who purposely drug children must be reported for the child's protection.

Medical care neglect. When a child with a treatable chronic disease has serious deterioration in his condition or frequent emergencies because the parents repeatedly ignore medical recommendations for home treatment, the case may require reporting for court-enforced supervision or even foster placement. An example would be a young child with diabetes who is not given his insulin. A court order to hospitalize and treat is also needed in situations in which an emergency exists that the parents will not acknowledge. Examples are a blood transfusion that is refused on religious grounds or a child with meningitis whom the parents refuse to hospitalize.

Emotional abuse. Emotional abuse can be defined as the continual scapegoating and rejection of a specific child by his caretakers. Severe verbal abuse and berating is always present. This condition is difficult to prove. Psychological terrorism is present in some cases (e.g., locking child in dark cellar or threats of mutilation). The diagnostic criteria of emotional abuse are severe psychopathology in the child documented by a psychiatrist plus the continued refusal by the parents of treatment for the child. Situations in which the only parent is floridly psychotic, and hence inadequate to care for the children, or severely depressed, and hence a danger to the children, should also be included and reported.

In addition, lack of supervision, abandonment, physical neglect (grossly inadequate hygiene, clothing and shelter) and school avoidance are also reportable, but usually do not involve physicians.

Statistics

Incidence. The incidence of child abuse and neglect is generally 1 per cent of children. The prevalence is approximately 650 cases per million population per year. The types of child abuse are 70 per cent physical abuse, 7 per cent sexual abuse, 3 per cent failure to thrive secondary to nutritional deprivation and 20 per cent neglect. Approximately 10 per cent of injuries seen in a hospital emergency room in children under five years of age are inflicted. The death rate is about 3 per cent, or 2000 deaths per year in this country.

The victim. Estimates of the average age for physical abuse show that one third occur under six months of age, one third from six months to three years of age, and one third over age three. Prematures are at a 3 to 1 greater risk. Stepchildren are also at increased risk.

The child with failure to thrive is usually less than two years of age, because he can usually obtain food for himself after that age. In bizarre circumstances, an older child may be confined to his room and slowly starved.

The abuser. The abuser is a related caretaker in 90 per cent of cases, a boyfriend in 5 per cent, an unrelated babysitter in 4 per cent and a sibling in 1 per cent. Parents who abuse their children come from all ethnic, geographic, religious, educational, occupational and socioeconomic groups. Poverty groups may have an increased incidence of child abuse because of the increased crises and the decreased resources available to them. Women are more likely to be involved in abuse than are men because mothers spend more time with their children. The difference is not present if the fathers are unemployed.

Etiology

Physical abuse. More than 90 per cent of abusing parents are neither psychotic nor sociopaths. They tend to be lonely, unhappy, angry adults under tremendous stress. They injure their children in a moment of anger after being provoked by some misbehavior. They usually have experienced physical abuse themselves as children. Their poor impulse control is thus a re-enactment of what happened to them.

For physical abuse to occur it requires not only the right parent but also the right child and the right day. The right child has characteristics that make him demanding and difficult. The right day usually is a day of crisis. The most common crises include losing a job, being evicted, having the car break down, birth of a sibling or an acute illness that leads to intractable crying.

Failure to thrive. The main cause of this disorder is that the baby is not fed enough. Certain factors in the mother, the baby and the environment contribute to this process. Most mothers involved in maternal deprivation feel deprived and unloved themselves. In the majority of cases the baby was unwanted. Multiple ongoing crises that overwhelm the mother are common. A frequent crisis is a physically absent father who is in the military, in shipping, a truckdriver or a traveling salesman.

Clinical History

Many cases of physical abuse are first suspected because of the implausible history that is offered to explain a child's injury.

Unexplained injury. Some parents will be reluctant to elaborate on how the injury might have happened, and others might say they have no idea about it. Some will give a vague explanation such as, "He might have fallen down." These explanations are self-incriminating. Normal parents know to the minute when and where their child was hurt.

Discrepant history. Sometimes there is a discrepancy between the histories offered by the two parents. Another common contradiction occurs between the history offered and the physical findings, such as a history of a minor accident and yet the findings of a major injury. Sometimes a discrepancy exists between the history and the child's developmental age.

Alleged self-inflicted injury. The child who is under six months of age is unlikely to be able to induce an accident. Absurd stories such as the baby rolled over on his arm and broke it or got his head caught in the crib and fractured it are pure nonsense. Histories of older children who deliberately injure themselves are also usually false (e.g., climbing up onto a hot radiator).

Delay in seeking medical care. Normal parents see a doctor immediately when their child is injured. Some abused children are not seen for a considerable period of time despite a major injury. In its extreme, children can be brought in nearly dead. Some 40 per cent of children do not see a doctor until the morning after an injury. Another 40 per cent are seen one to four days after the injury.

Failure to thrive. The diet history in caloric deprivation is usually not helpful because the parent reports that her baby consumes an abundance of calories. About 20 per cent of failure to thrive cases are due to errors in preparation of formula or errors in frequency or amount of feedings rather than maternal deprivation. These cases are diagnosed by a detailed diet history. Errors in formula preparation are especially likely with powdered milk. Breast-fed babies occasionally fail to thrive because the mother has been advised against all supplements.

Physical Examination

Bruises, welts, and scars. Bruises confined to the buttocks and lower back are almost always related to punishment. Finger and thumb prints may be found on the arms where the child was grabbed. Attempts to silence a screaming child with impatient, forced feedings may lead to bruising of the upper lip and frenulum. Human bite marks are distinctive, circular bruises with clear centers and some individual teeth marks. When a blunt instrument is used in punishment, a bruise or welt will often resemble it in shape. Loop marks on the skin are secondary to a doubled-over cord or rope. Lash marks are seen after beating with a belt, tree branch, or hard-edged ruler (Fig. 20–1). Choke marks may be seen on the neck, and circumferential tie marks on the ankles or wrists. Bruises and scars may be found at multiple stages of healing. One possible

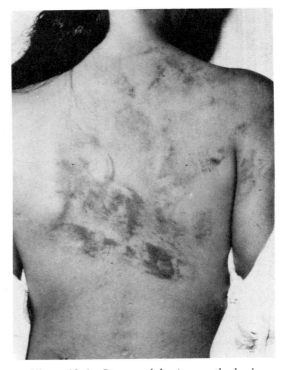

Figure 20–1   Strap mark bruises on the back.

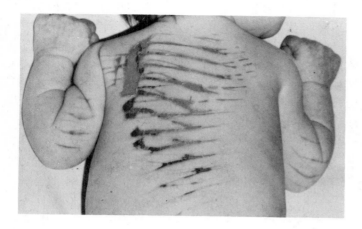

Figure 20–2 Heating grate burn of back and upper arms.

error is mistaking a Mongolian spot for a bruise.

Burns. Approximately 10 per cent of physical abuse cases involve burns. Cigarette burns are commonly inflicted. These are circular, punched-out areas of similar size. Lesions are often found on the palms or soles.

Dry contact burns can occur from forcibly holding the child against a heating device (e.g., a heating grate). These are usually second degree burns without any blister formation (Fig. 20–2). They usually involve only one surface of the body or both palms.

Hot water burns are of several types. A dunking burn occurs when a parent holds the thighs against the abdomen and dunks the buttocks and perineum into scalding water as punishment for enuresis or resistance to toilet training. This results in a circular type burn on the buttocks with a clear-cut water level. The hands and feet are spared, which is incompatible with falling into a tub or turning the hot water on while in the bathtub. The dunking burn accounts for half of inflicted burns. Forcible immersion of a hand or foot as punishment can be diagnosed by finding a burn scar that goes well above the wrist or ankle.

Eye damage. Ocular damage in the battered child syndrome includes acute hyphema, dislocated lens and detached retina. More than half of these result in permanent impairment of vision affecting one or both eyes.

Central nervous system damage. The worst injury in terms of death or serious sequelae is subdural hematoma. These children often are seen with coma and convulsions. Some of them have multiple skull fractures secondary to being hit against a wall or door. More than half the cases, however, have no skull fracture or scalp bruises. These were once called spontaneous subdural hematomas, but recent studies prove that the unexplained subdural hematoma is due to violent, shaking injuries. The rapid acceleration and deceleration of the head as it bobs about leads to tearing of the bridging veins with bleeding into the subdural space, usually bilaterally. Retinal hemorrhages are nearly always present and help to establish the diagnosis.

Abdominal visceral injuries. Intraabdominal injuries are the second most common cause of death in battered children. Children present with recurrent vomiting, abdominal distention, absent bowel sounds or localized tenderness. The most unique findings are tears or other injuries of the small intestine at sites of ligamental support such as the duodenum and proximal jejunum.

Failure to thrive. A failure-to-thrive child usually has a weight that is below the third percentile and a height that is above the third percentile. Although growth curves help, failure to thrive is diagnosed mainly by examining the patient and finding little subcutaneous tissue. Reduction in subcutaneous tissue leads to a pinched face from lack of buccal fat pads, prominent ribs, wasted buttocks with much redundant skin and spindly extremities.

Laboratory Data

If the child has unexplained bruises or the parents admit to inflicting the bruises but claim their child "bruises easily," special bleeding tests are in order. In most cases these are unnecessary. A child with failure to thrive and an otherwise normal physical examination requires very few baseline laboratory tests. A complete blood count, erythrocyte sedimentation rate, urine analysis, urine culture, stool pH, stool hematest, stool culture, serum electrolytes, BUN and tuberculin tests are adequate.

Radiological Findings

A radiological bone survey consisting of long bone, skull, thorax, pelvis and spine films will often clinch the diagnosis of physical abuse. A trauma survey should be obtained on all patients with suspected physical abuse or confirmed nutritional deprivation. These roentgenograms are of great diagnostic value, since the clinical findings of fracture often disappear in six or seven days even without orthopedic care. Sometimes no major fracture is present. Fortunately for the child who is too young to speak, wrenching injuries to the long bones usually tear off the periosteum plus a corner of metaphysis. Immediately after the injury, this chip fracture or corner fracture is visible on roentgenogram. From 10 to 14 days later the subperiosteal bleeding that has occurred will also begin to calcify (Fig. 20–3). The best diagnostic roentgenogram includes multiple bone injuries at different stages of healing. Such a roentgenogram implies repeated assault.

Rare bone disorders such as osteogenesis imperfecta, infantile cortical hyperostosis, scurvy, syphilis and neoplasms may resemble non-accidental trauma. However, a skilled radiologist can easily differentiate these entities.

Diagnosis of Physical Abuse

Physical abuse may be diagnosed if an injury is unexplained or inadequately explained. Certain bruises, burns and scars are pathognomonic. Subdural hematomas do not occur spontaneously and are often secondary to violent shaking. Radiographic findings of chip fractures or multiple bony injuries at different stages of healing are also diagnostic.

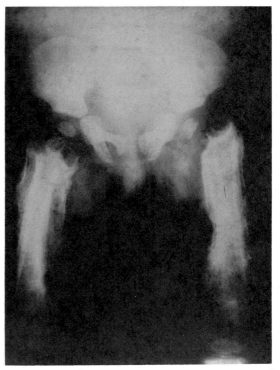

Figure 20–3 Severe subperiosteal bleeding and calcification of both femurs secondary to repeated trauma.

Diagnosis of Failure to Thrive Secondary to Nutritional Deprivation

An attempt at nutritional rehabilitation is the starting point for reaching a definitive diagnosis in infants with failure to thrive. The child should be hospitalized and placed on unlimited feedings of a regular diet for age. The formula should be identical to the one used at home. Rapid weight gain on a formula free of cow's milk protein or lactose would prove nothing. The daily caloric intake should approach 150 to 200 cal/kg/day. This therapeutic trial of feeding should last a maximum of two weeks. The underweight infant who gains rapidly and easily in the hospital is a victim of underfeeding at home. A rapid weight gain can be defined as greater than 1.5 oz/day sustained for two weeks. A gain of over 2.0 oz/day in a one-week period is also diagnostic. Sometimes hospital weight gain is less than this but if it is two to three times greater than a similar period at home it is diagnostic.

Treatment

The highest priority of treatment is to protect the child. Any child who is a suspected victim of abuse requires hospitalization until evaluations regarding the safety of the home are complete. All too often, a crying baby with a minor inflicted injury is sent home, only to return the next day with subdural hematoma or multiple fractures. The reason given to the parents for the hospitalization is that his "injuries need to be watched." Incriminating questions should be kept to a minimum in the outpatient setting. A more detailed history can be pursued once the child is safely admitted to the ward. If the parents refuse hospitalization, a court order can be obtained.

The physician is required by law to report these cases to the child protection service agency in the child's county of residence. This agency is made up of specially trained social workers. The report should be made by telephone within 24 hours and in writing within 48 hours. Unless these cases are reported, treatment will not occur, and abuse will probably continue. Reporting guarantees adequate evaluation, treatment and follow-up. The physician must tell the family what he is doing. He can simply state that he is obligated by state law to report any unusual injuries. He can reassure the parents that everyone involved will try to help them find better ways of dealing with their child. Maintaining a helping approach with these parents is often the hardest part of therapy. Feeling angry with these parents is natural, but expressing this anger is very damaging to parent cooperation. The physician should remember that the injury occurred in a moment of anger, it was not deliberate and these parents already feel inadequate and unloved. Confrontation, accusation and repeated interrogation must be avoided. The physician should encourage hospital visits by the parents and be certain that ward personnel treat them kindly.

Multidisciplinary teams, called Child Protection Teams, are needed to evaluate these complex cases and coordinate the numerous community agencies. Such a team is made up of physician, hospital social worker, protective service agency social worker, psychiatrist, psychologist, developmental specialist, lawyer, public health nurse, police representative and others. Within one week of admission and after all evaluations are completed, this interagency team holds a dispositional conference to decide the best immediate and long-range treatment plans for the family. Treatment modalities must be individually designed for the specific abusive family. These should be more expansive than traditional casework. Some modern types of treatment that have been shown to be successful are lay therapists or parenting aides, homemakers, parents anonymous groups, telephone hotlines, crisis nurseries, psychotherapy, marital counseling, vocational rehabilitation and child rearing counseling. The treatment needs of the child should also be considered and may require play therapy, a therapeutic preschool or day care. The child protective service agency also makes home visits and is responsible for assuring that therapy is in progress and that the family does not become "lost to follow-up." In about 20 per cent of cases the child must temporarily be placed in a foster home while his natural home is made safe. This requires a legal action in juvenile court.

Prognosis

Treated cases of child abuse and neglect. With comprehensive, intensive treatment of the entire family, 80 to 90 per cent of these families can be rehabilitated, and can thereafter provide adequate care for their child. Approximately 10 to 15 per cent of these families can only be stabilized, and require indefinite support services. Termination of parental rights and release of the child for adoption is required in 1 to 2 per cent of cases.

Untreated physical abuse. If the child is returned to his parents without any intervention, 5 per cent are killed and 35 per cent are seriously re-injured. Untreated families tend to produce children who grow up to be juvenile delinquents and violent members of society, as well as child abusers themselves. Child abuse has been correlated with playground violence, street violence, marital violence and criminal violence.

Untreated failure to thrive. Without detection and intervention, some children die of starvation. Others sustain superimposed physical abuse. Although weight loss and understature from malnutrition are entirely retrievable, brain growth and head circumference may not be. In addition to these physical problems, the child with nutritional deprivation usually suffers from prolonged emotional deprivation and subsequent personality disorders.

REFERENCES

Caffey, J.: The whiplash shaken infant syndrome. Pediatrics, 54:396, 1974.

Fontana, V. J.: The diagnosis of the maltreatment syndrome in children. Pediatrics, 51(Suppl.):780, 1973.

Hannaway, P. J.: Failure to thrive: A study of 100 infants and children. Clin. Pediatr., 9:96, 1970.

Helfer, R. E.: The responsibility and role of the physician. In Helfer, R. E., and Kempe, C. H. (Eds.): The Battered Child, 2nd ed. Chicago, University of Chicago Press, 1974, p. 25.

Helfer, R. E.: The etiology of child abuse. Pediatrics, 51(Suppl.):777, 1973.

Keen, J. H., Lendrum, J., and Wolman, B.: Inflicted burns and scalds in children. Brit. Med. J., 1:268, 1975.

Kempe, C. H., and Helfer, R. E.: Helping the Battered Child and His Family. Philadelphia, J. B. Lippincott Co., 1972.

Kempe, C. H., et al.: The battered child syndrome. J.A.M.A., 181:17, 1962.

Koel, B. S.: Failure to thrive and fatal injury as a continuum. Am. J. Dis. Child., 118:565, 1969.

Lansky, L. L.: An unusual case of childhood chloral hydrate poisoning. Am. J. Dis. Child., 127:275, 1974.

Lauer, B., Ten Broeck, E., and Grossman, M.: Battered child syndrome: Review of 130 patients with controls. Pediatrics, 54:67, 1974.

Sarles, R. M.: Incest. Pediatr. Clin. N. Am., 22:633, 1975.

Schmitt, B. D., and Kempe, C. H.: The pediatrician's role in child abuse and neglect. Curr. Probl. Pediatr., 5(5):3, 1975.

Sgroi, S. M.: Sexual molestation of children. Children Today, 4:18, 1975.

Silverman, F. N.: Unrecognized trauma in infants, the battered child syndrome, and the syndrome of Ambroise Tardieu. Radiology, 104:337, 1972.

Sussman, S. J.: Skin manifestations of the battered-child syndrome. J. Pediatr., 72:99, 1968.

Touloukian, R. J.: Abdominal visceral injuries in battered children. Pediatrics, 42:642, 1968.

Whitten, C. F., Pettit, M. G., and Fischoff, J.: Evidence that growth failure from maternal deprivation is secondary to undereating. J.A.M.A., 209:1675, 1969.

PART VII

DYSMORPHOLOGY DISORDERS

21 Congenital Postural Deformities*

P. M. Dunn

With few exceptions, congenital anomalies may be subdivided into "malformations," which arise as a result of primary errors in morphogenesis, and "deformations," which are alterations in the form or structure of a previously normally formed part. Malformations are discussed in Chapter 22. The great majority of deformations involve the musculoskeletal system and have been called the congenital postural deformities. The hypothesis that such deformities might be caused by mechanical factors operating during fetal life dates back to Hippocrates and was readvanced in recent times by Browne and by Chapple and Davidson.

This theory states that congenital postural deformities are caused by intrauterine moulding. While the pressure required to produce such moulding may occasionally arise intrinsically because of muscle imbalance secondary to neuromuscular disease, in most cases it is of extrinsic origin, arising in the later weeks of pregnancy as the volume of amniotic fluid diminishes and the still plastic and rapidly growing fetus becomes constrained within the uterus. All parts of the infant may be affected. The most important deformities are set forth in Table 21–1.

INCIDENCE AND ASSOCIATION WITH MALFORMATION

The data presented here are predominantly based on personal evaluation of 4754 infants born in the Birmingham (England) Maternity Hospital with information concerning the mother's medical and pregnancy history, the infant's follow-up record

TABLE 21–1 MUSCULOSKELETAL DEFORMATIONS OF MECHANICAL ORIGIN PRESENT AT BIRTH

Of the skull: dolichocephaly; plagiocephaly; depressions in skull.

Of the face: Potter's facies; nasal and oral deformities; mandibular asymmetry; retrognathia; midline cleft palate; facial nerve neurapraxia.

Of the neck: Sternomastoid contracture, 'tumour' and torticollis.

Of the upper limbs: dislocation of the shoulder; clubhand; compressed arm and hand (in Potter's syndrome); radial nerve neurapraxia.

Of the body: pigeon chest; pectus excavatum; postural scoliosis.

Of the lower limbs: dislocation of the hips; bowing of the long bones; genu recurvatum; various deformities of the feet including talipes equinovarus, calcaneovalgus, and metatarsus varus; sciatic and obturator nerve neurapraxias.

Of the whole body: arthrogryposis multiplex congenita, general compression (as in Potter's syndrome).

Note: Not all cases of some of the conditions noted here are due to mechanical factors (e.g., cleft palate and arthrogryposis)

*This chapter is largely based on an article: Dunn, P. M.: Congenital Postural Deformities. Br. Med. Bull., 32:71–76, 1976, and is partially reproduced by permission of the Medical Department, the British Council. This issue of the *British Medical Bulletin* was devoted to human malformations and contains a number of excellent papers in this regard. It is available from *British Medical Bulletin*, The British Council, 65 Davies St., London, WIY 2AA, England.

TABLE 21–2 SOME CONTRASTING CHARACTERISTICS OF CONGENITAL MALFORMATIONS AND CONGENITAL POSTURAL DEFORMITIES*

	Malformation	Deformation (postural)
Incidence before twentieth week	approximately 5.0	0.1
Incidence after twenty-eighth week	3.7	2.0
Perinatal mortality	41.0	6.0
Structural changes	Usual	Rare
Spontaneous correction	Very rare	Usual
Correction by posture	Not possible	Usually possible

*Based on Dunn and on Nishimura.

and post-mortem examinations. Some of the contrasting characteristics of congenital malformations and congenital postural deformities are shown in Table 21–2. The spectrum of severity from mild to severe moulding is another distinguishing feature of the postural deformities. Nishimura's observation, based on the examination of aborted fetuses, that deformities such as talipes and congenital dislocation of the hip (CDH) were exceedingly rare before the twentieth week of gestation, confirms the belief that these anomalies arise in late pregnancy.

If the various postural deformities have a common mechanical origin, one would expect to find infants with multiple deformities. Table 21–3 summarizes the highly significant clinical association between the main groups of postural deformities.

Deformation is much more common (7.6 per cent) among infants with malformation, especially in relation to particular types of malformation. The association between de-

formities and certain malformations may be readily explained within the mechanical theory. The legs of infants with meningomyelocele and other spinal anomalies may be partially paralyzed, and the resulting muscular imbalance may give rise to an intrinsic deforming force. In addition, paralysis of the lower limbs will deprive the fetus of its ability to kick and hence to change its position *in utero* and alter the direction along which potentially deforming extrinsic forces may be acting. This subject, and the high incidence of associated breech presentation that results, are discussed later. At this point, though, it should be mentioned that deformities are also found in association with other less common neuromuscular disorders of the fetus such as sacral agenesis or congenital myotonic dystrophy. Generalized disorders may result in congenital multiple arthrogryposis.

Oligohydramnios will also tend to prevent the fetus from moving and at the same time will expose it to extrinsic pressure. There can be no doubt that this is the cause of the compression of infants with bilateral renal anomalies; for oligohydramnios is almost always present in such cases. Multiple deformities include dislocation of the hip, congenital sternomastoid torticollis, talipes, compression of arms and hands and a characteristic facies first described by Potter. Potter's syndrome originally embraced the association between this facies and other limb deformities with bilateral renal agenesis, but similar signs of prenatal compression may be found in association with bilateral renal hypoplasia and multicystic kidneys, as well as with urethral atresia and urethral valves; the key factor is undoubtedly oligohydramnios due to fetal oliguria or anuria.

TABLE 21–3 STATISTICAL ANALYSIS OF STUDIES MADE DURING 1960–63 OF THE CLINICAL ASSOCIATION BETWEEN CERTAIN CONGENITAL POSTURAL DEFORMITIES

	Facial Deformities	Plagiocephaly	Mandibular Asymmetry	Sternomastoid Torticollis	Scoliosis — Postural	Congenital Dislocation of the Hip	Talipes
Facial Deformities	–	S	S°	S	S°	S°	S°
Plagiocephaly	S	–	S°	S°	S°	S°	N
Mandibular Asymmetry	S°	S°	–	S°	N	S°	S°
Sternomastoid Torticollis	S	S°	S°	–	S°	N	S°
Scoliosis — postural	S°	S°	N	S°	–	S°	S
Congenital Dislocation of the Hip	S°	S°	S°	N	S°	–	S°
Talipes	S°	N	S°	S°	S	S°	–

*Based on Dunn, 1972.
Abbreviations: N: not significant; S: $P < 0.05$; S°: $P < 0.001$.

FETAL GROWTH AND PLASTICITY

Anthropology provides many examples of deliberate postnatal deformation. For example, the curious shape of the skull of the Chinook Indians was achieved by splinting the head between boards during infancy, and the Chinese were accustomed to bind the feet of their girls in order to produce a crippling deformity that was regarded as beautiful. Both recognized the importance of applying constant pressure during infancy while the body was still relatively plastic and growing rapidly. Indeed, the orthopedic surgeon applies the same principle today in correcting deformities by postural means. If this is true for the infant, then the fetus must be much more vulnerable because of its greater plasticity and more rapid rate of growth. A child of five years requires six years to double his bodyweight. In contrast, a fetus of 28 weeks' gestation achieves the same feat in six weeks, while an embryo of eight weeks' gestation takes only six days. Thus, if the rate of growth were the only factor determining deformation, the fetus might be described as 52 times and the embryo 365 times more vulnerable than the five-year-old child. In addition, the fetus is closely confined within a small space and is exposed to the tone of the uterine and abdominal wall muscles.

The importance of fetal plasticity, which depends to a great extent on the rigidity of the skeleton, must be emphasized. During early gestation, when both the form and size of the embryo are changing rapidly, a rigid, well-developed skeleton would prove an embarrassment. Much of the calcification of the fetal skeleton is laid down during the second half of pregnancy. Thus the skeleton is barely visible radiographically at 20 weeks' gestation, but becomes increasingly radio-opaque in the succeeding months. Even at term, however, a considerable portion, particularly the growing ends of the bones, remains unossified and much more plastic than in later life.

Increased fetal plasticity may also be due to excessive joint laxity, a condition that has been reported in association with deformation and in particular with congenital dislocation of the hip. Both conditions may be familial. The influence of sex on fetal deformation must also be considered.

Among deformed infants, 73 per cent of those with CDH, but only 51 per cent of infants with other deformities, are girls. Thus, CDH alone among deformities appears to have a special predilection for girls. The probable explanation for this well-known phenomenon is that the pelvic ligaments of the female fetus tend to become softened and vulnerable to dislocation through the action of female hormones, including relaxin, probably produced by the ovaries and reproductive tract of the female fetus.

AMNIOTIC FLUID, OLIGOHYDRAMNIOS AND BIRTH-WEIGHT FOR GESTATION

During the early months of pregnancy, when the fetus is fragile and growing rapidly, it is protected from the pressure of the uterus by the amniotic fluid, which also permits the fetus to exercise freely and change its position. However, as pregnancy progresses, fetal growth takes place at the expense of this fluid. This difference is dramatically illustrated in Figure 21–1. While the fetus normally continues to grow until term, the volume of amniotic fluid usually starts to decrease after 37 weeks of gestation. The mean ratio of amniotic fluid volume to fetal volume falls steadily throughout pregnancy from a value of about three at 12 weeks' gestation to close to zero at 42 weeks. Fortunately, as the fetus becomes more exposed to extrinsic pressure, it becomes better able to resist deformation because of diminishing plasticity and slowing growth.

The terminal fall in amniotic fluid volume is thought to be related in part to aging of the placenta. There is certainly an association between oligohydramnios at or even well before term and a number of conditions that tend to impair uteroplacental circulation and placental function. These include an assocation between maternal hypertension, severe pre-eclampsia and oligohydramnios. If there is an association between oligohydramnios and placental insufficiency, then deformed infants might be expected to show signs of prenatal deprivation at birth. Indeed, deformed infants tend to be small for dates, and there is an increased incidence of fetal distress

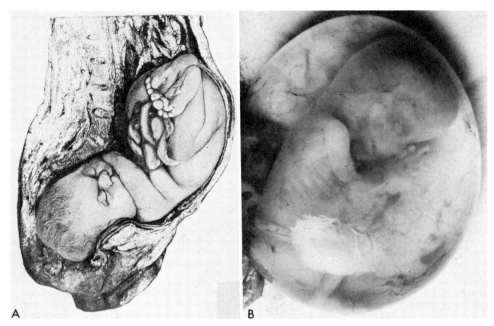

A   B

Figure 21–1 *A*, Frozen section of abdomen of a pregnant woman who died during labor. Note fetus flexed laterally around sacral promontory. *B*, Fetus of 13 weeks' gestation lying within amniotic sac removed at hysterectomy. The amniotic fluid completely protects the fragile fetus from pressure.

during labor and signs of wasting and malnutrition at birth.

Although exact measurements of amniotic fluid volume are rarely made, oligohydramnios may be readily diagnosed clinically and radiologically during pregnancy and may also be observed directly at cesarean delivery and at the time the membranes rupture. During the last 16 years it has been possible to document the association between oligohydramnios and deformation at birth on many occasions. Figure 21–2 shows one such example. It has also been possible to observe repeatedly the close correspondence between the posture of the fetus before delivery (as determined radiographically) and that assumed by the baby after birth, the "position of comfort" as it has been termed by Chapple and Davidson. Moreover, when such infants resume their prenatal posture, it can be seen that the moulded deformities reflect the shape of the uterine cavity. Often the deformities are reciprocal or mutually related, as in bilateral talipes equinovarus (Fig. 21–3), in talipes calcaneovalgus and CDH, in the close association between mandibular asymmetry, torticollis, upturned ear and plagiocephaly or in the laterality of deformations such as torticollis,

scoliosis and CDH in the "windswept baby." The moulding may be asymmetrical, as shown in Figure 21–4.

Perhaps, though, the most convincing evidence of the importance of oligohydramnios is the common occurrence of deformities among infants associated with a deficiency of amniotic fluid, whether by virtue of deficient urine flow into the amniotic space or because of chronic leakage of amniotic fluid. In this context, Poswillo showed that amniocentesis in rats at a certain stage of embryogenesis prior to palate closure led to micrognathia and midline cleft palate (100 per cent frequency) and to deformities of the limbs (30 per cent frequency). His work supports the suggestion that oligohydramnios in early pregnancy may be responsible for mandibular hypoplasia and retropositioning of the tongue with obstruction to palatal closure, the Robin anomalad, in the human infant. Support is lent to this hypothesis by the occurrence of other deformities in half the infants with this condition.

If oligohydramnios favors deformation, polyhydramnios should protect the fetus from extrinsic pressure. This is generally true. The impact on size is also important. Normally formed infants who have had

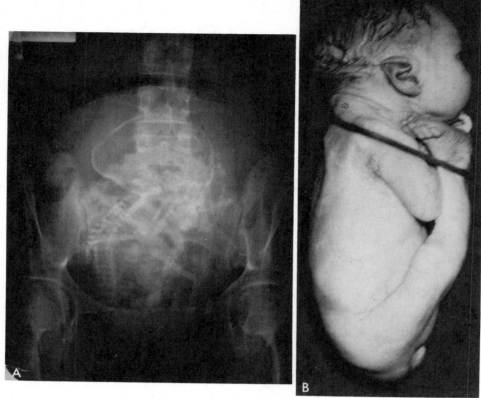

Figure 21–2 *A,* Prenatal and, *B,* postnatal views of female infant with bilateral renal agenesis with secondary oligohydramnios. Note oligohydramnios and compressed appearance with breech presentation and extended legs. Deformities included dolichocephaly, Potter's facies and bilateral congenital dislocation of the hips.

polyhydramnios tend to be large-for-dates, while infants born to women with oligohydramnios due to rupture of the membranes or with deficit of urine tend to be small-for-dates.

FETAL KICKING AND PRESENTATION

The strength of the legs of the fetus during the later weeks of pregnancy, which

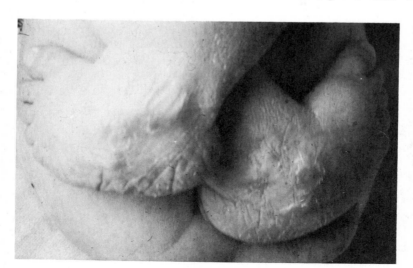

Figure 21–3 Bilateral talipes equinovarus deformity (club feet) associated with fetal cross-legged position and maternal oligohydramnios; note the characteristic pressure atrophy of skin over the external malleoli.

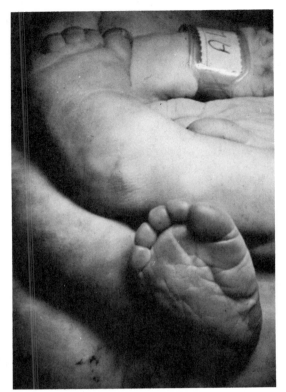

Figure 21–4 Asymmetric moulding deformities of the feet associated with prolonged maternal oligohydramnios.

enables it to kick, to change its position and to alter the direction along which potentially deforming extrinsic forces may be acting, is clearly of great importance. Certainly, conditions that impair or deprive the fetus of its ability to move may be shown to have a highly significant association with congenital deformation. The ability to kick may be impaired by malformations of the lower limbs, such as phocomelia and congenital amputation, or by paralysis secondary to meningomyelocele or other neuromuscular problem. The legs may be weak, either because of prematurity or as the result of disuse atrophy. Alternatively, the legs may be trapped in a position of mechanical disadvantage or have no room to move because of oligohydramnios or because of an abnormally shaped amniotic cavity.

Whether the legs are flexed or extended at the knees affects the ability of the fetus to kick and also alters the shape of its folded form. For both reasons, leg folding influences fetal presentation in the later weeks

of gestation. Thus the fetus with flexed legs is in a powerful kicking position that enables it to turn until its head lies in the smaller pelvic pole of the uterus, while the legs continue to exercise in the broader elastic upper pole. Such infants are much less often deformed than those with legs extended at the knee. An infant with extended legs tends to assume the breech position. The buttocks are toward the birth canal and form the narrow pole of the fetus that slips readily into the mother's pelvis, leaving the legs lying alongside the body and incapable of either flexing or kicking (Fig. 21–5). The fetus may remain for weeks in this predicament (in wrestlers' parlance termed "the folding body press"), becoming steadily moulded and deformed. The baby's hips, confined and growing within the mother's rigid and unyielding bony pelvis, are particularly at risk. Not surprisingly, infants presenting by the breech are approximately 10 times more likely to be deformed than those presenting by the more usual vertex cephalic position. However, it must be appreciated that the breech position of the fetus at term and the deformation may be of a common pathogenesis, as when both are the consequence of a neuromuscular disorder.

The importance of kicking in determining fetal presentation is shown by the raised incidence of breech delivery in various group of infants whose kick is likely

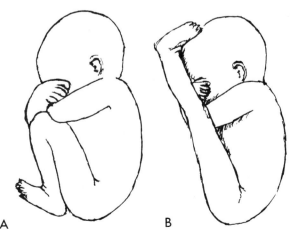

Figure 21–5 Lateral view of fetus with legs (A) flexed at knees, the normal posture, or (B) extended with feet alongside face. Diameter of "breech" is greater than that of vertex when legs are flexed, smaller when they are extended.

to have been impaired: all central nervous system malformations, 33 per cent; meningomyelocele, 48 per cent; reduction deformities of the lower limbs, 100 per cent; oligohydramnios with deformation, 50 to 64 per cent; and preterm infants, 25 per cent. Radiological studies have shown that 76 per cent of infants presenting by the breech after the thirty-fourth week of gestation have one or both legs extended at the knees.

Another way in which the legs of the fetus may become trapped at mechanical disadvantage is for them to be flexed and folded across each other, usually at the level of the ankles. Once again, the fetus may be rendered immobile and exposed to deformation. The feet are particularly exposed in this position and readily become moulded into the club-foot position. Usually both feet are affected, though characteristically the outer foot is the more severely deformed. Often there is pressure atrophy and skin dimpling over the external malleoli and outer borders of the feet.

Legs that have been trapped *in utero* for any length of time commonly show impaired power and movement for days or even weeks after birth. This is not surprising, for immobility and compression may be expected to lead to neural ischemia, impaired muscle nutrition and development and finally to weakness and even atrophy. In extreme cases, arthrogryposis may be caused by prolonged immobilization; of special interest is an infant with this condition who was born to a mother who, becauses of tetanus, had been treated with (+)tubocurarine immobilization for 19 days in early pregnancy.

SHAPE OF THE AMNIOTIC CAVITY

Another important factor in the etiology of prenatal deformation is the shape of the amniotic cavity within which the fetus lies. In part this will be determined by the shape of the uterus itself, which not only varies from person to person like any other part of the body, but may also be distorted by malformation such as unicornous uterus. The shape of the amniotic cavity will obviously also be influenced by the volume of amniotic fluid and the size and shape of the fetus. The latter will depend on the way it is folded as well as on its presentation and orientation within the uterus. Additional factors include the presence of more than one fetus, the site of placental implantation, the presence of uterine fibroids or other tumors and the shape of the abdominal cavity. The pelvis, sacral promontory and neighboring abdominal organs all exert an influence.

Clinical experience has provided many illustrations of the significance of the factors just mentioned so that one example will suffice. It has been possible to explain in terms of fetal position *in utero* the long-recognized observation that CDH is twice as common on the left side as it is on the right. Radiological studies have shown that the fetus tends to lie with its back towards the mother's left side nearly twice as often as towards her right. Further, it has been demonstrated that the leg of the fetus lying posteriorly is more likely to be dislocated than that lying anteriorly, whether the presentation is by the vertex or by the breech. It seems probable that because of the mother's spine, the leg of the fetus lying posteriorly is more likely to be adducted and hence to lie in a position in which the hip is more exposed to dislocation.

A further factor having a profound effect on the shape of the amniotic cavity is the degree of tightness of the mother's abdominal muscles. When these have not been stretched by previous pregnancies, their increased tone tends to compress the uterus backwards against the spine. As a result, the uterine cavity tends to become flattened in its anteroposterior diameter. This means that, for any given volume of amniotic fluid, the fetus will have relatively less room to move and therefore will be more exposed to pressure. First-born infants are more often deformed at birth than are those born to multipara. This observation holds true for each of the main individual deformities. Reports in the literature have also noted the increased tendency of first-born infants to exhibit the following deformities at birth; sternomastoid torticollis, various deformities of the feet and CDH. First pregnancies also have a raised incidence of maternal hypertension, breech presentation and small-for-dates infants.

In extrauterine pregnancy the amniotic sac may lie completely outside the uterus.

Malpresentation and oligohydramnios are frequently present. In such circumstances the fetus is especially exposed to pressure, and deformation is a common finding.

Three per cent of twins are deformed as compared with 2 per cent of singletons. This increased incidence might be expected in view of the associated uterine and abdominal distension and the raised incidence of maternal hypertension, breech presentation and fetal growth retardation. The reason that twins are not even more often deformed may be because there are two amniotic sacs and two pairs of fetal legs, because there is a deficit of multiple pregnancies in primigravid women and because multiple pregnancies often terminate prematurely before reaching the relative oligohydramnios of term.

CONCLUSIONS

Congenital postural deformities not only occur in association with each other but also share a number of pregnancy characteristics, including primigravidity, maternal hypertension, oligohydramnios, breech presentation and fetal growth retardation (Fig. 21–6). The way in which these factors may be interrelated is shown in Figure

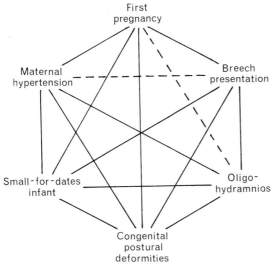

Figure 21–6 Congenital postural deformities and certain pregnancy factors. The unbroken lines represent statistically significant associations, whereas the interrupted lines represent probable but unproved associations. (From Dunn, P. M.: Br. Med. Bull., 32:71, 1976.)

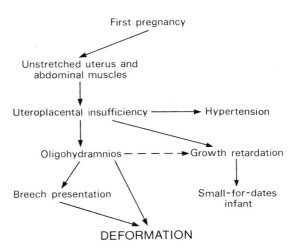

Figure 21–7 Possible interrelation of pregnancy associations with congenital postural deformation. The interrupted line represents a hypothetical association. (From Dunn, P. M.: Br. Med. Bull., 32:71, 1976.)

21–7. Uteroplacental insufficiency and pregnancy hypertension are known to occur more commonly in first pregnancies, perhaps because of the unstretched state of the uterus and abdominal wall muscles. Such uteroplacental insufficiency may be responsible for oligohydramnios, breech presentation and deformation on the one hand, and for fetal growth retardation on the other. Furthermore, the oligohydramnios itself may contribute to the growth retardation.

An attempt has also been made to indicate the way in which intrauterine forces capable of moulding the fetus increase throughout pregnancy as the infant grows, the mother's uterus and abdominal wall are stetched and the volume of amniotic fluid diminishes. At the same time, the ability of the infant to resist deformation also increases as the rate of fetal growth slows, the skeleton ossifies and leg movements become more powerful. These factors are, of course, directly or indirectly under the influence of heredity and are involved in a dynamic interplay throughout fetal life. Nature plays her hand to the limit. The price paid for a larger and more mature infant at birth, better able to withstand the stresses of extrauterine life, is a 2 per cent incidence of deformities. Perhaps we ought rather to marvel at the fact that 98 per cent of infants are *not* deformed at birth and that 90 per cent of those that are will correct spontaneously after birth; with early postural assistance this recovery rate may be brought near to 100 per cent.

REFERENCES

Bain, A. D., Smith, I. I., and Gauld, I. K.: Newborn after prolonged leakage of liquor amnii. Br. Med. J., 2:598, 1964.

Browne, D.: Congenital deformities of mechanical origin. Proc. R. Soc. Med., 29:1409, 1936.

Chapple, C. C., and Davidson, D. T.: Study of relationship between fetal position and certain congenital deformities. J. Pediatr., 18:483, 1941.

Dunn, P. M.: The influence of the intrauterine environment in the causation of congenital postural deformities, with special reference to congenital dislocation of the hip. M.D. Thesis, Cambridge (England), 1969.

Dunn, P. M.: Congenital postural deformities. Br. Med. Bull., 32:71, 1976.

Nishimura, H.: Incidence of malformations in abortions. In Fraser, F. C., and McKusick, V. A. (Eds.): Congenital Malformations. Amsterdam and London, International Congress Series, No. 204, Exerpta Medica, 1970, pp. 275–283.

Poswillo, D.: The aetiology and surgery of cleft palate with micrognathia. Ann. R. Coll. Surg. Engl., 43:61, 1968.

Potter, E. L.: Bilateral renal agenesis. J. Pediatr., 29:68, 1946.

Record, R. G., and Edwards, J. H.: Environmental influences related to the aetiology of congenital dislocation of the hip. Br. J. Prev. Soc. Med., 12:8, 1958.

Malformation

22

David W. Smith

The genetically determined, timely and interacting processes of controlled cellular mitosis, migration, death and association into organ tissues leave us to marvel at the relative infrequency of problems in morphogenesis. Actually, the great majority of problems in morphogenesis are early lethal ones, leading to unrecognized pregnancy, spontaneous abortion or stillbirth. It is important to distinguish between deformation problems, predominantly the consequence of postural molding in late fetal life and malformation, due to an intrinsic problem in the developing tissue. Deformations, covered in Chapter 21, occur in about 3 per cent of newborn babies. Serious malformation problems are recognized in about 2 per cent of liveborn babies, and this rises to around 4 per cent by one year of age, with the further recognition of central nervous system, cardiac, renal and other disorders not detected at birth. Many affected babies die early in life as a consequence of anomalies, such as anencephaly, certain cardiac defects and renal agenesis, which are not compatible with extrauterine life. Thus malformation ranks as the second most common cause of early death, after prematurity and its complications. One fifth of deaths related to malformation occur during the first day, half during the first month and three quarters by one year of age. Our major concern is the early detection of remediable defects of a lethal nature, such as intestinal atresia, or of a potentially handicapping nature, such as dislocation of the hip. For those infants with a non-remediable handicapping problem we should provide the best adaption toward an enjoyable and sociable life. When this is not possible because of severe defect in brain function, for example, we

should question whether life-perpetuating medical interference is merited. For all malformation problems management includes providing the parents with compassionate understanding and counsel, which is discussed at the end of this section.

Obviously, the initial task is recognition and an accurate total diagnosis of a malformation problem, especially in the newborn examination and throughout early infancy. You should be particularly alerted to the possibility of malformation in the high-risk categories set forth in Table 22–1.

Malformation problems may be crudely divided into two general categories: those that represent a single primary localized defect in morphogenesis in an otherwise normal individual, and those that represent multiple defects in one or more systems. The single primary defects, appearing in about three quarters of babies born with malformation, is considered first.

SINGLE LOCALIZED DEFECTS

It is important to appreciate that a single localized defect in early morphogenesis can upset the subsequent development of other structures and result in a baby with more than one anomaly at birth. Thus a failure of closure of the lip by 35 days may secondarily affect the closure of the palatal shelves at eight to nine weeks, or as illustrated in Figure 22–1, a primary defect of neural groove closure can prejudice the subsequent development of other tissues. The word anomalad (*anomaly*, which leads to d*iad*, tri*ad*, etc.) has been utilized to distinguish an initiating defect plus its secondary derived defects. For example, Robin anomalad designates small mandi-

TABLE 22–1 HIGHER RISK CATEGORIES FOR MALFORMATION PROBLEMS

Category	Anomalies	Comment
Prematurity or postmaturity	Any	Fetal malformation may alter gestational timing
"Small for dates" babies	Any	Hypoplasia of the fetus is often accompanied by other anomalies
Breech birth presentation	Any	Certain malformed fetuses are less likely to
	Dislocation of hip deformations	assume the proper birth position
Polyhydramnios	High intestinal atresia	Defective swallowing or intestinal resorbtion
	Anencephalus	of amniotic fluid
	Multiple defects	
Oligohydramnios	Severe kidney defect	Lack of urine flow into the amniotic space
	Urinary tract obstruction	
Twins in general	Club foot	Intrauterine crowding
Monozygotic twins	Any (2 to 3 times increased)	Probably due to same cause as monozygous twinning
Maternal diabetes mellitus	Any,	Maternal metabolic aberration
	Sacral and lower limb defects	
Baby has several minor anomalies	Any, especially a known syndrome	The baby with 2 or 3 or more minor anomalies frequently has a serious defect as well
Parent or previous sibling has a single common malformation	Same type of malformation as parent or sibling	Polygenic inheritance with recurrence risk about 5%
Parent or previous offspring has a genetically determined non-polygenic disorder	Same type of problem, with rare exceptions	Includes Mendelian inheritance and certain chromosomal abnormalities
Older maternal age	Autosomal trisomy syndromes	Risk of faults in chromosome distribution increases exponentially after 35 years, especially risk for 21 trisomy
Older paternal age	Single gene disorders	The likelihood of *fresh* gene mutation, though rare, increases about 10 fold from the paternal age of 30 to 60 years

ble, glossoptosis and posterior cleft of the palate. In this anomalad, the small mandible is considered the initiating defect, which resulted in posterior displacement of the tongue, which mechanically blocked the closure of the palatal shelves. The Robin anomalad may occur as a single defect in an otherwise normal individual or as one of multiple defects in a number of syndromes of variant etiology. This is one area in which knowledge of embryology will be of value in the determination as to

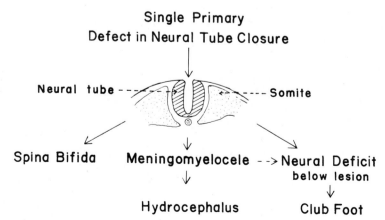

Figure 22–1 Schematic representation of how a single primary defect in neural groove closure, which must have occurred prior to 28 days development, can culminate in a baby with multiple secondary anomalies.

whether a child's malformation problem represented a single localized defect at its inception.

The most common single defects that occur in our population, each with an incidence of about 0.5 to 1.5 per 1000 babies, are defects of neural groove closure causing anencephaly or meningomyelocele; cleft lip with or without cleft palate; cleft palate alone; cardiac septal defects; dislocation of the hip; club foot; and pyloric stenosis. Together these include nearly half the babies recognized as having a serious defect in early life.

TABLE 22–2 SINGLE DEFECTS WITH AN INCIDENCE ABOVE 1 IN 5000 WHICH SHOULD BE DETECTED IN THE NEWBORN NURSERY

Anomaly	Clues Toward Early Initial Detection and Comment	
Central nervous system:		
Anencephaly	Amniocentesis may show alpha-fetoprotein in amniotic fluid for anencephaly and for meningomyelocele Polyhydramnios, roentgenogram of fetus, sonography	No medical intervention
Meningomyelocele	Mainly lumbosacral	Frequently develop hydrocephalus
Hydrocephalus	Full fontanel, spread sutures, transillumination	
Microcephalus	Small cranial circumference	
Eye:		
Cataract	Lack of red pupil reflex to light	
Blind	Blind eye may be turned in	
Face and Mouth:		
Cleft lip		Cleft palate a frequent association
Cleft palate alone	Visualization or palpation	Prone to otitis media and speech problems
Cardiac Defects (depending on degree, may not be noted until later):		
Ventricular septal	Murmur, may become continuous with patent ductus	
Auricular septal	+/– Failure to thrive and frequent respiratory infections	
Patent ductus arteriosus	+/– Cardiac failure with PDA, large VSD	
Transposition	Murmur, cyanosis, cardiac failure, failure to thrive	
Tetralogy of Fallot	Murmur, developing cyanosis, failure to thrive, limp spells	
Coarctation of aorta	+/– Murmur, higher pressure in upper limb, +/– cardiac failure	
Pulmonic stenosis	Murmur	
Intestinal:		
Esophageal atresia	Polyhydramnios because of inability to swallow amniotic fluid Bubbling of secretions, feedins return, aspirational choking	
Intestinal atresia	Bile stained vomiting, +/– abdominal distension	
Anal atresia	+/– No anal opening, abdominal distension	
Hernia:		
Diaphragmatic	Respiratory insufficiency, cyanosis, flat abdomen, heart shifted to right	
Renal:		
Bilateral renal agenesis	Oligohydramnios due to lack of urine flow into amniotic space, respiratory insufficiency due to immature lung	
Hydronephrosis	Large upper quadrant mass, best palpated at birth	
Ectopic kidney	Abdominal palpation, easiest at birth	
Genitalia:		
Hypospadias	If no testes palpable, always determine sex for question of masculinized female	
Cryptorchidism	More common in premature; testes normally descend in late fetal life	
Skeletal:		
Talipes equinovarus	Can result from fetal crowding or lack of function of foot	
Dislocation of hip	Abduction of hips for disturbing "click"; leg asymmetry	
Polydactyly	Most commonly ulnar, fibular	
Syndactyly	Most commonly 3rd to 4th fingers, 2nd to 3rd toes	
Skin:		
Sinus tracts	Sacral, preauricular, cervical (anterior to sternocleidomastoid)	
Nevi	Lipomata, angiomata, rarely melanomas Cavernous hemangiomas must be closely watched and can lead to secondary complications via sequestration of platelets, overgrowth of somatic area or local extension into vital regions	

Single localized defects, including anomalads, may have a variety of modes of etiology.

Indirect evidence implicates polygenic inheritance, the combined effect of many minor gene differences, as the predominant etiology for these anomalies. The X or Y chromosome appears to contain at least some of the genes that influence these anomalies, none of which has an equal sex incidence. For example, pyloric stenosis is five times as likely to occur in the male, whereas dislocation of the hip is five times as likely to occur in the female. Part of the evidence favoring polygenic inheritance is the non-random occurrence of the same type of defect in close relatives. The recurrence risk for normal parents who have one affected child is about 3 to 5 per cent, and the same risk applies for an affected parent having a child with the same type of defect. Although there are indications that environmental factors play a role, no single environmental factor has yet been implicated as a common major cause of any one of the above malformations. Hence at the present time you should be cautious about implying to a mother that any particular environ-

mental factor during her pregnancy was responsible for the occurrence of the single malformation in her child.

Whether polygenic inheritance is an important causal factor of many of the less common single defects of morphogenesis remains to be determined. Most of these also show unequal sex distribution and only occasional recurrence in a family. Be on guard, however, for some of the rare single gene or autosomal recessively inherited single anomalies. For example, ectrodactyly (split hand) may be inherited as an autosomal dominant, as may polydactyly. Primary microcephaly may be of autosomal recessive inheritance, and a rare instance of hydrocephalus may be of X-linked inheritance. Suffice it to conclude that you always wish to look closely at the family before you give genetic counsel about problems in morphogenesis.

Single defects that occur with a frequency greater than 1:5000 are summarized in Table 22–2, which details those anomalies that should be detected in the newborn nursery. Table 22–3 sets forth those seldom detected until a later age. Many of these defects are covered in more

TABLE 22–3   SINGLE DEFECTS WHICH ARE USUALLY NOT DETECTED UNTIL AFTER DISCHARGE FROM THE NEWBORN NURSERY

Anomaly	Clues Toward Early Detection, and Comment
Brain:	
Mental deficiency	Lag in developmental performance; neurologic and behavioral aberrations
Ear:	
Deafness	Limited monotonous vocalization; behavioral problems
Eye:	
Cataract	Lack of red ocular reflex
Blindness	Not following objects with eyes; developmental performance lag
Strabismus	Most commonly internal and alternating; if severe or persisting beyond 6 to 9 months, see ophthalmologist
Intestinal:	
Pyloric stenosis	Two- to six-week age onset of non-bile–stained vomiting, becoming projectile
Malrotation of colon	Bile-stained vomiting; abdominal distension
Meckel's diverticulum	Rarely symptomatic; GI bleeding, intussusception
Hernias:	
Umbilical hernia	Usually benign, generally close with time
Inguinal hernia	May incarcerate, merit early closure
Renal:	
Obstructive valves, etc.	Urinary tract infection, +/− failure to thrive
Hydronephrosis	Above, plus mass in upper quadrant
Skeletal:	
Inward tibial torsion	Mild degrees normal, serious degrees merit treatment
Malalignment of feet	Metatarsus adductus is one of most common
Malalignment at hip	Feet and knees noted to be in aberrant alignment
Skin:	
Hemangiomata	Strawberry hemangiomas may appear after birth and usually begin to recede by 9 to 18 months

detail in other sections of this book. There are also a host of rare defects that will not be considered.

MULTIPLE PRIMARY DEFECTS—MALFORMATION SYNDROMES

Examination of the patient with a malformation problem should *always* be complete. There is a tendency to act quickly when a serious correctable anomaly such as esophageal atresia is discovered, without completing a total evaluation. One such patient had successful surgery, only to be recognized later as having the 18 trisomy syndrome, a disorder that is usually an early lethal one for which we do not recommend surgical or medical intervention.

Once you have recognized that a patient has multiple primary defects the diagnosis

TABLE 22–4 FEATURES OF DOWN SYNDROME

Area	Common (50% or More of Patients)	<50% of Patients
General	Hypotonia; pouting expression when crying.* Usually happy and docile with a somewhat raucous voice. Tend to enjoy mimicry and listening to music	
Growth	Slower than normal	
Central nervous system	Mental deficiency, I.Q. = 25 to 50.* Most rapid period of developmental progress is during the first 2 years	Seizures†
Cranium	Relatively flat occiput*	
Eyes	Upward slanting palpebral fissures* Inner epicanthic folds Speckling of iris Short and sparse eyelashes	Strabismus Nystagmus Cataract†
Ears	Small; overlapping upper helices	Low-set ears†
Nose	Low nasal bridge; small nose	
Mouth	Hypoplasia of maxilla +/— narrow palate Protruding tongue +/— fissuring	
Neck	Broad or short in appearance	Laxity of skin
Hands	Short hands and fingers Clinodactyly, fifth finger Single upper palmar crease Dermal: distal palmar axial triradius	Single crease, fifth finger
Feet	Gap or furrow between first and second toes	Hallucal arch tibial dermatoglyphic pattern. Syndactyly second and third toes
Abdomen	Diastasis recti	Umbilical hernia
Genitals	Small penis	Cryptorchidism
Roentgen findings	Hypoplasia of midphalanx of fifth finger	Decrease acetabular, iliac angles
Cardiac		Atrioventricular communis Ventricular septal defect Tetralogy of Fallot†
Intestine		Duodenal atresia† Tracheo-esophageal fistula†

* Found in 80 per cent or more.
† Found in less than 10 per cent of patients.

TABLE 22–5 DISTINGUISHING FEATURES IN 25 OF THE MORE COMMON SYNDROMES OF MULTIPLE DEFECT (NOT ALL FEATURES PRESENT IN EVERY PATIENT)

Syndrome	Helpful Diagnostic Features			Mental Deficiency	Short Stature	Genetics
	Craniofacial	Limbs	Other			
1. XXY syndrome (Klinefelter syndrome)		Relatively long limbs, even in childhood	Small testes, incomplete virilization	+/−	−	XXY
2. Down syndrome	Upward slant to palpebral fissures, flat facies	Short hands with clinodactyly of fifth finger	Hypotonia	+	+/−	21 trisomy
3. 18 Trisomy syndrome	Microstomia, short palpebral fissure	Clenched hand, second finger over third; low arches on fingertips	Short sternum	+	+	18 trisomy
4. 13 Trisomy syndrome	Defects of eye, nose, lip and forebrain of holoprosencephaly type	Polydactyly, narrow hyperconvex fingernails	Skin defects, posterior scalp	+	+	13 trisomy
5. XO (Turner syndrome)	Heart-shaped facies, prominent ears, webbing of posterior neck, low posterior hairline	Congenital lymphedema or its residua	Broad chest with widely spaced nipples; hypogonadism	−	+	XO or variants
6. Turner-like syndrome (Noonan syndrome)	Webbing of posterior neck		Pectus excavatum, cryptorchidism, pulmonic stenosis	+/−	+	?
7. De Lange syndrome	Synophrys (continuous eyebrows), thin downturning upper lip	Small or malformed hands and feet, proximal thumb	Hirsutism	+	+	?
8. Rubinstein-Taybi syndrome	Microcephaly, slanting palpebral fissures, maxillary hypoplasia	Broad thumbs and toes		+	+	?
9. Russel-Silver syndrome	Triangular hypoplastic facies with downturning mouth	Skeletal asymmetry, clinodactyly of fifth finger	Underweight for length	−	+	?
10. Prader-Willi syndrome	+/− Upward slant to palpebral fissures	Hypotonia, especially in early infancy	Obesity from latter infancy, hypogenitalism	+	+	?
11. Myotonic dystrophy of Steinert	"Myopathic" facies; cataract, fine		Myotonia with muscle atrophy, hypogonadism	+/−	−	Aut. dom.
12. Treacher Collins syndrome (mandibulofacial dysostosis)	Malar and mandibular hypoplasia, defect in lower eyelid		Malformation of external ear	−	−	Aut. dom.

No. & Syndrome	Facial/craniofacial features	Skeletal features	Other features			Etiology
13. Sturge-Weber anomalad	Flat hemangiomas of face, most commonly in trigeminal region		Hemangiomas of meninges with seizures	+/-	-	?
14. Tuberous sclerosis (adenoma sebaceum)	Hamartomatous pink to brownish facial skin nodules	+/- Bone lesions	Seizures	+/-	-	Aut. dom.
15. Neurofibromatosis		+/- Bone lesions	Neurofibromas, café-au-lait spots	-/+	-	Aut. dom.
16. Hypohidrotic ectodermal dysplasia	Peg-shaped teeth, partial anodontia, midfacial hypoplasia		Hypoplasia to aplasia of sweat glands, hyperthermia, alopecia	-	-	X-linked
17. Achondroplasia	Low nasal bridge, +/- macrocephaly	Short limbs, short hands and feet, limited elbow extension	Caudal narrowing of spinal canal, short ilium	-	+	Aut. dom.
18. Apert syndrome (acrocephalosyndactyly)	Craniosynostosis, irregular midfacial hypoplasia and hypertelorism	Syndactyly, broad distal thumb and toe		+/-	-	Aut. dom.
19. Crouzon syndrome (craniofacial dysostosis)	Shallow orbits, maxillary hypoplasia, craniosynostosis			-	-	Aut. dom.
20. Hurler syndrome (MPS type I)	Coarse facies, cloudy cornea, early	Stiff joints by one year, kyphosis by 1–2 years	Valvular heart disease	+	+ Onset 6–18 mo.	Aut. rec.
21. Marfan's syndrome	Lens subluxation	Arachnodactyly	Aortic dilatation	-	-	Aut. dom.
22. Osteogenesis imperfecta	Bluish scleras, odontogenesis imperfecta	Fragile bone	+/- Deafness	-	+/-	Aut. dom.
23. Rubella syndrome	Cataract, deafness		Cardiac defect	+/-	+/-	rubella
24. Fetal alcohol syndrome	Short palpebral fissures, mild maxillary hypoplasia	Minor alterations	Cardiac defect	+	+	ethanol
25. Fetal hydantoin syndrome	Mild ocular hypertelevism, short nose, low nasal bridge	Hypoplastic distal digits, nail hypoplasia		+/-	+/-	hydantoins (Dilantin)

is no longer a purely anatomical one. Rather, you are searching to make an overall diagnosis for the total pattern of malformation. About 1 in 150 babies have multiple defects, and roughly half of them have a recognized clinical entity. There are over 150 such syndromes, and except for Down syndrome (21 trisomy), which has an incidence of 1:660, and XXY syndrome (1:500 males), no other syndrome, save fetal alcohol syndrome in populations with a high incidence of alcoholism in women of reproductive age, occurs with a frequency greater than 1:3000. Down syndrome is detailed in Table 22–4. Table 22–5 describes a few distinguishing features for 25 of the more common syndromes in the author's experience. Recognition of specific syndromes is critical in providing: (1) a rational further evaluation of the patient, (2) a prognosis and integrated program of management and (3) an understanding of etiology and risk for recurrence in future offspring. A specific diagnosis is dependent on recognition of multiple defects in the patient and then attempting through the use of textbooks and consultation to arrive at a specific diagnosis. The following general information, applicable to Down syndrome as well as many other syndromes, may assist in the recognition and understanding of such patients.

Growth. The same etiology that results in multiple defects in structural morphogenesis often has an adverse effect on skeletal development and leads to a general hypoplasia of the whole individual. Therefore, small size and altered skeletal morphology are frequent features in these syndromes, and such patients may initially present as a problem of deficient growth.

Central nervous system. The development and function of the brain are complex phenomena. Mental deficiency, behavioral aberrations and neurological abnormalities are frequent features in these multiple defect syndromes, and many such patients are initially evaluated for a problem in brain function.

Minor defects. Since, by definition, minor structural defects such as single upper palmar crease, inturned fifth finger or epicanthal fold are of little or no direct consequence to the patient, they are seldom noted by parents and often missed by the examiner unless he specifically searches for them. Before ascribing significance to a particular minor anomaly such as inturned fifth finger, it is important to determine whether this is a usual hereditary feature in that family. The finding of but a single minor defect is of little significance, but the discovery of three or more minor anomalies in a patient is highly indicative of a serious alteration in morphogenesis, and 90 per cent of such patients also have a major defect. As one example, the great majority of features upon which we base an early diagnosis of Down syndrome (Table 22–4) are minor alterations.

Most minor anomalies have been detected in the face, auricles, hands and feet, and are therefore readily available for inspection and familial comparison. One area that deserves routine inspection by direct magnified vision in the child with altered morphogenesis is the fine dermal ridges of the hands and feet, especially the hands. Alterations in the dermatoglyphic patterning may add significant clues in establishing the total pattern of malformation.

Non-specificity of individual defects. With rare exception, a clinical diagnosis of one of these malformation syndromes cannot be made on the basis of a single defect. Rather, the diagnosis is usually dependent on the total *pattern of defect.* Such minor anomalies as inner epicanthal fold, incomplete development of the upper ear, a single upper palmar crease, inturned fifth fingers and syndactyly between the second and third toes are very non-specific indicators of altered morphogenesis and may be found as features in syndromes of widely variant etiology.

Variance in expression. Variance in expression (severity) among individuals with the same etiological syndrome is the rule, rather than the exception. Except for such non-specific general features as mental deficiency or small stature, it is unusual to find a given defect in 100 per cent of patients with the same etiological syndrome. For example, in Down syndrome only mental deficiency is ubiquitous, hypotonia is a usual feature and most of the other individual clinical features are found in 80 per cent or less of patients; however, it is rare that a specific clinical diagnosis of Down syndrome cannot be made in the affected newborn, based on the *total pattern of anomalies.*

Etiologies

Genetic alterations appear to be the predominant cause for the recognized malformation syndromes, though there are an unfortunate number of environmentally determined syndromes as well.

Chromosomal abnormalities. The vast majority of chromosomal abnormalities are altered chromosomal number (aneuploidy) as a consequence of faulty distribution of chromosomes at cell division. More than 4 per cent of early conceptuses are aneuploid. Most of the genetically imbalanced conceptuses abort, and only some of the sex chromosome aneuploidies and three of the autosomal trisomies (13, 18 and 21 trisomies) allow for viable offspring, collectively comprising about 1 in 200 newborn babies. Faulty chromosomal distribution is more likely at advanced maternal age, about half the babies with Down syndrome having been born of mothers over the age of 35 years. Chromosomal breakage is a less common cause of genetic imbalance, but it is important to recognize when a parent is a balanced translocation carrier and is at significant risk of having another abnormal offspring. Chromosome study for genetic counseling is usually indicated for the Down syndrome child of a mother under 30 years of age; 6 per cent of such babies will be translocation cases, and in one third of such instances a parent will be found to be a translocation carrier with a higher recurrence risk.

A single **mutant gene etiology** (dominant, X-linked in the male) or a pair of mutant gene etiology (autosomal recessive) has been implicated as the cause for a number of multiple defect syndromes. Some of these result in multiple system defects, whereas others adversely affect predominantly one system (osteochondrodysplasias, ectodermal dysplasias). It is important to appreciate that the *majority* of autosomal dominant serious syndromes represent a *fresh* gene mutation from unaffected parents whose recurrence risk is negligible. Of course, the affected child in that case has a 50 per cent risk of any offspring being affected.

Environmental teratogens. Thalidomide and aminopterine are hopefully now of historic significance. Only in recent years have the fetal alcohol syndrome, fetal hydantoin syndrome, fetal tridione syndrome and fetal warfarin syndrome been recognized as serious preventable disorders. The first occurs in offspring of chronically alcoholic women, the next two in offspring of women taking these anticonvulsive medications and the last in offspring of women taking this anticoagulant. Each gives rise to prenatal growth deficiency with mental deficiency and a relatively specific pattern of malformation. The rubella viral agent continues to be a serious potential threat to the conceptus when acquired by the mother during the first four months of gestation.

Evaluation of the Patient with Multiple Defects

The following approach merits consideration in the evaluation of a patient who appears to have a multiple defect problem.

Obtain a family history for similar physical features or a similar entity. It is important to note abortions, stillbirths, parental ages and consanguinity.

Obtain the complete phenotype including minor defects and appropriate roentgenograms. Then try to identify the syndrome (see Table 22–5 and references). If you are unable to reach a diagnosis, obtain consultation.

Sex chromatin studies are indicated only when you suspect a sex chromosome abnormality such as XO, XXY or XXX.

Chromosome studies are merited for confirmation of a suspected diagnosis or to exclude chromosomal breakage with or without rearrangement. If a patient has the latter, then both parents should be studied to determine whether either is a balanced translocation carrier. Also consider a chromosomal study for the unknown multiple defect case; the likelihood of finding an unusual chromosomal abnormality in such cases is about 5 to 8 per cent.

Management and Counsel

Known syndromes. Read about the condition and carry out the indicated evaluation. Corrective procedures should only be utilized when indicated, forestalling such measures when the general prognosis is grim; for example, the majority of babies with 18 trisomy or 13 trisomy syndromes expire within the first three months. Start your counseling with the etiology (when known), and proceed with what is usual to expect for that condition. Then become specific in terms of the problems for this child and how one can best adapt the child within the family and society, if this is possible. Finally, discuss the risk for recurrence for the parents and the risk of the patient having similarly affected offspring, when indicated.

Unknown syndromes. Appropriate roentgenograms, including a pyelogram, are often indicated if there is multisystem involvement. Follow-up should be cautious. No accurate genetic counsel can be rendered, but parents can be told that the lowest recurrence risk would be zero and the highest 25 per cent.

SUMMARY

As a summary, and to give an appreciation of the general manner in which the author counsels parents who have a child with a malformation problem, the following three examples are set forth. The first is an example of a defect that need not seriously interfere with the individual's leading a normal life; the second is an example of a chronic handicapping disorder that will alter the life of the individual; the third example is a severe problem for which the parents should be given the early option of no medical or surgical intervention toward survival of the patient.

COUNSELING APPROACH

An Otherwise Normal Child with Unilateral Cleft Lip, of Normal Parents

1. Tell the parents that the *child* is normal, that the *lip* did not close completely. This is important in helping them to *accept* the child and not think of the child as being malformed, since only the lip is malformed. Such an approach is applicable when a correctable anomaly need not interfere seriously with the sociability and function of the child.

2. Explain how this cleft represents a normal stage in development of the lip and

that a problem existed in that region prior to 35 days, when the lip would have normally been fused. The mother can thereby be reassured that the anomaly could not have been related to any environmental problem after 35 days, even though we do not know of *any* single environmental factor, with the exception of hydantoins (Dilantin), which are thought to cause cleft lip in the human.

3. Explain how closure of the lip depends on a number of genes and that "the set of genes" that the baby derived from *both* parents did not allow for complete closure of the lip, but the baby seems normal in every other respect. Explain that the chance of a future baby being affected is about 5 per cent, or 95 per cent chance of not having a cleft lip with or without cleft palate.

4. Finally, explain how the surgeon will bring about the lip closure. If the result is not quite satisfactory he can carry out further cosmetic surgery in the future.

A Baby with Down Syndrome, 21 Trisomy by Chromosome Study

1. Explain to the parents what a chromosome is and how usual development depends on having two sets of genes, two sets of chromosomes. Explain that one chromosome of each pair is present in the egg and one in the sperm. When they come together a new and unique individual develops with a full set of genes. Tell them how, by a simple error in distribution of chromosomes to the egg or sperm, or in the first cell division after they join, the baby can start life with an extra chromosome, an extra set of genes.

2. Then tell them that their baby started life with an extra 21 chromosome. There is no abnormal gene, but a whole extra set of normal genes that altered the pattern of the baby's development. Explain to them what is *usual* for Down syndrome, the natural history of the condition, including the brain function. Try to arrange for them to talk with several parents of children with Down syndrome so they can see some older Down syndrome children and gain insight from the experience of the families.

3. Counsel them, if young parents, that since the baby has a whole extra 21 chro-

mosome the chance for any future child being affected is very low, about 1 in 200. Also tell them there is no need for relatives or their other children to be unusually concerned about having a child with Down syndrome.

A Baby with 18 Trisomy Syndrome, Full Trisomy by Chromosome Study

1. Same as point 1 for Down's syndrome.
2. Explain that at least 3 per cent of pregnancies begin with an altered number of chromosomes. Most of these have a very serious effect on early development, and the great majority abort spontaneously. Tell them that their baby has an extra 18 chromosome. I then make the following statement to the mother: "You must have provided the baby with excellent genetic background and you must be very good at carrying babies, because most developing babies with an extra 18 chromosome set of genes do not survive to be liveborn. Having survived to be born, these babies have a very limited capacity for surviving on their own and the majority pass on within the first weeks or months, even with optimal care. If they do survive they have very limited growth and function. I feel the kindest approach for us to take is to keep the baby comfortable and fed, but not interfere by utilizing any medical or surgical life-saving measures. Is this the approach you would like us to take?"

The manner in which this is presented is designed to assist the mother in apprecia-ting the situation as a "late miscarriage," which is realistic. The same type of approach can be utilized for certain other early lethal disorders such as 13 trisomy syndrome and also for anencephaly.

The foregoing examples provide you with the spectrum of approaches toward malformation problems. These range from the disorder which need not seriously affect the child's life, for which the attitude conveyed is of a *normal* child, to the chronically handicapping disorder, for which the parents must realign their thinking about what will be usual for this child, to the disorders for which medical interference toward survival should be questioned.

REFERENCES

General

Gorlin, R. J., Pindborg, J. J., and Cohen, M. M.: *Syndromes of the Head and Neck.* New York, McGraw-Hill Book Co., 1976.
McKusick, V. A.: *Mendelian Inheritance in Man.* Baltimore, The Johns Hopkins Press, 1970.
Smith, D. W.: *Recognizable Patterns of Human Malformation,* 2nd ed. Philadelphia, W. B. Saunders Co., 1976.
Vaughn, V. C., III, and McKay, R. J. (Eds.): *Textbook of Pediatrics,* 10th ed. Philadelphia, W. B. Saunders Co., 1975.

Connective Tissue

McKusick, V. A.: *Hereditary Disorders of Connective Tissue,* 4th ed. St. Louis, C. V. Mosby Co., 1972.

Skeletal

Spranger, J. W., Langer, L. O., and Wiedemann, H. R.: *Bone Dysplasias.* Philadelphia, W. B. Saunders Co., 1974.

PART VIII

GROWTH AND ENDOCRINE DISORDERS

23

Growth Disorders

David W. Smith

Linear growth is predominantly an expression of skeletal development, which does not near completion until 15 to 18 years. During the growth period the child should be considered in relation to his maturational age (bone age) as well as his chronological age. For example, a six-year-old child with the average height of a four-year-old and osseous maturation of a four-year-old is *not* short for biological age. He may continue to grow for a longer period of time than usual and achieve a final adult stature within the normal range.

Since there are several hundred different disorders in which growth deficiency is one feature, it is important to have a general approach toward the evaluation and diagnosis of a patient with this clinical sign. The following approach may assist the reader in this regard.

A particular diagnosis derives from an appropriate history and physical evaluation, the important aspects of which are summarized here.

History

FAMILY HISTORY

The stature of the parents and siblings should be obtained as well as their pace of maturation, as suggested by their ages of puberty. For the mother the age of menarche is a standard usually remembered, whereas it may require several questions to elicit the approximate age of puberty in the father. These may include such general inquiries as: "Were you small as a child but of normal stature in your teens?" "Did your adolescent development occur sooner, later or at about the same time as your classmates?" "How old were you when you had your fastest period of growth (peak growth velocity, mean age 14.1 years)?" "How old were you when you began to shave?—reached your final height?" Depending on the nature of the problem, it may also be pertinent to inquire about the size and maturational rate of other close relatives such as aunts, uncles and grandparents.

MATERNAL AND PREGNANCY HISTORY

The prepregnant height and weight of the mother are pertinent information to the size of the infant at birth. Gestational timing should ideally be calculated from presumed date of conception, two weeks after the beginning of the last menstrual period, in order to be more representative of the age of the infant at birth. Unfortunately, most of the present standards count gestational age from the first day of the last menstrual period. Birth size should be interpreted for gestational age. If there was evidence of prenatal onset of growth deficiency—also termed *small for gestational age* or *small-for-dates*—then a number of questions pertaining to the mother's socioeconomic status, health and nutrition before and during the pregnancy and ingestion of medications and ethanol and cigarette smoking during the pregnancy may be pertinent. The history of maternal weight gain during the pregnancy may also be of interest. The gestational weight gain normally relates to fetal size, being about three times the fetal weight or more. Questions concerning fetal status and function may also be merited, such as the age of onset and consistency and vigor of fetal movements, the amount of amniotic fluid and whether or not the fetus rotated into the usual vertex position prior to delivery.

PATIENT HISTORY

Adequacy of adaptation at birth, progress in developmental performance, general vigor, general health and specific serious illnesses, gastrointestinal function, diet and appetite and social and home care situation are variably important, depending on the nature of the growth problem. Whenever possible, data on linear and weight growth should be obtained in an effort to determine the *age of onset of the growth problem*, the recent *growth velocity* and whether the velocity of growth has changed. If the patient is at or beyond the age of adolescence or has shown any sign of adolescent change, then the age of onset and stage of adolescent development should be recorded.

Physical Evaluation

Patient evaluation. Stature may be interpreted in terms of the growth percentile for age. Between the ages of two and nine years it should be interpreted in relation to mid-parental height. *Weight* should be interpreted as a particular percentile for age but may also be related as the percentile for *stature*. Prior to adolescence this is determined by taking the age for which the stature of the patient is the fiftieth percentile, the "height age," and figuring the weight percentile for that height age. It is helpful to indicate the apparent reason for any deficiency or excess of weight. Is it due to variance in one or more of the major weight components of adipose tissue, muscle and skeletal mass? *Head circumference* may be interpreted as a particular percentile for chronological age as well as percentile for height age.

Should any of the foregoing values be below the third percentile, or above the ninety seventh percentile, it is helpful to express the measurement values in *standard deviations* below or above the mean for age. This allows a better perspective of the relative degree of aberration for each feature of growth. It also allows a comparison of the relative severity of growth aberration between such parameters as height and head circumference.

If there is any apparent or suspected malproportionment of a particular aspect of growth such as trunk versus limbs, or un-usual size of facial features, auricles, hands, feet or genitalia, these should be measured and contrasted to normal standards for chronological age and height age such as those set forth in Chapter 7 of Smith, D. W.: *Recognizable Patterns of Human Malformation*. A careful search should also be made for evidence of asymmetry.

A crude attempt should be made to judge the maturational age of the individual. In the young infant the size of the fontanels may be a helpful indicator. Also, during this time and throughout childhood, the facial bony maturation may be assessed by judging the level of development of the nasal bridge, malar eminences and mandible. How old does the patient appear? As with evaluating roentgenograms for bone age, the clinician must be careful not to misinterpret evidence of a basic osteochondrodysplasia, for example, as being evidence of a lag in osseous maturation. Thus the larger than usual fontanels and low nasal bridge in infants with achondroplasia are not signs of lag in maturation of the bone. Dental assessment is merited, but the level of tooth development does not appear to be a good general indicator of the level of osseous maturation. Signs of adolescent development should be assessed in the older child and adolescent as an added indicator of level of maturation. In the male the effect of gonadotrophin may be directly assessed via the growth of the testes, which can be measured. For the female, only the indirect effects of the gonadotrophin-induced production of estrogens can be assessed via breast development and estrinization of the vaginal mucosa.

The physical examination should include a cautious search for evidence of altered morphogenesis, especially minor anomalies, which may not be readily evident. Such anomalies may provide helpful clues to a specific pattern of malformation or a syndrome.

In a number of growth disorders there is an effect on brain growth as well as skeletal growth. Hence, a developmental and neurological assessment is often merited. This should include an evaluation of the retina, the one area of the brain that can be visualized.

Laboratory studies. There is no laboratory test that is indicated in every patient with a growth disorder. Rather, as Andrea Prader of Zürich has emphasized, "only

TABLE 23–1 CLASSIFICATION OF GROWTH DEFICIENCY

Normal Variants

Features	Familial Short Stature	Familial Slow Maturation
Onset of growth deficiency	Postnatal	Postnatal (early childhood)
Rate of maturation	Normal	Slow
Family history	Short stature	Slow maturation
Final stature	Short	Normal limits
Therapy to increase eventual stature	None	None

Abnormal Growth

Features	Primary Skeletal Growth Deficiency	Secondary Growth Deficiency	
		Prenatal Onset	Postnatal Onset
Onset of growth deficiency	Usually prenatal	—	—
Rate of maturation	Variable, usually normal	Variable, slow to normal	Usually slow
Malproportion	Frequent	Variable	Unusual, except rickets
Associated anomalies	Frequent	Variable	Unusual, except causative anomaly
General modes of etiology	Chromosomal abnormalities Mutant gene disorders, including osteochondrodysplasias Syndromes of unknown etiology	Crowding (twins) Maternal: Small mother Low socioeconomic level Malnutrition Hypertension Toxemia Renal disease Heart disease Cigarette smoking Heroin addiction Ethanol intake Hydantoin therapy Warfarin therapy Rubella Cytomegalic inclusion disease Toxoplasmosis Syphilis	Nutritional deficiency, neglect, poor absorption Mental deficiency Cardiac defect Renal dysfunction Respiratory insufficiency Growth hormone deficiency Thyroid hormone deficiency Still's disease Metabolic disorders
Therapy to increase eventual stature	None to date	May or may not show postnatal catch-up growth	Specific treatment yields catch-up growth

tests aimed at confirming a suspected diagnosis should actually be performed." There should also be a specific indication for roentgenograms. A bone age determination is not indicated in all, or even the majority, of children with a growth problem. Should the possibility of a skeletal dysplasia be indicated, the most appropriate roentgenograms include a view of the hand and wrist, the knee (area of most rapid epiphyseal plate growth), anterior-posterior view of the hip (shows molding under stress of weight bearing on "weak" bone) and lateral of the lumbothoracic spine (T-12 to L-1 are the most likely vertebrae to show compression changes).

The findings from the history and examination, sometimes supplemented by roentgenograms, usually allow placement of the patient into a general diagnostic category. The largest categories are the normal variants of *familial small stature* and *familial slow maturation*, which are summarized in Table 23–1 and discussed here.

VARIANTS OF NORMAL

Familial Short Stature

This is characterized by a small child who is maturing at an otherwise normal rate, as indicated by bone age, with a family history of small stature in otherwise normal close relatives. Such individuals are usually within normal limits for size at birth, have a consistently slow pace of linear growth during childhood, reach adolescence at a usual age and are relatively short in final stature.

Familial Slow Maturation

This is characterized by a slowly maturing child, who is short for chronological age but not for maturational age (bone age), with a family history of slow maturation. The latter is indicated by a late advent of adolescence and final height attainment in one or more close relatives. Such individuals are usually within normal limits for size at birth, with slowing in the pace of growth and maturation becoming evident during late infancy or early childhood. They have late onset of normal adolescence and usually achieve final height within the normal range, but at a late chronological age.

ABERRANT GROWTH

Patients with truly aberrant growth may be divided into predominantly two categories on the basis of the age of onset of the slow growth and whether the cause appears to be *primary* within the skeletal

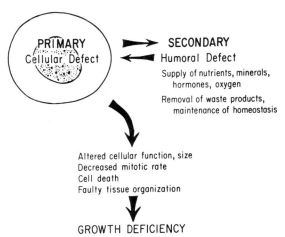

Figure 23–1 Growth deficiency may be either the consequence of a primary problem within the skeletal cells or secondary to a problem outside the skeletal cell.

cells or a problem which is exogenous to the skeletal cells and *secondarily* affects their growth, as summarized in Table 23–1. The latter concept is depicted in Figure 23–1.

Prenatal Onset Growth Deficiency

Growth deficiency of prenatal onset means small-for-gestational-age babies. Excluding multiple births, about 0.43 per cent of newborn infants weigh less than 2.5 kg at full term gestation. The small size is generally due to a deficient number of cells and hence represents congenital hypoplasia, which should be considered as a *congenital malformation.* The same cause that gave rise to the skeletal growth deficiency has often caused growth deficiency in other tissues as well, such as the brain. The growth deficiency will often be disharmonic or asymmetrical, resulting in malproportionment or asymmetry. The disproportionate growth deficiency may result in "anomalies." Examples include short palpebral fissures secondary to small eye size in the fetal alcohol syndrome and unduly small distal phalanges with small nails in the fetal hydantoin syndrome. Anomalies such as ventricular septal defect in the fetal alcohol syndrome may simply represent early deficiency in the growth of the cardiac septum, which may continue to grow and close postnatally. Thus most of the more serious congenital hypoplasia disorders present as a *pattern of multiple malformations.* Many of these syndromes may be recognizable and are set forth in Smith, D. W.: *Recognizable Patterns of Human Malformation.*

The causes of prenatal onset growth deficiency may be divided into two gross categories:

Primary prenatal onset growth deficiency. The implication in this category is of a primary problem in the skeletal cells that affects their capacity for growth, even in the placental situation with its ready delivery of nutrients and oxygen. The growth deficiency is frequently disharmonic with features such as malproportion, asymmetry and malformations in non-skeletal tissues as well. The majority of such disorders for which the mode of etiology is known have a genetic basis. This includes genetic imbalance due to chromosomal abnormality.

Most chromosomal abnormalities give rise to prenatal growth deficiency. There is also a number of mutant gene disorders that adversely affect cell number in terms of growth. They vary from those in which the predominant problem is in the skeletal cells — the osteochondrodysplasias — to those in which multiple tissues are affected.

Caution should be exercised in interpreting roentgenograms for bone age in patients with primary prenatal onset growth deficiency. The basic aberration that has affected skeletal growth and morphogenesis may affect the timing, sequence and form of secondary centers of ossification. Such aberrations may not be indicative of the maturational rate by comparison to normal standards such as in the Greulich and Pyle atlas.

The diagnosis is usually dependent on recognition of the total pattern of malformation and may be confirmed in the case of chromosomal abnormalities. Postnatally, there is seldom any improvement in growth rate in terms of catch-up growth. The rate of childhood growth and the eventual height can best be implied by empiric knowledge of the range of stature for a specific known disorder coupled with knowledge of the stature of the child's parents. Brook, et al. found that the parent-child correlation still held for both the XO Turner syndrome and for Down syndrome individuals: the taller parents still had the tallest children. Thus these two genetic imbalance disorders have a blunting impact on growth, but the genetic background still exerts a role in the relative stature of affected individuals.

To date there has been no effective mode of therapy to increase the stature of individuals with primary cellular growth deficiency disorders. Deficient growth has not been shown to be the consequence of a known endocrine disorder.

Secondary prenatal onset growth deficiency. Skeletal growth deficiency is considered to be *secondary* to an exogenous cause outside the skeletal system in this category. The cause may be uterine crowding, such as with twins. More commonly the cause is maternal-related, such as those summarized in Table 23–1. The growth deficiency is most commonly mild in babies born of mothers with malnutrition, toxemia, hypertension, renal disease, cardiac disease, moderate ethanol intake or heavy cigarette smoking, and affects weight more than length, without obvious malproportionment or anomalies. However, for the other causes listed in Table 23–1, in which the degree of congenital hypoplasia may be more severe, there is often malproportionment in growth with a pattern of associated anomalies.

Postnatal growth is variable in these disorders. In twins, for whom the growth deficiency most commonly is secondary to uterine constraint due to crowding, the extent of catch-up growth is variable. Most of them show catch-up growth postnatally. However, those with more severe prenatal growth deficiency may not show appreciable catch-up growth. For other mild exogenously caused prenatal growth deficiency there is often some postnatal catch-up growth. Rapid catch-up within the first three to six months is a favorable sign for the subsequent health and growth of the patient. There may also be a slow, insidious catch-up over many years. For those with more serious degrees of prenatal growth deficiency, especially those presenting as a pattern of malformation, there is rarely postnatal catch-up growth and only occasionally a mild to moderate insidious catch-up lasting into later childhood. In general, the deficiency of postnatal growth is proportionate to the relative size of the infant at birth. For example, the smallest full-term babies with fetal alcohol syndrome grow at the slowest rate in childhood. Thus, despite the fact that the fetus is removed from the cause of growth deficiency, there is a failure of catch-up growth to occur in serious prenatal growth deficiency.

Postnatal Onset Growth Deficiency

Primary postnatal onset growth deficiency. There are a few primary skeletal growth deficiency disorders in which slow growth does not become obvious until after birth. These include an occasional patient with XO Turner syndrome, most patients with mucopolysaccharide storage disorders, such as Hurler syndrome and Hunter syndrome, and those with Progeria and X-linked spondyloepiphyseal dysplasia.

Secondary postnatal onset growth deficiency. The majority of postnatal onset

TABLE 23–2   SECONDARY GROWTH DEFICIENCY, POSTNATAL ONSET

Problem	Reason for Growth Deficiency	Diagnostic Studies
Nutritional a. Inadequate intake b. Partial intestinal obstruction c. Malabsorption	Nutritional deficiency	Response to adequate caloric intake GI radiographic studies Absorption, GI enzyme studies, intestinal biopsy
Deprivation syndrome	Neglect, abuse, nutritional	Response to environmental change Home and family investigation
Mental deficiency, usually severe	Unknown	Exclude other causes in mentally defective individual
Cardiac defect a. Large left to right shunt b. Cyanotic type	?Rapid circulation time ?Hypoxia, sluggish circulation	Cardiac evaluation
Respiratory insufficiency	?Hypoxia	Usually obvious
Renal dysfunction	Acidosis Polyuria with dehydration Rickets	Urine pH, serum electrolytes, CO_2, urine concentrating ability Serum calcium, phosphorus
Pituitary growth hormone deficiency	Diminished somatomedin	Stimulated serum growth hormone values
Hypothyroidism	Deficit in energy metabolism	Serum thyroxin or protein-bound iodine
Chronic serious infectious disease (not upper respiratory)	Unknown	

Metabolic disorders such as hypercalcemia, hypophosphatemic rickets, hypokalemia, galactosemia, glycogen storage disease and salt-losing congenital adrenal hyperplasia.

growth deficiency disorders represents conditions in which there is no primary problem in the skeletal cells that affects their capacity for growth. Rather, the growth deficiency is *secondary* to a problem outside the skeletal system that affects its growth. The problem may reside in the delivery of nutrients, hormones or oxygen to the skeletal cells or the maintenance of extracellular homeostasis. Specific types of secondary growth deficiency are summarized in Table 23–2. Included are defects in development and function of the brain, pituitary, thyroid, heart, lung, liver, intestine or kidney that seldom have a serious effect on prenatal growth because of the placental situation, as illustrated in Figure 23–2, but can cause postnatal growth deficiency. Thus onset of deficient growth is usually postnatal and there are seldom associated malformations, save a malformation that may be responsible for the growth deficiency. Furthermore, the skeletal system is normally proportioned and modeled, except in rickets.

Skeletal maturation is usually retarded to about the same extent as linear growth, except in primary hypothyroidism, in which the secondary spondyloepiphyseal dysplasia-like lag in skeletal development is more profound.

When the cause of secondary postnatal onset growth deficiency is recognized and rectified, one may witness the amazing phenomenon of catch-up growth toward expectancy for age. This dramatically empha-

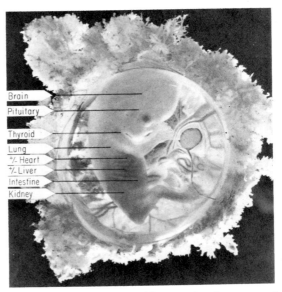

Figure 23–2   Serious problems in development and function of the labeled tissues usually do not have an adverse effect on prenatal growth, whereas each can be the cause of serious postnatal secondary growth deficiency.

sizes the fact that there is no primary growth problem in the skeletal system. The extent of catch-up growth varies in accordance with age of onset, duration and nature of the growth problem plus the adequacy of the therapy.

NATURE OF GROWTH DEFICIENCY IN A GENERAL POPULATION OF 10-YEAR-OLD CHILDREN

Very few studies have been done to determine the actual frequency and nature of growth deficiency disorders within the general population. One English study was carried out by Lacey and Parkin, who evaluated all 10-year-old children in Newcastle-upon-Tyne who were at or below the third percentile for stature. These children were born in 1960–1962. Obviously, all early-lethal disorders such as thanatophoric dwarfism and trisomy 18 syndrome have been excluded. The 98 children below the third percentile corresponded closely to 3 per cent of the 10-year-old children. The majority of these, 82 per cent, were considered to be variants of normal, relating to the independent contribution of one or more of three factors presented in order of frequency: (1) *small parentage*, (2) *slow maturation* and (3) *lower birth size*, often related to *smaller maternal size*. In about one third of instances the small size related to poor social environment. Therefore, Lacey and Parkin considered small size to be partially a "disease of social environment." It is difficult to disassociate the cause and effect relationship between stature and social status, however. Are the parents and children smaller because of their poor social environment? Or are they more likely to be in a poor social environment because of their smaller size?

Eighteen per cent of those below the third percentile in stature were considered to have an organic cause for growth deficiency. These consisted of five children with Down syndrome, four with idiopathic mental deficiency and one each with Hurler syndrome, Still's disease, tetralogy of Fallot, chronic renal disease, cystic fibrosis of the pancreas, a questionable instance of growth hormone deficiency and an unknown multiple defect disorder. The reader will note the relative rarity of endocrine disorders as a cause for growth deficiency. This, despite the fact that about 40 per cent of patients evaluated in a pediatric endocrine clinic are seeking advice about short stature.

PSYCHOLOGICAL ADAPTATION TO SHORT STATURE

Finally, a brief commentary about the psychological adaptation of the child with growth deficiency. Virtually all short children will be treated as younger than their age and will be teased. Their behavioral response may vary from the "Peter Pan" persistence of immature ways to resentment and fighting, denial, social isolation or mascotism. The latter response, the "Tom Thumb" type of behavior, in which the child accepts the relative fame of being short, does not resent being noticed, and acts the "court jester" role, is often the most wholesome response. It requires self-confidence and a sense of humor, traits which seem to be more common in children with achondroplasia than in other growth disorders. Management should include frank discussions, realistic guides for prognosis and life planning and special attention to age-related dress.

This author is strongly opposed to branding the whole individual on the basis of one non-specific physical feature such as short stature. The use of terms such as "dwarf" or "midget" seem quite unnecessary and may only enhance the serious danger of a short child developing a deformed self-image out of proportion to the real situation. Today, when we can usually arrive at a specific diagnosis for the child who has growth deficiency, we should counsel with regard to the natural history of that particular disorder and hopefully never again retreat to the use of such non-specific terms as "dwarf" or "midget."

The following poem should be self-explanatory:

I met a little Elfman once,
Down where the lilies blow.
I asked him why he was so small,
and why he didn't grow.

He slightly frowned, and with his eye
He looked me through and through.
"I'm just as big for me," said he,
"As you are big for you!"

JOHN KENDRICK BANGS

REFERENCES

General:

Faulkner, F.: *Human Development.* Philadelphia, W. B. Saunders Co., 1966.

Smith, D. W.: *Recognizable Patterns of Human Malformation,* 2nd ed. Philadelphia, W. B. Saunders Co., 1976.

Smith, D. W.: *Growth and Its Disorders.* Philadelphia, W. B. Saunders Co., 1977.

Specific:

Brook, C. G. D., Van der Schreien-Lodeweickx, M. A., Werder, E. A., and Prader, A.: Parent-child correlations of stature in normal subjects and in subjects with Turner's, Klinefelter's and Down's syndromes. In press, 1975.

Jarvinen, P. A., Pankamaa, P., and Kinunen, O.: The full-term underdeveloped liveborn infant. Études Neo-Natales, 6:3, 1957.

Lacey, K. A., and Parkin, J. M.: Causes of short stature. A community study of children in Newcastle upon Tyne. Lancet, 1:42, 1974.

Lacey, K. A., and Parkin, J. M.: The normal short child. Arch. Dis. Child., 49:417, 1974.

Money, J.: Dwarfism, questions and answers in counseling. Rehabil. Lit., 28:134, 1967.

Tanner, J. H., Goldstein, H., and Whitehouse, R. H.: Standards for children's height at ages two to nine years allowing for height of parents. Arch. Dis. Child., 45:755, 1970.

Endocrine Disorders, Including Diabetes Mellitus

Frank J. Gareis

Endocrine disorders, although rare in a general pediatric practice, warrant prompt recognition and treatment because of the profound effect of some of these diseases on the growing and developing child. This chapter highlights some of the more frequently encountered endocrine disorders of infancy and childhood with emphasis on those conditions that significantly alter growth and maturation.

CONGENITAL HYPOTHYROIDISM

Defects in either the development of the thyroid gland or the biosynthesis of thyroid hormone may give rise to congenital hypothyroidism. The central nervous system is especially dependent upon thyroid hormone during its period of rapid development from fetal life through infancy, and for this reason early diagnosis and adequate thyroid hormone replacement is critical to the intellectual prognosis for infants with hypothyroidism.

For reasons that are not well understood, the diagnosis of hypothyroidism is seldom made at birth. Infants with this disorder are usually of normal birth length and weight. The clinician, therefore, should be particularly aware of the often subtle features of early hypothyroidism, many of which are evident in the newborn baby with hypothyroidism. Table 24–1 summarizes the alterations that follow thyroid hormone deficit in early life, and Figure 24–1 shows the facial appearance of a hypothyroid infant.

Routine screening of the newborn for either serum thyroxine (T4) or thyroid stimulating hormone (TSH) is now being carried out in some regions in an effort to provide early detection of this serious disorder.

Osseous maturation is particularly sensitive to the effects of thyroid hormone, and infants with athyrotic hypothyroidism usually have prenatal retardation of enchondral ossification as evidenced by delay in "bone age." Retardation in membranous ossification gives rise to large fontanels that are easily palpable and may be an early clue towards the diagnosis. A low nasal bridge is further evidence of osseous immaturity.

With partial defects in the organogenesis of the thyroid gland the signs of hypothyroidism are milder, with slow growth and maturation and relatively sluggish activity being the predominant features. Acquired hypothyroidism in later childhood is often heralded by an abrupt slowing of growth and physical activity.

Laboratory studies necessary to confirm a diagnosis of hypothyroidism usually involve measurement of circulating thyroid hormone (serum thyroxine) and thyrotropin stimulating hormone as well. The latter measurement is particularly useful in mild hypothyroidism (low or low normal serum T4, elevated serum TSH) or when the hypothyroidism is on a central nervous system basis with a low serum T4 and TSH. Additionally, the location and functional capacity of the thyroid gland can be assessed by radioactive ^{131}I studies.

Treatment consists of full replacement therapy with thyroid hormone, following which there is rapid catch-up growth and restoration toward physical normalcy. Treatment results in a cessation of the adverse effects of thyroxine deficiency on early brain development.

A standard reliable preparation of desiccated thyroid or a synthetic form of L-thyroxine may be used.

HYPERTHYROIDISM AND THYROIDITIS IN CHILDREN

Hyperthyroidism is rare in children before the age of 10 years. This disorder is

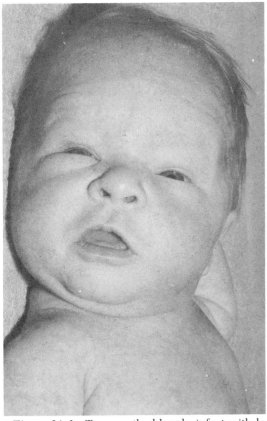

Figure 24–1 Two-month-old male infant with hypothyroidism. Note the immature facies with low nasal bridge, characteristic puffiness of the lower lids and mottled skin.

TABLE 24–1

A. Signs and Symptoms of Hypothyroidism that May Be Manifest by the First Week after Birth

Evidence of Osseous Immaturity	Large fontanels, especially the posterior fontanel. Immature facies with low nasal bridge and short nose. Retarded ossification of secondary centers, sometimes with epiphyseal dysgenesis.
Other Lag in Evidence of Maturation	Respiratory distress. Occasional persistence of patent ductus arteriosus.
Physiological Alterations	Hypothermia. Peripheral cyanosis. Hypotonia. Hypoactivity with poor feeding. Lag in advent of stooling. Abdominal distention with or without vomiting. Persisting indirect bilirubinemia. Edema, occasionally large tongue.

B. Additional Signs and Symptoms Evident by One to Three Months of Age

Immaturity	Umbilical hernia. Immature upper/lower segment ratio.
Physiological Myxedema	Constipation Prominent supraclavicular pads, enlarged muscle mass with prominent gastrocnemii and large tongue.
Growth	Slow growth.

C. Additional Signs Evident by One Year

Immaturity	Lag in advent of dentition.

more prevalent in females, and there is frequently a family history of thyroid disease. The thyroid gland is consistently enlarged (see Fig. 24–2) and the majority of the clinical findings can be related to excessive thyroid hormone production. The onset of hyperthyroidism is heralded by *change* in function and behavior and other indicators of increased metabolic rate. Hyperactivity and restlessness, along with poor concentration, often lead to poor school performance. Decreased heat tolerance, tachycardia and increased skin temperature and sweating are common findings. Appetite increases, but food intake rarely keeps pace with the increased metabolic rate, and weight gain lags behind linear growth. Eye signs of exophthalmos are usually minimal to mild early in the clinical course.

Treatment consists of administration of drugs such as propylthiouracil or methimazole, which act to block the production of thyroid hormone. Partial thyroidectomy may be undertaken if remission is not

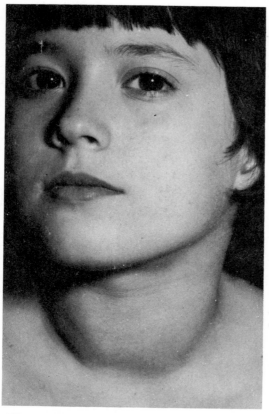

Figure 24–2 Ten-year-old girl with hyperthyroidism. Eyes are somewhat prominent and have a shiny or "pretty" appearance. Note the fullness in the lower neck due to the enlarged thyroid.

achieved after a period of prolonged medical therapy.

Autoimmune thyroiditis (Hashimoto's thyroiditis) is a more common occurrence in childhood and occasionally presents with symptoms of mild hypo- or hyperthyroidism. Children with autoimmune thyroiditis are usually asymptomatic, however, and the only physical finding is an enlarged, firm, non-tender thyroid gland. Diagnosis may be difficult because thyroid antibodies may not be present in the early stages of Hashimoto's thyroiditis in children. Continued follow-up is indicated, and thyroid hormone replacement therapy may be warranted if there are chemical or clinical signs of hypothyroidism.

CONGENITAL ADRENAL HYPERPLASIA

Congenital adrenal hyperplasia is a genetically determined inborn error of steroid-

ogenesis that is inherited as an autosomal recessive trait. It is estimated to occur once in 10,000 births. There are several types of congenital adrenal hyperplasia, each resulting from deficient enzyme activity at a particular stage in the cortisol biosynthesis pathway. Only the most common form, which involves defective hydroxylation of the steroid molecule at the 21 carbon position, will be discussed. Figure 24–3 depicts the pathogenesis of virilizing congenital adrenal hyperplasia. Cortisol acts as a negative feedback control on the release of pituitary adrenocorticotropin (ACTH). Deficient cortisol production results in increased ACTH release and consequent adrenal hyperplasia with the production of increased androgenic steroids. Since the metabolic block exists *in utero*, at birth the female infant with congenital adrenal hyperplasia will show varying degrees of masculinization of the external genitalia (Fig. 24–4). Without treatment, accelerated growth and maturation with progressive virilization ensues. Deficient mineralocorticoid production leads to a salt-losing state with failure to thrive in early infancy in some patients.

Total replacement therapy with cortisol or one of its analogues effectively sup-

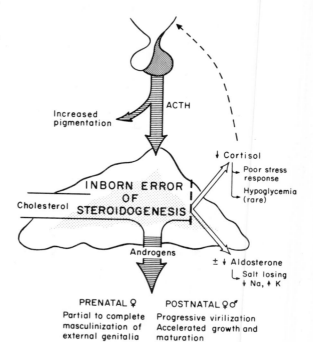

Figure 24–3 Pathogenesis of congenital adrenal hyperplasia.

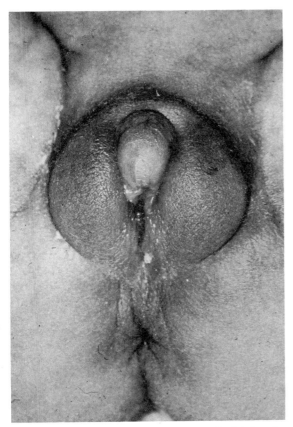

Figure 24-4 Genitalia of a two-week-old female infant with congenital adrenal hyperplasia. Note the enlargement of the clitoris and labia majora and hyperpigmentation.

estrogenizing granulosa cell tumor in the female and virilizing Leydig cell tumors in the male. The earliest signs and progression of precocious puberty generally follow the usual sequence of pubertal development outlined in Chapter 9 on adolescence.

Far more common than these are the occurrence of certain secondary sex characteristics that are isolated phenomena and relatively benign. In the neonate, breast enlargement can occur in either sex and usually subsides within several weeks. Transient breast enlargement occasionally occurs between six months and two years of age in infant girls. This type of breast hyperplasia may initially be unilateral and is seldom accompanied by nipple or areolar changes. In some cases it may persist until a normal advent of puberty, after which further progressive enlargement occurs. The normal adolescent male may have some transient mammary duct hyperplasia as a normal finding during the period of rapid virilization. Growth of axillary or pubic hair before the usual age of puberty occurs more commonly in females, especially those with central nervous system disorders. Mild acceleration of growth and maturation may be accompanying features, and although the etiology is unknown, early stimulus of adrenal androgen production is suspected.

presses ACTH and thereby stops excessive androgen production. If salt loss is a problem, mineralocorticoid replacement with desoxycorticosterone acetate in a long-acting intramuscular form (Percorten pivalate) or other mineralocorticoid therapy should be instituted.

PRECOCIOUS SEXUAL DEVELOPMENT

Early production of increased pituitary gonadotropins, most commonly seen in females, is the major cause of premature onset of puberty. This condition is most often idiopathic, but consideration should be given to the possibility of a central nervous system lesion such as a tumor, especially in males. Early advent of secondary sex characteristics and acceleration of growth and maturation can also result from a number of very rare neoplasms such as

OBESITY

Obesity in childhood rarely has an endocrine cause. The vast majority of cases appears to be based on a complex of genetic and environmental factors. Such obese children are generally tall and strong for their age and easily distinguishable from the very rare child with obesity secondary to excessive production of cortisol (Cushing syndrome), in which growth deficiency and weakness are prominent features. The problem of obesity is discussed further in Chapter 9 on adolescence.

GROWTH HORMONE DEFICIENCY AND HYPOPITUITARISM

Growth deficiency in children seldom results from pituitary growth hormone (PGH) deficiency. However, the rare possibility of hypopituitarism or isolated growth hormone deficiency should be kept in mind when evaluating any child with *progressive* growth failure. Although the diagnosis can be difficult, the following clinical features are frequently encountered: Infants with PGH deficiency are usually of normal birth weight and length, even when there is maternal growth hormone deficiency, indicating that growth *in utero* is not dependent upon PGH. Growth deficiency is variable in onset but generally occurs within the first year or two of life and usually leads to serious stunting of growth. The facies is characteristically immature, being round and doll-like, with premature wrinkling common in older individuals. Weight retardation does not occur to the same degree as height retardation, and there is an increase in subcutaneous fat, particularly around the pelvic and pectoral regions, giving an overall pudgy appearance. Skeletal proportions and head circumference are usually near normal for age.

In children it is generally not possible to differentiate isolated PGH deficiency from more generalized hypopituitarism on clinical grounds alone, and for this reason measurements of PGH followed by assessment of other pituitary tropic hormones are indicated. In hypopituitarism there is a variable degree of multiple tropic hormone deficiency. Males are affected more frequently than females, and there is an increased incidence of breech birth. In most instances the etiology is unknown but birth trauma may play a role.

Hypopituitarism may also result from the presence of a central nervous system tumor, especially *craniopharyngioma.* The combination of growth failure, suprasellar calcification on skull roentgenogram, with or without diabetes insipidus (posterior pituitary involvement), is virtually diagnostic of this type of neoplasm. In testing pituitary function it must be kept in mind that PGH is not secreted in a continuous manner, and random blood samples in normal children may show low serum PGH. Maneuvers to provoke PGH release such as insulin-induced hypoglycemia, infusion of the amino acid arginine, and oral administration of L-dopa, are utilized to test the PGH response. ACTH function may be determined by inducing a block in the cor-

tisol biosynthesis pathway by means of metyrapone and noting the presence or absence of an increase in 17-hydroxycorticosteroid excretion over baseline values. Serum thyrotropic stimulating hormone (TSH) can be determined directly, and pituitary TSH reserve can be evaluated by measuring TSH response to exogenous thyrotropin releasing hormone (TRH). Gonadotropins may also be measured in serum. At the present time the only PGH available for clinical use is derived postmortem from human pituitaries.

JUVENILE DIABETES MELLITUS

Diabetes mellitus occurs in about 1 in 1000 children with a peak incidence that roughly coincides with the early adolescent growth spurt.

The etiology of diabetes remains obscure, with hereditary factors known to be important in determining susceptibility. It is generally not transmitted as an autosomal recessive trait as was once thought. Polygenic inheritance is considered the most likely mode of determination.

Symptoms

Onset of diabetes mellitus in children is generally insidious, with symptoms of excessive thirst, increased appetite, polyuria and lethargy. Gradually over a period of days or weeks weight loss and dehydration become evident. At times the presentation is abrupt, especially when there is concomitant infectious illness. A greater awareness of the early signs of diabetes mellitus has resulted in speedier recognition of the disorder, and fewer children present with severe diabetic ketoacidosis and coma.

Diagnosis

Glycosuria along with blood glucose elevation is the essential laboratory feature of diabetes mellitus. Rarely is it necessary to perform a glucose tolerance test to establish the diagnosis in children. The typical clinical picture, with glycosuria and a serum glucose in excess of 200 mg/dl, is usually indicative of juvenile diabetes mellitus. An exception is the infant or young child who, in response to stress or an acute illness, becomes transiently hyperglycemic and glycosuric. This is especially true if intravenous fluids containing glucose are being administered or if there has been treatment with drugs of the sympathomimetic amine type.

Management

Acute. Intravenous fluid therapy with prompt correction of fluid and electrolyte disturbances and judicious use of insulin is the key to the initial management of the newly diagnosed child with diabetes mellitus. (See Chapter 38 on fluid and electrolyte disorders). Insulin may be given subcutaneously, intravenously or in a combination of the two, depending on the clinical situation. It is hazardous to rely on the uptake of insulin from a subcutaneous site in a severely dehydrated patient. Initial insulin dosage usually ranges from 0.2 to 2 u/kg of regular insulin, depending on the severity of the ketoacidosis. Continuous low dose infusion of insulin (0.1 u/kg/hr) provides an alternative to this and has the advantage of posing a lesser risk of precipitous blood sugar fall during therapy. With either method, careful monitoring of the ketoacidosis is important.

Long term. DIET. As a rule, 1000 plus 100 calories per year of age with allowance for approximately 2 gm/kg/day of protein will provide an adequate intake for growth and energy needs.

A combination of intermediate-acting (NPH or Lente) and regular (crystalline, short-acting) insulin provides flexibility of insulin dosage, especially when given in combination twice daily. We find the following partition of insulin to be particularly useful in the teenage diabetic.

	A.M. Dose	P.M. Dose
NPH	2/3	1/2
Regular	1/3	1/2
	2/3	1/3
	of total insulin dose (approx.)	of total insulin dose (approx.)

Example: A teenage child with diabetes requiring a total of 45 units of insulin daily would receive 30 units in the morning as a 20/10 mixture of NPH/regular insulin and 15 units before the evening meal as an 8/7 NPH/regular mixture.

Younger children with diabetes, especially if in partial remission ("diabetic honeymoon"), will usually be easily managed on a single morning dose of intermediate-acting insulin. Unfortunately, virtually all children with diabetes eventually manifest complete Beta cell failure and are dependent on insulin therapy for life.

Although never completely satisfactory, testing for glycosuria preprandially and at bedtime is an important aspect of monitoring control of the diabetes. In school-age children the noontime test for glucose may be omitted, but a minimum of three tests (before breakfast, before the evening meal and at bedtime) is recommended.

Patients are encouraged to carry some form of identification (e.g., Medic-Alert bracelet obtained from the Medic-Alert Foundation, Turlock, CA 95380). In addition, parents should be instructed in the use of glucagon injection (1 mg vial) for emergency treatment of hypoglycemia in the unconscious child.

The absence of significant nocturia, a feeling of general well-being, and in particular, normal growth and weight gain are among the best guides to the adequacy of the management of the diabetes mellitus.

REFERENCES

Standard Texts

Gardner, L. I.: *Endocrine and Genetic Diseases of Childhood and Adolescence,* 2nd ed. Philadelphia, W. B. Saunders Co., 1975.
Wilkins, L.: *The Diagnosis and Treatment of Endocrine Disorders in Childhood and Adolescence,* 3rd ed. Springfield, Charles C Thomas, 1965.
Williams, R. H.: *Textbook of Endocrinology,* 5th ed. Philadelphia, W. B. Saunders Co., 1974.

Articles

Andersen, H. J.: Studies of hypothyroidism in children. Acta Pediatr. Scand., 50(Suppl. 125):1, 1961.
Bongiovanni, A. M.: Care of the critically ill child: Acute adrenal insufficiency. Pediatrics, 44:109, 1969.
Drash, A.: Diabetes mellitus in childhood: A review. J. Pediatr., 78:919, 1971.

Fisher, D. A.: Advances in the laboratory diagnosis of thyroid disease. Part I. J. Pediatr., 82:1, 1973.

Fisher, D. A.: Advances in the laboratory diagnosis of thyroid disease. Part II. J. Pediatr., 82:187, 1973.

French, F. S., and Van Wyk, J. J.: Fetal hypothyroidism. J. Pediatr., 64:589, 1964.

Goodman, H. G., Grumbach, M. M., and Kaplan, S. L.: Growth and growth hormone. N. Engl. J. Med., 278:57, 1968.

Kaufman, I. A., Keller, M. A., and Nyhan, W. L.: Diabetic ketosis and acidosis: The continuous infusion of low doses of insulin. J. Pediatr., 87:846, 1975.

Rallison, M. L., et al.: Occurrence and natural history of chronic lymphocytic thyroiditis in childhood. J. Pediatr., 86:675, 1975.

Root, A. W., Bongiovanni, A. M., Harvie, F. H., and Eberlein, W. R.: Treatment of juvenile thyrotoxicosis. J. Pediatr., 63:402, 1963.

Sigurjonsdottir, T. J., and Hayles, A. B.: Precocious puberty: A report of 96 cases. Am. J. Dis. Child., 115:309, 1968.

Smith, D. W., Blizzard, R. M., and Wilkins, L.: The mental prognosis in hypothyroidism of infancy and childhood: Review of 128 cases. Pediatrics, 19:1011, 1957.

PART IX

BRAIN DYSFUNCTION DISORDERS

25 Neurological Disorders

Robert H. A. Haslam

Children with disorders of the central nervous system (CNS) are an important segment of pediatric practice. The pediatrician constantly encounters symptoms of CNS dysfunction, including mental retardation, convulsions, headache, learning difficulties and abnormalities of gait and posture, all of which demand a keen appreciation of the developing nervous system.

HISTORY AND EXAMINATION

A precise history is the foundation of neurological assessment. Particular attention is directed to the clinical features of the pregnancy and the behavior of the infant during the perinatal and neonatal periods. Abnormalities of sucking and feeding, body tone, temperature control or sleep may signify malfunction of the CNS. The neurological history is incomplete without a thorough evaluation of the child's developmental milestones. These may be categorized into four major groups; motor, adaptive, social and communication skills (Table 25–1). In the normal infant, developmental milestones are interdependent and predictable. Significant deviation from the expected pattern of growth may involve only one sector of development (e.g., motor) or a more uniform delay in the acquisition of all skills. Important clues to the extent and localization of neurological dysfunction may be derived from careful evaluation of these growth parameters. The physician utilizes this information to determine whether the neurological problem is static or progressive.

The history must establish the symptoms in chronological order, as the physician may never witness a seizure or observe the child during time of headache and vertigo. All family members become important during this phase of the evaluation. The mother's information may be extremely detailed and inclusive, the father's the most dispassionate and the child's often the most enlightening. Review of the salient features of the history following the physical examination may assist in clarification of certain fundamental issues. Inspection of baby books, portraits or discussions with relatives or teachers can provide additional important information about the time of onset and rate of progression of the disorder.

The neurological examination seeks to localize the process within the central or peripheral nervous system, to determine the extent and character of the lesion and finally to suggest possible causes and mechanisms of dysfunction. It is evident that the evaluation differs significantly among infants, children and adults. Because the newborn neurological examination so frequently tests the ingenuity of the physician, a format for investigation of the infant nervous system will be summarized. It is important to recall that the time of the last feeding (hungry — alert, just fed — lethargic) and the room temperature (cool — alert, warm — lethargic) may materially influence the infant's wakefulness.

Observation of the infant is the most significant aspect of the neurological examination. Does the baby assume a normal flexed position or is there extreme extension, opisthotonus or hypotonia? Are the extremity movements symmetrical or asymmetrical, thus implying a localized abnormality? Excessive tremulousness or frequent twitching movements may herald the onset of a seizure disorder. Aberrations of the

234

TABLE 25–1   DEVELOPMENTAL MILESTONES

Age of Acquisition	Fine Motor	Gross Motor	Adaptive	Social	Communication
1 month		Good head control when held erect	Occasional eye following	Recognizes facial form	Guttural sounds
2 months		Head up when lying prone	Follows regularly	Smiles	Early cooing
3 months	Opens hands, grasps at objects	Assumes portion of body weight with arms when prone	Looks at objects in hand	Reaches for familiar objects Plays with hands	Coos, laughs
6 months	Uses the hand in a raking motion	Rolling over for 2 to 3 months Sits unsupported	Transfers from hand to hand Successfully picks up various toys	Plays with feet Clearly shows joy and displeasure	Babbles
9 months	Picks up object using fingers and thumb	Crawling for 1 to 2 months Pulls to stand, may be cruising	Feeds from a cup Holds own bottle	Finger feeds Plays peek-a-boo	Imitates sounds Ma-Ma (no meaning)
12 months	Well developed pincer grasp	Stands unsupported Walks with a minimum of assistance	Builds tower of 2 cubes	Understands yes and no	One or two meaningful words
18 months	Simultaneously turns 2 to 3 pages of a book	Runs well Walks up stairs with assistance	Feeds self with utensils Scribbles	Pulls a wheeled toy Mimics mother during household tasks Points out some facial body parts	Gestures, jargons 4 to 6 recognizable words Beginning 2-word phrases
24 months	Turns pages one at a time Builds a 6-cube tower	Walks up and down stairs Kicks a ball	Removes some articles of clothing	Beginning to enjoy play, occasionally with other children	Well developed 2 to 3 word phrases Follows one step commands

respiratory cycle, including prolonged apnea, ataxic breathing, paradoxical movement and unilateral expansion of the thoracic wall, may have a primary neurological cause. What is the color and texture of the skin and hair? Inspection of the skin may uncover diagnostically important findings including hemangiomas, café au lait spots and vitiliginous lesions. The child's facial features may suggest a specific syndrome. The cry, if high-pitched and piercing, is consistent with a disorder of CNS origin. Constant urinary dribbling may indicate denervation of the bladder, and defects or masses overlying the bony spine may point to a congenital abnormality of neural tube closure.

The shape and circumference of the cranium deserves special attention. The sutures normally override at the time of birth. The skull may assume peculiar shapes in conjunction with premature closure of one or more sutures. Position and prominence of the scalp veins and the size and configuration as well as tension and pulsation of the anterior fontanel should be noted on inspection of the cranium. Palpation may help to detect cranial defects, fractures or abnormally separated sutures. Auscultation of the skull is an important adjunct to the physical examination. Although soft symmetric bruits are common in children less than four years of age, loud, localized bruits are highly significant and warrant further investigation. Transillumination of the skull is a useful screening procedure, in that hydranencephaly, severe hydrocephalus, porencephalic cysts, Dandy-Walker syndrome and subdural effusions may be demonstrated by this rapid, simple technique.

Cranial nerve examination in the newborn is much less refined than in the older patient. Nevertheless, invaluable information may be retrieved by diligent evaluation of cranial nerve function. Although most infants have not developed conjugate eye movements by the time of birth, vision in some may be documented by the finding of opticokinetic nystagmus when a striped drum is rotated through the field of vision. Inspection of the retina is mandatory, though it may be delayed until the conclusion of the exam. If the retina is difficult to visualize through the undilated pupil, a mydriatic agent such as 10 per cent phenylephrine can be used. The optic nerve is normally pale in the newborn. Retinal hemorrhages may be apparent but are usually of no consequence in this age group. An area of chorioretinitis, particularly in the macular region, is suggestive of intrauterine infection.

Disorders of ocular movement may be assessed by the doll's head maneuver in which the infant's head is turned on a horizontal and vertical axis. When the head is passively moved to the left, the eyes will momentarily deviate to the right. A right abducens nerve palsy is characterized by incomplete lateral movement of that eye to the right during head rotation to the left. Weakness of the facial nerve is often inapparent but should be suspected in an infant whose eyes remain open while crying or when the child is unable to suck.

Evaluation of the auditory nerve is difficult in the newborn. Asymmetrical movement of the palate and nasal regurgitation of milk may indicate glossopharyngeal or vagal nerve involvement. Stridor may result from bilateral vagus nerve impairment. Wasting and fasciculation of the tongue is noted when an abnormality of the hypoglossal nerve exists.

Finally, neurological examination of the primitive reflexes is often helpful. Their absence or prolonged persistence, although of little localizing value should alert the physician to the possibility of a CNS lesion (Table 25–2). It is interesting to note that primitive reflexes are controlled for the most part by the brain stem and do not require the cerebral cortex for their elaboration.

The following examples of some common pediatric neurological conditions were chosen as an introduction to this vitally important area of child health. The symptoms and signs of the various entities are emphasized in order to provide the student with a frame of reference upon which to build further physiological, biochemical and pharmacological knowledge.

CONGENITAL MALFORMATIONS OF THE CENTRAL NERVOUS SYSTEM

Malformations of the central nervous system are relatively common. Their cause is often undetermined, but a host of genetic and intrauterine environmental factors, including exposure to certain drugs, toxins, ionizing radiation and infections, are important etiological agents. Certain malformations result from faulty closure of the neural tube during embryogenesis, others from deranged migration of cell populations within the developing brain and still others occasionally result from an arrest in the differentiation of vital structures. The severity of the abnormality is variable; some are incompatible with an extrauterine existence, others result in significant lifelong handicap and, rarely, the consequences of the defect are considered minimal.

Hydrocephalus

Hydrocephalus is a complex disorder that results from overproduction or incomplete absorption of cerebrospinal fluid (CSF). The process may be subtle and slowly progressive or relentlessly rapid and destructive. The excessive accumulation of CSF may be secondary to an obstruction within the ventricular system (non-communicating hydrocephalus) or may arise from a lesion that restricts or impedes the circulation and absorption of CSF within the subarachnoid space (communicating hydrocephalus). Hydrocephalus of both types may be congenital or acquired.

In rare circumstances, hydrocephalus may become evident during a prolonged labor because of cephalopelvic disproportion, but more commonly it is discovered

TABLE 25–2 SELECTED PRIMITIVE REFLEXES

Reflex	Description of Reflex	Appears	Disappears
Root	The infant turns its head to follow a stimulus applied to the lips	Birth	3–4 months
Moro	With sudden controlled extension of the head the arms extend, the fingers spread and then the arms flex over the surface of the chest	Birth	2–4 months
Grasp	The infant's fingers or toes reflexly grasp an object	Birth	1–2 months
Tonic neck	Rotation of an infant's head causes extension of the extremities to the side he is looking while flexion occurs in the opposite extremities	Birth to 1 month	4–5 months

because of the too rapid enlargement of the infant's head during the initial months of life. The most dependable normal correlate of head growth is the child's height. If the head circumference should cross the grid lines while linear growth proceeds along a predictable curve, hydrocephalus must be considered (Fig. 25–1).

In addition to an enlarged head, the hydrocephalic infant may show a bulging anterior fontanel, downward displacement of the eyes (the setting sun sign due to pressure upon the colliculus), dilated scalp veins, prominent forehead, irritability, high-pitched cry and feeding difficulties. The toddler or older child may only experience symptoms and signs of increased intracranial pressure because fusion of the

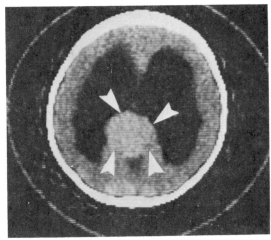

Figure 25–2 A CAT (computerized axial tomography) scan with contrast material showing a large arteriovenous malformation of the vein of Galen (arrows) producing massive hydrocephalus.

cranial bones prevents abnormal expansion of the skull.

It is imperative that every infant with a too rapidly expanding head undergo a comprehensive diagnostic evaluation to discover the cause of enlargement. Rarely, a papilloma of the choroid plexus, causing an overproduction of CSF, will be discovered. Non-communicating hydrocephalus may be caused by occlusion of the foramen of Monro, aqueductal stenosis or atresia, the Arnold-Chiari malformation, the Dandy-Walker syndrome, vascular malformations of the vein of Galen (Fig. 25–2) and mass lesions of the posterior fossa that distort or obstruct the aqueduct of Sylvius or the fourth ventricle. Communicating hydrocephalus may result from subarachnoid bleeding (particularly in the premature), meningitis (pneumococcal, tuberculous) or other processes that may obliterate the subarachnoid spaces, such as leukemic infiltration of the leptomeninges.

Investigation includes a thorough neurological examination, transillumination of the head, radiographs of the skull, visualization of the ventricular cavities by computerized axial tomography (CAT scan) or pneumoencephalography (PEG) and cerebral angiography if vascular malformation, subdural hematoma or thrombosis of a major venous sinus is suspected. In selected cases, radioactive isotope study of CSF circulation is extremely useful.

BOYS' HEAD CIRCUMFERENCE

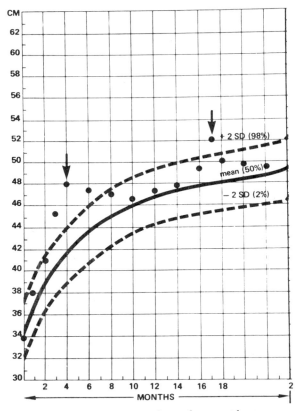

Figure 25–1 A 22-month infant with communicating hydrocephalus. A ventriculo-peritoneal shunt was performed at four months (arrow). The head circumference followed the expected curve until the shunt became nonfunctional. Revision at 17 months (arrow) corrected the obstruction. *From* Nellhaus, G.: Pediatrics, *41*:106, 1968.)

Hydranencephaly

Hydranencephaly represents a striking CNS malformation characterized by absence of the cerebral hemispheres. Large CSF-filled cavities lined by a thin glial membrane and conglomerates of cerebral tissue occupy the cerebral hemisphere areas. Hydranencephaly probably results from several causes including intrauterine infection, obliteration or thrombosis of the fetal carotid artery system or a defect in cellular migration during the early stages of CNS development.

The hydranencephalic infant may appear quite normal at birth. The head circumference and shape is not unusual. However, the infant soon demonstrates idiosyncrasies in neurodevelopment including irritability, poor feeding habits, a piercing cry and lack of attentiveness. The head may begin to grow at an excessive rate. Certain primitive reflexes including the Moro and tonic neck are exaggerated and persistent. The child does not follow objects with his eyes or smile and is not interested in the environment. Neurological examination may show optic atrophy and spastic quadriparesis. A hydranencephalic infant rarely survives beyond one year of age.

Transillumination of the hydranencephalic skull illuminates the entire cranial cavity irrespective of placement of the light source (Fig. 25–3). Not infrequently, severe hydrocephaly or large bilateral subdural effusions may transilluminate to the same degree as hydranencephaly. A PEG or CAT scan becomes useful for differentiation of these conditions and assists in the management of the structural defect. Occasionally, a patient with severe hydranencephaly is shunted to simplify nursing care, but results of treatment are uniformly unsuccessful.

Microcephaly

Microcephaly may be defined as an abnormally small brain, in which the head circumference measures more than two standard deviations below the mean when the child's age, sex and height are considered. It is usually associated with mental retardation. Microcephaly must not be confused with craniosynostosis, which is the result of premature fusion of the cranial bones. In the latter condition the brain development and size are usually normal.

Microcephaly may be inherited as an autosomal recessive. Children present a rather typical clinical picture with long sloping foreheads and significant mental retardation. Other causes include Down, cri-du-chat, and deLange syndromes. In other infants arrested brain growth is secondary to malformations of gyrus formation or disordered cytoarchitectural develop-

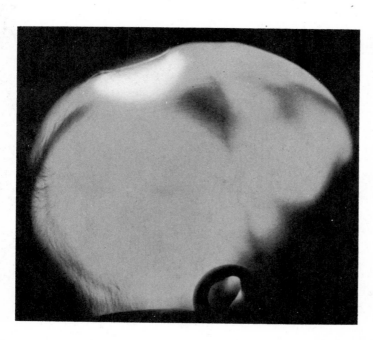

Figure 25–3 Transillumination of the entire intracranial cavity of an hydranencephalic infant.

ment including microgyria and agyria (lissencephaly).

Various antenatal insults may interfere with cerebral maturation. These include excessive radiation, drugs and intrauterine infections (toxoplasmosis, cytomegalic inclusion disease and rubella). Anoxia or significant perinatal CNS trauma, inborn errors of metabolism, neonatal meningitis and degenerative diseases of the brain are examples of postnatal factors that may have a detrimental effect on brain growth, causing microcephaly. Many syndromes characterized by mental retardation, short stature and unusual facial features are also associated with microcephaly.

Small head circumference at birth would suggest a genetic or intrauterine cause for the arrested brain growth, whereas a normally sized skull with a subsequent delay in growth points to an insult occurring after birth. Examination of a microcephalic infant should include a thorough inspection of the retina for evidence of chorioretinitis. A skull radiograph may show calcifications that may also suggest an intrauterine infection. This may be documented by elevated antibody titres or cultivation of a virus. Chromosomal studies are often indicated. Specific biochemical tests are accomplished if a metabolic disease is entertained (e.g., phenylketonuria, maple syrup urine disease).

Macrocephaly

The average weight of the newborn brain approximates 350 gm. By adulthood the weight has quadrupled, reaching 1400 gm. Occasionally, a patient is encountered with an enlarged skull circumference who does not have hydrocephalus, abnormal collections of subdural fluid or markedly thickened cranial bones. Macrocephaly may be suspected if these conditions are systematically eliminated and the skull circumference is more than two standard deviations above the mean while the patient's linear growth rate approximates the mean for sex and age. The brains in most of these patients are large and heavy, sometimes weighing more than twice normal. Macrocephaly may be inherited as an autosomal dominant. Parent and child may have normal intelligence or show significant mental retardation. Convulsions are relatively

frequent. Certain degenerative diseases of the central nervous system may cause macrocephaly because of the abnormal accumulation of ganglioside or myelin products. The neurocutaneous syndromes, particularly neurofibromatosis and tuberous sclerosis are often accompanied by macrocephaly.

CEREBRAL PALSY

Cerebral palsy is a complex disorder of CNS function characterized by abnormalities of movement, intellect, speech and sensation. It is a relatively common condition occurring in approximately 2 per 1000 of the population. The severity of cerebral palsy is extremely variable, dependent in part on the nature and degree of the initial cerebral insult. Cerebral palsy is a *static disturbance* but the disability can vary immensely with emotional duress, growth, medication and environmental factors.

The pathogenesis of cerebral palsy has not been completely delineated. Although symptoms and signs of cerebral palsy may follow almost any significant incident to the brain during the first several years of life, it appears that in the majority of affected children an injurious process occurs during the perinatal period. Improved obstetric techniques have substantially reduced the frequency of severe traumatic birth injuries. However, prolongation of the second stage of labor, too rapid delivery, abnormal presentation, faulty forceps application and cephalopelvic disproportion undoubtedly enhance the possibility of cerebral damage. This may result in tearing of the falx cerebri or intracranial bleeding, particularly into the ventricles and subarachnoid space. Premature infants are especially at risk because of their increased propensity to intracranial bleeding. Some children with cerebral palsy have congenital malformations of the brain. Other factors that may produce significant injury to the immature brain during the perinatal period include hypoglycemia, severe acidosis, icterus, anoxia and maternal hypotension during labor.

Infants at Risk For Cerebral Palsy

The infant who ultimately manifests the clinical parameters of cerebral palsy frequently shows many abnormal characteristics during the neonatal period. The cry may be high-pitched and piercing, and the child appears agitated. The suck is often uncoordinated, and feeding disinterests the infant. The child tends to be excessively sleepy and must be awakened and then continuously stimulated during feeding. Later, tongue thrust supervenes, augmenting the feeding difficulty. Various procedures such as artificially enlarging the nipple opening may facilitate feeding. Abnormalities of posture should alert the physician to the possibility of a CNS insult, including persistent cortical fisting, opisthotonus and marked hypotonia or spasticity. A bulging fontanel, prolonged apnea or convulsions are obvious signs of CNS malfunction. Finally, the absence or protraction of the primitive reflexes such as the root, Moro, tonic neck and stepping reaction strongly suggest an aberration of brain function.

Classification of Cerebral Palsy

There are two major clinical types of cerebral palsy: spastic (or pyramidal) and extrapyramidal. A third form (mixed) is reserved for those children with a combination of pyramidal and extrapyramidal signs, although careful neurological examination usually shows an admixture of the two clinical types in every cerebral palsied child. The spastic group may be subdivided into at least three entities.

Spastic (Pyramidal) Cerebral Palsy

Hemiplegia. Hemiplegic cerebral palsy is the most common type and accounts for approximately 40 per cent of all cases. The parents may be unaware of the condition until the child attempts to crawl. In other instances the patient is noted to reach exclusively with one hand. Some hemiplegics are unrecognized until they attempt to walk. The upper extremity is involved to a greater extent than the lower. The affected limbs, particularly the hand, often show impressive growth arrest, the result of parietal lobe injury. In time, contractures develop, causing the child to walk on his toes. Eventually, many individuals complain of movement disorders such as dystonia in the affected limbs as well as sensory disturbances, including astereognosis and inattention. Approximately 50 per cent develop seizure disorders, but fortunately, most are controlled by anticonvulsants. About two thirds of the children are found to be intellectually impaired and one third have a homonomous hemanopsia due to destruction of the optic radiation.

Quadriplegia. In most series, quadriplegic cerebral palsy accounts for 20 per cent of the affected population. Patients with this form of cerebral palsy are the most severely incapacitated. The child tends to assume a decerebrate posture, and the tone is markedly increased. Contractures and dislocated hips may result because of spasticity. Seizures are inordinately common and difficult to control. Many children have microcephaly, implying an arrest of cerebral maturation, and most are severely mentally retarded. The life span of these patients is curtailed primarily owing to recurrent pulmonary infections.

Diplegia. Patients with spastic diplegia have upper motor neuron signs, principally in the lower extremities. These children tend to "scissor" when walking is attempted because of the increased tone. Neurological examination will show clonus, enhanced deep tendon reflexes and extensor plantar responses in the lower extremities. Contractures may develop, and toe-walking is common. Approximately one third develop seizures, some are retarded and many have speech defects. By adulthood, the lower portion of the body is often underdeveloped as compared to the upper torso.

Extrapyramidal Cerebral Palsy

The extrapyramidal type accounts for approximately 15 to 20 per cent of cases. The outstanding clinical abnormality is delayed motor development. Most infants with this form of cerebral palsy are markedly hypotonic at birth. The tendon reflexes are variable, but usually difficult to elicit. Neurological findings change with time, and by the age of one year athetosis becomes evident in most affected children. In addition, careful examination may show chorea and dystonic posturing as well as occasional tremors, all of which suggest a lesion within the basal ganglia. Incoordination of speech and drooling are common features of extrapyramidal cerebral palsy. The incidence of convulsions is surprisingly low in this group of patients, and normal or near normal intelligence is to be expected, particularly in children who lack upper motor neuron signs.

Treatment

A recent advance in the management of children with chronic disorders of the central nervous system such as cerebral palsy has been the introduction of the interdisciplinary concept, a method in which a variety of professionals interact with a patient and his family, ultimately formulating a plan of habilitation that strives to elevate the patient to his greatest potential.

The pediatrician must be responsible for a thorough history and examination of the child. He should pay particular attention to the events of the perinatal period, searching for possible historical clues to assist in the diagnosis. One of the pediatrician's prime responsibilities is to ensure that the physical disability is in fact secondary to a static process and not the result of a progressive organic disturbance. Careful scrutiny during repeated examinations is the only means to determine non-progression.

The psychologist is an important member of the team, as children with cerebral palsy are at risk for mental retardation or a learning disability. Test results provide a baseline for further assessment, and if a drastic decline in function is noted at a later date, an active process must be suspected. Assignment of the level of intellectual functioning allows realistic counseling, and appropriate educational facilities may be sought. The psychologist may be of assistance in the management of severe behavior disorders, such as head banging, food idiosyncrasies, temper tantrums and severe irritability by the use of behavior modification techniques.

Occupational and physical therapists have developed procedures that enhance certain motor activities such as rolling over, sitting, reaching, feeding and walking. They, with the orthopedist, must investigate and work with children who display a lag in walking. The ultimate program developed for the individual patient depends upon whether or not independent ambulation is the goal, or whether or not assistant devices, canes or crutches will be utilized. In addition, the physical therapist practices preventive techniques by the prescription of various exercises to prevent the development of joint contractures. Finally, the occupational therapist is concerned with the development of self-help skills ranging from toilet training to the provision of a special typewriter for the college student with cerebral palsy.

Many drugs, including diazepam, dantrolene sodium, Artane, and L-dopa, have been investigated to determine their usefulness in the management of children with cerebral palsy complicated by marked spasticity or athetosis. For the most part, those agents studied either have not demonstrated a persistent desirable effect or their discontinuance was imperative because of CNS depression, the emergence of ataxia, seizures or motor weakness.

The spastic child may benefit from bracing in order to correct the deformity produced by increased muscle tone. Surgical procedures in selected patients are warranted to relieve joint deformities caused by excessive muscular forces (e.g., dislocated hips secondary to severe adductor spasm) or Achilles tendon lengthening to provide a more functional gait. Because of the high frequency of strabismus in cerebral palsied children, the ophthalmologist becomes an integral member of the team. In many instances, following a suitable period of patching or other conservative methods of treatment, surgery is indicated primarily for cosmetic purposes. Some patients with severe athetosis have undergone thalamotomy with limited success.

The speech therapist may provide ongoing therapy for the child with a severe language disorder, and of course, the school system becomes responsible for the provision of an educational program that will meet the needs of the individual child. Finally, the pediatrician must act as the ombudsman for his patient, interpreting the evaluation results of others as well as providing a continuum of care.

SEIZURES OF CHILDHOOD

Convulsions during infancy and childhood are the most prominent neurological disorder encountered by the physician. They may occur as a singular event, in which case normal intellectual and neurological development and function are expected, or a repetitive, modified seizure pattern may emerge, signifying a complex fundamental neurophysiological disturbance. Approximately 0.5 per cent of children fall into the latter group, whereas some 3 to 4 per cent of all children experience a convulsion if extreme pyrexia and systemic diseases are included as causative factors.

Seizures are merely a symptom of an underlying CNS disturbance. Convulsions that are classified as primary or idiopathic tend to be associated with genetic etiological factors. They rarely evolve prior to two years of age, and pathological changes within the brain are infrequent. Secondary seizures are the consequence of a basic disease process, and therefore, may develop at any age including the neonatal period. Examples of "seizure-related" diseases include CNS infections (both antenatal and acquired), congenital and structural malformations of the brain, CNS degenerative diseases, inborn errors of metabolism, birth injury or trauma, disturbances of water and electrolyte metabolism, vascular disease and exogenous poisons.

A clinical classification of seizures is important. The seizure type may provide valuable information about cerebral location, thereby influencing the investigation and management of the patient. A precise description of a seizure is of considerable assistance in the choice of the most efficacious anticonvulsant.

International Classification of the Epilepsies (After Merlis)

Generalized epilepsies
  a. Primary generalized epilepsies (includes grand mal and petit mal seizures)
  b. Secondary generalized epilepsies
  c. Undetermined generalized epilepsies
Partial epilepsies. (focal, local; includes Jacksonian, temporal lobe or psychomotor epilepsies).
Unclassifiable epilepsies. For practical purposes, convulsive disorders may be grouped into four major categories: grand mal (major motor), petit mal (absence), psychomotor (temporal lobe) and minor motor (akinetic). A brief description of each type follows, accompanied by a representative electroencephalogram (EEG) (Fig. 25–4).

GRAND MAL. Major motor convulsions are the most common and most frightening form of epilepsy. On occasion, the patient can anticipate a seizure. The aura may consist of a severe headache, lassitude, abdominal discomfort or perhaps clouding of the sensorium.

The convulsion may be initiated by a sudden piercing cry and simultaneous loss of consciousness. The child may fall, the eyes roll upwards, respirations momentarily cease, urinary sphincter control is lost and the face becomes slightly dusky. During this phase of the convulsion the child's arms and legs are rigid (tonic). Rhythmic synchronous movements of the entire body ensue (clonic activity) that usually persist for a few minutes but in the rare situation may continue for hours. The seizure is terminated by diminishing frequency, and finally, cessation of the tonic-clonic motion, followed by the appearance of spontaneous purposeful movements. In most instances, the patient is drowsy following a convulsion and prefers to sleep.

PETIT MAL. Petit mal seizures rarely occur prior to five years of age. The seizure classically consists of brief episodes of staring. The child momentarily appears to be disinterested, daydreaming and out of contact with reality. There may be lapses of speech and fluttering of the eyelids, but there is no loss or change in body tone. If these attacks are repetitive, school performance may deteriorate as the result of an altered state of concentration. The physician may precipitate a series of petit mal seizures by asking the patient to hyperventilate for three to four minutes.

PSYCHOMOTOR. Psychomotor seizures may be extremely difficult to perceive and recognize because of their bizarre nature and variable modes of presentation. Onset is rare prior to two years of age and much more usual after age 10 or during early adolescence. The initial symptom is often an obscure visual or auditory hallucination. In addition, the child may experience the déjà vu phenomenon or note distortion of body shapes or images. Some children complain of abdominal discomfort or headache at the

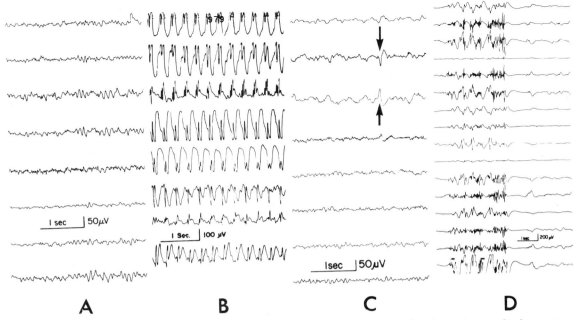

Figure 25-4 *A*, A normal electroencephalogram. *B*, Typical three per second spike and wave discharges in a patient with petit mal epilepsy. *C*, A 10-year-old boy with psychomotor epilepsy. Spike discharges from the left anterior temporal region are shown by arrows. *D*, Minor motor epilepsy. Bursts of synchronous spikes followed by a period of suppression.

onset of the seizure. Unusual movements of the tongue, smacking of the lips or repetitive motor activity such as rubbing or clasping the hands or writhing motions of the extremities may be observed. The child may also stare during this phase of the convulsion, incorrectly suggesting a diagnosis of petit mal epilepsy. Most demonstrate excessive perspiration, tachycardia, perioral pallor, salivation or marked blushing during a psychomotor seizure. The child does not show altered body tone and thus rarely falls. For the most part, psychomotor seizure duration is a matter of a few minutes, but on occasion may progress to a grand mal convulsion.

MINOR MOTOR. Minor motor seizures are characterized by brief alterations of consciousness and loss of body tone so that the head drops or, if the child is standing, he falls. They tend to occur in series. It is not uncommon for some children to experience several hundred minor motor seizures per day. The child usually has no forewarning of an impending convulsion, thus, facial abrasions, cut lips and bruised foreheads often result. Minor motor seizures have many causes. The treatment and prognosis of this type of epilepsy depends, to a

great extent, upon the underlying disorder. A thorough medical investigation, including a search for metabolic, toxic and infectious agents, is mandatory.

Investigation

Investigation must progress in an orderly fashion. The history and physical examination are without question the most important components of the work-up. The physician rarely observes the seizure, so that an accurate account of the convulsion must be secured in order to establish the seizure type and initiate the appropriate diagnostic steps. The physical examination gives particular attention to localizing neurological signs, examination of the retina, cutaneous abnormalities (suggesting a neurocutaneous syndrome), hepatosplenomegaly or an unusual respiratory pattern (degenerative CNS disease, inborn error of metabolism), meningeal signs, congenital malformations and other clues of an underlying disease process.

The extent of the initial laboratory investigation is dictated by the seizure type and frequency, age of the patient and history and neurological examination. For example, although a focal seizure is of little localizing value in the infant, it becomes extremely significant in the older child. A fasting serum glucose and calcium should be performed routinely. A skull radiograph is desirable in most instances. The EEG is most useful in confirming a clinical impression of a specific seizure type, particularly petit mal, or localizing the convulsion to a given cortical area. Examination of the CSF must always be achieved if an infection is suspected, if a subarachnoid hemorrhage is a possibility, if an immunological disorder of the central nervous system is considered or when a degenerative disease may exist. More specific neuroradiological investigation including brain scan, arteriography, PEG, myelography and CAT scan may be carried out in selected patients depending on the findings, as may more intense metabolic and genetic investigations of the patient.

Management

Certain factors that enhance or increase seizure frequency in a child with a convulsive disorder include illness, particularly when associated with a fever, immunization, severe emotional upset, erratic anticonvulsant compliance, ingestion of certain drugs (alcohol, chlorpromazine) and perhaps hormonal changes during adolescence. Children with epilepsy require constant guidance and understanding.

The principles of anticonvulsant therapy are similar to other well-established pharmacological protocols. A single drug is chosen that is considered effective for the particular convulsive disorder (Table 25–3). The drug dosage is slowly increased until toxic symptoms appear or the desired therapeutic influence is achieved. Measurement of serum anticonvulsant levels is useful, particularly if the seizures remain uncontrolled in spite of a seemingly adequate dosage. If a single drug achieves only partial control, another suitable anticonvulsant is added to the therapeutic regimen. In desperation, some patients are maintained on as many as five or six drugs at one time, often to the detriment of their intellectual and locomotor function. Approximately one half of all children with seizures can be completely controlled by anticonvulsants, and an additional substan-

tial number can be at least partially regulated.

The physician must be familiar with the short-term and more prolonged side effects of the anticonvulsant drugs. Knowledge of the pharmacokinetics of each agent is essential for calculation of the appropriate dose and scheduling of the medication. For example, during the first several days after birth the half-life of phenobarbital in an infant is prolonged so that the injudicious use of the drug may cause severe depression. Certain drug combinations may compete for similar degradation pathways, thereby producing toxicity (e.g., occasionally with diphenylhydantoin-diazepam). Although anticonvulsant therapy must be individualized, most children will be maintained on a drug for a significant period, varying from years to a lifetime. A drug should never be discontinued suddenly but gradually tapered when the anticonvulsant is no longer deemed necessary, as abrupt withdrawal of anticonvulsant medication may precipitate status epilepticus.

Status Epilepticus

Status epilepticus is a series of convulsive episodes during which the patient does not regain consciousness. A patient in status epilepticus must be treated as a medical emergency. Initial therapeutic efforts are directed toward establishing an adequate airway, clearing secretions, maintaining respiratory effort (with mechanical assistance if necessary) and supporting the cardiovascular system.

There are several useful pharmacological approaches to the patient in status, but the physician should be fully cognizant of the drugs he has chosen, including their cumulative effect and toxic side reactions, as the morbidity and mortality of status epilepticus is intensified by the imprudent use of antiepileptic agents.

Diazepam at a dose of 0.3 mg/kg slowly IV (not to exceed 10 mg/dose) is probably the most effective drug for arresting status epilepticus. Unfortunately, its anticonvulsant activity is short-lived. Therefore, a longer acting drug such as phenobarbital must be given following the use of diazepam. If diazepam fails to control the seizure, phenobarbital (5 to 10 mg/kg IM) or

TABLE 25–3   COMMON ANTICONVULSANTS

	Seizure Type	Usual Daily Dose (Oral)	Usual Therapeutic Serum Level (μg/ml)	Major Side Effects
ACTH gel	Infantile spasms	20–30 units IM		Similar to the oral steroids
Barbiturates Phenobarbital	Grand mal Focal motor Temporal lobe Petit mal	5–10 mg/kg	15–25	Drowsiness, lethargy and hyperactivity Rarely, hypersensitivity (fever, lymphadenopathy and morbilliform rash within two weeks of onset
Mephobarbital	Grand mal Focal motor	5–15 mg/kg	Adjust according to phenobarbital level	Less toxic than phenobarbital Skin eruptions
Primidone	Temporal lobe Grand mal Focal motor	10–25 mg/kg	5–10	Nausea, vomiting, fatigue Nystagmus, vertigo, diplopia and ataxia Morbilliform rash, megaloblastic anemia
Benzodiazepines Clonazepam	Minor motor	0.05 mg/kg increased to 0.25–0.5 mg/kg	15–70 ng/ml	Drowsiness, dysarthria, ataxia, irritability, hyperactivity, potentiation of major seizures
Diazepam	Status Epilepticus	0.3 mg/kg IV slowly	0.1–1	Drowsiness, dysarthria, ataxia, skin rash, jaundice
Carbamazepine	Grand mal Temporal lobe	10–30 mg/kg	4–10	Drowsiness, vertigo, diplopia, confusion and headache, nausea, vomiting, abdominal discomfort, abnormal liver function, skin rashes and rarely bone marrow depression
Hydantoins Diphenylhydantoin	Grand mal Focal motor Temporal lobe	5–10 mg/kg	10–20	Nystagmus, ataxia, dysarthria, vomiting, neuropathy, gingival hyperplasia, hirsutism, morbilliform rash, fever, lymphadenopathy, megaloblastic anemia, rickets
Mephenytoin	Grand mal Focal motor Temporal lobe	5–15 mg/kg	–	Ataxia, drowsiness, lymphadenopathy, bone marrow depression, skin rash, lupus erythematosus
Succinimides Ethosuximide	Petit mal	10–30 mg/kg	40–100	Skin rashes, bone marrow depression, drowsiness, fatigue and ataxia
Methsuximide	Petit mal Minor motor	5–20 mg/kg	10–40	Nausea, vomiting, anorexia, weight loss, drowsiness, ataxia, vertigo, skin rashes, bone marrow depression

paraldehyde (0.15 ml/kg deep IM) can be utilized. Diphenylhydantoin is an excellent drug for the management of unresponsive status epilepticus. The drug is given undiluted slowly IV (15 to 30 minutes) in a dosage of 12 to 15 mg/kg not to exceed 1000 mg. The patient is placed on a maintenance dose of diphenylhydantoin once the seizures have subsided.

DISTINCTIVE PAROXYSMAL DISORDERS OF INFANCY

Neonatal Seizures

In the neonate, seizures are often difficult to recognize. They usually signify a potentially serious underlying disorder, and therefore, demand immediate investigation in an effort to disclose a treatable cause so irreversible CNS injury may be prevented. The convulsion may be focal clonic, multifocal clonic, tonic, myoclonic or generalized. The symptoms and signs (Table 25–4) are extremely variable, probably in part related to the immaturely developed brain.

The etiologies of neonatal seizures are listed in Table 25–5. Possible metabolic or infectious causes must be dealt with immediately, as prompt therapy may result in immediate cessation of the convulsions. Management of the seizure disorder will depend on the cause.

Breath Holding Spells

Breath-holding spells are a common pediatric disorder that must not be confused with epilepsy. They most frequently begin during the latter half of the first year of life, although they have been noted in the neonate. The episodes are *always* provoked, usually by a reprimand or conflict with a parent. The child holds his breath for 10 to 20 seconds in expiration, becomes cyanotic and loses consciousness. Body tone varies from flaccidity to rigidity, and a brief major motor seizure may ensue, probably the result of cerebral hypoxia. The child may experience several incidents per day. The neurological examination and the EEG are normal except during the actual spell. There is no effective medical management, but parents must be reassured and informed of the excellent prognosis with usual cessation of the breath-holding spells by three or four years of age.

Febrile Convulsions

Febrile convulsions are the most common seizure disorders of childhood. Ap-

TABLE 25–4 SYMPTOMS AND SIGNS OF NEONATAL SEIZURES

1. Poor feeding, mouthing movements, excessive salivation, "colic"
2. Lethargy, irritability and excessive tremor
3. Asymmetrical extremity movements, abnormal body posture
4. Eye blinking, nystagmus, staring
5. Vasomotor disturbances, color change
6. Variable body tone (e.g., hypotonia, spasticity)
7. Apnea

TABLE 25–5 ETIOLOGIES OF NEONATAL SEIZURES

Electrolyte Abnormalities
  a. Hypocalcemia (<7.0 mg/100 ml)
  b. Hypomagnesemia
  c. Hypo or Hypernatremia

Metabolic Disturbances
  a. Hypoglycemia (<30 mg/100 ml in full term)
  b. Aminoacid abnormalities
  c. Pyridoxine dependency
  d. Urea-cycle abnormalities

Anoxia and Intracranial Hemorrhage
  a. Subarachnoid
  b. Intracerebral
  c. Intraventricular
  d. Subdural

Infections of the CNS
  a. Congenital
  b. Bacterial
  c. Viral

Congenital Malformations (e.g., porencephaly, polymicrogyria)

Drug Withdrawal (e.g., maternal heroin addiction)

Degeneration Diseases (e.g., tuberous sclerosis)

Unknown

proximately 3 per cent of children experience a convulsion with significant pyrexia. Fever convulsions may be defined as generalized convulsions associated with a high fever, occurring in a child aged six months to five years, lasting five minutes or less. The diagnosis of febrile convulsion excludes CNS infection and those children with idiopathic epilepsy who may undergo a prolonged convulsion with a mild temperature elevation.

The cause of febrile convulsions is not entirely understood, but there appears to be a direct relationship to the ultimate fever elevation and its rate of climb. Approximately 50 per cent of children with febrile convulsions have a family history for similar seizures among close relatives suggesting a genetic predisposition (single dominant gene with incomplete penetrance). Febrile convulsions are most frequently associated with viral illnesses such as roseola and upper respiratory tract infections. The recurrence rate approximates 40 per cent.

The immediate management of a febrile convulsion is straightforward. If the child is convulsing, an appropriate antiepileptic drug is given parenterally. Antipyretics are administered to lessen the fever. Examination of the cerebrospinal fluid is mandatory in the infant less than 18 months old as well as the older child with suspected meningeal signs or when a cause for the fever is not forthcoming. The EEG is normal except for several days immediately following the seizure when non-specific transient abnormalities are present, representing the postictal stage.

Considerable controversy continues over the most appropriate long-term therapy. The major question is the ultimate effect of repetitive convulsions on the developing nervous system. At the present time, the introduction of prophylactic phenobarbital (5 mg/kg/day) following the second febrile convulsion appears justifiable. The child should be examined at regular intervals, with the occasional measurement of serum phenobarbital levels to ensure a degree of drug compliance. The anticonvulsant is gradually tapered following the fifth birthday. The likelihood of additional seizures at a later age is not much greater than for an individual who remained seizure free during the first five years of life.

DISORDERS OF LOCOMOTION PECULIAR TO THE CHILD

Abnormalities of the neuromuscular system may result from a host of factors including certain infectious diseases, genetic conditions, trauma and metabolic disorders. The process may be self-limited and reversible or progressive and ultimately fatal. The following examples of neuromuscular diseases are provided to illustrate the variable modes of presentation, particularly in relation to the age of the child.

Werdnig-Hoffmann Disease (Spinal Muscular Atrophy)

Werdnig-Hoffmann disease is a progressive degenerative disorder of the anterior horn cells that usually results in death within the first year of life. In the majority of instances, neurological signs are evident during the neonatal period. It is not un-common to elicit a history of diminished fetal movements during the third trimester, particularly in infants with a rapidly fatal course.

The child is hypotonic and immobile, with a striking lack of spontaneous motor activity due to generalized weakness. There is a remarkable delay or absence of motor development. The weakness is symmetrical and the deep tendon reflexes are lost, but sensation, sphincter function and intellect are preserved. Any movement that does occur is most evident distally (hands and feet). The respiratory effort is characterized by a "see-saw" or paradoxical pattern secondary to intercostal muscle weakness that increases diaphragmatic ventilatory activity. The muscle mass is markedly diminished. Inspection of the tongue may show atrophy and fasciculations indicating involvement of the hypoglossal nucleus. The diagnosis is substantiated by a neurogenic pattern on electromyography (EMG), and the muscle biopsy shows evidence of neurogenic atrophy. Ascertainment of the correct diagnosis is vital since Werdnig-Hoffmann disease is inherited as an autosomal recessive. To date, prenatal diagnosis is not available.

Acute Cerebellar Ataxia

Acute cerebellar ataxia principally affects children aged one to three. In some instances it appears that the physical findings are the result of direct viral invasion of the brain stem or cerebellum (e.g., Echovirus). In others, an autoimmune mechanism is suggested, as the syndrome may follow a viral exanthem, particularly varicella and measles.

Acute cerebellar ataxia classically begins with a sudden disturbance of locomotion. The child may be so severely affected that walking or sitting becomes impossible. Examination shows truncal ataxia, intention tremor, horizontal nystagmus and abnormal coordination. The speech may be dysarthric. The child does not appear ill, and there is a surprising lack of constitutional signs. The cerebrospinal fluid is normal, although a modest elevation of protein may occur during the recovery phase of the illness.

For the majority of children, complete recovery is accomplished without specific therapy over a two- to three-month period. However, approximately 30 per cent of patients show some evidence of irreversible CNS injury, including tremor, abnormal eye movements and gait disturbances, most of which do not appreciably interfere with a normal existence.

Duchenne Muscular Dystrophy

The muscular dystrophies are inherited diseases characterized by progressive symmetrical weakness and muscle wasting. There are several forms of muscular dystrophy that are discerned by the mode of inheritance, the distribution of initial muscle involvement, the age of onset and the natural course of the disease.

Duchenne dystrophy is the most common and most severe form of dystrophy and is almost exclusively limited to males since it is inherited as an X-linked recessive. The incidence rate is approximately 1 in 20,000 live births, excluding fresh mutations.

The initial concern of the parent may be a delay in the onset of walking, averaging approximately 18 months. The child displays a waddling gait, falls frequently and appears clumsy. Most children experience considerable difficulty in negotiating stairs and are unable to run normally. The progressively abnormal gait is secondary to weakness of the pelvic girdle muscles. Gower's sign (the child "crawls up" his legs using his hands in order to assume an erect position) is usually evident in the early stages of the disease and is the result of pelvic muscle weakness, particularly the gluteal group. Pseudohypertrophy is a common feature and need not be limited to the gastrocnemii (Fig. 25–5). It results primarily from abnormally enlarged muscle fibers. Weakness of the trunk muscles produces an exaggerated lordosis and a protuberant abdomen. A progressive scoliosis develops with the continued muscle wasting and weakness. The patellar deep tendon reflexes are lost early, but the ankle jerks are maintained until the terminal stages.

By the age of 10 years the child becomes non-ambulatory and is confined to a wheelchair. Severe contractures evolve, particularly within the hip flexors. Mental retardation is a common accompaniment occurring

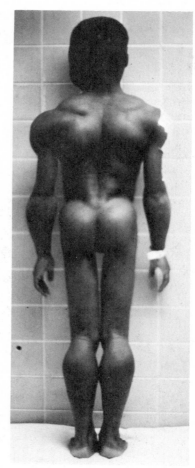

Figure 25–5 Diffuse pseudohypertrophy in an eight-year-old boy with Duchenne muscular dystrophy.

in approximately 50 per cent of patients and does not appear to correlate with the severity of the disease. Hypertrophy of the heart, congestive heart failure and electrocardiographic abnormalities are frequent. Death usually occurs by the third decade owing to susceptibility to pulmonary infections, cardiac arrhythmia and hypercapnic episodes.

The diagnosis of Duchenne dystrophy may be established by the history and clinical findings in conjunction with a markedly elevated serum creatine phosphokinase (CPK) and a myopathic picture on EMG and muscle biopsy. Approximately 60 to 70 per cent of female carriers of the abnormal gene will have an elevated serum CPK. Various techniques have been attempted, with a minimum of success, to enhance the detection of carriers, including physical exercise prior to obtaining serum for CPK determination. Some investigators suggest that the chances of a carrier-state are very unlikely if the CPK levels are normal and the physical examination including muscle testing, EMG and muscle biopsy show no abnormality.

Management consists of physical therapy to retard the development of contractures, the appropriate use of wheelchairs and other assistant devices and comprehensive genetic counseling to the family members. Rigorous physical therapy directed towards "muscle strengthening" is contraindicated.

NEUROCUTANEOUS SYNDROMES

The neurocutaneous syndromes are heritable disorders of unknown etiology. Abnormalities of the integument and central nervous system as well as a propensity to multiorgan embryonal defects are common to each. The student must be familiar with their diagnostic features so that the various associated anomalies and complications may be anticipated and important genetic counseling provided. Although there are at least six well known neurocutaneous syndromes (Table 25–6) only the more common pediatric subtypes will be described.

Neurofibromatosis (Von Recklinghausen's Disease)

Neurofibromatosis is the most prevalent neurocutaneous syndrome, occurring with a frequency of approximately 1 in 3,000 live births. The clinical parameters include characteristic lesions of the integument and tumors of the central and peripheral nervous system, as well as abnormalities of many unrelated structures, particularly the skeleton. Mental retardation is present in a small number of patients.

Café au lait spots are the most conspicuous cutaneous finding in the affected child (Fig. 25–6). They may be present at birth, but typically increase in size and number with time. The café au lait spots are distributed primarily on the trunk. Five or more lesions measuring more than 1.5 cm in diameter strongly suggest the diagnosis of neurofibromatosis. Cutaneous tumors tend to appear as the child matures. Plexiform neurofibromata may be associated with hypertrophy of a body part such as an extremity.

Tumors of neural origin occur with some frequency in patients with neurofibromatosis. A glioma of the optic nerve is the most common intracranial neoplasm. The child may present with progressive visual loss and exophthalmos if the lesion is situated within the orbit, and hypothalamic signs (diabetes insipidus, aberrations of growth) when the tumor extends posteriorly. Rarely, bilateral acoustic neuromas and meningiomas are discovered. Occasionally, intramedullary spinal cord tumors are detected, often associated with syringomyelia. A pheochromocytoma should be suspected in a patient with significant hy-

TABLE 25–6 NEUROCUTANEOUS SYNDROMES

	Cutaneous Lesions	CNS Involvement	Seizures	Mental Retardation	Intra-cranial Calcification	Pattern of Inheritance
Neurofibromatosis	Café au lait spots Axillary freckling	Optic nerve glioma Acoustic neuroma Meningioma Spinal cord tumor	Rare	Occasional	No	Autosomal dominant
Tuberous Sclerosis	Depigmented lesions Adenoma sebaceum Shagreen patches Subungual fibromas Café au lait spots	Glial nodules (may cause increased intracranial pressure) Retinal lesions (phacoma)	Common	Common	Common	Autosomal dominant [85% result of a fresh mutation]
Sturge-Weber Syndrome	Facial vascular nevus	Leptomeningeal angiomata	Common	Common	Common	?
Linear Nevus Sebaceous Syndrome	Linear scalp nevus present at birth	Hydrocephalus Several disorders of the eye	Common	Common	No	Not established

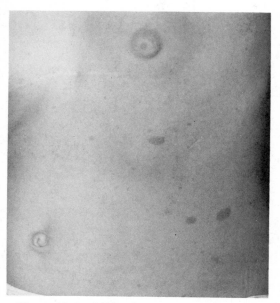

Figure 26–6 Café au lait spots in a preadolescent girl with neurofibromatosis.

pertension. Although seizures tend to occur in patients with neurofibromatosis with a slightly greater frequency than the general population, their presence suggests the possibility of an underlying CNS tumor.

Abnormalities of the skeleton are numerous and include a high incidence of scoliosis due to scalloping of the posterior vertebral bodies or an underlying intraspinal tumor.

Tuberous Sclerosis

Tuberous sclerosis is a multisystem disorder that when originally described was limited to the triad of adenoma sebaceum, convulsions and mental retardation. The clinical features have subsequently been expanded so that lesions may be demonstrated in skin, eye, brain, bone, heart, kidney and occasionally the lung parenchyma. Tuberous sclerosis is a protean syndrome; the ultimate severity is usually determined by the age of onset of the symptoms and signs.

Infantile spasms (hypsarrhythmia) are common early manifestations of tuberous sclerosis in the infant. These children should be carefully examined for depigmented skin lesions, which are most prominent on the trunk. The lesions assume the shape of an "ash" leaf and measure approximately 1.0 cm in diameter. Examination of

the skin with a Wood's lamp may highlight the vitiliginous areas. The prognosis for these patients is poor; many become severely retarded. The convulsions may be difficult to control.

More commonly, the child with tuberous sclerosis presents during the preschool period with a major motor convulsion (either focal or generalized) or because of mental retardation. Inspection of the skin may show several characteristic abnormalities. Adenoma sebaceum are the most typical, but may not appear prior to four years of age. They are red colored papules that cluster at the nasolabial junction (Fig. 25–7). Biopsy demonstrates a benign hamartomatous tumor. Subungal fibromas and café au lait spots are frequently discovered.

Abnormal conglomerates of glial nodules are found within the central nervous system. Approximately 50 per cent of patients over five years of age demonstrate calcification, particularly of the basal ganglia. In addition, abnormalities of the retina are very prominent (Fig. 25–8).

Sturge-Weber Syndrome

The Sturge-Weber syndrome may be suspected at the time of the newborn examina-

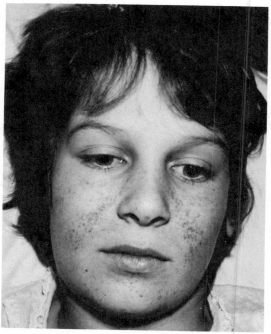

Figure 25–7 Adenoma sebaceum. A 12-year-old girl with tuberous sclerosis.

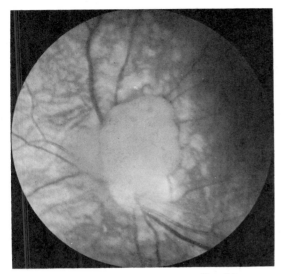

Figure 25-8 A retinal tumor partially obliterating the optic disc in a child with tuberous sclerosis. (Courtesy of Dr. Warren Hindle.)

tion with the finding of a facial portwine vascular nevus (nevus flammeus, cavernous angioma). The nevus usually occurs in the distribution of the trigeminal nerve (most commonly the ophthalmic division) and is usually unilateral (Fig. 25–9). The angiomatous process may also involve the mucous membranes of the oral cavity and the choroid membrane of the eye. In the latter situation, glaucoma and buphthalmos are frequent complications.

Most patients develop intracranial calcifications by the time of adulthood. They are seldom present in the newborn period. Intracerebral calcifications assume a typical radiographic appearance and location (Fig. 25–10). Neuropathological findings include leptomeningeal angiomata, which result in anoxic and degenerative changes in the underlying cerebral cortex. Calcification of the affected cerebral tissue is the end result.

Seizures become evident in the majority of patients within the first two years of life. The seizures are often difficult to control with anticonvulsants. On occasion, if the convulsions are focal and unresponsive to medical management, a hemispherectomy is indicated. Approximately one third of affected children manifest a progressive hemiparesis, contralateral to the intracerebral calcifications, during the course of the disease, possibly the result of the localized cerebral degeneration. Although not initially apparent, mental retardation is prominent in the majority of patients.

INCREASED INTRACRANIAL PRESSURE

The early signs of increased intracranial pressure in an infant or child are often subtle. Increased intracranial pressure assumes many patterns determined by the age of the child and the pathophysiological abnormality. The infant with significant increased intracranial pressure invariably demonstrates a persistent, tense, bulging anterior fontanel, whereas the fontanel in a normal child who is not crying is slightly depressed and pulsatile. Symptoms of raised intracranial pressure in the older child include nausea, vomiting, irritability, fatigue, headache, behavioral changes and diplopia. Headache tends to occur during the early morning hours or shortly after arising and may be associated with vomiting. Headache is poorly localized by most young children, but tends to be a diffuse, generalized throbbing pain that is more prominent frontally or over the occipital region of the skull. The headache is often enhanced by activity that normally raises the intracranial pressure such as coughing, sneezing or straining during a bowel move-

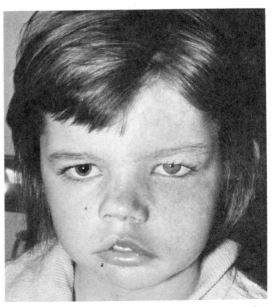

Figure 25-9 The facial nevus of Sturge-Weber syndrome. The left pupil is constricted with pilocarpine.

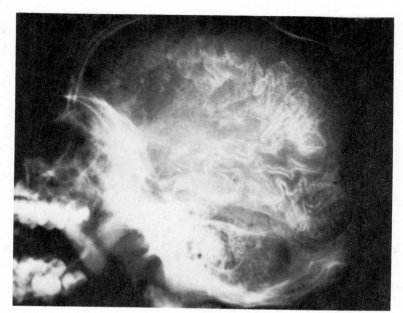

Figure 25–10 A lateral skull radiograph showing the characteristic unilateral double-lined or "railroad-track" cerebral calcification in a patient with the Sturge-Weber syndrome.

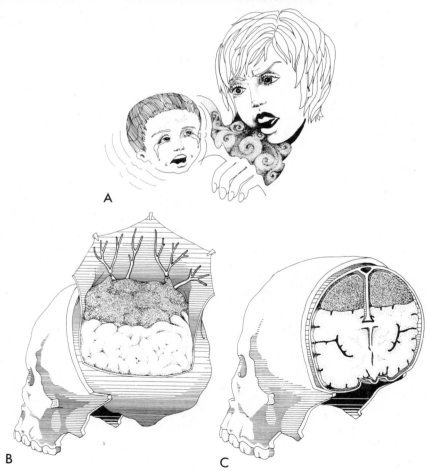

A

B   C

Figure 25–11   Subdural hematoma. *A*, The physically abused child is at greater risk. *B*, Trauma results in rupture of bridging cortical veins. *C*, Venous blood aggregates in the subdural space (often bilaterally) causing an increase in intracranial pressure. (*From* Haslam, R. H. A., and Valletutti, P. J.: *Medical Problems in the Classroom.* Baltimore, University Park Press, 1975.)

ment. Papilledema is the most reliable sign of increased intracranial pressure beyond infancy.

Investigation must include a thorough history and physical and neurological examinations, mindful of the multiple causes of increased intracranial pressure. The following conditions are presented in a condensed fashion in order to introduce the student to the common causes of elevated intracranial pressure during childhood.

Subdural and Epidural Hematoma

A subdural hematoma is the consequence of a rupture of bridging cortical veins that traverse the subdural space (Fig. 25–11). Acute subdural hematomas result from severe trauma and are associated with significant mortality. Although any form of head trauma may produce subacute or chronic subdural collections of blood prod-

ucts, the physically abused child is particularly susceptible to this type of head injury. Clinical findings include convulsions, vomiting, changing levels of consciousness, an enlarging head, bulging fontanel or papilledema, retinal hemorrhages and fractures of long bones. Skull fractures are relatively uncommon. Transillumination of the head is positive when the fluid collections are long-standing, but is of little use in the acute situation because of the viscosity of fresh blood. Cerebral arteriography is the most precise diagnostic procedure for the detection and localization of subdural collections.

An epidural hematoma results from traumatic disruption of the middle meningeal artery, usually by a fracture of the overlying bone (Fig. 25–12). The child may initially respond quite normally and be considered fit except for nausea, vomiting and perhaps a headache. Rather suddenly, progressive neurological signs supervene in-

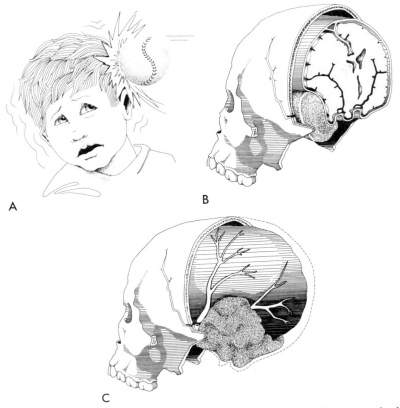

Figure 25–12 Epidural hematoma. *A,* The most common cause is a forceful injury to the lateral part of the skull. *B,* The trauma may result in a fracture, causing disruption of the middle meningeal artery and arterial bleeding within the epidural space. *C,* The arterial bleeding results in a rapidly expanding mass lesion, which may cause compression of the brain stem. (*From* Haslam, R. H. A., and Valletutti, P. J.: *Medical Problems in the Classroom.* Baltimore, University Park Press, 1975.)

cluding a diminishing level of consciousness, a dilated pupil (oculomotor nerve paresis) and contralateral hemiparesis. The prognosis is very favorable if the correct diagnosis is made and surgical therapy is implemented immediately. If treatment is significantly delayed, the child may expire, or as a consequence, significant neurological deficits will result.

Hydrocephalus

Hydrocephalus is, with rare exception, associated with increased intracranial pressure. Although hydrocephalus is usually immediately evident in the infant, its presence can be deceptive in the older age group. A more detailed description is included within the section on Congenital Malformations of the Central Nervous System.

Brain Tumors

It is not within the scope of this chapter to outline the various childhood brain tumors, but rather to briefly describe those tumors characterized by increased intracranial pressure. CNS tumors are among the most common of all childhood malignancies. The majority of brain neoplasms in this age group are situated within the posterior fossa (70 per cent), whereas in the

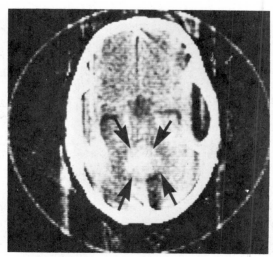

Figure 25–14 A CAT scan with infusion of contrast material showing a medulloblastoma (arrows) in an eight-year-old patient.

adult most tumors are located supratentorially.

Posterior fossa tumors characteristically produce elevated intracranial pressure owing to their encroachment on the fourth ventricle and aqueduct, thereby producing obstructive hydrocephalus. Specific neurological signs may not be evident even when papilledema exists.

Three tumors comprise the majority of posterior fossa tumors of childhood: cerebellar astrocytoma, medulloblastoma and ependymoma. Cerebellar astrocytomas are slow-growing, often cystic tumors located within a cerebellar hemisphere or in the region of the vermis (Fig. 25–13). Neurological signs including ipsilateral dysmetria, head tilt, irregular speech and unsteady gait are common when the tumor is confined to a cerebellar hemisphere. If the lesion is midline, neurological findings may be minimal or absent. Surgical removal of a cerebellar astrocytoma is associated with an excellent prognosis. The medulloblastoma is a midline, solid, invasive tumor that probably originates from embryonal cell rests in the posterior medullary velum. These tumors show a propensity to metastasize to the spinal cord and vertebral bodies. Complete surgical removal is unusual, and chemotherapy is ineffective, so treatment consists of radiation to the cranial-spinal axis. The five-year survival rate approaches 70 per cent in some series (Fig. 25–14). Ependymomas are slow-growing tumors that stem from the floor of the

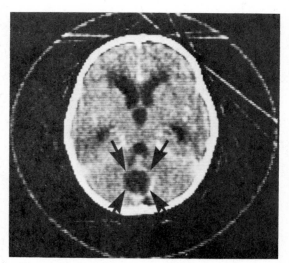

Figure 25–13 A CAT scan showing a midline cystic cerebellar astrocytoma (arrows) in a relatively asymptomatic two-year-old. Note the ventricular dilation.

fourth ventricle. Their growth eventually obstructs the egress of cerebrospinal fluid from the ventricular system so that hydrocephalus results. Treatment consists primarily of radiotherapy, and the long-term results are similar to those for medulloblastoma.

Cerebral Abscess

Cerebral abscesses are difficult to diagnose because of their subtle evolution and insidious course. Discovery of an abscess may be significantly delayed because of the paucity of clinical signs and the often imprudent practice of antibiotic usage for the treatment of fever of unknown origin. Cerebral abscess occurs in all age groups but is most prevalent during the preadolescent years.

The majority of brain abscesses are located supratentorially in one of the cerebral hemispheres (particularly the frontal lobe). Most abscesses lie in close proximity to the distribution of the middle cerebral artery and appear to originate at the junction of the white and gray matter, where the blood flow and perfusion are reduced relative to other areas within the cerebral hemispheres. Cerebellar abscesses usually represent complications of chronic mastoiditis or otitis by direct extension through the dura. The most common organisms are aerobic bacteria (*Staphylococcus aureus, Streptococcus viridans* and gram negative rods). The mortality rate remains alarmingly high (25 to 50 per cent), as death results either from rupture of an abscess cavity into the ventricular system or from the consequences of the mass lesion.

All children with known congenital heart disease, particularly if a right to left shunt exists, should be examined thoroughly if the symptoms and signs noted here are un-

covered. Skull radiograph may show separation of the sutures or, in the older child, erosion of the dorsum sellae and the EEG a focal area of slowing corresponding to the underlying area of cerebritis. The brain scan is diagnostic when a circumscribed doughnut-shaped lesion is discovered. If precise localization is necessary or the diagnosis uncertain, cerebral arteriography and CAT scanning should be undertaken. A lumbar puncture is contraindicated if there is a high degree of suspicion that a cerebral abscess is present.

Management of cerebral abscess involves surgical drainage of the cavity and the parenteral use of the appropriate antibiotic for an *absolute* minimum of four weeks. It is evident that the location and extent of the abscess cavity as well as its pretreatment duration play an important role in the eventual neurological outcome. Complications include seizures, mental retardation, hemiparesis, aphasia, visual defects and hydrocephalus.

Meningitis and Encephalitis

Significant cerebral edema may develop during the acute phase of meningoencephalitis, probably the result of disturbed cerebrospinal absorption. Complications of bacterial meningitis including subdural effusion and hydrocephalus may produce a slowly progressive elevation in intracranial pressure.

Pseudotumor Cerebri (Benign Intracranial Hypertension)

Pseudotumor cerebri is a clinical syndrome with many causes, characterized by increased intracranial pressure. The ventricular size and position is normal and the

Etiologies	Symptoms	Signs
Hematogenous	Headache	Focal neurological signs
Congenital heart disease	Fever	Papilledema
Chronic lung disease	Nausea, vomiting	Nuchal rigidity
Septicemia	Weight loss	Ataxia, dysmetria
Sinusitis, mastoiditis	Lethargy and obtundation	Impending herniation (irregular respiration)
Trauma, penetrating injury	Convulsions	
Unknown		

cerebrospinal fluid unaltered, except for the elevated pressure.

Symptoms	Signs
Headache	Bulging fontanel in infant
Vomiting	Papilledema
Diplopia	Abducens nerve paralysis
Visual blurring	
Absence of constitutional symptoms	Occasional inferior nasal field defects

As noted, the causes are multiple and include metabolic disorders (galactosemia, hypo- or pseudohypoparathyroidism, vitamin A deficiency, hypervitaminosis A, Addison's disease, hypophosphatasia, obesity, menarche, pregnancy and oral contraceptives); infections (roseola infantum, Guillain-Barré syndrome); hematological disorders (severe anemia, polycythemia); drugs (nalidixic acid and tetracyclines, sudden withdrawal of long-term corticosteroids); obstruction by thrombosis of intracranial venous channels (lateral sinus, posterior sagittal sinus); and a significant number in which a causative factor is not established.

A clear understanding of the pathogenesis of pseudotumor cerebri is unavailable because of the lack of pathological material and the incomplete understanding of cerebrospinal fluid mechanics and physiology.

It is quite probable that many factors operate simultaneously (Fig. 25–15). One possible cause is an alteration in absorption or increased production of CSF. In many patients increased CSF volume with a decreased protein content suggests a dilutional effect. Demonstration of small ventricles by neuroradiological techniques raises the possibility of cerebral edema as a cause of the increased pressure. Changes in the intracranial vessels may result from disturbances of vasomotor control, and obstruction of the venous sinuses by infection or trauma may lead to an elevation of the intracranial pressure. Diagnosis of pseudotumor cerebri is established by excluding all known causes of intracranial hypertension discussed here.

The prime goal of management is directed at the discovery of the underlying cause of the increased intracranial pressure. For the most part pseudotumor cerebri is a self-limited condition, but optic atrophy and blindness may complicate prolonged increased pressure. It is imperative, therefore, that frequent visual acuity determinations be recorded. Several appropriately timed lumbar punctures to decrease the pressure may be the only form of therapy required. Osmolar agents (urea, mannitol) are not practical for prolonged use because of their "rebound phenome-

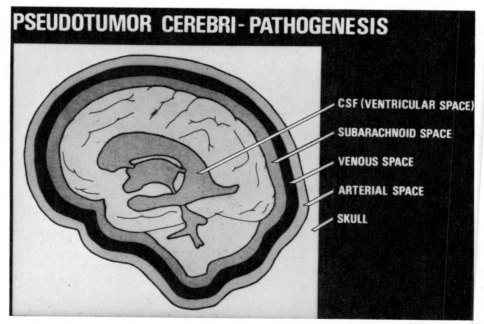

Figure 25–15 The brain and its interrelated compartments are tightly confined by the skull. The enlargement of any intracranial component (brain, subarachnoid, venous or arterial space) may produce increased pressure.

non." Corticosteroids may be beneficial. Dexamethasone is the most commonly used steroid for the management of acute cerebral edema. The recommended dose is 0.25 to 0.5 mg/kg/day parenterally in four divided doses. Later, if indicated, it may be given orally for long-term management. The prognosis for full recovery is excellent.

Lead Poisoning

Cerebral edema and increased intracranial pressure may complicate lead poisoning in children. Early stages of lead intoxication are difficult to recognize because of the vagueness of symptoms, which include abdominal pain, nausea and vomiting, constipation, failure to grow and irritability. The onset of cerebral involvement is often abrupt, with lethargy, convulsions, coma and signs of increased intracranial pressure including papilledema. In spite of aggressive management, the morbidity and mortality rates following lead encephalopathy are extremely significant. Continued efforts must be directed toward the preventative aspects and early detection of this dreaded condition.

REFERENCES

Bell, W. E., and McCormick, W. F.: *Increased Intracranial Pressure in Children*. Philadelphia, W. B. Saunders Co., 1972.

Chao, D. H.: Congenital neurocutaneous syndromes in childhood. J. Pediatr., 55:189, 447, 635, 1959.

Crothers, B., and Paine, R. S.: *The Natural History of Cerebral Palsy*. Cambridge, Mass., Harvard University Press, 1959.

Ford, F. R.: *Diseases of the Nervous System in Infancy, Childhood and Adolescence*, 6th ed. Springfield, Ill., Charles C Thomas, 1973.

Livingston, S.: *Comprehensive Management of Epilepsy in Infancy, Childhood and Adolescence*. Springfield, Ill., Charles C Thomas, 1972.

Menkes, J. H.: *Textbook of Child Neurology*. Philadelphia, Lea and Febiger, 1974.

Merlis, J. K.: Proposal for an international classification of the epilepsies. Epilepsia, *11*:114, 1970.

Warkany, J.: *Congenital Malformations*. Chicago, Year Book Medical Publishers, 1971.

26

Mental Deficiency*

David W. Smith

Given the complexity of brain development, it is not surprising that about 3 per cent of individuals have deficiencies in mental capabilities with intelligence quotients below 75. Table 26–1 shows a rough breakdown of mental deficiency in terms of IQ values. It is often difficult to be secure about the delineation of mental deficiency in early infancy. Mild degrees of slowness in major motor progress do *not* correlate well with future intelligence quotients. However, gross degrees of lag in developmental performance *do* correlate with a lower IQ in the future. It is often possible to imply mental deficiency in early infancy by recognizing the infant's total disorder. This is true for Down syndrome and for a host of other disorders in which mental deficiency is but one part of a pattern of malformation. The advantage of such early recognition is that family adaptation and special training for the infant can begin early, as delineated in Chapter 27.

Mental deficiency most commonly implies a problem in function of the central nervous system. The lower IQ is but one sign of the problem in brain function. Behavioral functioning is also determined by the central nervous system, and behavior is frequently affected. Some behavioral components likely to be found in the more severely mentally deficient children include perseveration with a lack of change in responsiveness, dependency on routine, stimulus-bound and therefore easily distractable, fear, lack of spontaneity, and diminished ability to maintain a chain of thought, and, therefore, poor judgment. Such children are liable to manifest repetitive physical activities that are disturbing to other people, such as oral preoccupation, rocking, head banging, hyperactivity and temper tantrums. Neurological functioning is also frequently altered, as evidenced by such signs as hypertonicity, hypotonicity, ataxia, altered reflexes, poor coordination and a variety of minor and major motor types of seizures. Furthermore, aberrant development or function of the brain may result in secondary physical signs and symptoms, some of which will be discussed in the next section.

APPROACH TO PROBLEMS IN WHICH MENTAL DEFICIENCY IS A FEATURE

Mental deficiency is but a sign, never a total diagnosis. It is well to strive for a total diagnosis since this will usually provide the best answers in terms of the natural history, management, etiology and recurrence risk for the particular disorder. Though the primary diagnosis is often unknown, there are several hundred recognized disorders in which mental deficiency is but one feature. The following section provides a clin-

TABLE 26–1 CATEGORIES OF MENTAL DEFICIENCY BY IQ

IQ	Category
50–75	Mild mental deficiency, "educable"
35–50	Moderate mental deficiency, "trainable," self-care
less than 35	Severe mental deficiency, seldom trainable
less than 20	Profound mental deficiency, dependent on others for care

*The more commonly used term is mental retardation. The experience of the author indicates that mental deficiency is the more realistic terminology.

258

ical approach toward the diagnosis and classification of such disorders. The approach begins with an appropriate history and physical evaluation, some features of which are emphasized here.

History and Physical Evaluation°

Family (genetic) history: This is of increasing importance, both for diagnosis and counseling. It is estimated that about half of seriously mentally deficient patients have genetically determined disorders.

Pedigree: Search specifically for a problem similar to that of the patient in first-degree relatives (siblings and parents) and second-degree relatives (aunts, uncles and grandparents). For autosomal dominant and X-linked disorders and for chromosomal translocation disorders, the pedigree should be more extensive. Miscarriages and still-births should be noted and consanguinity excluded.

Parental Ages at Birth of Patient: Older maternal age is a factor in chromosomal trisomy syndromes, and older paternal age is a factor in certain fresh mutant gene disorders such as the Apert syndrome and acrodysostosis.

Parental Levels of Intelligence and Head Circumference: This information is especially important for instances of mild mental deficiency or mild microcephaly, which may be familial.

Cultural-social history: Low socioeconomic status may play a role in mild degrees of mental deficiency. It may also be a factor in the occurrence of prematurity, prenatal cytomegalovirus infection, maternal alcoholism and environmental and emotional deprivation, each of which may be associated with mental deficiency in the offspring.

Prenatal history:
Fetal activity should be noted, both in terms of time of onset and vigor.
Gestational problems, such as early threatened miscarriage, severe toxemia, diabetes mellitus with ketoacidosis, chronic alcoholism or rubella exposure or disease

during the first four months, may be relevant.
Duration of gestation is pertinent.
Perinatal history:
Birth presentation is noteworthy, since problems of morphogenesis and neurological function are more common in fetuses who fail to assume the vertex position.
The amount and character of amniotic fluid is of interest. Polyhydramnios may occur with neurological deficits resulting in impaired swallowing, and meconium-stained fluid may be evidence of perinatal distress.
Head circumference and body length and weight at birth are important. Fetal growth deficiency represents a congenital anomaly of overall size and is not uncommonly accompanied by other problems in morphogenesis, including that of the brain.
Note the Apgar scores and early function in terms of crying and sucking.
Perinatal problems such as placenta previa, traumatic delivery, prolonged hypoxia, apneic spells, seizures, hyperbilirubinemia, symptomatic hypoglycemia or sepsis should be recorded.
Postnatal history:
Describe developmental progress and central nervous system (CNS) function, including presence or absence of behavior problems, seizures and neurological aberrations, and the patient's age at onset of slow or deteriorating developmental progress.
Postnatal events that might have been a cause of the developmental lag should be recorded.
General growth rate, changes in physical features and illnesses also merit inquiry.
Examination: Length and weight as related to normal standards should be noted. The remaining examination should be divided into the indirect evaluation of brain and brain function and the non-CNS evaluation.
Indirect assessment of brain and brain function: Measure head circumference and relate it to normal standards. Transilluminate, note shape of cranium and evaluate scalp hair patterning. Recent studies have implied that scalp hair directional patterning is determined at 10 to 16 weeks of fetal life by the growth and shape of the underlying brain; hence, aberrant scalp hair patterning may be used as a clue toward an early fetal problem in brain morphogenesis. Examine the ocular fundus following

---

°Part of this section is taken from Smith and Simons. See References.

dilation of the pupils, as this is the one area in which neural tissue can be directly viewed. Assess CNS function and record developmental age, neurological status and behavioral patterns.

Complete non-CNS examination for major and minor anomalies: Scrutinize the entire body carefully for anomalies, including sensory deficiencies. For any given minor anomaly, including unusual dermatoglyphic findings, determine whether it is a usual feature in otherwise normal family members before ascribing importance to the anomaly. For any major anomaly, an effort should be made to interpret whether it was of prenatal onset or not. Finally, when there is a pattern of altered morphogenesis in the patient, an attempt should be made to determine whether the non-CNS anomalies are *secondary* to a primary brain defect, or whether they represent multiple primary defects of morphogenesis. Hand and foot positional deformities and scoliosis, for example, may be secondary to neurological deficits. Prominent lateral palatine ridges in the infant may be a sign of long-term tongue thrust into the hard palate, secondary to neurological deficiencies.

Clinical Sub-Categorization of Mental Deficiency

A majority of children with milder degrees of mental deficiency, with IQs in the range of 50 to 75, come from mentally dull or socioeconomically deprived parentage, related to polygenic and environmental factors. This group also contains some XXY boys, an occasional XXX girl, some children with malformation syndromes and some patients with inborn errors of metabolism, milder defects of central nervous system (CNS) development or residual CNS insults. Among the more severely mentally deficient patients, with IQs below 50, the clinician is more likely to arrive at a precise overall diagnosis. Though the following categorical breakdown of mental deficiency is especially relevant for patients with moderate to severe mental deficiency, it is applicable to all degrees of mental deficiency.

This general subcategorization of mental deficiency is designed to be of clinical value in the rational diagnostic evaluation

of a given patient with mental deficiency. It is based on findings derived from an appropriate family history, prenatal and birth history, postnatal history and physical examination that includes a cautious search for associated major and minor malformations. It is the authors' contention that there is no single laboratory study indicated for all patients with evidence of mental deficiency. Rather, further diagnostic evaluation should be individualized in accordance with the findings from the history and physical examination. This subcategorization is predominantly based on the apparent *age of onset* of the problem.

Category I: prenatal problem in morphogenesis of the brain. This group is the largest, making up 44 per cent of 1224 seriously mentally deficient patients evaluated by Kaveggia, Durkin, Pendleton and Opitz, and 53 per cent of a less severely mentally deficient group reported by Smith and Simons. About one third of this subcategory of patients was considered to have a single primary defect in brain morphogenesis such as primary microcephaly, hydrocephalus, hydranencephaly, a defect of neural tube closure or other types of cerebral dysmorphogenesis. The other two thirds had multiple major or minor malformations of non-CNS structures, and by inference, the mental deficiency was also considered the consequence of a defect in morphogenesis of the brain. This discrimination is often dependent on a cautious total physical examination to detect minor as well as major anomalies. For example, Smith and Bostian evaluated 50 consecutive patients with idiopathic mental deficiency and found that 42 per cent of them had three or more extra-CNS major or minor anomalies of prenatal onset, versus none with three or more associated anomalies in 100 concomitantly examined control children without mental deficiency. Within Kaveggia's multiple defect subcategory, 41 per cent of patients had a chromosomal abnormality, mostly Down syndrome; 18 per cent had known syndromes of non-chromosomal etiology; and 41 per cent had unknown patterns of malformation.

Category II: perinatal insult to brain. This group includes kernicterus due to indirect hyperbilirubinemia, severe neonatal hypoglycemia, intracerebral hemorrhage; perinatal hypoxia and meningitis and sepsis—all more common in the premature infant. Caution should be exercised before assuming that problems of birth and perinatal adaptation are the *primary* cause of mental deficiency in patients who have evidence of prenatal onset of a problem in morphogenesis. Such patients, especially those who have a severe defect of early brain development and those with prenatal onset of growth deficiency, are more likely to have problems in neonatal adaptation.

Category III: postnatal onset of problem in brain function. These patients generally appear normal as newborns. After a variable period of time, during which they have normal appearance and function, there is a slowing or deterioration in developmental progress and performance. This group includes patients who have experienced environmental insults such as trauma, meningitis, encephalitis, hypernatremia, water intoxication, severe hypoglycemia, severe hypoxemia and lead encephalopathy, plus those with certain enzymatic defects of amino acid, carbohydrate, uric acid, mucopolysaccharide and brain lipid metabolism. Though some of these latter inborn errors of metabolism may have a prenatal onset, only a few such as the Leroy I-Cell syndrome or generalized gangliosidosis have gross clinical manifestations by the time of birth. Thus the *clinical* implication is usually that of a postnatal onset of the problem. Kaveggia, *et al.* found that 4.3 per cent of the 1224 seriously mentally deficient patients had established inborn errors of metabolism, of which one third had phenylketonuria.

One of the most common disorders in this category is X-linked recessive mental deficiency, which is at least partially responsible for the excess of males with mental deficiency. These individuals most commonly have IQs in the 30 to 50 range and are characterized by *not* having any physical abnormalities and being pleasant socially. Thus they often stand out among the more serious mental deficiency patients because they look normal.

Category IV: undecided age of onset of the problem in brain function. These patients show no obvious evidence of a prenatal problem in morphogenesis, have no established history of a gross insult to the brain in the perinatal period and have been consistently slow in postnatal developmental progress, without evident cause. They may or may not have other evidence of CNS dysfunction such as spasticity, hypotonia, seizures and aberrant behavior. This is the second largest group, making up 41 per cent of the series studied by Kaveggia, *et al.*

DISORDERS THAT MAY PRESENT CLINICALLY IN SEVERAL OF THE FOREGOING CATEGORIES

Prenatal infectious disease. The patient with mental deficiency as a consequence of prenatally acquired infectious disease, such as rubella, cytomegalic inclusion disease or toxoplasmosis, may have obvious historical and physical indications of prenatal onset of the disorder, may have had serious problems in perinatal adaptation or may have had no obvious problems until a later age. Thus clinical presentation may be in any one of the categories noted.

Congenital hypothyroidism. Early detection of congenital hypothyroidism, with thyroid hormone replacement, is critical in preventing, or at least limiting, the adverse effects of hypothyroidism on early brain development. Signs of prenatal onset of osseous immaturity, such as unusually large fontanels and facial immaturity, are usually present at birth, and perinatal problems not uncommonly include persisting indirect bilirubinemia, lethargy and poor feeding. Unfortunately, congenital hypothyroidism is seldom detected on the basis of these early signs and symptoms. Most commonly, it is not suspected until postnatal onset of slow growth, sluggish activity, myxedematous fullness of tissues and lag of developmental progression become evident. Patients with partial degrees of congenital hypothyroidism may not show signs of myxedema and may have very subtle postnatal onset of slowness in growth, maturation and developmental progress with borderline sluggishness in activity. Thus the clinician could interpret the patient as belonging in any of the above categories, although they obviously belong in Category I (prenatal onset).

Diagnostic Studies in Patients with Mental Deficiency: Their Rational Usage

Studies that may resolve the diagnosis:

Chromosomal and X-chromatin studies: Indications for chromosome studies are largely limited to appropriate patients in Category I who have multiple malformations. Buccal smear for X-chromatin is merited for patients in Category IV (undecided) when the clinical findings do not *exclude* the possibility of XXY or XXX syndromes. Should the findings be suggestive of XYY syndrome, a chromosome study or Y-chromatin study is merited.

Studies for inborn errors of metabolism: Patients with mental deficiency due to an inborn error of metabolic function, most commonly the consequence of a recessively inherited enzyme defect, often have one or more additional clues besides mental deficiency alone. Some of these are set forth in Table 26–2. These patients usually fit into Category III. They appear normal at birth, and at variable postnatal ages develop diffuse non-lateralizing evidence of central nervous system deficit or deterioration of function. A history of intermittent lapses of consciousness, inanition, unexplained hypoglycemia or recurrent acidosis should each be potential clues to an inborn error of metabolism. For example, acidosis may be a feature of lactic acidemia, and intermittent loss of consciousness may occur in the severe form of maple syrup urine disease or in hyperammonemia.

Phenylpyruvic oligophrenia may be difficult to suspect from the clinical findings. When it cannot be excluded as a possibility by the overall features, a urine ferric chloride test or a serum phenylalanine determination should be done.

Studies for prenatal infectious disease: Patients with mental deficiency as the result of congenital rubella, cytomegalic inclusion or toxoplasmosis disease usually also have one or more of the following features: microcephaly, chorioretinitis, prenatal onset growth deficiency, hepatosplenomegaly, neonatal petechiae and jaundice or deafness. Patients with congenital rubella may also have cataract, cardiac defect and other anomalies. Mentally deficient patients who have one or more of these additional findings and whose total findings do not *exclude* the possibility of the disorder being due to prenatal infectious disease should be considered for one or more of the following studies: direct culture of the infectious agent (in early infancy), specific

TABLE 26–2   EXAMPLES OF FEATURES IN ADDITION TO MENTAL DEFICIENCY WHICH OFTEN OCCUR POSTNATALLY IN CERTAIN INBORN ERRORS OF METABOLISM

Disorder	Features
Phenylketonuria, classical Autosomal recessive	Light pigmentation, eczema (1/3), poor coordination, seizures (1/4), autistic behavior
Sanfilippo syndrome (MPS III) Autosomal recessive	Developmental lag after 1 year with deterioration toward restless behavior, clumsiness by age 6–7 years; development of coarse facies and hair by 2–3 years; gum hypertrophy, mild limitation in finger extension
Hurler syndrome (MPS I) Autosomal recessive	Developmental lag after 6–10 months with deterioration and growth deficiency, coarse facies, stiff joints, gibbus, hepatosplenomegaly, cloudy corneas, rhinitis
Hunter syndrome (MPS II) severe type X-linked recessive	Developmental lag after 6–12 months with growth deficiency, coarse facies, stiff joints, hepatosplenomegaly; no gibbus or cloudy corneas
Galactosemia, severe type Autosomal recessive	Development in early infancy (on cow's milk feeds) of lethargy, hypotonia, hepatomegaly, icterus, hypoglycemia, cataract, with failure to thrive
Lesch-Nyhan syndrome X-linked recessive	Development after 6–8 months of spasticity, choreoathetosis, self-mutation, autistic behavior, growth deficiency; tophi in late childhood
Homocystinuria Autosomal recessive	Mild arachnodactyly, pectus, genu valgus, pes cavus, mild limitation of finger extension. Downward lens dislocation, usually by age 10 years; wide facial pores, malar flush; thrombotic phenomena, contributing to CNS problems
Argininosuccinicaciduria Autosomal recessive	Onset in first 1–2 years of growth deficiency, mild hepatomegaly, skin lesions, dry brittle hair with trichorrexis nodosa, seizures

fluorescent IgM antibody determination and complement-fixation antibody determination.

Thyroid studies: A protein-bound iodine or serum thyroxine determination is merited for the mentally deficient patient who shows evidence of osseous immaturity, slow postnatal growth, sluggish physical activity and myxedematous fullness in the tissues. Thyroid studies are *not* indicated in the patient with mental deficiency and short stature who does not show any other clinical indication of being hypothyroid.

Ancillary studies that may assist in the diagnosis

EMI scanning or pneumoencephalography may occasionally be indicated in a Category I patient with a primary defect in brain morphogenesis in an effort to better delineate the nature and extent of the brain malformation. This may be of particular relevance for hydrocephalus. For other defects the study may provide a better perspective for prognosis as well as genetic counseling.

Skull roentgenograms merit consideration in a patient with clinical signs of craniosynostosis, evidence of increased intracranial pressure, cutaneous signs of tuberous sclerosis or Sturge-Weber syndrome or evidence of prenatal infectious disease, especially toxoplasmosis. Otherwise, there is seldom any clinically relevant information to be derived from this study.

Long bone roentgenograms may be indicated by clinical findings such as skeletal abnormalities. Bone age determination may be indicated in patients with decelerating growth, especially those in whom the overall findings are compatible with hypothyroidism and in patients with excessive rate of growth, but is of little practical value in patients with prenatal onset of growth deficiency.

Electroencephalograms may be warranted in patients with a history of seizures or suspected seizure–equivalent.

Fasting blood glucose merits consideration in patients with histories suggestive of hypoglycemic signs and symptoms, but is not necessarily indicated for all patients with seizures.

Other serum chemistries, blood studies and urinalyses should be performed only as prompted by findings other than mental deficiency in history or examination.

ADAPTATION IN THE FAMILY AND SOCIETY

It is difficult to inform parents about mental deficiency in their child. Ideally, both parents should be present, and the counselor should have adequate time to discuss the entire situation with them. Throughout the discussion the child should be discussed as a human being who has capabilities and potential, but whose potential will be less than the parents would usually be expecting. Any special needs should be emphasized, such as special training and education, which are discussed in the next chapter. When a diagnosis has been made, such as Down syndrome, the counseling should relate specifically to that disorder, as set forth in Chapter 22. Initial parental response is often one of grief or shock and disbelief. This grief response may at least partially relate to the "loss" of the anticipated normal child. Such grief responses may last for a long time, sometimes months, during which the parents need support. It is often helpful to rediscuss the entire situation for a few days or weeks after the initial presentation, as much may not be remembered or accepted. It takes time before the parents come to accept the mentally deficient child as he or she really is. Without acceptance there is a greater likelihood of overprotection or rejection, and the normal flow of affection and stimulus may be thwarted.

Often the most helpful individuals for the parents are *other parents* of children with a similar problem. It is often quite helpful for the parents to meet with them and to see other children with the same problem. Parents not uncommonly develop a concept of the child that is far worse than the actual situation. They sometimes do not appreciate that a mentally deficient child can be truly loved and loveable, and that the term "special child" is realistic for some families. There are organizations such as the National Association for Mental Retardation that can assist parents in this regard. Basically, the physician should almost always extend his counsel outside his office for the problem of mental deficiency. Because of their special problems in brain function, mentally deficient children generally need specialized training and education in order to achieve their best potential (see Chapter 27).

PREVENTION

Obviously, we would like to prevent as much mental deficiency as possible. Today it *is* possible to prevent a significant proportion of mental deficiency, and the promise for tomorrow is even better.

The majority of mental deficiency caused by PKU is now being prevented by routine testing for homozygotes in newborns who are unable to convert phenylalanine to tyrosine. These individuals are treated with a special diet to prevent a high phenylalanine blood level and its consequences on the developing brain. Routine screening of blood spots is also utilized in a few regions to detect congenital hypothyroidism at birth and begin thyroid replacement therapy soon thereafter. Such babies may also be recognized by signs and symptoms of hypothyroidism during the newborn period, as emphasized by Smith, *et al.* Hopefully, earlier recognition and therapy of hypothyroidism will prevent mental deficiency in this disorder.

The above disorders are relatively rare, about 1 in 7 to 15 thousand noted for each. It is now becoming possible, however, to prevent some of the more common causes of mental deficiency. If amniocentesis can be made sufficiently safe to allow routine evaluation of the early developing fetus, then "nature's way" could be slightly extended to allow for early termination of *all* chromosomal abnormalities and the majority of neural tube defects. The former would be determined by chromosomal studies of fetal amnion cells, and the latter by the presence of alpha fetoprotein in the amniotic fluid. At present, these studies are made in higher risk pregnancies such as older women and women who have had one offspring with a chromosomal abnormality in the former case and regions of high frequency of neural tube defect and families with one affected child in the latter case. Genetic counseling may result in prevention of the less common disorders of high recurrence risk, and occasionally early amniocentesis studies might allow selective termination in such disorders.

Removal of environmental agents that can cause mental deficiency in the offspring of exposed women is especially important. Methyl mercury and lead are chemical examples. Maternal alcoholism can cause serious problems in morphogenesis of the brain in offspring, as can Dilantin or Tridione, two anticonvulsant medications. Warfarin (Coumadin), an anticoagulant medication, also poses a serious threat to the developing brain. Any woman receiving these agents or having chronic ethanol ingestion, should know the risk to a developing fetus. Ideally she should not be using such agents when pregnant and should have the opportunity to terminate an unplanned pregnancy that occurred while she was receiving one of these agents.

Prevention of fetal infectious diseases, most of which adversely affect the development of the brain, is also quite important. Syphilis should be effectively treated prior to pregnancy and actively treated the moment it is recognized in the pregnant woman. Congenital rubella can hopefully be prevented through mass vaccination against rubella. Cytomegalic inclusion disease (CID) of the fetus, derived from the mother, who is rarely recognized as having the disease, is now the most serious recognized viral cause of mental deficiency. The incidence of CID in newborns is as high as 1 per cent in lower socioeconomic populations, and it is estimated that about one fourth to one half of these babies have variable degrees of mental deficiency as a consequence of this viral agent. Hopefully, some means of prevention of CID, such as vaccination, may be developed.

REFERENCES

General

Fischer-Williams, M.: The neurological aspects of mental subnormality. J. Mental Subnormality, *15*:21, 63, 1969.

Holmes, L. B., *et al.*: *Mental Retardation: An Atlas of Diseases with Associated Physical Abnormalities.* New York, The Macmillan Co., 1972.

Smith, D. W., and Simons, F. E. R.: Rational diagnostic evaluation of the child with mental deficiency. Am. J. Dis. Child., *129*:1285, 1975.

Specific

Drillen, C. M., Jameson, S., and Wilkinson, E. M.: Studies in mental handicap. Part I: Prevalence and distribution by clinical type and severity of defect. Arch. Dis. Child., *41*:528, 1966.

Fisher, R. L., Johnstone, W. T., Fisher, W. H., and Goldkamp, O. G.: Arthrogryposis multiplex congenita, a clinical investigation. J. Pediatr., *76*: 255, 1970.

Kaveggia, E. G., Durkin, M. V., Pendleton, E., and Opitz, J. M.: Diagnostic genetic studies on 1,224 patients with severe mental retardation. Proceedings of the Third Congress of the International Association for Scientific Study of Mental Deficiency. Held at The Hague, Holland, September 4–12, 1973.

Smith, D. W., Blizzard, R. M., and Wilkins, L.: The mental prognosis in hypothyroidism in infancy and childhood: A review of 128 cases. Pediatrics, 19:1011, 1957.

Smith, D. W., and Bostian, K. D.: Congenital anomalies associated with idiopathic mental retardation. J. Pediatr., 65:189, 1964.

Smith, D. W., Klein, A. M., Henderson, J. R., and Myrianthopoulos, N. C.: Congenital hypothyroidism—signs and symptoms in the newborn period. J. Pediatr., 87:958, 1975.

27

Educational Intervention for the Mentally Retarded Child

Nancy M. Robinson

The physician plays a pivotal role with many families who have mentally handicapped children. Often he or she is the first to note delays in development, retention of primitive reflexes or the infant's lack of responsiveness to sights around him. It is to the child's physician that parents first voice tentative concerns about their baby, toddler or preschool child or report subtle cues easily missed or discounted. It is, then, the physician who weathers with the parents the pangs of recognition that a serious problem may exist, who shepherds the family through diagnostic studies, if needed and who introduces them to a network of supportive people and services, of whose existence they are likely to be unaware. Even in very small communities today there are usually professionals and other parents of handicapped children who can help families meet their children's special needs while maintaining equilibrium.

As the parents proceed beyond their initial uncertainties, they begin to make a long series of choices about their child's training and care that may extend for the rest of their lives. It is essential that each physician either become personally acquainted with the available local resources or establish effective relationships with knowledgeable professionals who can serve as reliable matchmakers between families and services. Such matches are, however, never settled once and for all.

New bridges have to be crossed as the child grows older and his developmental patterns clarify and mature, as family circumstances shift and as available personnel and programs change. Sometimes battle must be done to guarantee that the legal rights of family and child are respected. The physician who is effective as counselor and advocate may be called on many times in the course of the child's upbringing and education.

Efficacy of Educational Intervention

There is a strong consensus among professionals in many disciplines that intervention for mentally handicapped children should begin as early as possible. It should be carefully designed to meet individual needs and should continue at least into early adulthood, provided that the individual continues to function at a retarded level. This position is now axiomatic, and services are proliferating rapidly to provide such intervention.

Yet, unequivocal empiric evidence in favor of special programming is sparse. Except for children living in extremely deprived circumstances such as understaffed institutions or disintegrated families, or those experiencing deprivation through impairment of hearing or sight, it is a mistake to expect dramatic improvement as a result

266

of the child's participation in special programs. Seldom are "cures" obtained. Little increments, little victories may be important, nevertheless, and many of the most valuable results of special programs lie in the rather nebulous areas of the child's self-image and orientation to learning and the quality of family relationships.

Special Characteristics of Retarded Children as Learners

Aside from their overall developmental delays, what is "different" about retarded children that requires their education and training to diverge from that of other children? This question constitutes a controversial battleground between those who maintain that most retarded children are primarily developmentally immature and those who posit any of a variety of underlying deficits or distortions of the central nervous system. There are, of course, enormous differences among children. Indeed, retarded children are as heterogeneous as any other group of children, aside from their limited intelligence. A few children exhibit identifiable syndromes; some others have sustained demonstrable central nervous system damage; many others show no such signs at all. Even in intellectual competence the children vary widely, with most children showing only mild retardation, which may be much more apparent in schoolwork than anywhere else. Even so, there remain some frequent behavioral characteristics and conditions that seem to demand special intervention when they occur.

Parents seldom know what to expect of slow-learning children day by day, sometimes setting expectations too high, but more often failing to demand enough growth and independence. Mistaking slow learning for hopeless lack of capacity, many parents find it easier to do for the child than to wait out his clumsy efforts. As a result, many retarded children are overprotected and fail to achieve the best of which they are capable.

Second, many retarded children seem not to acquire new skills and knowledge incidentally, as non-retarded children often seem to do almost by osmosis. They must be taught each step quite deliberately, in part because they have difficulty centering on the most relevant cues or aspects of the environment. Once locked into the right cues and functioning within the limits of their capacity, learning proceeds rather well. Teaching then requires clever engineering, catching and holding the children's attention on "pay dirt," sequencing carefully the skills being taught and taking nothing for granted.

Because one cannot rely on learning to be automatic and since complex skills develop from simpler components, even very basic mental and motor behavior must often be taught and practiced in careful sequence. Where there are neurological problems such as persistent infantile reflexes, "natural" patterns may interfere with mastery of more complex skills. Some children acquire habitual self-defeating responses such as throwing everything they touch, head banging or misbehaving to get attention.

From work with older children and adults there is considerable evidence that retarded persons tend not to play active roles as learners or to employ the strategies at their disposal for mastering new tasks. They may have to be alerted to the challenge presented and reminded many times how to go about the task. Once having acquired a new skill, they may have to be taught explicitly to generalize it to new situations and to adapt it to changing circumstances.

Once of school age, many handicapped children acquire debilitating self-images after repeated failures with schoolwork and unfortunate encounters with peers. For a vulnerable child, protracted failure may be devastating. School systems have devised a variety of means of dealing with these problems, but there is no perfect solution because the discrepancies are built in: retarded children must live in the society of the non-retarded. Even among children of normal intelligence with subtle kinds of learning disabilities, special attention is likely to be essential to avert the discouragement and disturbance that result from protracted school failure.

Finally, early and continued intervention is needed to support families in meeting their responsibilities to the special child while leading reasonable lives themselves. While they usually need guidance for the skilled and active instruction required by the child, families also need the personal support a professional can offer by sharing responsibility for care, recognizing the burden that the child's care implies and assuring that the family receives the most appropriate services available. In recent years, the vigorous trend away from institutional placement has created a broad spectrum of programs—often uncoordinated to the point of chaos—including parent organizations, school classes, home helpers, day care, recreation, non-institutional residential placement, specialized medical clinics, speech and occupational and physical therapy resources. These may make the difference between a disrupted family and an effective one, between a child who can live amicably and productively at home or elsewhere in the community and a child who can function only in a restrictive institution.

Ends and Means

The goals of intervention are preventive, educational and supportive: to prevent maladaptive patterns before they become entrenched; to provide specialized, sequential and carefully engineered learning experiences geared to and not underestimating the capabilities of the child; and to provide personal and practical support to families. Among the qualities to look for in an effective program will be the following:

Careful analysis of learning goals. Teaching is sequential, step-by-step, with meticulous attention to reinforcement of appropriate behavior and non-reinforcement of that which is unwanted. The sophisticated tools of behavior modification are nowhere more relevant than in the special classroom (Krumboltz and Krumboltz).

Parent involvement. The most effective early childhood programs involve parents in a central, purposive role as the child's principal educators rather than as amateur adjuncts to "experts" (Bronfenbrenner). Children with special needs demand extraordinary parental skills and resolve and an unusual degree of consistency between home and school.

Overall view. A total view of child and family should provide "education" as well

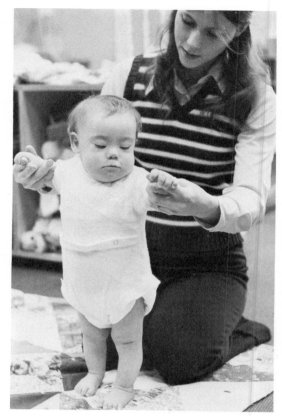

Figure 27–1 Step-by-step learning. (Courtesy of University of Washington Child Development and Mental Retardation Center.)

as treatment as needed in motor and language spheres. A spirit of cooperation with the child's physician and other professionals involved with the family is essential. Although the intensity of appropriate services may wax and wane, mental handicap is a chronic condition, which implies that the individual may need an integrated network of services on a continuing basis.

Optimism and realistic expectations. These should not undercut development by demanding too little or too much. While retarded children, of course, progress more slowly than other children, their teachers are as prey to underexpectation as are parents, with the result that in many special education settings retarded children achieve less than equally retarded children in regular classes. Parents and teachers need to maintain perspective, taking pleasure in the small victories, yet recognizing that, except in circumscribed areas, retarded children remain behind their nonretarded peers.

Education and Training Programs

It was once accepted that, unless a child was "educable," that is, capable of academic learning, public schools had no responsibility. Gradually, through the efforts of concerned parents and other citizens and, more recently, on the basis of judicial decisions and legislation, the right of every handicapped child in the United States to publicly supported training and education appropriate to his needs has been firmly established. While in many areas this compulsory responsibility is restricted to the common school age of 5 or 6 to 18 years, permissive legislation has made possible not only services for infants and preschool children but also continued training for young adults.

Infant programs. The past few years have seen a very rapid increase in programs designed to identify handicapped infants (birth to age three) as early as possible and to provide stimulation and parent education, together with treatment for specific disorders as needed. The infants enrolled tend to be either those whose developmental handicap is spotted early because of dysmorphic features or severe pathology, or those known to be at unusual risk, such as prematures or postmatures. Some programs involve home visits by staff personnel; some require the mother to bring the child to a clinic or center; some handicapped infants are given physical therapy. These programs tend to be quite expensive and are unlikely ever to be available for large numbers of children. They offer a unique opportunity, however, for family support during the particularly critical time of coming to terms with the facts of their child's developmental handicaps. Early intervention hopefully also provides the opportunity for effective reduction of maladaptive patterns.

Preschool programs. Although some programs for preschool children, three to five years of age, include or consist of home visits, group facilities at this age are more common. Since mild learning handicaps in preschool children tend to be missed, the programs tend to be slanted, on the one hand, toward a few children with easily discernible generalized delays or severe specific sensory, motor or language problems, or on the other, toward larger groups at socioeconomic risk, e.g., Project Head Start. Head Start is required to include in its enrollment about 10 per cent handicapped children, but appropriately trained teachers are very often missing. School districts are recognizing with increasing frequency the advisability of providing for developmentally delayed children in this age group; other programs are to be found under the auspices of parent or church groups, clinics and other voluntary agencies. Proprietary special programs, which have proliferated for non-handicapped children in this age range, are almost non-existent because of their prohibitive costs.

Programs for school-age children. All public school systems provide special arrangements and reduced-size classes for a large proportion of their retarded children. There are a variety of plans for *educable mentally retarded* (EMR) children, generally defined as having IQs from 50 or 55 to 70 or 80; these children are expected eventually to achieve academic work of third to sixth grade level. *Trainable mentally retarded* (TMR) children, with IQs from 25 or 35 to 50 or 55, are not expected to achieve useful academic skills. They are almost always taught in self-contained classes in which self-care and social adjustment within a restricted environment are the goals, although some TMR children are capable of more advanced academic skills. Children with still lower IQs are known by a variety of terms, such as *right-to-education* children, for whom training programs usually have very limited goals oriented primarily toward enabling the child to live amicably at home. Because there are very few such children in any geographic vicinity, schools must often improvise programming, including home visits, placement in classes for younger TMR children and so on.

Contemporary sentiment tends to staunchly oppose institutional placement of retarded children, largely because life in large, understaffed institutions tends to depress development without marked benefit to children or families, indeed without recognition of the important relationships among family members and retarded children. There clearly are situations, however, in which out-of-home care should be seriously considered by the family. A variety of such arrangements is possible, ranging from care in another family, through group homes and mini-institutions within the community, to self-contained institutions. However handicapped the child may be, placement outside the family in no way reduces his or her right to appropriate training.

EDUCATION FOR THE EDUCABLE MENTALLY RETARDED [EMR] CHILD. Children with mild mental handicaps pose difficult questions for educators attempting to optimize their placement. Many such children are to be found in regular classes, especially in the early school grades, while teachers sometimes make heroic efforts to "bring them up to norm." With the move toward individualized instruction for all children, it is often feasible in the early grades to accommodate the deviant child. Supportive services can be provided by a resource teacher who takes the child for part of the day, by tutors and by specialists such as speech therapists or physical therapists. The most common approach, however, is eventually to transfer a child from a regular classroom in which he is failing to a special classroom that may be completely self-contained or may interact part of the day with regular classes.

The *elementary primary* class for EMR children 6 to 10 years of age is generally a preacademic program; the *elementary intermediate* class, for children aged 9 to 13 with mental ages roughly of 6 to 9 years, often covers the academic work expected during the regular primary grades as well as enriching the child's knowledge of his environment and his capacity for healthy social relationships. Children who transfer into the intermediate class are often burdened with negative self-concepts, dislike for school and self-defeating behavior patterns born of repeated failure.

Secondary school classes for EMR children tend to diverge more markedly from classes for non-retarded children, as the latter become more adept at conceptualizing subject matter far removed from their concrete experience and their immediate needs. Special programs tend to emphasize vocational and domestic skills needed for independent living. Instruction in school subjects is continued, while occupational education is generally aimed less at acquiring salable skills that can be learned on the job than at the development of appropriate job-related attitudes such as courtesy, punctuality and ability to follow directions. *Post-school* classes are provided in many school districts but are seldom taken advantage of by retarded persons. In recognition of the continuing vocational, social and recreational needs of retarded adults in our complex society, these are often coordinated with non-school agencies such as sheltered workshops, state employment services and rehabilitation facilities.

Questions about the effectiveness of the various forms of special education are for the most part unresolved. Seldom are children randomly assigned to one arrangement or another; those placed in the least contact with non-retarded children tend to include those whose failures have been most obvious both from an academic and a social point of view. It is hardly surprising, then, that retarded children in regular classes often gain higher academic achievement than those in special classes, though there is some evidence pointing to the superior social adjustment of EMR children in self-contained classrooms. In neither setting, though, do retarded children tend to achieve academically at the level predicted by their mental ages, suggesting that adult expectations may be too low and that teaching methods and content may also need improvement. In many school systems, teachers and parents now agree periodically on short-term goals; these contracts also contain an agreement that both will monitor the child's progress and will make explicit contributions to the child's training. Legislation passed in 1976 indeed mandates such goal-setting in all special education programs supported by federal funds.

TRAINING FOR THE TRAINABLE MENTALLY RETARDED (TMR) CHILD. Trainable mentally retarded children constitute only a small group, perhaps 1 in 500. Because it is the rare TMR child who achieves a significant degree of social or economic independence as an adult (though he or she may certainly engage in economically useful work and may get along quite well in a family setting), educational goals center on the development of skills that normal and mildly retarded young children learn at home as a matter of course: self-care, communication, work habits, following directions and the rudiments of social participation. Many of these

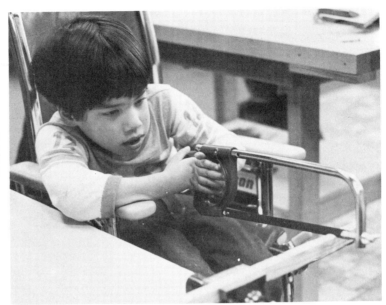

Figure 27–2 Practical skills as well as academic tasks are emphasized. (Courtesy of University of Washington Child Development and Mental Retardation Center.)

children have physical, sensory and perceptual handicaps that require special attention. While special programs for TMR children have not been spectacularly successful as measured by tests of academic achievement, it is important to keep in mind that some seemingly small accomplishments may make a great deal of difference in the quality of family life. In addition, classes may provide essential relief for the parents and help with developing realistic expectations about the child's achievement. The fact that many families place TMR adolescents outside the home when they outgrow school classes is perhaps proof enough of the value of programs. It is easy to underestimate the capabilities of TMR children. Indeed, if one visualizes a moderately retarded adult as an individual with the intellectual capabilities of a child of, say, six to eight and a half years, but with the practice and strength developed from added maturity one sees that there is indeed hope that such an individual may make a real contribution to and be an integral member of society.

TRAINING FOR THE SEVERELY AND PROFOUNDLY HANDICAPPED. Expectations for children with more severe handicaps are, of course, quite restricted. Most of these children have sustained significant central nervous system impairment. Their care is often very demanding, and even such matters as toileting and feeding skills require detailed task analysis and step-by-step training. Expert guidance is, of course, valuable, but training requires many hours of repetition that blend into every interaction with the child. Family relief from daily care constitutes an important contribution of any training program, for, unlike TMR children, these individuals even as adults will not be expected to be able to care for their own needs or to avoid common dangers. They may seldom be left unsupervised. Even with these severe limitations, however, there are varying degrees of social competence and self-care skills that may make an enormous difference in caretaking demands and the quality of personal relationships.

Issues and Controversies

Labeling. There is a widespread conviction that labeling a child as mentally retarded by placing him in a special program should be avoided if possible. In addition to other handicaps, the label is seen as another cross to bear, as lowering expectations of others, as leading to rejection by peers and as affecting the child's self-concept and aspirations. This controversy may appear a bit foreign to those accustomed to a diagnostic approach, but mental retardation does not exist alone but only as a symptom of some underlying lack of integrity of structure or function, constitutional or experiential in origin. Particularly for mildly retarded children, the school years are often the most demanding and demeaning. Many such children function adequately outside of school hours and can be expected to blend into society at large once the school years are over. The question of labeling, then, is a real one, for if an individual is coping adequately and responsibly with the demands of a relatively normal environment, he cannot legitimately be called mentally retarded. Classification rests not only on general intelligence but on adaptive behavior as well (Grossman).

Neither children nor adults like to be called retarded, but it is not at all clear whether special class placement increases or decreases the chances of peer rejection or leads to healthier or less healthy self-concepts and social relationships. Children who reach special classrooms have been selected because they have not coped adequately in one way or another. Sometimes the label serves a protective or explanatory function, as when another child on the playground accepts the retarded child's behavior "because she is retarded," or the employer refuses to lay off the retarded worker even in times of economic stress.

The IQ required for special class placement is, like any other test score, subject to error. Referral to an EMR class usually follows intensive observation by at least one teacher, the concurrence of the school principal and a comprehensive examination not only of the child but of all his school records by the school psychologist. If special placement seems appropriate, the parents are consulted. There are always, then, several adults involved, each of whom may be presumed to have the child's best interests at heart.

Much of the controversy about labeling has stemmed from recognition of the large numbers of minority children in special classes and from the struggle to eliminate racial segregation in the schools. The over-representation of minority group children does not, of course, by itself prove that they have been misclassified, but one must be careful not to perceive children as retarded when their major problem is that they come from non-English-speaking homes or culturally different ethnic groups.

Mainstreaming. The concept of *normalization* or *mainstreaming* in educational placement of handicapped children is much in vogue. The concept is interpreted as the part-day or whole-day integration of handicapped and non-handicapped children, under conditions as normal as possible. Contrary to the argument that retarded children need small classes, special curricula and materials and specialized teachers, the contemporary philosophy of normalization holds that isolation or homogeneous grouping in itself encourages deviant behavior, that the "real world" provides more appropriate models and a more natural growth setting. Mainstreaming applies, of course, only to those EMR children who can to some degree adapt to a regular classroom; it is not applied to TMR children. The evidence for and against mainstreaming is unclear. What is clear, however, is that there is much danger of using it as an excuse for budget-cutting and the subsequent underattention to children with special needs.

REFERENCES

Bronfenbrenner, U.: Is early intervention effective? *In* Ryan, S. (Ed.): *A Report on Longitudinal Evaluations of Preschool Programs. Vol 1.* Washington, D.C., Office of Child Development, 1974.

Grossman, H. (Ed.): *Manual on Terminology and Classification in Mental Retardation.* Washington, D.C., American Association on Mental Deficiency, 1973 revision.

Hobbs, N.: *The Futures of Children.* San Francisco, Jossey-Bass, 1975.

Krumboltz, J. D., and Krumboltz, H. B.: *Changing Children's Behavior.* Englewood Cliffs, N.J., Prentice-Hall, 1972.

Linde, T. F., and Kopp, T.: *Training Retarded Babies and Pre-schoolers.* Springfield, Ill., Charles C Thomas, 1973.

Robinson, N. M., and Robinson, H. B.: *The Mentally Retarded Child: A Psychological Approach,* 2nd ed. New York, McGraw-Hill, 1976.

Developmental Issues and Psychosocial Problems in Childhood

II. More Serious Behavioral and Performance Disorders

William Hetznecker
and Marc A. Forman

28

It is recommended that the reader become familiar with Chapter 12 on normal development and minor behavioral problems prior to reading this chapter, which deals predominantly with the more serious or chronic problems of behavioral function and performance.

LEARNING DISABILITY

Learning disability is a term that denotes a problem in learning academic skills, most often reading. In a smaller percentage of children, mathematical learning is impaired as well. Spelling and handwriting are also frequently poor. "Learning disability" connotes different notions, depending upon its use. Some pediatricians and neurologists make the term synonymous with the hyperkinetic syndrome. Psychiatrists of a psychological persuasion imply that learning disability is closely allied with psychologically induced learning inhibition. Educators use the term to mean children of normal intelligence who have great difficulty learning to read, write, spell or calculate when taught by the usual means.

Present knowledge indicates that learning disability is not primarily a psychiatric or emotional disorder. Psychiatric difficulties arise as a consequence of the child's inability to learn. He subsequently experiences frustration, discouragement, repeated failure, onerous comparison with siblings and peers and the disappointment of his parents. Symptoms can be primarily subjective in the form of anxiety, depression and withdrawal or behavioral, in the form of disruption in school, defiance and passive resistance to school work. It is currently thought that learning disability is the result of subtle neurophysiological and neuropsychological disturbances in the handling of verbal or written material. These disturbances can occur in one or a combination of the following processes: perception of visual or auditory information, central nervous system symbolization of either visual or auditory information, and expression of information either in verbal or written form.

Learning disability is thought to affect about 10 per cent of the elementary school population. It occurs about six times more frequently in boys. There are no well-established socioeconomic differences. These children have scores on standard IQ tests that range from average to superior. There is a greater than expected family history of learning difficulties, slowness to read and poor spelling.

Children with a learning disability may have early difficulty with the alphabet, especially writing or recalling letters or in learning numerals. Often, the first signs may not be evident until the child tries to read words or spell simple words. Reversal of letters—*d* for *b* or *p* for *q*—which normally disappears by age seven, persists in these children. Whole words are often reversed or inverted: *saw* for *was*. Certain children exchange the position of letters in the middle of words; others have problems with initial or final consonants or have significant difficulty with diphthongs and unusual spellings. Children who have difficulty in the visual sphere will encounter serious trouble if the look-see whole word method of reading is used. Children who have difficulty in the auditory sphere (they usually have normal response to audiometric tests) will not be able to learn adequately by a phonetic approach to reading. Many of these children may also show some features of the hyperkinetic syndrome, primarily the short attention span, inability to concentrate and low frustration tolerance.

The condition is almost always first detected in school but often not before the third grade. Neurological examination may reveal "soft signs." These are difficulties in performing rapidly alternating finger and hand movements, hopping, standing on one foot and tandem walking. Clumsiness and poorly developed coordination in throwing, catching or kicking a ball are often present.

Standard IQ tests such as the WISC (Wechsler Intelligence Scale for Children) may show discrepancies between verbal and performance scale—the latter usually higher. Certain subtests may be particularly sensitive. The Raven progressive matrices, the Bender-Gestalt, the Frostig test of perceptual ability and the Illinois Test of Psycholinguistic Abilities all may help establish the presence of learning disability and define the specific areas of difficulty.

These children need special approaches to education. Children with major learning disabilities often require small-sized classes with specially trained teachers, emphasizing a highly individualized curriculum. Extraneous and distracting stimuli are kept to a minimum. Methods of teaching that utilize multisensory approaches, overlearning of material and concentration exercises are employed.

Parents of these children need help to be patient, to support small gains and to recognize that some of these children will be handicapped in learning throughout their academic careers. Expectations should be adjusted accordingly. This does not mean a bleak prognosis. With early detection and application of remedial approaches, many of these children will be able to attend high school, vocational schools, colleges and professional schools.

Concomitant or associated emotional difficulties usually develop when the condition has persisted for several years and the child has experienced failure into fourth or fifth grade. When psychiatric disturbances do occur, they will require treatment that should include the parents. Psychiatric treatment is not sufficient by itself, however, and must be accompanied by special educational programs of the kind outlined here. Occasionally, medication such as prescribed for the hyperactive child (methylphenidate, dextroamphetamine or thioridazine) is indicated. This is primarily the situation if restlessness, inattentiveness and a high level of distractibility are prominent.

HYPERACTIVE SYNDROME

The term *hyperactive child* is one of the most widely used and abused in the fields of pediatrics, psychiatry and education as well as in the ordinary lives of children and families. Hyperactivity is a designation of a particular form of behavior. It is quantitative, not qualitative, implying a context within which it is judged. Constant running in an open playground while playing would not be considered hyperactivity. Constantly moving from chair to chair, then to floor and then in and out of the room while purportedly "watching television" could well be construed as hyperactivity. The hyperactive (hyperkinetic) child tends to demonstrate a cluster of behavior types, of which the excessive amount of movement from one place to another is only one. Controlled studies of various sorts have been unable to demonstrate consistently that hyperactive children do engage in more movement than controls. Nevertheless, truly hyperactive children do appear to move about with less specific purpose for each move. In addition, such children are fidgety and fiddle constantly with their fingers whether it be itching, pulling at themselves or playing with a pencil, silverware, knobs and switches. These children demonstrate a short attention span, are easily distracted by spurious stimuli and tend to act quickly without much reflection. They are frequently neutral or positive in mood and in their approach to people. However, their frustration tolerance is low. They expect to get what they want immediately, and they can be obstinate and emotionally volatile.

The combination of these traits often puts them at odds with parental and adult expectations and interferes with cooperative play with peers. Frequently, negative reactions of others to the hyperactive child's behavior lay the groundwork for emotional difficulties, whether minor or severe.

Although some of these children are identified shortly after they begin to walk, the more likely point of discovery is upon entrance to school. The demands of the school environment for attention, concentration, control of motor behavior and impulses may conflict with these very limitations in the child. It is in school that the secondary psychosocial problems and learning difficulties begin to emerge.

There is much dispute about the etiology of this disorder. A strongly held view is that the signs and symptoms of hyperkinetic syndrome are the result of subtle neurophysiological or neuropathological disturbances in the central nervous system. Minimal cerebral dysfunction, minimal brain damage and minimal brain syndrome are a few of the common diagnostic terms applied to these children. At present, there is no evidence that demonstrates whether or not or where and how the brain is affected.

Diagnostic steps include the following:

1. A detailed history, including careful attention to mother's reproductive history, nature of her pregnancy, labor and delivery, whether the infant was premature or below weight and presence of any complicating factors at delivery or in immediate postnatal period. Information should be obtained about temperamental characteristics, early neonatal adjustment, illness history, when hyperactivity began, when it occurs and what, if any, other symptoms and behavior are associated with it.

2. A careful physical examination should include functional neurological examination, specific for children and designed to identify so called "soft signs."

3. Other supplementary examinations as indicated include psychological examination, psychoeducational testing procedure and classroom observational visit.

Treatment is first directed at interpreting the nature of the child's problem to the parent. The parents should be helped to recognize and accept that the child is not just defiant, oppositional and willfully destructive. They should also understand clearly that whatever diagnostic label is used, the child does *not* have a progressive neurological disease or an organic defect in his brain structure. Frequently, the concept of developmental hyperactivity is helpful in this regard. The parent should be helped to realize that the environment can be "structured" in ways that minimize the child's handicap and help him learn to concentrate, attend and develop controls on his behavior.

Management of Hyperactivity

Environmental structure and manipulation

1. It is important for the child to have a regular daily routine.

2. Parents should enunciate clearly defined behavioral expectations coupled with firm but fairly imposed limits, including restrictions or deprivations for behavioral transgressions. Rules should be clear and simple. Enforcement should be carried out with a minimum of discussion.

3. Overstimulation and excessive fatigue should be avoided. The child needs time to slow down after play. Time before bed should be quiet, and exciting television shows or rough-and-tumble games should be avoided.

4. For the young child, the home should be arranged so that valuable, dangerous and breakable objects are out of the child's reach or locked away.

5. Parents need to be supported and advised that these procedures will not psychologically damage or inhibit the child. Rather they should be clearly instructed that as adults and parents, it is their responsibility to provide such an environment so that the child will be happier and more effective and avoid becoming the "brat" of the family or neighborhood. It is also extremely important that affection, acceptance and regular praise and reward for acceptable behavior be dispensed by the parents.

6. School: classroom management requires the application of the same principles described for the home. The child should be given an extensive trial in one or more regular classrooms before a decision is made to place him in special class. When the decision is made, it should be based on educational, not merely behavioral, criteria. The hyperactive child often manifests a learning disability and therefore may need the special educational approaches described for this condition. Frequently, special classes employ some type of contingency or operant behavior modification system. When carefully planned and carried out by a teacher who is well-grounded in theory and practice, such an approach can be quite helpful to these children.

Medication. Pharmacotherapy is often used for the control of hyperactive behavior and the more fundamental disturbances in concentration, attention span and impulsivity.

1. The sympathomimetic amines, dextroamphetamine and methylphenidate, are currently the most commonly used, with the latter the drug of choice because of fewer side effects.

2. Phenothiazine medications have also been used extensively but the side effects of somnolence, irritability and dystonias make these medications less attractive, generally.

3. Children should have a three- to four-week trial of medication combined with regular reports from the teacher and parents about which effects and side effects are evident. These drugs may be used for prolonged periods of time. Because they are primarily employed to enhance the child's ability to perform school tasks, drug holidays may be taken on weekends, during the summer vacation and even intermittently during the school year.

4. If the child is under the care of a psychiatrist or other mental health professional, psychotherapy, behavior therapy or family therapy may be employed. In any case, continued regular guidance of parents in management of the child is essential.

PSYCHOSOMATIC DISORDERS

Psychological conflict and distress may produce alterations in somatic functioning. These "psychosomatic" illnesses are of two types: conversion ("hysterical") reactions and psychophysiological disorders.

In the conversion reaction, onset is generally sudden and frequently precipitated by a traumatic environmental event. Voluntary musculature and special sense organs are the most common target sites for the expression of a specific symbolic conflict in physical terms (e.g., the child who develops hysterical blindness because he unconsciously does not wish to "see" a family disturbance). Physical examination of affected parts fails to indicate any objective signs of damage. For example, normal deep tendon reflexes may be present in a paralyzed limb. Past history often reveals a tendency towards overdramatization in the child and his family, as well as a history of previous conversion episodes and hypochondriasis.

In the psychophysiological disorders onset is more insidious. States of chronic anxiety lead to disturbances in the functioning of the autonomic nervous system and finally to the production of actual tissue damage. Ulcerative colitis, bronchial asthma, migraine and eczema are examples of potential psychophysiological disorders. In each, there is presumed to be an interplay between underlying biological vulnerability in the affected organ system and the presence of chronic non-specific psychological stress. Children with psychophysiological disorders have a history of obsessive-compulsive, perfectionistic and constricted character traits. They tend to be pseudomature, high achievers and compliant "good children."

Management of children with psychosomatic disorders is dependent on the following principles: (1) These children are not malingerers and should not be treated as such. There is a real physical-psychological problem present over which they have no conscious control. (2) Joint pediatric-psychiatric management is essential. The primary physician should ask for a mental health consultation promptly. The psychiatric consultant should not be seen as the "last resort" to be called in after exhaustive studies are done but rather as an early contributing member of the treatment team. (3) In similar fashion, the parents must be helped to accept and understand the role of the emotions in the development of the disorder before any effective intervention can take hold. (4) Ongoing psychotherapy is often indicated, along with medical supervision and treatment. Small amounts of tranquilizing medication may be helpful in some instances. (5) Early return to normal activities of daily life should be encouraged. The child should not be shamed or made to lose face, nor should he be permitted to use his condition as a way of obtaining excessive dependency, sympathy and "special citizen" treatment. There should be a minimum of discussion or focus on the symptom or condition. Parents and teachers should avoid having the illness or the symptom become the major way of "doing business" with the child.

PSYCHONEUROSES

The definition of the neuroses derives from psychoanalytic theory as developed by Freud. The theory posits that unconscious conflicts between unacceptable wishes, sexual and aggressive, and the cultural restrictions against their expression give rise to anxiety. This anxiety can be consciously expressed as a free floating distressing affect or by the development of symptoms. Technically, the neuroses are characterized by the presence of significant overt anxiety, or by the development of symptoms that serve to disguise or mask underlying anxiety (e.g., conversion reactions, phobia, obsessive-compulsive neurosis). Unlike the psychoses, there is no disruption in the child's ability to test or appreciate reality. In practice, pure or classical psychoneuroses are not commonly seen in childhood. Rather, the child displays mixed behavioral and emotional patterns. A number of these clinical entities have been described in Chapter 12, e.g., tics, enuresis, school phobia.

DEPRESSION

Depression has been referred to in several sections of this chapter. Depression in children, as in adults, can be a symptom or a definitive psychiatric syndrome. Depression is primarily an emotional state or mood characterized by feelings of sadness, worthlessness, ineffectiveness, loss of positive view of the future and loss of pleasure and engagement in day-to-day activities. Depression is often missed in children because psychiatric theory, literature and research have neglected or minimized its occurrence in children. The cultural perspective emphasizes childhood as happy, and adults recoil at the notion of a child being depressed.

Children do not manifest the "classical" syndromes associated with adult illness: severe psychotic depression, involutional, or manic-depressive depression. Children are more prone to action, both from a developmental perspective as well as in attempts to cope with unpleasant feelings. Denial, avoidance and excess activity can be used by a child to avoid or cope with feelings of depression. Reacting against the environment in an angry or provocative manner, with constant demands or recurrent expressions of disappointment can manifest the depressed state. Some children do withdraw, cry more easily, become less effective at school and have trouble in their relationships in family and with peers. The main problems to look for when these various behavior patterns occur are situations in which the child has experienced separation, loss, failure, rejection and criticism. Depression in a parent may precipitate a depressive reaction in a child as a result of the psychological unavailability and perplexing sadness of the parent that colors his or her relationship with the child.

Most depressions in children are short-lived. Parent or teacher awareness of the child's condition can by itself increase the child's sense of importance and esteem. Parents should be encouraged to help the child express his sad, unhappy feelings and should not try to "Pollyanna" or "kid" the child out of them. Psychological availability, spending time with the child in a mutually pleasurable activity and helping him understand the reasons for a particular rejection or loss can be helpful. Most important is helping the child identify what can be done about the situation. For example, if he feels athletically incompetent, the child should be helped to find sports or athletic activities in which he can begin to experience success and competence. If the situation is one the child can not rectify by his own individual actions, such as rejection by a friend, then he needs help to find ways to talk about his feelings in a nonjudgmental setting and to gain the confidence to develop other relationships.

Grief and mourning are closely allied to depression and are seen as a normal response to the disruption of a significant relationship. If the child continues to grieve or remain depressed after two to three months, or if his functioning is affected, he should be referred to a mental health professional for evaluation and treatment. Chronic and recurrent depression is seen in some children who have experienced multiple separations from or losses of siblings, parents and other caretakers in their early years. These children are more vulnerable to depression, in response to a variety of emotional stresses. They require early identification and referral for psychiatric evaluation and treatment. Such children may in fact have a yet undiscovered biological propensity for depression.

The standard medications employed in treating adult depressions, the tricyclic compounds and monoamine oxidase inhibitors, have not been approved by the FDA for use in children under 12 years of age. Depression in children should be treated by significant doses of human involvement since the condition is most frequently a reaction to a disturbance in significant human relationships.

CHILDHOOD PSYCHOSES

Early Onset Psychoses

Early infantile autism is a major psychological disturbance of unknown etiology. Fortunately, it is a rare disorder, with a prevalence rate of approximately 1 to 2 per 10,000. Autism was first described by Kanner in 1943 and is characterized by profound impairment in the child's ability to relate to people, including his parents. As infants, autistic children are not "cuddly," the social smile may be absent or delayed and they frequently do not assume an anticipatory posture prior to being picked up. Language development is impaired and the emergence of speech is seriously delayed or absent. If speech is present, echolalia (parrot-like repetition), confusion in pronoun-usage and nonsense rhyming may predominate. Autistic children display extreme withdrawal, appear to prefer inanimate objects over affectional relationships with family members and demonstrate marked ritualistic behavior in an attempt to preserve environmental sameness. Eye contact is fleeting, and attempts to engage the autistic child in any playful activity may be met with total indifference. Temper tantrums and rage reactions may occur if the child's self-imposed compulsive routines are disturbed (e.g., touching objects or singing songs in the same sequence each time). Episodes of anxiety to the point of panic can occur without external cause. Repetitive rocking or spinning is noted. The child can engage in repeated head banging, cause serious excoriations of his skin and may attempt self-mutilation that can endanger his life. Deficits in language and interpersonal relationships make it difficult to test autistic children, and their functional intelligence quotient usually falls in the retarded range. However, some autistic children perform adequately on non-verbal tests, and in others, especially those with speech, good intellectual potential can be observed.

Numerous etiological speculations have been made concerning autism. Imputed causative agents have included parental rejection, brain injury, constitutional vulnerability, developmental aphasia and reticular activating system deficits. Recent evidence appears to indicate that autism is not parent-induced, but probably neurophysiological in origin. Various therapeutic measures have been tried, including intensive psychotherapy, medication and residential treatment away from home, but success has been quite limited. Modest gains in speech acquisition and development have been reported with behavior therapy operant conditioning approaches. These methods have also been used to control or extinguish destructive and non-functional repetitive behavior. The prognosis remains guarded, however. Some autistic children may grow up to lead marginal lives in the community, but for many chronic placement in state institutions is the ultimate outcome. There is no clearly evident relationship between autism and disorders of later childhood and adult life included in the schizophrenias.

Symbiotic Psychosis

This disorder, originally described by Mahler in 1952, has onset between the ages of two to five years. (The existence of this condition as a separate, clinically defined entity is disputed by many child psychiatrists.) Early development frequently appears to be normal, although the children are sometimes described as having been "oversensitive" infants. The threat of separation from mother, e.g., by the birth of a sibling or by nursery school attendance, usually serves as the precipitating event. Acute panic-like anxiety ensues, together with marked deterioration in behavior and cognitive functioning. The child clings intensely to his mother, but may also transfer this same attachment in an indiscriminate manner to many other persons. Speech that has been present may become idiosyncratic, jargonistic and no longer used for communicative purposes. Bizarre behavior occurs, and the child becomes a serious management problem for parents. Following an acute phase, the child may lapse into a chronically withdrawn state, closely resembling that of autism. Constitutional vulnerability, organicity, and parental psychopathology have all been suggested as causative agents, but the etiology of the symbiotic psychosis remains unknown. As with autism, various treatment modalities have been attempted, but prognosis remains guarded, especially if a chronic state is reached.

Late Onset Psychoses

In contrast to those of early childhood, the psychoses of late childhood more closely resemble adult schizophrenic reactions. Late onset psychoses are characterized by severe thought disorder, delusions and hallucinations, disorganized and re-gressed behavior, withdrawal from interpersonal relations and failure of reality testing. The etiology of these disorders is also unclear. There is a high rate of schizophrenia in families of these children, unlike the early onset types. Treatment approaches include individual psychotherapy, family therapy and behavior therapy, and these are most often employed together with the administration of major tranquilizing medications. Hospitalization or residential treatment for weeks to as long as several years may be employed. Prognosis appears to be somewhat more favorable than in early onset types.

HANDICAPPED CHILDREN

Handicapped children are those with congenital or acquired defects affecting the central nervous system, orthopedically impaired children, mentally retarded children and children who are visually impaired or hard of hearing. For each type of handicap or function deficit, the psychosocial risks are different, but some general statements can be made.

The stigma of being different and not being able to do what age mates can do puts these children at risk of developing low self-esteem. Self-esteem has several dimensions, including the feelings of being valued, competent and powerful. For children with handicaps, each of these dimensions can be affected. A child with cerebral palsy or an orthopedic defect who cannot control his arms or legs may feel inferior, incompetent and helpless. Similarly, a child who is mentally retarded can be acutely aware of the inability to learn as effectively as other children. He knows that he is in a class that is different from the rest of the classes at school. He starts to know the pain of words such as "retarded," "dummy" and "stupid," and knows that he will be isolated from the mainstream of school achievement and possibly of social and personal acceptance.

The emotional reactions of a child with a handicap are as varied as those of a child without such handicap and are conditioned by temperamental characteristics, the nature of the handicap and most important, the attitude, behavior and emotional reactions of parents, siblings, peers, neighbors and teachers. A major difference is that the handicapped child may be limited in the manner in which he can cope with or express his emotional reactions. Society has incorporated traditional biases and reactions to blind, deaf, retarded and crippled individuals. These reactions are a combination of sympathy, helplessness, avoidance, rejection, fear and disgust, as well as genuine care and concern. Parents, siblings and teachers will be affected by these emotions to varying degrees, and the particular mixture will be manifest in their behavior toward the child.

The risks for the child from well-intentioned and loving parents are different at varying ages and always conditioned by the specific nature and extent of the handicap. In the first two to three years, the greatest risk may be overindulgence and an excess of sympathy, leading the parents to do too much for and expect too little from the child. By four or five years, the risk can be the reverse. Since these children have handicaps that set some limits on their physical, intellectual or social attainment, they require early enrollment in special education programs geared to their specific needs, physical, cognitive and social. Because of the early indulgence and excessive catering to the child, he or she may not be socially or emotionally prepared for a nursery school program in which teachers and other adults must be responsive to the needs of all children. In addition, demands will be placed on the child for conforming to social expectations and attempting to accomplish the tasks and activities of the particular program. It is at this time the opposite hazard can face the child. He or she may be expected to do too much too soon. This is particularly true for the child who was previously kept too dependent and was overprotected or indulged out of sympathy, anxiety and guilt.

The other major psychosocial hazard for the handicapped child is that the combination of his handicap and the attitudes and behavior of family, peers and teachers may enhance and promote passivity and helplessness. This is probably the most insidious and pernicious complication of a handicapping condition. Along with the negative self-esteem and lack of familial acceptance and support, passivity can lead to a variety of maladaptive psychological and behavioral reactions.

The physician needs to spend a good deal of time and effort with parents and often siblings. He needs to be able to provide or emphasize the following:

1. Adequate and accurate information about the nature of the child's condition, the etiology if known, its general prognosis and the sorts of intervention that will be needed as the child grows and develops. These can range in diversity from medication to a special recreational program.

2. Parents need to have the opportunity to express *if they can and wish to* the anger, resentment, disgust, guilt and other negative emotions they may feel about the child, his condition and the effects on them and their family. Parents should not, however, be pushed into or expected to express all their negative feelings. For some people, denial, avoidance, reaction formation and compensation are the most adaptive ways of coping. The physician should not see himself in the role of performing radical emotional exploration or surgery. He needs to respect the style, personality and judgment of the parents as to when, how and if they wish to discuss these feelings. They may prefer to do this with a clergyman. They should not be automatically referred to a psychiatrist on the assumption that all parents of a handicapped child necessarily will have emotional reactions and problems that require psychiatric help.

3. Parents need guidance from the physician, in encouraging and stimulating the child to the basic tasks of socialization. Motor and language development, sphincter control, appropriate expression of anger and social experience with age mates are basic tasks for all children within the limits of their handicap.

4. The physician can help parents encourage the child by identifying and promoting development of the child's strengths. Small successes and accomplishments should be recognized and praised, not taken for granted. Most important, as the child becomes of elementary school age and older, he or she needs help at becoming "good at something." This may take a good deal of energy and effort on the part of the parents and other adults to help the child identify and work at some skill or develop some ability that will provide intrinsic reward and a sense of competence.

5. Parents will need help in facing the child's unhappy, discouraged and resentful feelings connected with his handicap and its social or emotional implications. Pollyanna and "count your blessings" attitudes are very provocative and tend to

make the child feel guilty and resentful. Even though no one can take away, cure or make up for the handicap, the important adults can face and stand by the child when he is tormented and overwhelmed by his feelings. The physician can support parents and help them with their feelings so they, in turn, can deal with the child's feelings and be psychologically available.

As parents and siblings accept and encourage the child he will accept himself with a realistic recognition of his limitations yet with an equally realistic appreciation of his strengths, abilities and intrinsic worth as a person.

THE POOR CHILD

Children from poor families are at risk of developing a diversity of physical, psychosocial and educational disabilities. Poverty is not associated with the occurrence of one particular kind of problem, but with many interrelated problems. From the outset, poor children begin their lives at a disadvantage, and the circumstances of poverty compound their disadvantaged position. Poorly nourished mothers who have had multiple pregnancies and inadequate obstetrical care tend to give birth to premature infants. Prematurity increases the risk of neurological impairment and subsequent behavioral problems. The child's development is further jeopardized by poor control of infections, risk of lead intoxication, dietary deficiencies and accidental or deliberate injuries. The devastating effects of chronic unemployment and densely crowded, substandard living conditions produce states of despair that lead to family disorganization, child neglect and abandonment. Lack of intellectual stimulation restricts the child's cognitive development and limits his educational motivation. Precocious exposure to overstimulating sexual and aggressive experiences creates intense anxiety and provides the child with models for subsequent acting out behavior. As he grows older, the poor child encounters a local school system in which resources are more limited than its affluent counterpart. The longer he is in school, the farther behind he may fall academically. A gang-oriented subculture provides an attractive, though illusory, remedy to his diminished self-esteem. In adolescence, school dropout, unemployment and pregnancy ensue.

The poverty cycle continues with the next generation.

This description is admittedly a rather fatalistic overgeneralization. Many poor families have formidable adaptive strengths and coping skills. Confronting major obstacles, they maintain family stability and provide their children with opportunities for the full expression of developmental potential. Frankly, we know less about how these families and children survive and overcome while others are overwhelmed. We cannot expect that the risk for poor children will lessen, however, until major changes are made in social policy and the allocation of national resources.

MEDICATIONS FOR EMOTIONAL AND BEHAVIORAL CONDITIONS OF CHILDHOOD

There are numerous psychopharmaceutical preparations available. Many are not recommended for children under six years of age and some not for children under 12. We will describe only a few for which there is extensive literature documenting their use in a variety of psychiatric and behavioral conditions of childhood. The medications listed in Table 28–1 are those found useful in our own clinical experience. We recognize that responsible clinicians may disagree with the use of certain medications for certain conditions. For instance, there is a continuing controversy about the indication for, and even the use of, the stimulant medications methylphenidate and dextroamphetamine for the hyperkinetic syndrome.

We also recognize that other clinicians may have their own "favorite" medication not listed here that they have used successfully for certain conditions. It is our contention that, as in other areas of medicine, a clinician should learn to use one or two medications from each of the major groups. He should become familiar with the indications, contraindications, side effects and varying dose levels for children of different ages, as well as schedules of administration. The initial dosage of any drug should be small and gradually increased until desired effects occur. The clinician should be alert for, and ask parents and teachers about, general signs of toxicity. These can be excessive lethargy, behavioral deterioration, marked anorexia, weight loss and

TABLE 28-1

Medication	Indications	Outpatient Dosage Range	Side Effects and Toxicity
Major Tranquilizers chlorpromazine (Thorazine) thioridazine (Mellaril)	Severe anxiety, agitation, hyperactivity, aggressiveness, psychosis	Total daily dose: 30–150 mg, in divided doses	Sleepiness, irritability, dry mouth, tympanies, parkinsonism, dystonia, blood dyscrasias, hepatic findings, cutaneous reactions, photosensitivity, alteration in pigment metabolism with high doses over prolonged time, cataracts
haloperidol (Haldol)	Tics, psychotic conditions marked by agitation and aggressiveness; not approved for children under 12	Total daily dose: 1–6 mg, in divided doses	
Stimulants methylphenidate (Ritalin)	Hyperkinetic syndrome; Neither drug approved for children under 6 years	Total daily dose: 10–30 mg/day in two divided doses	Anorexia, weight loss, irritability, abdominal pain, headache, insomnia, variable blood pressure response, tachycardia, increased hyperactivity; to date, addiction has not been reported; tolerance is rare
dextroamphetamine (Dexedrine)		5–15 mg/day in two divided doses; may also be given in elixir form	
Antidepressants imipramine (Tofranil)	Depressive states (not approved in children under 12); enuresis (imipramine only)	For depression, 30–75 mg/day in divided doses; for enuresis, 25–50 mg h.s.	Hypotension, hypertension, tachycardia, insomnia, restlessness, nightmares, ataxia, parkinsonism, dry mouth, blurred vision, blood dyscrasias
amitriptyline (Elavil)		30–50 mg/day in divided doses	
Miscellaneous diphenhydramine (Benadryl)	Hyperactivity, anxiety, sleep disorders	For hyperactivity, 25–150 mg/day in divided doses. For sleep disorders, 25–50 mg h.s.; can be given as elixir	Dry mucous membranes, skin rash

During treatment with major tranquilizers and antidepressants, baseline and periodic laboratory examinations should be obtained. These include CBC, differential, platelet count, liver enzyme studies and urine urobilinogen.

central nervous system reactions such as spasm, tremors and dystonias.

As in therapy for other conditions or infectious diseases, the clinician should avoid using multiple medications at the same time or shifting from one medication to another when a favorable response does not occur immediately. This usually represents a response to a clinician's own anxiety and insecurity or to pressure from parents and teachers rather than reasoned judgments based on the child's condition and the clinician's knowledge of the disturbance. Nowhere else in medicine is there so great a propensity for reliance on drugs to cure everything and "change" the child. These medications have significant biochemical effects on the developing child. Beyond this intrinsic hazard is the risk that by the introduction of drugs for treatment of childhood behavioral conditions the significant adults—doctor, parent, teacher—

will feel less responsibility for using human interaction as a major therapeutic tool.

REFERENCES

Brutten, M.: *Something's Wrong with my Child: A Parent's Book for Children with Learning Disabilities.* New York, Harcourt, Brace and Jovanovich, 1973.

Freedman, A. M., Kaplan, H. I., and Sadock, B. J. (Eds.): *Modern Synopsis of Comprehensive Textbook of Psychiatry.* Baltimore, Williams & Wilkins, 1972, p. 574–673.

Freeman, R. D.: Emotional reactions of handicapped children. *In* Chess, S., and Thomas, A. (Eds.): *Annual Progress in Child Psychiatry and Child Development.* New York, Bruner Mazel, 1968, p. 379–395.

Glaser, K.: Masked depression in childhood and adolescence. *In* Chess, S., and Thomas, A. (Eds.): *Annual Progress in Child Psychiatry and Child Development.* New York, Bruner Mazel, 1968, p. 345–355.

Werry, J. S.: Developmental hyperactivity. *In* Chess, S., and Thomas, A. (Eds.): *Annual Progress in Child Psychiatry and Child Development.* New York, Bruner Mazel, 1969, p. 485–505.

PART X

SPECIAL SENSE
DISORDERS

Ocular Disorders

Robert E. Kalina

The care of vision in childhood is a responsibility shared by the ophthalmologist and all health professionals. Some disorders are related to systemic diseases for which the ophthalmologist may not be consulted unless a high index of suspicion exists, while other disorders cause no symptoms and may be detected best through screening techniques administered by those offering generalized care. All too frequently, eye examination is omitted because of the erroneous belief that sophisticated instrumentation is required. In fact, most ocular disorders can be detected with readily available facilities and equipment. When dealing with the eyes of children, one is reminded constantly that either omission or commission may be rewarded by responsibility for a lifetime of blindness.

It is helpful to be familiar with the designations of persons in the eye care field:

An *ophthalmologist* (oculist) is a doctor of medicine (M.D.), a physician licensed to practice medicine and surgery, who specializes in the diagnosis and treatment of diseases and defects of the eye. In treatment, the ophthalmologist prescribes medicines, glasses, contact lenses, prisms, exercises and other therapies and performs surgery. Some ophthalmologists, often after additional training, may elect to limit their practices to children, but additional specialty certification is not implied.

An *optometrist* is a doctor of optometry (O.D.), a licensed non-medical practitioner, who measures refractive errors and eye muscle disturbances. In treatment, the optometrist prescribes glasses, contact lenses, prisms and exercises.

An *optician* is one who fits, adjusts and dispenses glasses and other optical devices on the written prescription of a licensed physician or optometrist.

A comprehensive review of diseases of the eye in childhood cannot be provided in a chapter such as this. Certain disorders occurring with greatest frequency during childhood have been selected for discussion here, using the organizational format of the recently published *Ophthalmology Study Guide for Students and Practitioners of Medicine.*

VISUAL ACUITY

Visual acuity is the most sensitive indicator of visual function, and testing should be part of every periodic well-child examination. Visual acuity testing is indicated for any child with suspected ocular or neurological disease. No infant is too young for some estimate of visual acuity.

Visual Acuity Testing Methods
(Test Each Eye Separately)

Birth	Pupillary responses and facial responses
3 months	Follow light or large objects
1 year	Grasp small objects
2 years	Identify pictures
3 years	Illiterate "E"
4 years	Snellen chart

WHEN TO REFER. Children with apparent poor vision or anatomic ocular defects should be referred to an ophthalmologist. If the child can be tested with the illiterate "E" or the Snellen chart, failure to reach 20/40 with either eye should be cause for referral. In addition, there are clues suggesting poor vision that should lead to prompt referral of children, even when visual acuity cannot be measured precisely:

1. Resistance to covering one eye but not the other
2. Pupillary abnormalities
3. Nystagmus
4. Strabismus

OPHTHALMOSCOPY

Fundus examination by ophthalmoscopy may provide valuable clues to systemic disease and to ocular disorders affecting the retina and optic nerve. Examination of a great number of normal fundi will be required in order to appreciate the many normal variations that exist.

Technique. Fundus examination through an undilated pupil is difficult in an adult and often impossible in an uncooperative child. Recommended mydriatics are 1 per cent cyclopentolate (Cyclogyl) or 1 per cent tropicamide (Mydriacyl) or 10 per cent phenylephrine (Neo-Synephrine). One drop of any of these agents in each eye repeated once in five minutes will provide satisfactory pupillary dilation in 20 minutes. Concentrations should be halved for infants less than one year old. Pharmacological dilation of the pupil with these agents is entirely without risk in children.

Retrolental Fibroplasia

The retina of the newborn infant (especially the premature) is incompletely vascularized. The developing retinal blood vessels constrict markedly in response to increased arterial oxygen tension. If vasoconstriction is prolonged, the peripheral retinal blood vessels may become obliterated, later stimulating neovascularization of the peripheral retina that may lead to retinal detachment and blindness. Once this sequence of events is initiated, no proven treatment exists, and the disease may either regress spontaneously or progress to cicatrization (Fig. 29–1) with marked reduction in vision, or blindness. Effective management of the critically ill, premature infant in order to prevent the development of retrolental fibroplasia while administering sufficient oxygen to sustain life is a difficult task. It requires mature clinical judgment assisted by information gathered by arterial blood gas monitoring. Although a marked reduction in incidence of retrolental fibroplasia has occurred since the recognition of the relationship of oxygen abuse to retrolental fibroplasia, occasional cases continue to occur especially among infants of very low birth weight.

The White Pupil in Infancy and Childhood

The presence of a white pupillary reflex (cat's eye) (Fig. 29–2) at any time in infancy or childhood may be due to a variety of causes, all of which are a threat to either life or vision and require immediate refer-

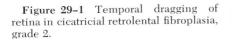
Figure 29–1 Temporal dragging of retina in cicatricial retrolental fibroplasia, grade 2.

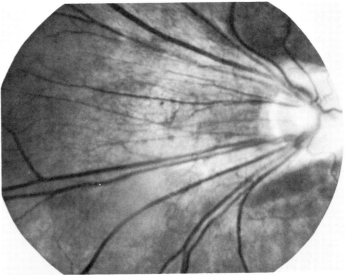

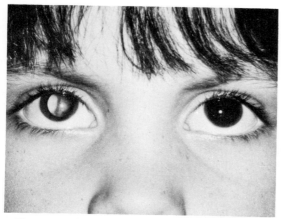

Figure 29–2 White pupillary reflex (retinoblastoma).

ral to an ophthalmologist. Retinoblastoma is a primary malignant tumor of the retinal neuroepithelium that is present at birth but may not become noticeable for months or years. Extraocular spread is by hematogenous metastases or by direct extension along the optic nerve to the brain and meninges. The tumor is often bilateral and may occur either sporadically on the basis of mutation or as an inherited autosomal dominant trait. Treatment is urgent and consists of enucleation of grossly involved eyes. Smaller tumors may be treated with irradiation, chemotherapy, cryotherapy or a combination of these entities. Parents and survivors should receive genetic counseling. Other causes of the white pupil in infancy and childhood are not described here since differentiation among them is not the province of the non-ophthalmologist.

GLAUCOMA

Glaucoma may become apparent at birth or at any time thereafter. It is manifested by progressive enlargement of one or both eyes due to increased intraocular pressure. Tearing and photophobia are prominent early signs of glaucoma in infants and children that also should call for examination by an ophthalmologist. Intraocular pressure screening (tonometry) is not a routine part of well-child examinations because of apprehension and the low incidence of glaucoma that might be detected by this method. Tactile tension measurements are entirely without value.

THE INFLAMED EYE

Neonatal conjunctivitis (ophthalmia neonatorum). Because of the frequency with which ocular infections occur due to contamination of the conjunctiva during passage through the birth canal, most states now require instillation of an antibacterial agent into the eyes of newborn infants immediately following delivery. The most frequently used and only proven agent for prevention of gonococcal conjunctivitis is 1 per cent silver nitrate (Credé method), but antibiotic solutions also are used and probably are effective. Silver nitrate often causes mild chemical conjunctivitis that resolves promptly without treatment. Silver nitrate (1 per cent solution) is supplied in ampules expressly for delivery room use. *Never* use any other form or concentration of silver nitrate or permanent corneal damage may result.

Gonorrheal conjunctivitis. This occurs owing to conjunctival contamination during passage through the infected genital tract. The usual onset is explosive between ages two and six days. There is copious purulent discharge, and diagnosis is by demonstration of intraepithelial gram negative diplococci in conjunctival scrapings. Appropriate culture techniques should be used to differentiate gonococcal conjunctivitis from the rare case of meningococcal conjunctivitis. Prompt treatment with topical and systemic penicillin is essential in order to avoid corneal infection. Urgent ophthalmic consultation is indicated. Failure by hospital personnel to instill the silver nitrate drops or other prophylactic preparation competently accounts for most cases of gonorrheal ophthalmia. One must be alert, however, to the possibility of prenatal infection in cases of prematurely ruptured membranes or reinfection after birth. In these situations, the time of onset may be outside the usual limits of two to six days after birth.

Bacterial conjunctivitis. This is most commonly due to *Staphylococcus*, but other organisms may be implicated. Onset and signs are similar to those of gonorrheal ophthalmia but less marked. Diagnosis is by demonstration of bacteria in Gram stained scrapings from the conjunctiva. Antibiotic therapy appropriate to the organism is instituted in order to avoid corneal involvement. Bacterial infection of the cornea (corneal ulcer) appears as a white or yellow opacity in the cornea and requires immediate ophthalmic consultation. Pseudomonas conjunctivitis, a severe form with frequent corneal complications, is of special significance in the compromised premature infant in whom it may lead to septicemia and death.

Inclusion conjunctivitis (inclusion blenorrhea). This is caused by contamination of the conjunctiva with the causative agent (chlamydia oculogenitalis) during passage through the birth canal and is not prevented by silver nitrate. Now the most common form of neonatal conjunctivitis, onset usually is between the fifth and fourteenth day of life. There is copious purulent discharge and conjunctival injection. Conjunctival scrapings show inclusion bodies in the cytoplasm of epithelial cells in Giemsa stained smears. Symptoms usually respond promptly to 10 per cent sulfacetamide drops or ointment applied four times daily, but relapses are common if treatment is not continued for three weeks or more. Parents should be examined for evidence of genital or ocular infection.

Ocular inflammations after the newborn period. After the neonatal period, *bacterial conjunctivitis* continues to be a frequent cause of ocular inflammation, but gonococcal and chlamydial infections are rare. Conjunctival injection and mucopurulent discharge are prominent signs. The eyelids frequently are matted together upon awakening. Most cases of bacterial conjunctivitis will respond promptly to removal of the discharge and instillation of 10 per cent sulfacetamide drops applied four times daily. Viral conjunctivitis may occur independently but often is associated with viral syndromes. Symptoms, signs and treatment are similar to bacterial conjunctivitis. If any corneal abnormality is suspected, the patient should be seen by an ophthalmologist immediately. Topical corticosteroid preparations should *never* be used either alone or in combination with an antibacterial agent by the non-ophthalmologist since these agents do not hasten recovery significantly and may cause blinding ocular complications.

BLEPHARITIS (inflammation of the eyelids). This is manifested by redness, crusting and scaling of the eyelid margins. The underlying cause most often is seborrhea, and seborrhea of the scalp, eyebrows and face often is associated. Treatment of this chronic condition includes attention to the scalp and face and especially diligent cleansing of the lid margins and eyelashes once or twice daily. Topical 10 per cent sulfacetamide drops may be helpful initially in severe cases, but lid hygiene is most important in long-term management.

STYE (hordeolum). This is a staphylococcal infection of a hair follicle or gland of the eyelid that may occur independently or as a complication of chronic blepharitis. Most such inflammatory masses will resolve spontaneously, aided by the application of frequent warm compresses. Topical 10 per cent sulfacetamide drops may be used to treat or prevent a secondary conjunctivitis, but time and warm compresses are the mainstays of therapy. Occasionally, a Meibomian gland in the margin of the eyelid may become obstructed, leading to a chronic localized granulomatous nodule called a chalazion. If symptomatic, the mass can be excised by an ophthalmologist.

IMPERFORATE NASOLACRIMAL DUCT. Stagnation of tears may result with chronic discharge and tearing. Finger pressure over the area of the lacrimal sac may express purulent material and control the chronic discharge when combined with topical sulfacetamide or antibiotics. Most imperforate nasolacrimal ducts will become patent either spontaneously or by use of massage of the lacrimal sac. The child should be seen by an ophthalmologist for definitive ther-

| | | **Neonatal Conjunctivitis** | |
| | | Conjunctival | |
Agent	Onset	Scrapings	Treatment
AgNO₃	24 hrs	No organisms	None
Gonococcus	2–6 days	Gram negative intracellular diplococci	Topical and systemic penicillin
Bacteria	3+ days	Cocci or rods	Topical antibiotic
Chlamydia	5–14 days	Intracytoplasmic inclusions	Topical sulfa

apy (probing) if patency is not established prior to the age of six months or if acute inflammation of the lacrimal sac occurs.

IRITIS. This is a sterile inflammation of the iris and adjacent intraocular structures that may result in irreversible ocular damage and blindness if not treated. Children frequently fail to report ocular symptoms until such changes have occurred, and external signs (e.g., injection) may be minimal. Therefore, it is important to be alert to ocular signs of iritis, especially alterations in size or shape of the pupil. Many cases of iritis in childhood occur in association with juvenile rheumatoid arthritis, and special attention should be given to the eyes in the periodic examination of such patients.

INJURIES

The eye tolerates injury poorly, since the processes involved in repair of injuries may lead to destruction and opacification of the normally transparent ocular media with resultant permanent decrease in vision. Unfortunately, children are particularly prone to injuries. Spectacles are of great protective value, and most children who have lost vision in one eye should wear protective lenses (at least in hazardous situations) to protect vision in the remaining eye. In the past, many serious eye injuries were related to laceration of the globe by broken spectacles, but modern lenses are produced from specially treated glass. Only through the cooperation of legislative bodies, thoughtful parents and others will the terrible toll in children's vision taken by fireworks, air rifles, arrows and other missiles be reduced.

Specific suggestions for the initial management of several injuries follows. Remember that a single instillation of topical anesthetic (e.g., 0.5 per cent proparacaine) is often necessary and always permissible to facilitate examination, but that repeated instillations damage the cornea. Topical anesthetics should never be prescribed for continued use.

Corneal abrasion. When the surface epithelium of the cornea is damaged, the patient experiences tearing, photophobia and severe pain. The pain usually is described as a foreign body sensation, usually under the upper eyelid. The corneal epi-thelial defect often can be seen with a flashlight, especially if highlighted by staining with sodium fluorescein applied from a sterile paper strip. Do not use fluorescein solutions, as they are apt to be contaminated with bacteria. The mainstay of treatment is immobilization of the eyelid by a tight patch so that the eyelid does not remove the epithelial cells as they slide to fill the defect. A single dose of a sulfa or antibiotic solution usually is instilled, as is a drop of short-acting cycloplegic (1 per cent Cyclogyl or 2 per cent Homatropine). The patient should be given an analgesic and told to remain at rest with both eyes closed until healing is complete, usually within 24 hours. Over-wearing of contact lenses and exposure to ultraviolet energy (sunlamps, arc welders) also produce corneal epithelial injury, which should be treated in the same manner.

Foreign bodies. Foreign bodies of low velocity such as cinders that can be seen on the surface of the cornea or conjunctiva can be removed easily after topical anesthesia by irrigation with a sterile solution or by a moist cotton applicator. Foreign bodies lodged more securely in the cornea may require removal by the use of a spud or hypodermic needle directed tangentially to the cornea. If the corneal epithelium is disrupted by the foreign body or its removal, treatment should be instituted as described above for a corneal abrasion.

Contusions. Blunt injuries to the globe may result in ecchymoses of the lids and conjunctiva. These are of little consequence and clear spontaneously. Reduction of visual acuity, however, should alert the examiner that intraocular damage may exist, and ophthalmic consultation should be requested. Of particular danger is blood in the anterior chamber (hyphema), because of the propensity for secondary hemorrhage with development of glaucoma and other complications. Be alert also to complaints of double vision after a blow to the eye, since acute compression of the orbital contents may lead to a fracture of the orbital floor (blowout fracture) with entrapment of extraocular muscles.

Penetrating wounds. Although microsurgical techniques and the development of better suture materials have improved the prognosis for lacerations of the globe, prevention of such injuries is the only really satisfactory solution at present. Initial treatment by the non-ophthalmologist for a penetrating injury of the globe consists of application of a protective dressing and immediate consultation. Similar advice is appropriate for lacerations of the eyelids that involve lid margins.

Chemical injuries. The eye is subject to a variety of chemical insults, both accidentally and intentionally inflicted. The most devastating of these are alkaline solutions, particularly lye. Urgent treatment consists of copious irrigation with any available non-toxic irrigating solution, most commonly tap water. The child will resist such treatment, and the lids must be forcibly separated in order to let the running water contact the eye directly. Irrigation should be continued for a minimum of five minutes by the clock, at which time the patient should be evacuated to the nearest emergency center for repeated irrigation and further care. Chemical eye injuries represent one of the most urgent situations in all of medical practice, and one in which the initial treatment (irrigation) is a major determinant of the visual result.

AMBLYOPIA AND STRABISMUS

Strabismus includes all situations in which the eyes are not parallel with one another, including crossed eyes (esotropia), eyes that deviate outwardly (exotropia), and eyes that deviate vertically (hypertropia). Some cases of strabismus are due to a palsy of one or more of the extraocular muscles, but most ocular deviations in childhood have no demonstrable neuromuscular deficit. Children with strabismus may use either eye equally well and equally frequently (alternating strabismus). Some children, however, use one eye to the exclusion of the other, and therein lies the risk for development of amblyopia since the developing visual system requires stimulation in order to achieve normal vision.

Amblyopia refers to any reduction in visual acuity, but most commonly is used to refer to reduction of visual acuity due to non-use of the eye that occurs in non-alternating strabismus, prolonged occlusion of an eye, or pronounced difference in refrac-

tive error. If proper therapy is not instituted prior to maturity of the visual system, which occurs at approximately six years of age, future treatment will be to little avail, and the child will face a lifetime of reduced vision in one eye. Treatment consists of occlusion of the non-amblyopic eye, forcing use of the amblyopic eye. Surgical correction of strabismus often produces cosmetic improvement and may improve the capacity for binocular single vision (fusion), but usually has no effect upon amblyopia.

WHEN TO REFER. Visual acuity testing as described in this chapter should be part of the well-child examination regardless of age. Reduced vision may indicate amblyopia and requires prompt referral to an ophthalmologist if treatment is to be effective.

Random movements of the eyes may be seen before the age of six months, but constant strabismus at any age or intermittent strabismus after the age of six months should be cause for referral to an ophthalmologist without delay. Strabismus accounts for more than one half of all cases of amblyopia. Note that the other cases of amblyopia will have no easily detectable outward signs, however, and will be discovered only through visual acuity testing.

NEURO-OPHTHALMOLOGY

The eye is an extension of the brain, and many neurological disorders have eye manifestations. Selected comments relative to neuro-ophthalmology in children follow.

Pupils. The normal pupil should be round, regular and responsive to light. Pupillary inequality in size may be due to neurological or ocular disease requiring further investigation, but such pupils generally have altered responsiveness as well as abnormal size. Be especially alert to:

1. Small differences in pupillary size with normal reactivity in a healthy child. A small difference in the size of normal pupils is not unusual, and further investigation may be delayed if there are no other neurological or ocular signs.

2. A fixed, dilated pupil that has appeared suddenly as the only sign of ocular or neurological disease. Most often this

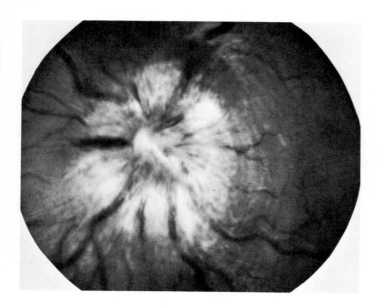

Figure 29–3   Swelling of optic disc due to increased cerebrospinal fluid pressure (papilledema).

pupillary abnormality occurs from accidental or intentional exposure to a pharmacological agent (e.g., atropine) or a naturally occurring alkaloid (e.g., Jimson weed). This diagnosis usually can be made by an ophthalmologist by pharmacological testing (pilocarpine), and confirmation of all isolated pupillary abnormalities by an ophthalmologist prior to invasive neurological investigation usually is wise.

Eye movements.   Although most cases of strabismus in childhood are of developmental origin, cranial nerve palsies also may lead to strabismus. Children quickly learn to suppress the image from one eye to avoid the expected double vision, and chronic cranial nerve palsies may be difficult to distinguish from non-paralytic strabismus.

Optic disc.   Swelling of the optic disc due to increased cerebrospinal fluid pressure (papilledema) is an ophthalmoscopic finding of great importance (Fig. 29–3). Fully developed papilledema is detected easily, but early papilledema may be difficult to differentiate from normal. In such cases, serial observation may be warranted. Also, since papilledema may be mimicked by developmental variations, confirmation of any but typical cases by an ophthalmologist prior to detailed neurological investigation generally is desirable.

Visual fields.   Although young children will not submit to formal perimetry, neurologically significant field loss often can be detected by observing the child's response or lack of response to movements or objects in various positions in the field of vision.

REFERENCES

General

Ophthalmology Study Guide for Students and Practitioners of Medicine, 2nd ed. Rochester, Minn., American Academy of Ophthalmology, 1976.
Harley, R. D.: *Pediatric Ophthalmology.* Philadelphia, W. B. Saunders Company, 1975.
Newell, F. W., and Ernest, J. T.: *Ophthalmology: Principles and Concepts.* 3rd ed. St. Louis, C. V. Mosby Company, 1974.

Ophthalmoscopy

Bishop, J. O., and Madsen, E. C.: Retinoblastoma. Review of the current status. Surv. Ophthalmol., 19:342, 1975.
Patz, A.: Retrolental fibroplasia. Surv. Ophthalmol., 14:1, 1969.

Glaucoma

Shaffer, R. N., and Weiss, D. I.: *Congenital and Pediatric Glaucoma.* St. Louis, C. V. Mosby Company, 1970.

Inflamed Eye

Ostler, H. B.: Oculo-genital disease. Surv. Ophthalmol., 20:233, 1976.
Thompson, T. R., Swanson, R. E., and Wiesner, P. J.: Gonococcal ophthalmia neonatorum. J.A.M.A., 288:186, 1974.

Injuries

Paton, D., and Goldberg, M. F.: *Management of Ocular Injuries.* Philadelphia, W. B. Saunders Company, 1976.

Amblyopia and Strabismus

Burian, H., and von Noorden, G.: *Binocular Vision and Ocular Motility.* St. Louis, C. V. Mosby Company, 1974.

Neuro-ophthalmology

Walsh, F. B., and Hoyt, W. F.: *Clinical Neuro-ophthalmology.* Volumes 1–3, 3rd ed. Baltimore, The Williams & Wilkins Company, 1969.

Hearing, Language, and Speech Disorders

30

LuVern H. Kunze and Gary Thompson

Health professionals are frequently asked for an opinion concerning a child's ability to communicate, including the adequacy of his hearing and the degree to which his language and speech are developing normally. Because this occurs, health professionals need some understanding of the skills involved in communication, the way in which these skills develop in children and the disorders related to these skills that are common among children in order to screen young patients and make appropriate referrals.

Communication can be divided into receptive and expressive skills. Disorders may effect the child's function in any one or more of these skills.

RECEPTIVE SKILLS AND DISORDERS

Hearing Loss

Hearing loss interferes with the communication process to various degrees depending upon the extent and type of impairment present. The nature of hearing loss can best be understood through discussion of commonly used testing procedures.

Pure-tone audiometry. The two most important attributes of sound are frequency (measured in hertz [Hz]) and intensity (measured in decibels [dB]). Frequency and intensity are perceived by the auditory system as pitch and loudness. The normal ear is capable of responding to a wide range of frequencies, but only a portion of this range is important for hearing and understanding speech. Accordingly, the typi-

cal hearing assessment of a child includes measurement at 250, 500, 1000, 2000, 3000 and 4000 Hz. Hearing loss is measured in dB relative to a standard reference. The standard reference (O-dB hearing level [HL]) represents the amount of sound pressure required by the average normal ear to detect a sound. An audiometer is used to present tones in a controlled manner to the child via ear phones, a loudspeaker or a bone oscillator. When ear phones are used to deliver test signals, the process is called *air-conduction* testing. When a bone oscillator is used, the process is called *bone-conduction* testing. The use and interpretation of hearing tests are summarized in Table 30-1.

Audiometric responses can be classified as falling in the normal range (0 to 20 dB), mild hearing-loss range (20 to 40 dB), moderate hearing-loss range (40 to 60 dB) and severe hearing-loss range (60 dB and greater). Hearing levels of 30, 45 and 60 dB HL correspond roughly to soft, medium and loud conversational levels. It follows that if a child has a hearing loss in excess of 60 dB, he hears very little speech without the use of amplification. Even a relatively mild sensorineural or conductive hearing loss can have a significant effect on communication skills. For example, children with fluctuating conductive hearing impairment have poorer speech and language skills than matched controls without a history of middle-ear involvement (Holm and Kunze).

Some children have selective hearing loss, in which low frequency sounds are heard normally but middle and high frequency sounds are heard poorly. These

291

TABLE 30–1   HEARING LOSS TYPES AND LOCATION OF PATHOLOGY WITHIN AUDITORY SYSTEM

Conductive loss.........................Pathology:	Outer ear or middle ear, or both
	Audiometric results: Loss for air conduction
	Normal bone conduction
Sensorineural loss.....................Pathology:	Cochlea or 8th nerve, or both
	Audiometric results: Loss for air conduction
	Similar loss for bone conduction
Mixed loss.............................Pathology:	Outer ear or middle ear *and* cochlea or 8th nerve
	Audiometric results: Loss for air conduction
	Loss for bone conduction, but less than for air conduction

children appear to hear well because they are able to respond to many sounds including low-frequency components of speech at very soft levels. Speech understanding is severely impaired, however, since many speech sounds are heard either poorly or not at all.

Children with selective hearing loss are often misdiagnosed as being emotionally disturbed, brain injured or mentally retarded. Early identification of these children can lead to appropriate diagnosis and optimal educational management.

Tympanometry. Tympanometry is a procedure by which compliance of the ear drum is measured as a function of varying air pressure in the external ear canal. The normal ear shows greatest compliance when the ear canal is at normal atmospheric pressure. As positive or negative pressure is applied, compliance of the ear drum is reduced. In contrast, if the middle ear contains fluid, compliance of the ear drum does not vary significantly as a function of air pressure changes in the ear canal. If there is negative pressure in the middle ear with perhaps retracted drums, a compliance peak may be observed, but only when negative pressure is applied to the ear canal. Tympanometry has become a sensitive indicator of the physical characteristics of the ear drum and middle ear. In combination with direct physical examination and audiometry, it represents a powerful diagnostic tool. For a more complete description of tympanometry and other procedures designed to measure impedance characteristics of the auditory system, the reader is referred to Northern and Downs (see References at the close of this chapter).

Speech audiometry. Speech audiometry provides direct information about the reception and discrimination of speech. *Speech reception* testing determines the softest level at which speech can "just be heard." *Speech discrimination* testing assesses how well speech can be understood when it is presented at various levels above threshold.

Test methods vary according to the questions the examiner is attempting to answer. For example, sometimes it is important to determine the intensity required for maximum discrimination performance even if that level reaches 100 dB on the hearing loss dial. This information can be used to make predictions about benefit from hearing-aid use. Or the examiner may be interested in testing discrimination performance at levels corresponding to soft, medium and loud conversation. Results allow inference about how a child understands speech in his everyday environment, particularly if testing is done in the presence of competing noise designed to simulate a real-life setting.

Sensorineural hearing loss often produces impaired speech discrimination performance regardless of speech level. As a result, some persons believe that hearing aids are not beneficial for children with severe cochlear damage. This is simply not the case. The amplified speech may not be perceived clearly but, nevertheless, provides the child with auditory cues he otherwise would not hear. These auditory cues in combination with visual cues (lip reading), parent counseling, language and speech training and appropriate educational placement provide the basis for proper management of the severely hearing-impaired child.

Symptoms of hearing loss. For expected auditory behaviors of the infant and young child, refer to the section about the schedule of receptive language development later in this chapter. If such behavior is not present, be alert to the possibility of hearing loss and subsequent referral.

The following symptoms suggest the possibility of hearing loss in school-age children:

Case History Information

1. High-risk infancy: maternal rubella, birth trauma, hearing loss in family.
2. History of upper respiratory infections including middle-ear problems
3. Poor vocabulary and speech development
4. Parental and teacher concern
5. Inconsistent response to soft speech
6. Inappropriate response to questions
7. Inconsistent response to environmental sounds, e.g., responds to a door closing but not to a telephone (could suggest selective high-frequency hearing loss)
8. Difficulty locating the source of sound (could suggest a hearing loss in one ear)
9. Poor schoolwork, particularly in class discussion
10. Poor attention and behavior problems

Direct Observations

1. No response when child's name is called softly
2. Inability to follow simple instructions
3. No response to environmental sounds or noisemakers such as bells, jingling keys or crinkling paper. Note: If gross tests are attempted with noisemakers, make sure that visual cues are not presented to the child. Also, be aware that many noisemakers produce considerable intensity. A child with a mild-to-moderate hearing loss would be expected to respond to many noisemakers. Consequently, only relatively severe hearing loss can be detected with gross noisemaker tests.
4. If tuning-fork tests are used, be aware of their limitations. Young children often respond poorly to pure tones even if their hearing is normal. Furthermore, children often have trouble telling which ear a sound is in or whether a sound is louder or soften than another one. Many fork tests require these kinds of responses, which are difficult for youngsters to make. Considerable experience and careful interpretation are essential to proper administration of tuning-fork tests on children.
5. Audiometric pure-tone screening is probably the most effective method for identifying hearing loss, provided it is done by someone who has adequate knowledge of basic screening procedures. Children who have sufficient language ability to follow verbal instructions can ordinarily be screened with little difficulty. Very young children or children with limited communication skills often must be referred to a clinical audiologist for evaluation.

Referral. The sooner hearing loss is detected, the better it is for the child because early management maximizes speech and language development and educational success. When a hearing loss is suspected—regardless of the age of the child—referral should be made for audiological testing. Management of the disorder depends on the type and extent of the impairment. Many conductive losses can be eliminated or at least substantially improved by otological procedures. Sensorineural hearing loss, which is generally not responsive to medical treatment, is responsive to educational management. Educational management includes consideration of amplification, auditory training, lip reading, speech and language therapy, special classroom considerations either in a regular classroom or a classroom for the hearing-impaired, and parental counseling.

Understanding

A child must acquire the ability to understand what is said to him. He achieves this by relating words to objects, actions and ideas in his environment. The meaning that a child assigns to a word represents the sum of all of his experiences with that word. As a result, the meaning of a given word changes over time. Meaning would be expected to develop from the specific to the general, e.g., "dog" is first applied to a family pet, then to a class of animals. He may also generalize the use of a word; e.g., "dog" may be applied to all animals. With further experience, he adjusts to a class that is consistent with common use.

Understanding phrases and sentences is a more complex matter. The sum of experiences continues to determine meanings assigned to individual words in the sentences. Meaning is added or altered on the basis of other factors, however, e.g., word order, conceptual relationships between words, prefixes and suffixes added to words and inflectional patterns.

Unfortunately, not all children learn to assign meaning to words and word combinations. With the hearing-handicapped child this can readily be understood. Not all children who hear adequately learn to assign meaning to words and sentences which they hear, however, e.g., the child who will echo an instruction precisely but not understand what he is to do. Because words have no meaning for them, some of these children stop attending when they are spoken to and may appear to have a hearing impairment. Some children, who are able to assign appropriate meaning to single words but who lack the ability to relate words in a sentence, will respond to a single word in an instruction but not respond to the instruction itself in an appropriate manner; e.g., he may identify the object named but not carry out the designated action.

Because receptive language skills are acquired in a predictable order, a child can be evaluated by comparison with his peers. The following is a schedule of expected receptive behavior characteristics at six-month intervals. The behavior types listed at each age level are selected from those found by Hedrick and Prather to be correctly used by 75 per cent of the children in their samples.

Schedule of Receptive Language Development

6 Months
1. Turns head (but may not locate), quiets, alerts or makes other consistent change in behavior when sound (e.g., doorbell, rattle, human voice) occurs.

12 Months
1. Locates speaker quickly and accurately when his name is called at conversational level
2. Looks at or goes to person named when asked, "Where's Daddy (Mama)?"
3. Responds to "No, no" spoken sharply

18 Months
1. Identifies when asked two body parts, favorite foods, toys, etc.
2. Follows one- and two-word commands when given *with gestures* (e.g., look, sit down, come here, get the _____)

24 Months
1. Correctly identifies four body parts, six objects and members of the family when instructed, "Show me the _____" or "Point to the _____," *without gesture*
2. Follows instruction containing preposition "in" (e.g., "Put it in the _____.")
3. Responds with appropriate behavior to questions (e.g., gets coat or goes to door when asked, "Are you ready to go?" or "Ready to go bye-bye?")

30 Months
1. Understands prepositions "in" and "on," pronouns "I," "you" and "me"
2. Identifies five body parts named for him

36 Months
1. Understands (may not use) names of games, taking turns, comparisons (e.g., big–little, fast–slow, hard–soft), prepositions "in," "on" and "beside," and penny (not other coins)
2. Follows instruction involving two objects and two actions (e.g., "Put the cup on the table and give me your plate")
3. Identifies two colors and objects or pictures from descriptions (e.g., "Show me what mama cooks on")

40 Months
1. Identifies five or six colors
2. Understands prepositions, "in," "on," "beside" and "under"

48 Months
1. Has number concepts to three (e.g., will give one, two or three objects on command)
2. Follows commands involving three objects and three actions (e.g., "Put the car on the floor, give me the bear and open the book")

Any child who fails all of the items at his age level and the immediately preceding level should be referred for evaluation.

EXPRESSIVE SKILLS AND DISORDERS

Expressive skills can be divided into language functions and speech functions.

Language

Use of expressive language includes a number of tasks not necessarily performed in any specified sequence: (1) the child selects the words which he will employ to express his ideas (vocabulary); (2) he chooses the form of the word he wishes to use (grammar); and (3) he determines the order in which the words will appear (syntax).

Children who experience disabilities in expressive language may be deficient in any or all of these skills. Word-finding problems are observed in children who can describe an object or occurrence in detail but cannot think of the name usually attached to it; e.g., the child who, when shown a picture of a stove, can say, "It's hot and mother cooks on it," but cannot name it. Other children appear to have vocabulary readily available but do not use the correct forms of the words they select, e.g., the child who uses only present tense verbs or who has no plural nouns. These children seem to have failed to acquire the rules that govern grammatical functions of the language. Still other children seem able to select the vocabulary and may or may not use the correct grammatical forms but seem unable to learn to order the parts of a sentence in acceptable sequence, e.g., the child who states "Climb Mama mountain" for "Mama climbed the mountain." As demonstrated by this example, these children also tend to omit words from sentences. Omitted words are usually those that carry little or no meaning, such as articles, conjunctions and prepositions.

Like receptive skills, expressive language skills are acquired in a predictable order, and evaluation of a child must be made in relation to his peers. The behavior characteristics listed at each age level in the schedule below are slected from those found by Hedrick and Prather to be correctly used by 75 per cent of the children in their sample.

Schedule of Expressive Language Development

6 Months
1. Laughs aloud
2. Cries in response to environment or bodily needs

3. Babbles and makes repeated sounds (e.g., "da-da-da") Note: Be concerned about the "good baby," i.e., one who lies quietly when awake, making no vocal sounds
12 Months
1. Increases his vocalization
2. Imitates sound and inflectional patterns
3. Objects by crying or vocalization when toy is taken from him
18 Months
1. Points and vocalizes to get what he wants (may not use intelligible words)
2. Uses consistent combinations of sounds to stand for words (may not be correct)
3. Says "no" when interfered with
24 Months
1. Asks "What's that?"
2. Names objects and people when asked, "What's (Who's) that?"
3. Uses recognizable words to get some things he wants (names of people and objects)
4. Uses two- and three-word combinations
30 Months
1. Asks "Why?" or "How come?"
2. Uses pronoun "I," descriptive words (e.g., pretty, big), present tense and "-ing" forms of verbs, regular pleurals and contractions (I'm, I'll, don't)
3. Tells about experiences from immediate past (e.g., what he did outdoors, what a sibling did, what happened on television)
4. Uses four- and five-word sentences
36 Months
1. Asks "why" questions in complete form (e.g., "Why does he do that?")
2. Responds to questions
   a. "Do you want _____?" with "yes" or "no"
   b. "What are you playing?" by naming toy or game
   c. "How are you?" with "fine" or "OK"
   d. "What do you wear on your feet?" by showing shoes or saying "shoes"
   e. "What do you do when you're hungry?" with appropriate verbal response
   f. "If you had a penny, what would you do?" with appropriate verbal response
3. Uses five- and six-word sentences *correctly*

40 Months
1. Answers questions
   a. "What says meow?" with "cat" or "kitty"
   b. "What animals do you see at the zoo?" by naming two or three
2. Uses seven- and eight-word sentences *correctly*
3. Talks in paragraphs (i.e., ideas strung together in sentence-like constructions)

48 Months
1. Uses future tense of verbs (e.g., I will do it), irregular plurals (e.g., men, women), past tense verbs (e.g., walked, ran) and possessive pronouns (e.g., my, his, hers)
2. Uses sentences having dependent clauses (complex sentences)

If a child does not display any of the behavior for his age level or the immediately previous level, he should be referred for evaluation.

Speech

Speech activities include motor functions that make it possible for the child to produce words in an intelligible manner, including phonation, articulation and rhythmic production.

Phonation is defined as the production of sound by the vocal folds. Most children phonate easily, producing a broad variety of sounds in terms of pitch and loudness without trauma to the vocal folds. A few have abnormal vocal folds or develop habits of phonation that result in vocal abuse, however. The primary symptom of these problems is an unusual voice characteristic, e.g., harshness, hoarseness or breathiness. When such characteristics are present, they not only interfere with communication but also suggest the need for treatment to prevent further trauma and danger to the child's health. Children exhibiting phonation problems should be referred for thorough medical examination.

The sound produced in phonation is amplified differentially to produce the sounds that are combined to form words. This articulation requires very rapid and precise movement of the velum, jaw, tongue and lips. Like all other motor skills, articulation develops fairly predictably over time. The order in which sounds are mastered is also fairly predictable. The most common articulatory disorders involve sounds learned in the later stages of development. Articulatory disorders are usually classified as functional (those that are learned) and organic (those that result from structural defects or lack of neuromuscular control of the articulators). A child whose parents are concerned about his articulation after 48 months of age should be referred for evaluation.

Normally, speech is produced in a smooth, rhythmic manner with the speaker controlling rate and rhythm patterns. There are exceptions, however, some of which are considered normal, some of which are considered normal at certain stages of development and some of which are considered abnormal. Most speakers will break their rhythm pattern while searching for words. At these times they may vocalize "ah" or "um" or some other syllable or may repeat syllables, words or phrases previously used. Children from four to six years of age are particularly likely to do this. These years are frequently referred to as a period of normal dysfluency.

The abnormal form of dysfluency is commonly referred to as stuttering or stammering. Parents sometimes view normal dysfluency with anxiety, fearing that their child is becoming a stutterer. A child should be referred for evaluation anytime the parents express concern about stuttering.

Referral

Early identification and treatment of language and speech disorders is vital to the social growth and academic success of the child. When a child fails to meet the criteria for satisfactory language development or when he exhibits voice, articulation or dysfluency problems, he should be referred to a clinical speech pathologist or communication disorders specialist for evaluation and treatment.

REFERENCES

Holm, V. A., and Kunze, L. H.: Effects of chronic otitis media on language and speech development. Pediatrics, *43*:833, 1969.

Hedrick, D. L., and Prather, E. M.: *Sequenced Inventory of Language Development*, Experimental Edition. Seattle, Child Development and Mental Retardation Center, University of Washington, 1970.

General Reading

Davis, H., and Silverman, S. R.: *Hearing and Deafness*, 3rd ed. New York, Holt, Rinehart and Winston, 1970.

Frisina, D. R.: Measurement of hearing in children. *In* Jerger, J.: *Modern Developments in Audiology.* New York, Academic Press, 1963.

Northern, J. L., and Downs, M. P.: *Hearing in Children.* Baltimore, The Williams & Wilkins Company, 1974.

Van Riper, C. (Ed.), *The Foundations of Speech Pathology Series.* Inglewood Cliffs, N.J., Prentice Hall.

Carrell, J. A.: *Disorders of Articulation*, 1968.

Moore, G. P.: *Organic Voice Disorders*, 1971.

Murphy, A. T.: *Functional Voice Disorders*, 1964.

O'Neill, J. J.: *The Hard of Hearing*, 1964.

Robinson, F. B.: *Introduction to Stuttering*, 1964.

Wood, N. E.: *Delayed Speech and Language Development*, 1964.

PART XI

OTHER DISORDERS

31

Cardiovascular Disorders

Beverly C. Morgan and Isamu Kawabori

The purpose of this chapter is to provide information that may be helpful in the routine evaluation and care of infants and children with cardiac problems.

HEART DISEASE IN INFANCY

Six of every 1000 infants are born with congenital heart disease. It is estimated that, without surgical intervention, half of these children die during the first year of life. More than 70 per cent of these infants may now be aided by corrective or palliative surgery if warranted by their symptoms. A positive outlook, therefore, should be assumed toward severely ill infants with congenital heart defects.

Serious heart disease in infants is indicated by the development of congestive heart failure or hypoxia, and the onset of these complications warrants prompt cardiac consultation.

Congestive heart failure has relatively rapid onset in infants. The history often reveals rapid respirations, weak cry, easy fatigability (most notable in poor feeding) and failure to gain weight. The physical examination typically discloses the classic triad of findings in infants with congestive heart failure: tachypnea, tachycardia and hepatomegaly. Venous distention is difficult to evaluate in infants, and liver size is more helpful in evaluating right-sided heart failure. Pulmonary rales usually indicate pneumonia, although left ventricular failure and pulmonary venous congestion are not rare. Peripheral and periorbital edema are uncommon and suggest severe failure. Cardiomegaly is virtually always present. In the presence of relatively mild congestive heart failure the physician may choose to refer the infant for medical therapy, as well as for definitive diagnosis and possible surgery. Severe, progressive congestive heart failure, however, presents a medical emergency, and immediate therapy may be required while arrangements for transfer are in progress.

Digoxin is recommended for digitalization of pediatric patients for several reasons. The use of a single digitalis preparation avoids potentially lethal dosage errors associated with confusion between drugs with similar names, and digoxin has the advantage of relatively rapid excretion, thereby decreasing the hazards of digitalis intoxication. Table 31–1 outlines pediatric dosage. The intramuscular route of digoxin administration results in less predictable absorption from the injection site both in time and amount, as well as causing local pain. Digoxin studies indicate that intramuscular digoxin has only about 80 per cent of the bioavailability as intravenous digoxin. Diuretics are frequently necessary in severe congestion, but the associated reduction in serum potassium may precipitate digitalis intoxication unless supplemental potassium is provided. Supportive measures, including rest, oxygen administration, and low sodium formula, may be required.

Digitalis intoxication is a potentially fatal complication, and the therapeutic advantage to be gained from digitalization in congenital heart disease is relatively small; therefore, digitalis should be used only in moderate doses with electrocardiographic monitoring. A predigitalization electrocardiogram is important in evaluating sub-

TABLE 31-1 DIGITALIS DOSAGE AND DURATION

Drug	Route	Digitalization	Maintenance	Onset of Effect	Maximal Effect	Duration
Digoxin	Oral	<2 yrs: 0.07 mg/kg >2 yrs and prematures: 0.05 mg/kg	25–30% daily 25–30% daily	1 hr	7 hr	3 days
	IV	75% above	—	10 min	4 hr	3 days

sequent tracings. There is no proof that "pushing" digitalis is more effective than a moderate dose in pediatric patients. The principle symptoms of digitalis intoxication are gastrointestinal, such as anorexia, nausea, vomiting, and diarrhea, and cardiac, including increasing congestive heart failure, bradycardia, heart block greater than first degree, paroxysmal atrial tachycardia with block, nodal tachycardia and ventricular premature beats. The presence of first degree atrioventricular block as evidenced by prolongation of the P-R interval warrants extreme caution in the administration of additional digitalis. For non-life–threatening arrhythmias induced by digitalis intoxication, withholding one to several doses of digoxin and reinstitution of maintenance digoxin at a reduced level is therapeutic. For severe digitalis-induced arrhythmias, particularly the tachyarrhythmias, intravenous administration of potassium with electrocardiographic monitoring is the treatment of choice, assuming normal renal function. Intravenous diphenylhydantoin and lidocaine are also effective for digitalis arrhythmias, particularly with a high-grade block. Infants and children require larger doses per kilogram than do adult cardiac patients. Normal therapeutic serum digoxin levels in infants and children may be at levels that would be considered toxic in adults.

Paroxysmal hyperpnea with hypoxic or blue spells may complicate the course of infants with heart defects. Infants with cyanotic congenital heart defects and decreased pulmonary blood flow may have these episodes, characterized by paroxysms of increasing rate and depth of breathing, with increasing cyanosis and limpness. These spells may lead to permanent brain damage or death. Improvement usually results if the infant is placed in the knee-chest position, which older infants may spontaneously assume. Intramuscular administration of morphine (1 mg/5 kg) is necessary in more severe cases, and rarely, general anesthesia is required to interrupt the attack. Oral propranolol (0.5 to 2.0 mg/kg/dose qid) has been advocated for longer periods of relief, but surgical intervention is usually necessary.

Additional indications for early cardiological consultation include significant cyanosis, failure to thrive or repeated pulmonary infections in an infant with a murmur. Abnormalities of chest roentgenogram or electrocardiogram are not in themselves indications for special studies in an asymptomatic infant, although occasional exceptions occur, particularly with cardiomegaly. The presence of a murmur alone is rarely, if ever, an indication for catheterization in an asymptomatic infant with a normal electrocardiogram and heart size.

Paroxysmal supraventricular tachycardia (atrial or nodal) may occur in infants without structural cardiac anomalies, but it is infrequent in those with congenital heart disease. Since untreated paroxysmal supraventricular tachycardia may progress to congestive heart failure with relative rapidity, therapy should be instituted promptly. Vagal stimulation by unilateral carotid massage or gagging may be attempted but is usually not successful unless the patient is given digitalis. Orbital pressure should not be attempted. Digitalization is successful in abolishing the arrhythmia in most infants. For the rare patient who does not respond to digitalization, phenylephrine (Neo-Synephrine) 0.01 mg/kg diluted and given slowly intravenously to raise the blood pressure by 50 per cent will almost invariably restore normal sinus rhythm. Digitalis, propranolol and reserpine have been used effectively for supraventricular tachyarrhythmias for long-term management.

HEART DISEASE IN CHILDHOOD

Management of the older child with heart disease is simpler in many respects than that of the infant. If he has survived the first year without significant symptoms, his progress throughout childhood is usually good. Nevertheless, additional problems may present in older children, such as evaluation of the significance of heart murmurs and management of episodes of chest pain or ectopic beats. Decisions may need to be made about prophylaxis against bacterial endocarditis, as well as the imposition of exercise restrictions for the child with a cardiac defect.

The incidence of murmurs in normal infants, children and adolescents is as high as 50 per cent. Murmurs are graded on a scale from 1 to 6; a grade 1/6 murmur is very soft and difficult to hear, grade 2/6 murmur is soft, grade 3/6 murmur is easily heard, grade 4/6 and louder murmurs are always associated with a thrill (a palpable murmur), grade 5/6 murmur can be heard with the edge of the stethoscope just touching the chest and a grade 6/6 murmur is audible with the stethoscope off the chest wall. Because of the high incidence of murmurs in normal children, it is obviously necessary to differentiate a significant murmur from an innocent one. An approach suggested by Dr. Alexander Nadas has been to use the following criteria to aid in this diagnosis:

Major	Minor
Systolic murmur louder than 3/6	Systolic murmur less than 3/6
Diastolic murmur	Abnormal electrocardiogram
Congestive heart failure	Abnormal roentgenogram appearance
Cyanosis	Abnormal pulmonary second sound
	Abnormal blood pressure

One major or two minor criteria strongly suggest a diagnosis of congenital heart disease.

The three most common innocent or insignificant murmurs are (1) the physiological ejection murmur at the second left interspace, (2) the jugular venous hum and (3) the vibratory or "twanging string" left sternal border systolic murmur. The physiological ejection murmur in the second left interspace is similar to the murmur of a secundum atrial septal defect, but differentiation can be aided by careful auscultation of the second heart sound in the pulmonic area and confirmed by radiological changes. With the innocent physiological ejection murmur, normal splitting of the second heart sound occurs with a narrowing or obliteration of the splitting during expiration, while with an atrial septal defect, the second heart sound is widely split through all phases of the respiratory cycle. A normal heart size with normal pulmonary vascular markings rules out a significant atrial defect. Although the murmur of a jugular venous hum occurring throughout systole and diastole may be confused initially with a patent ductus arteriosus, the venous hum disappears or dramatically diminishes in intensity in the supine position.

Once a murmur is thought organic or significant or a serious cardiac problem is considered present in the absence of murmurs, a decision needs to be made about when to refer the patient to a pediatric cardiologist for evaluation. If significant symptoms are present, the patient should, of course, be referred for consultation without delay. If the patient is asymptomatic, no urgency exists, and the referral may be made at the convenience of the family.

A cardiac evaluation includes a complete history, a thorough physical examination, an electrocardiogram and chest roentgenograms. The history should include inquiry into the presence of cyanosis, exercise tolerance, dyspnea, repeated pulmonary infections and chest pain. As with all pediatric patients, the family and prenatal histories are important. The history is most useful for clues concerning the severity of the disorder and is rarely diagnostic.

The physical examination should begin with attention to evidence of variations in normal growth and development. The presence or absence of cyanosis and clubbing should be noted. Blood pressures are measured routinely in the upper and lower extremities in the initial cardiac evaluation, even if palpable lower extremity pulses are present. Observation of respiratory effort is important, as is auscultation of the lungs.

Although palpation of the heart is informative in regard to the presence and location of thrills and determination of the point of maximum impulse, percussion is rarely rewarding in infants and children.

Careful auscultation should be performed while observing the first and particularly the second heart sound and recording the presence or absence of splitting and intensity of the second heart sound. The presence of murmurs and their timing and intensity with the point of maximum impulse and transmission should be reported.

A complete cardiac evaluation includes 12- or 13-lead electrocardiograms and frontal and lateral chest films, preferably a cardiac series with barium swallow. In the older child, the studies outlined here will provide an accurate diagnosis in approximately 80 to 90 per cent of patients.

The indications for catheterization in the older child are less stringent than in the infant, since the associated hazards are less. Significant symptoms, cardiomegaly or significant abnormality of the electrocardiogram may be adequate indication for diagnostic evaluation. A more difficult problem is the asymptomatic child with an organic murmur whose electrocardiogram and chest roentgenogram are normal. The decision for elective catheterization in such patients must be individualized and depends upon many factors, including the anxiety of the parents and the lesion clinically suspected. Occasionally, catheterization may be justified so that decisions can be made about insurability or participation in competitive athletics. Generally, however, diagnostic studies are only performed to establish whether or not operation is indicated. Certain congenital cardiovascular lesions, such as patent ductus arteriosus and coarctation of the aorta, can be diagnosed with sufficient assurance by clinical findings alone. Although the risk of catheterization is extremely small, potentially fatal complications may occur, and therefore, catheterization is not recommended as a routine procedure for all children with congenital heart disease.

Non-invasive procedures for evaluation include the application of ultrasound. Echocardiography, a procedure without risk, can contribute information not obtainable by other non-invasive techniques. Such data include chamber and vessel dimensions, wall thickness and motion, contractility, presence of pericardial fluid, valve motion, valvular thickening, discontinuities in structure such as overriding aorta discontinuous with the interventricular septum because of a ventricular septal defect, and abnormal structures. Cardiac catheterization and angiocardiography remain the standards by which other techniques are judged.

Decisions about surgical intervention in congenital heart disease should be based upon considerable knowledge of the natural history of various defects and the local surgical morbidity and mortality. When cardiovascular surgery is indicated as an elective procedure, it is generally recommended shortly before entry into school. There are several reasons for this, including the fact that surgery is well tolerated emotionally and physically by the young patient. This program allows the child to enter school without the stigma of heart disease. For these reasons, elective cardiac catheterization and angiocardiography are often performed at the age of four to six years.

Bacterial endocarditis is uncommon in the pediatric group. It may occur in older children, although it is rare in infancy. Since prophylactic antibiotic therapy decreases the incidence of this potentially disastrous complication, prophylaxis is indicated for dental extractions and manipulation of infected tissue in children with organic heart disease.

The question of exercise restriction is frequently raised. Children with severe congenital heart disease usually limit themselves in activity, and restriction in milder cases is generally not indicated. The exception is the teenage child with aortic stenosis for whom sudden death has been reported. The child with aortic stenosis who is asymptomatic and has a normal electrocardiogram and chest roentgenogram is generally allowed full activity except for continuously strenuous sports such as basketball or soccer. The presence of angina, syncope or significant abnormalities of the electrocardiogram warrants further limitation and the consideration of catheterization and surgery. The decision must be made for each individual in an attempt to allow optimum management of the cardiac lesion, without producing emotional or psychiatric problems for the child. Fortunately, moderate activity is healthy, even in children with significant heart disease.

Certain symptoms related to the cardiovascular system occur frequently in children without heart disease. Chest pain may cause great anxiety to the child and his parents. Although a careful history is usually adequate to rule out a cardiac origin, occasionally a chest roentgenogram, electrocardiogram and exercise tolerance test are indicated to rule out organic heart disease. Precordial pain is unusual in children with heart disease, although it occasionally occurs with severe aortic or pulmonic stenosis or pulmonary hypertension. Vague complaints of chest pain not associated with exertion in a child with an insignificant murmur and a normal electrocardiogram and roentgenogram are virtually always benign. Pericarditis may produce precordial pain, but associated clinical findings such as friction rub and S-T changes on the electrocardiogram aid in diagnosis.

Abnormalities of heart rate and rhythm are not uncommon in childhood and often occur in children without heart disease. Extrasystoles may be atrial, nodal or ventricular. They occur most commonly in normal children, but their presence may warrant evaluation. Increased frequency of ectopic beats with exercise suggests heart disease, whereas benign extrasystoles tend to disappear with exercise. Therapy, beyond reassurance, is rarely required.

DIFFERENTIAL DIAGNOSIS OF CONGENITAL HEART DISEASE

The differential diagnosis of congenital heart disease should be approached in a systematic, organized manner, with consideration of the physical findings, electrocardiogram and chest roentgenograms. An outline of such an approach is given in Table 31-3 and the pertinent pediatric cardiology abbreviations are set forth in Table 31-2.

The history is of less importance in the diagnosis, but of considerable value in assessing the severity of the disorder. Auscultation is absolutely essential in the acyanotic forms such as a patent ductus arteriosus, but is much less specific in the cyanotic type of congenital heart disease. An increase in hemoglobin or hematocrit value may confirm cyanosis, and serial determinations are useful to follow the course of hypoxia in cyanotic heart disease. The electrocardiogram is an excellent predictor of severity in disorders involving pressure overload such as pulmonic stenosis; the roentgenograms, however, usually show no cardiac enlargement in pressure overload unless failure supervenes. Roentgenograms are excellent predictors of volume overload as in atrial septal defect, whereas the electrocardiogram provides little correlation with the size of the shunt. Angiocardiograms are indispensable in the precise diagnosis of cyanotic disease but are only occasionally essential in the acyanotic, left-to-right shunts.

A synopsis of the findings in 10 of the most common forms of congenital heart defects included in the systematic approach to such defects in Table 31-3 is discussed in Tables 31-4 and 31-5. In the interest of brevity, only the more typical findings are presented for each lesion.

GENETICS OF CONGENITAL HEART DEFECTS

Approximately 5 per cent of children examined with heart disease have known as-

TABLE 31-2   TABLE OF ABBREVIATIONS

ASD	Atrial septal defect		PBF	Pulmonary blood flow
CHD	Congenital heart disease or defect		PDA	Patent ductus arteriosus
CHF	Congestive heart failure		RAD	Right axis deviation
CVH	Combined ventricular hypertrophy		R→L	Right to left
IVC	Inferior vena cava		RA	Right atrium
L→R	Left to right		RAE	Right atrial enlargement
LA	Left atrium		RV	Right ventricle
LAE	Left atrial enlargement		RVE	Right ventricular enlargement
LV	Left ventricle		RVH	Right ventricular hypertrophy
LVE	Left ventricular enlargement		RVP	Right ventricular pressure
LVH	Left ventricular hypertrophy		SBE	Subacute bacterial endocarditis
LVP	Left ventricular pressure		SVC	Superior vena cava
PA	Pulmonary artery		VSD	Ventricular septal defect
PAP	Pulmonary artery pressure			

TABLE 31–3 CLINICAL AND PHYSIOLOGICAL CLASSIFICATION
OF CONGENITAL HEART DISEASE*

Acyanotic			Cyanotic		
X-ray	ECG (EKG)	Suggested Diagnosis	X-ray	ECG (EKG)	Suggested Diagnosis
A. Normal pulmonary blood flow (No shunt)	RVH LVH	Pulmonic stenosis Mitral regurgitation Aortic stenosis Aortic regurgitation Coarctation Primary myocardial disease (including subendocardial sclerosis, anomalous coronary artery, glycogen storage disease, etc.)	A. Decreased pulmonary blood flow	RVH LVH CVH or R or LVH	Severe pulmonic stenosis with VSD (i.e., tetrad), ASD or PFO Severe pulmonary vascular obstruction ("Eisen- menger's physiology") with ASD, VSD, ductus, etc. Tricuspid atresia Truncus arteriosus with hypoplastic pulmonary arteries Ebstein's anomaly (severe conduction disturbances) Transposition with pulmonic stenosis
B. Increased pulmonary blood flow (L→R shunt)	RVH LVH	ASD, secundum type Partial anomalous pulmonary venous return (Incom- plete transposition of pulmonary veins) All L→R shunts with increased RV pressure VSD, small to moderate size PDA, small to moderate size ASD, primum type Arteriovenous fistula	B. Increased pulmonary blood flow	RVH CVH or R or LVH	Preductal coarctation with systemic RV (includes aortic atresia, hypoplastic LV syn- drome, etc.) Total anomalous pulmonary venous return (complete transposition of the pul- monary veins) Transposition of the great vessels Single ventricle Truncus arteriosus Pulmonary vascular obstruc- tion with bidirectional shunting

*A systematic approach to CHD is outlined in this table. By asking the proper questions one can utilize the clinical and simple laboratory tools to arrive at a logical differential diagnosis. One first needs to determine whether the patient is acyanotic or cyanotic. Next, by determining whether the pulmonary blood flow on the chest x-ray is normal, increased or decreased, one further narrows the range of possible abnormalities. Interpretation of the ECG as RVH, LVH or CVH brings one to a logical differential diagnosis in the majority of patients.

sociations with chromosomal abnormalities or other associated factors. Examples are patients with Down syndrome and with disorders due to congenital rubella or viral myocarditis. Occasionally a single gene etiology is implied. For example, asymmetrical septal hypertrophy has an autosomal dominant mode of inheritance associated with a family history of sudden death.

In the vast majority of patients with congenital heart disease (95 per cent), no direct cause can be identified. Family studies have shown that the frequency of having additional affected children is increased if one offspring (or one parent) is affected. This frequency of recurrence varies up to 4 to 5 per cent for the common

defects. These children usually are normal except for the congenital heart disease. This enhanced recurrence risk is considered to be the result of multiple gene effects, polygenic inheritance.

RHEUMATIC HEART DISEASE

Diseases, like society, undergo change; rheumatic fever in the United States appears to be less severe now and has a diminished recurrence risk, probably as a result of social factors, adequate treatment of early streptococcal infections and prophylaxis. Statistics show no change in incidence of first attacks of rheumatic fever,

TABLE 31-4 OPERABLE ACYANOTIC CONGENITAL HEART DISEASE: 6 MOST COMMON TYPES

Definition and Pathology	Incidence: % of CHD	Clinical Findings		
		History	*Physical Findings*	*Major Complications*
VENTRICULAR SEPTAL DEFECT (VSD) 1. Usually in the membranous septum, but size is more important than location in determining natural history 2. Position of the aorta is usually normal, but some overriding may occur, particularly if defect is large	20–25%	1. Dyspnea, exercise intolerance, pulmonary infections and congestive heart failure (CHF) occur with large defects 2. Pulmonary vascular disease occurs early with large defects, but rare otherwise 3. Spectrum varies from death in infancy to normal life span; size of defect determines course 4. Spontaneous closure occurs in up to one third	1. Loud harsh systolic murmur at low left sternal border 2. Apical diastolic rumble with large shunts 3. S_2 pulmonic area dependent on PA pressure; with high pressure, is loud and unsplit	1. CHF 2. Subacute bacterial endocarditis (SBE) 3. Pulmonary vascular disease 4. Evolution into "tetralogy" by development of RV outflow obstruction
ATRIAL SEPTAL DEFECT (secundum type) 1. Occurs in the mid or upper portion of the atrial septum 2. Partial anomalous pulmonary venous drainage occurs in 20–25% of cases	10–15%	1. Symptoms rare in infancy, unusual in childhood 2. Dyspnea, exercise intolerance may occur later in life	1. Ejection murmur at left base, may be soft 2. Mid-diastolic murmur at low left sternal border with large shunts 3. Wide fixed splitting of second heart sound	1. SBE extremely rare 2. Pulmonary vascular disease, CHF are late, uncommon complications
PATENT DUCTUS ARTERIOSUS Persistence of the normal fetal communication between the left pulmonary artery and the aorta just distal to the left subclavian artery	10% Females 3:1 > males ↑ incidence in premature	1. Patients may be asymptomatic with small ductus 2. Dyspnea, exercise intolerance and pulmonary infections most common symptoms 3. Late spontaneous closure, particularly in young premature, occurs occasionally	1. Crescendo-decrescendo murmur throughout systole and diastole is loudest at left base ("machinery") murmur 2. Wide pulse pressure, S_2 may be accentuated with large ducts	1. SBE 2. CHF 3. Pulmonary vascular disease
PULMONIC STENOSIS Obstruction to right ventricular outflow resulting in pressure gradient across obstructive site a) Valvular in 90% b) Subvalvular or infundibular in <10% (usually seen with tetralogy of Fallot) c) Supravalvular or peripheral uncommon	8%	1. Patient may be asymptomatic with normal life span 2. Dyspnea, exercise intolerance in moderate cases 3. Above, plus CHF and cyanosis in severe forms	1. Loud ejection murmur, "diamond-shaped," maximal at left base, transmitted to back 2. S_2 in pulmonic area ↓, splitting usually not audible 3. Cyanosis unusual, indicates R to L shunt via foramen ovale	1. SBE 2. CHF
COARCTATION OF THE AORTA 1. Narrowing usually occurs beyond the left subclavian artery near the insertion of the ductus ("adult" or postductal coarctation) 2. The "infantile" or preductal coarctation may be generalized hypoplasia of the aortic arch or may be localized narrowing proximal to the ductus 3. Bicuspid aortic valve or aortic stenosis in 50% or more	5% Males 4:1 > females	1. CHF in infancy occurs, but is not common later 2. Leg pains, headaches, exercise intolerance occur in adults, but symptoms not common during childhood	1. Hypertension in arms; pressure in legs usually ↓ 2. Pulses in legs delayed, ↓ 3. Systolic murmur is well heard over upper back	1. SBE (on bicuspid or stenotic aortic valve) or endarteritis 2. CHF in infancy 3. Intracranial bleeding 4. Dissecting aneurysm or rupture 5. Hypertensive cardiovascular disease
AORTIC STENOSIS Obstruction to left ventricular outflow resulting in pressure gradient across obstructive site a) Valvular >90%; valve bicuspid or tricuspid b) Subvalvular; may be muscular or diaphragmatic c) Supravalvular; annular constriction above valve	5%	1. Patient asymptomatic in mild cases 2. Dyspnea, exercise intolerance in moderate and severe cases 3. Chest pain, syncope ominous 4. LV failure rare, but ominous 5. Sudden death occurs, rare, in severe cases 6. Severity of stenosis may progress	1. Loud systolic ejection murmur, maximal at right base, transmitted to neck 2. Diastolic murmur of aortic insufficiency may be present 3. Ejection click (split 1st sound) may be present 4. Blood pressure usually normal; narrow pulse pressure in severe cases	1. Sudden death 2. SBE 3. LV failure 4. Arrhythmias 5. Coronary insufficiency

TABLE 31-4 (CONTINUED)

| | Laboratory Data | | | |
Electrocardiogram	Radiologic Findings	Cardiac Catheterization	Surgery	Summary
1. LVH or CVH if defect large 2. RVH with pulmonary hypertension or pulmonary outflow obstruction	1. ↑ Pulmonary blood flow (PBF) unless defect is small 2. Cardiac enlargement and with large VSD, left atrial enlargement (LAE), LVE characteristic 3. Relatively ↓ vasculature peripherally suggests pulmonary vascular disease	1. ↑ O₂ saturation in RV 2. PA pressure may be ↑ with large VSD 3. Angiocardiography generally not necessary for diagnosis	1. Not indicated for small shunts, with or without pulmonary hypertension 2. Surgical closure indicated if pulmonary blood flow 2 × systemic	1. Clinical course highly variable from death in infancy to normal life span; size of defect critical factor 2. Progression of pulmonary vascular disease uncommon except in large VSD 3. Spontaneous closure may occur in up to one third of cases
1. RVH occurs with large defects 2. RAD, right bundle branch block (RBBB) in majority	1. PBF ↑ unless ASD small 2. Enlargement of right atrium (RA) and RV (LA *not* enlarged)	1. ↑ O₂ saturation in RA 2. Pulmonary artery (PA) pressure usually normal 3. Angiocardiography generally unnecessary for diagnosis	Surgical closure indicated if pulmonary blood flow 2 × systemic	1. Course usually benign in childhood; symptoms often develop in 3rd–5th decade, resulting in death from CHF or progressive pulmonary vascular disease 2. The heart murmur may be soft, but wide relatively fixed splitting of S₂ suggests diagnosis in presence of cardiac enlargement and ↑ PBF
1. LVH may be present 2. RVH suggests pulmonary vascular disease	1. PBF ↑ unless ductus small 2. LAH, LVH, if ductus large 3. Aorta enlarged proximal to ductus 4. ↓ PBF peripherally if pulmonary vascular disease present	1. Not required in typical cases 2. ↑ O₂ saturation in pulmonary artery 3. PAP variable, normal with small ductus	Anatomic existence of ductus with L to R shunt is indication for surgical division	1. "Machinery" murmur characteristic, bounding pulses suggestive 2. Cardiac catheterization usually not required 3. Surgical division indicated in virtually all cases
1. May be normal 2. RAD; RVH: degree of RVH correlates well with degree of obstruction 3. Severe cases show RVH with "strain" (wide QRS–T angle); may have p-pulmonale	1. PBF normal, but RVE, RAE seen in more severe cases 2. Poststenotic dilatation of main pulmonary artery common	1. ↑ Pressure in RV, normal pressure in PA 2. Angiocardiography helpful in demonstrating site and nature of obstruction	Surgical repair indicated if peak gradient > 70 mm Hg	1. Severity and symptoms dependent on degree of obstruction 2. Amount of RVH on EKG correlates well with elevation of RV pressure 3. Pressure gradient > 70 mm Hg warrants surgery
1. RBBB in infancy 2. LVH if severe 3. RVH suggests "infantile" coarctation	1. PBF normal 2. Heart size usually normal 3. Coarctation may be visualized, particularly if barium in esophagus (E-sign) 4. Rib notching in older patients	Not required in typical cases	Surgical resection indicated if significant hypertension occurs	1. Patient generally asymptomatic with hypertension in arms, relative hypotension in legs 2. Comparison of upper versus lower extremity pulses should suggest diagnosis 3. Surgery indicated if narrowing is significant, since life expectancy ↓ by lesion
1. LVH frequent 2. LV "strain" (wide QRS–T angle) may be present in severe form	1. May be normal, even in severe forms 2. Dilatation of ascending aorta frequent	1. LV pressure elevated 2. Angiocardiography may be necessary to document site of obstruction and confirm severity	1. Significant symptoms (chest, pain, syncope, CHF) warrant surgical relief of severe stenosis 2. Mean gradient > 50 mm Hg, valve area < 0.7 cm²/M² warrants consideration of surgery	1. Patient often asymptomatic with loud systolic ejection murmur at left base 2. Significant symptoms or LV "strain" on EKG warrants catheterization 3. No ideal operation yet available; therefore surgery reserved for moderately severe cases 4. Restrictions, particularly for competitive sports, indicated for moderate and severe cases

TABLE 31-5 OPERABLE CYANOTIC CONGENITAL HEART DISEASE: 4 MOST COMMON TYPES

Definition and Pathology	Incidence; % of CHD	Clinical Findings		
		History	Physical Findings	Major Complications
FALLOT'S TETRAD (Tetralogy of Fallot) 1. Complex with RVP = LVP = aortic P due to VSD with obstruction to RV outflow 2. Pulmonic stenosis: 10% valvular 50% infundibular 30% combined 10% atretic valve 3. Overriding of aorta variable 4. Right aortic arch in 25%	10% (50–70% of cyanotic CHD in non-operated patients)	1. Cyanosis; onset generally after 2–3 months of age unless atresia present 2. Dyspnea 3. Exercise intolerance 4. Squatting 5. Mild form ("pink" tetrad) may have few symptoms	1. Cyanosis 2. Clubbing 3. ↓ S_2 pulmonic area without audible splitting 4. Loud systolic murmur along left sternal border (with pulmonary atresia may be no murmur)	1. Hypoxic spells (paroxysmal hyperpnea with severe cyanosis; may lead to unconsciousness) 2. Brain abscess 3. Embolism 4. Thrombosis 5. SBE NOTE: CHF rare in childhood
TRANSPOSITION OF THE GREAT ARTERIES 1. Aorta arises anteriorly from RV, pulmonary artery arises posteriorly from LV 2. Communication (ASD, VSD or PDA) essential for mixing and survival	3–5% Males 3:1 > females	1. Cyanosis, tachypnea develop in neonatal period and are progressive 2. CHF develops early 3. Survival beyond 3–6 mo. in "uncomplicated" cases rare without therapy 4. Symptoms may progress rapidly to death—immediate diagnostic studies indicated	1. Cyanosis 2. Systolic murmur may or may not be present 3. Tachypnea common	1. CHF 2. Hypoxia
TRICUSPID ATRESIA 1. Tricuspid valve imperforate or absent (resulting in total R to L shunt via ASD) and right ventricle markedly hypoplastic 2. VSD present in majority 3. Transposition of great arteries 30% 4. Pulmonary atresia or hypoplasia present in majority	1–2%	1. Cyanosis, tachypnea develop early in infancy 2. Hypoxic spells common	1. Cyanosis 2. Clubbing 3. Systolic murmur (VSD)	1. Hypoxia if PBF inadequate 2. Embolism 3. Thrombosis 4. CHF if atrial communication inadequate
TOTALLY ANOMALOUS PULMONARY VENOUS RETURN (Complete transposition of the pulmonary veins) 1. All pulmonary veins enter the right atrium or one of its tributaries 2. Pathologic types a) supracardiac (via SVC) = 60% b) cardiac (via coronary sinus or direct to RA) = 30% c) infracardiac (via portal vein or ductus venosus) = 10% 3. Atrial communication an integral part of complex	1%	1. Cyanosis, mild to moderate 2. CHF common in infancy may progress rapidly, particularly if obstruction to pulmonary venous return exists 3. Dyspnea, exercise intolerance and pulmonary infections common 4. Occasional patients survive to adult life with few symptoms	1. Cyanosis, not severe, may appear "grayish" 2. Systolic murmur generally soft; diastolic murmur low LSB common; 3rd and 4th heart sounds ("quadruple rhythm")	1. CHF 2. Pulmonary vascular obstruction

although carditis appears to be less frequent. Carditis is the only manifestation that can result in permanent damage. Carditis is found in a decreasing proportion of individuals as the joint symptoms become more pronounced. The early murmurs found in rheumatic heart disease are due to mitral insufficiency, apical mid-diastolic murmur and aortic insufficiency.

The revised Jones' Criteria for the diagnosis of rheumatic fever require the presence of two major criteria, or of one major and two minor criteria, plus supporting evidence of preceding streptococcal infection,

TABLE 31–5 (CONTINUED)

| | Laboratory Data | | | |
Electrocardiogram	Radiologic Findings	Cardiac Catheterization	Surgery	Summary
RAD, RVH	1. ↓ PBF 2. Small heart; apex elevated + small pulmonary conus = "boot shape" 3. R. aortic arch in 25%	1. Pressure = in RV, LV and aorta, ↓ in PA 2. Shunt in ventricle: R to L with ↓ arterial O_2 saturation; may be L to R only in mild form 3. Angiocardiography required to demonstrate anatomy	1. Infants: palliation aortic-pulmonary or subclavian-pulmonary artery anastomosis; in selected older infants total repair possible as initial procedure 2. Over age 2–3, open-heart correction	1. With RVH on EKG, ↓ PBF on x-ray – tetralogy until disproved 2. Hypoxia, not CHF, is main threat during infancy and childhood 3. Surgical procedures are palliative or corrective, depending on age and anatomy
RAD, RVH usual	1. ↑ PBF 2. Large heart 3. Narrow base of heart; may give "egg shape" appearance	1. Pressure systemic level in RV, variable in LV 2. Arterial desaturation usually considerable, = RV saturation 3. Balloon catheter atrial septostomy (Rashkind procedure) may be life-saving palliation 4. Angiocardiography required to demonstrate anatomy	1. Palliation by production of ASD if Rashkind fails 2. Complete correction by intra-atrial venous transposition possible at any age in "uncomplicated" cases	1. Early development of severe cyanosis, cardiomegaly, pulmonary plethora suggests diagnosis of transposition 2. Angiocardiography diagnostic method of choice 3. Since symptoms may progress rapidly and lesion is correctable, diagnostic studies should not be delayed
LAD, LVH, RAH	1. ↓ PBF 2. Small heart common 3. Similar appearance to tetralogy	1. Course of catheter from RA to LA to LV 2. Arterial desaturation usually considerable, depending upon PBF 3. Angiocardiography required to demonstrate anatomy	1. Hypoplasia of RV makes complex uncorrectable 2. Palliation: aortic-pulmonary, subclavian-pulmonary artery or superior vena caval-pulmonary shunt (latter preferred after 6 months)	1. Cyanosis and dyspnea occur early 2. X-ray findings variable, often simulate tetralogy 3. LVH, LAD in patients with cyanotic CHD usually = tricuspid atresia 4. Underdevelopment of RV makes complex uncorrectable, but palliation often possible
RAD, RAH, RVH	1. ↑ PBF 2. RA and RV enlarged; LA *not* enlarged 3. Supracardiac form has "figure 8" or "snowman" appearance after infancy 4. Obstructed form (often infradiaphragmatic) has small heart, severe pulmonary congestion	1. Complete mixing in RA of all venous blood (RA O_2 saturation = PA = aorta) 2. RV, PA pressure normal to moderately ↑ except in obstructed form when PAP ↑↑ 3. Angiocardiography necessary to determine anatomy of pulmonary venous return	1. Palliation unsatisfactory 2. Complete correction can be done in most cases	1. Mild cyanosis, CHF and death in 1st year common 2. EKG, x.ray show RV overload 3. Cardiac catheterization reveals approximately equal O_2 saturation in all cardiac chambers and both great vessels 4. Surgical correction required in all cases

either by elevated antistreptococcal antibodies, positive throat culture for Group A streptococcus or recent scarlet fever. The criteria are as follows:

Major	Minor
Carditis	Fever
Polyarthritis	Arthralgia
Chorea	Previous rheumatic fever
Erythema marginatum	or rheumatic heart
Subcutaneous nodules	disease
	Acute phase reaction
	(ESR, CRP, leuko-
	cytosis)
	Prolonged P-R interval

Following establishment of the diagnosis, anti-inflammatory therapy is indicated. Aspirin is the drug of choice for rheumatic fever without carditis. With carditis, particularly with cardiac enlargement or heart failure, corticosteroid therapy is indicated. Individuals who have had rheumatic fever should be placed on continuous antistreptococcal prophylaxis, following an initial therapeutic course of antibiotics.

PREVENTIVE CARDIOLOGY

Pediatricians have been leaders in practicing preventive medicine, promoting normal emotional and physical development of their patients and demonstrating leadership in accident prevention and immunization against infectious diseases. Early diagnosis and management of hypertension can be of great benefit in reducing cardiovascular problems in adults. At this time it is not yet clear whether or not reduction in blood lipid levels in adults will reduce the occurrence of myocardial infarction. It will be a full generation before information is available regarding the effect of early diagnosis and treatment of hyperlipidemia in children upon the incidence or age of onset of coronary artery disease in adults.

Hypertension

Previously it was thought that most hypertensive children had secondary hypertension, and that essential hypertension was rare in children. It is now apparent that a significant percentage of hypertensive children, particularly adolescents, have essential hypertension. The diagnosis of essential hypertension is no longer one of exclusion. A careful history and physical examination will help separate most of the organic causes. The clinical challenge is to determine which child warrants a full-scale diagnostic work-up. Our abbreviated evaluation consists of a urinalysis, urine culture, creatinine test and an intravenous urogram with very early filming. Two groups of patients need to be singled out for special comment. Infants and young children who are hypertensive and older children and adolescents who have severe hypertension with a diastolic pressure greater than 100 mm Hg should have a complete work-up to rule out a treatable cause. Excessive blood pressures for age would be at or above:

Age	Blood Pressure
1 to 3 months	100/65
3/12 to 1 year	110/70
1 to 10 years	130/85
10 to 15 years	140/85

There is suggestive evidence that some young patients with labile hypertension or with blood pressure at the upper limits of normal may become the adult hypertensive patients. Hypertension is found in familial clusters.

The use of the proper cuff size is important in the accurate measurement of the blood pressure. Regardless of the age and size of the patient, a cuff that is too small will falsely elevate the blood pressure and a cuff that is too large will lower it. The proper cuff is one in which the width of the bladder is 20 per cent wider than the average diameter of the arm for upper limb and 25 per cent wider than the average diameter of the thigh for lower limb, with a cuff bladder that is long enough to encircle at least three-fourths of the circumference of the limb and fits snugly around the limb. If a choice must be made between a cuff that is too small or one too large, select the larger sized cuff, since it will better reflect the true intra-arterial pressure.

Reserpine and propranolol, for physiological and pharmacological reasons, are excellent drugs for young essential hypertensive patients who have labile increases in blood pressure during stressful situations, or who exhibit a hyperkinetic state. Thiazide diuretics are usually the second class of drugs to be added, if necessary. Dietary treatment consists of limiting salt intake and maintaining an optimal weight for height.

Hyperlipidemia

Increased cholesterol is associated with increased risk of coronary artery disease. At this time, there is no substantial evidence that by maintaining lower serum lipid levels in children the subsequent development of ischemic heart disease can be delayed or prevented. However, fatty streaks are present in aortas of all children after three years of age and in nearly all coronary arteries after 20 years of age. Gross evidence of coronary atherosclerosis was found in 45 to 77 per cent of autopsies of American soldiers in the 18 to 35 year old age group.

The cholesterol measurement should be made with the patient in a steady state. There is a fair amount of intraindividual variability for cholesterol values, and a single sample may be inadequate to establish a diagnosis. The upper limits of normal are:

Age	Serum Cholesterol, Upper Limit
1 to 6 months	180 mg/100 ml
1/2 to 8 years	205 mg/100 ml
9 to 19 years	210 mg/100 ml

National Institutes of Health values of upper limits for serum cholesterol are 230 mg/100 ml and for triglyceride 140 mg/100 ml up to 19 years of age. Secondary hyperlipoproteinemia due to hypothyroidism, diabetes mellitus, chronic renal disease and hepatic disease rarely presents a diagnostic problem but must always be excluded.

Because of the present lack of data to confirm the prevention of coronary artery disease with treatment, any therapeutic modality involving diet and drugs needs to be safe and acceptable.

Other Risk Factors Relative to Future Heart Disease

Premature cardiovascular events are related to hypertension, diabetes and to the hyperlipidemias. Other factors include cigarette smoking, obesity, positive family history and maleness. Exercise will not, unfortunately, prevent myocardial infarctions, but it will improve the likelihood of survival.

REFERENCES

1. Goldberg, S. J., Allen, H. D., and Sahn, D. J.: *Pediatric and Adolescent Echocardiography*, Chicago, Yearbook Medical Publishers, 1975.
2. Gould, S. E.: *Pathology of the Heart and Blood Vessels*, 3rd ed. Springfield, Ill., Charles C Thomas Co., 1968.
3. Guntheroth, W. G.: *Pediatric Electrocardiography*. Philadelphia, W. B. Saunders Co., 1965.
4. Markowitz, M., and Gordis, L.: *Rheumatic Fever*, 2nd ed. Philadelphia, W. B. Saunders Co., 1972.
5. Morgan, B. C., Guntheroth, W. G., Figley, M. M., Dillard, D. H., and Merendino, K. A.: Operable congenital heart disease. Pediatr. Clin. N. Am., *13*:105, 1966.
6. Nadas, A. S., and Fyler, D. C.: *Pediatric Cardiology*, 3rd ed. Philadelphia, W. B. Saunders Co., 1972.

32

Rheumatic Diseases (Inflammatory Diseases of Connective Tissues, Collagen Diseases)

Jane Green Schaller

The rheumatic diseases (inflammatory diseases of connective tissue, collagen diseases) are diseases of unknown cause that are grouped together; it is not known whether these diseases have common etiological or pathogenic mechanisms, however. They are characterized by non-suppurative inflammation of various connective tissues throughout the body and are associated with varying clinical pictures and diverse symptoms and signs. Diagnosis of the various rheumatic diseases rests almost solely on their distinctive clinical pictures; there are no precise diagnostic criteria and no diagnostic laboratory tests.

Speculation about causes of the rheumatic diseases continues. The theory that rheumatic diseases are caused by some sort of an infectious process with as yet unidentified organisms, such as viruses, mycoplasma or bacterial variants, remains attractive. The concept of aberrant immune mechanisms or "autoimmunity" as basic mechanisms in the rheumatic diseases has been popular since the discovery of certain antibodies that react with body constituents: rheumatoid factors (antibodies reactive with gamma globulin), antinuclear antibodies (antibodies reactive with nuclear constituents, including deoxyribonucleic acid and deoxyribonucleoprotein) and LE cells (caused by antibodies to deoxyribonucleoprotein). Such "autoantibodies" are found not only in the rheumatic diseases but also in non-rheumatic conditions such

as chronic infections. None is diagnostic or has been proved causative of any disease. It may be, however, that such antibodies sometimes contribute to tissue damage through mechanisms such as immune complex formation. For example, it has been demonstrated that the nephritis of lupus erythematosus is caused by deposition of antinuclear antibodies complexed with their antigens. The association of various immunodeficiency states with rheumatic disease syndromes, autoantibody formation and certain "autoimmune" states (such as hemolytic anemia and thyroiditis) also suggests that defective immune mechanisms, either primary or acquired, might underlie some rheumatic disease states. The role of the individual's genetic background in susceptibility to rheumatic diseases is currently of great interest since the recent demonstration of highly significant associations between the histocompatibility antigen HLA-B27 and ankylosing spondylitis and certain other types of seronegative arthritis.

An understanding of the rheumatic diseases may help the physician beginning clinical medicine for several reasons. First, because diagnosis of the rheumatic diseases rests solely on accurate interpretation of the patient's history and physical examination, the physician must learn to synthesize his observations accurately. Second, the rheumatic diseases provide an important example of chronic diseases that can

312

benefit from early diagnosis and good medical care. Caring for a patient with a chronic illness such as rheumatoid arthritis is a true test of the complete physician. Third, the rheumatic diseases, particularly rheumatoid arthritis and acute rheumatic fever, are common causes of disability in the United States today. Rheumatoid arthritis affects about 1 per cent of the adult population, primarily young adults; juvenile rheumatoid arthritis (JRA) is one of the most common chronic debilitating diseases of childhood. Rheumatic fever is the most common cause of acquired heart disease in children and young adults.

The rheumatic diseases considered in this chapter include juvenile rheumatoid arthritis, rheumatic fever and lupus erythematosus. Other rheumatic diseases, including dermatomyositis, scleroderma and the vasculitis syndromes (polyarteritis nodosa, Schönlein-Henoch vasculitis, Wegener's granulomatosis) are not described here.

JUVENILE RHEUMATOID ARTHRITIS (JRA)

Rheumatoid arthritis (RA) is a disease characterized by chronic synovitis; numerous extra-articular manifestations may also occur. About 5 per cent of cases of RA begin in individuals less than 15 years old; it has been estimated that there are about 200,000 children with JRA in the United States today. Chronic arthritis in children was first described by an English pediatrician, George Frederick Still, in 1897, and the disease is often referred to as Still's disease. Still thought that JRA was a different disease from adult-onset RA; this question has not yet been settled. It is probable that what we call JRA is in fact more than a single disease.

Clinical manifestations. From analyses of large groups of patients, it appears that several distinct clinical subgroups exist within JRA (Table 32–1). These subgroups differ in sex, age of onset, patterns and severity of articular and extra-articular manifestations, serological and genetic studies and prognosis. The polyarticular type of JRA resembles adult RA in many ways; the systemic onset and pauciarticular types of disease occur rarely in adults. Ankylosing spondylitis, a disease characterized by arthritis of the lumbodorsal spine, is well recognized as a distinct rheumatic disease in adults; a significant number of children with what seems to be JRA in fact have early ankylosing spondylitis. Recognition of these disease patterns is useful in diagnosis and care of children with JRA. Whether these differences signify multiple different diseases or multiple distinct host reactions to similar disease processes remains to be determined.

Onset of arthritis may be insidious, with gradual development of joint stiffness and loss of motion, or fulminant, with the sudden appearance of symptomatic disease. Affected joints may be swollen, warm, tender, painful on motion and limited in motion. Joint swelling results from periarticular edema, joint effusion and synovial thickening. Some patients have pain and joint stiffness initially before objective changes are present. A significant percentage of children do not complain of pain in affected joints. Muscle spasm and guarding of joints are common. Young children with polyarthritis often assume a characteristic posture: irritable, anxious and protecting their joints from movement. Stiffness of joints after inactivity, notably in the morning, is common. The synovitis in JRA is characteristically chronic, lasting many weeks or even years in an affected joint. If chronic synovitis persists long enough, articular cartilage and subchondral bone may be damaged, causing permanent joint damage and sometimes permanent deformities such as subluxation or fusion of joints. Fortunately, most children with JRA escape permanent joint damage or deformity. Growth disturbances adjacent to inflamed joints may result in overgrowth or undergrowth of the affected part; this occurs because of proximity of epiphyseal growth plates to the inflamed synovium.

"Systemic" JRA almost always begins with systemic symptoms, particularly high fevers and rheumatoid rash; joint manifestations usually begin soon after systemic manifestations. Early ankylosing spondylitis generally begins as pauciarticular arthritis in late childhood; early hip and hip girdle symptoms are common, and radiographic sacroiliitis is frequent on follow-up, although it may be years before changes in the lumbodorsal spine permit diagnosis of ankylosing spondylitis.

Course and prognosis. The outlook for most children with JRA is good; at least 75

TABLE 32–1 JUVENILE RHEUMATOID ARTHRITIS: CLINICAL PATTERNS OF DISEASE

Disease Pattern	Per cent of JRA Patients	Girls/Boys	Arthritis	Laboratory Findings	Extra-articular Manifestations	Outcome
Polyarticular Rheumatoid factor– negative	30	8/1	Multiple joints involved: Any synovial joint (except lumbothoracic spine) Often symmetrical Small joints of hands characteristic	ANA 25% RF negative	Malaise, anorexia, irritability Mild anemia Low grade fever Rheumatoid nodules rare	10% significant disability from arthritis
Rheumatoid factor– positive	10	6/1	Same as above	ANA 75% RF 100%	Same as above Rheumatoid nodules common Rheumatoid vasculitis occasional	>50% significant disability from arthritis
Pauciarticular Young age onset, predominantly girls	25	7/1	Arthritis confined to 1-5 joints: Large joints: knees, ankles, elbows most frequent Small joints generally spared, Hips spared	ANA 50% RF negative	Chronic iridocyclitis in 50% Slit lamp examinations mandatory for early detection	Disability from arthritis rare 10–20% visual loss from iridocyclitis
Older age onset, mostly boys	15	1/10	Same as above except hip girdle involvement and sacroiliitis common	ANA negative RF negative HLA–B27 associated	Acute iridocyclitis in 10%	Ankylosing spondylitis in some at follow-up
Systemic (characterized by fever, usually with one or more additional systemic manifestations)	20	8/10	Multiple joints usually involved Arthritis usually occurs within 6 months of onset Arthritis may initially be overshadowed by systemic manifestations	ANA negative RF negative	1. *Fever:* 1 or 2 daily elevations to 102–107° with rapid return to normal or subnormal 2. *Rash:* small, pale red macules, evanescent and recurrent 3. *Pleuritis and pericarditis:* usually mild 4. *Lymphadenopathy and hepatosplenomegaly:* may be marked suggesting malignancy 5. *Leukocytosis:* may exceed 50,000/mm^3 6. Malaise, anorexia, irritability, anemia, abdominal pain	Systemic manifestation transient (months), not a cause of permanent disability 20% significant disability from chronic arthritis

per cent eventually enter long remissions with no significant disability. There are, however, three causes of permanent disability in JRA. The major cause of disability is musculoskeletal, occurring in patients who have arthritis severe enough to cause permanent joint damage. Severe destructive arthritis occurs most often in patients with rheumatoid factor positive polyarticular disease and systemic onset disease and also in some children who have early ankylosing spondylitis. Many deformities of JRA, such as joint contractures, can be prevented with adequate therapy during periods of active disease. A second permanent disability in JRA is loss of vision caused by iridocyclitis; this condition can also be ameliorated by early recognition and appropriate therapy. A third permanent disability in JRA occurs if patients are allowed to develop an image of chronic invalidism and incur emotional damage from chronic illness; this, too, should be preventable with sympathetic and comprehensive medical care. Unfortunately, another important cause of morbidity in JRA in recent years has been the side effects of toxic drugs, particularly corticosteroids.

The severity and duration of JRA are not predictable for the individual patient. This chronic illness can pursue several courses: (1) one attack of disease followed by long, perhaps permanent, remission; (2) periodic exacerbations and remissions of disease; (3) long-lasting though relatively mild disease without disabling permanent damage; or (4) severe progressive disease with joint destruction and disability despite currently available forms of therapy. Fortunately, most patients follow one of the first three courses; severe progressive disease is uncommon in children. A few patients who have had JRA followed by long remission again have recurrences of the disease in adulthood.

Laboratory tests. There are *no* diagnostic laboratory tests for rheumatoid arthritis. Classic rheumatoid factors (IgM antibodies reactive with gamma globulin) are demonstrable by agglutination techniques (such as the latex fixation test) in 80 per cent of adults with RA, but in few children with JRA. Positive agglutination tests for rheumatoid factors are related to the age of the patient at onset of disease; they are rarely found in children with JRA beginning before eight years of age and do not become positive in young-onset patients even when active disease continues for years. It has recently been noted that some children with JRA have IgG or IgA antiglobulin factors that may be detected by different techniques; their significance is not known. Antinuclear antibodies are demonstrable in 25 per cent of children with JRA, most frequently in patients with chronic iridocyclitis, in girls and in children with early childhood onset of disease. Serum immunoglobulin levels are frequently elevated.

Joint fluid changes are not diagnostic but may be helpful, particularly in excluding septic arthritis. Rheumatoid joint fluid contains an increased number of white cells, predominantly polys (5,000 to 75,000/cu mm). The synovial fluid sugar may be low. Phagocytic cells containing immunoglobulin inclusions may be found; joint fluid complement may be normal or low. Serum complement levels are usually normal or high. Collections of lymphocytes and plasma cells are found in synovial tissues. Although this histological picture is not specific, synovial biopsy may be helpful in excluding infectious arthritis.

Acute phase phenomena such as elevated sedimentation rates and C reactive protein may appear in the blood during active inflammatory disease but are of no diagnostic usefulness since they do not distinguish various causes of inflammation. Since acute phase phenomena are not invariably found during active inflammation, their absence does not exclude an active rheumatic process. There is seldom virtue in ordering more than one acute phase reactant test; the sedimentation rate is the easiest and most readily available.

Radiographs may provide useful diagnostic information and are important in documenting the extent of joint damage. Films taken within the first year of disease generally show only soft tissue swelling, osteoporosis and sometimes periostitis. Films taken later in severe disease may show characteristic changes of articular damage including loss of cartilage space, erosions into subchondral bone and varying destruction of bones and joints. Such radiographic changes, particularly in the hands and wrists, are diagnostic. Many children with JRA never incur enough articular damage to be visible radiographically.

Diagnosis. As noted, diagnosis of JRA rests solely on clinical grounds, by recognition of the disease manifestations described here and by exclusion of other diseases associated with arthritis, including septic arthritis, osteomyelitis, other rheumatic diseases, post-infectious arthritis, leukemia and malignancies. Aside from the radiographic changes occurring with joint destruction late in severe disease, there are no diagnostic laboratory tests. It is particularly important to consider and exclude potentially treatable diseases such as septic arthritis and osteomyelitis before concluding that a patient with arthritis has JRA.

Therapy. In designing therapy it is important to realize that the overall prognosis for the majority of children with JRA is good, although the outcome is uncertain in any given patient, and the disease may last a long time. With adequate care during periods of active disease, 75 per cent of children with JRA will incur no lasting disability from their disease. The physician must therefore avoid harmful drugs if possible and remember to use a good measure of optimism and reassurance in helping children and families cope with this discouraging, but by no means hopeless, disease. Optimum treatment requires a knowledgeable primary physician and often the help of several specialists including a rheumatologist, a specialist in physical medicine, an orthopedist, a physical therapist, an ophthalmologist and occasionally a social worker or psychiatrist. Such coordinated medical care is unfortunately expensive and often impossible to obtain. It is of paramount importance for the primary physician to establish good rapport with the patient and family and to work closely with them.

Since etiology and pathogenesis of JRA are not understood, therapy is necessarily symptomatic and not curative; since the natural history of the disease is unpredictable and spontaneous remissions frequent, the physician must be wary of claiming miraculous "cures." Adequate control of arthritis means that the patient is reasonably comfortable, can function adequately, and is not developing progressive deformities; unfortunately, it is not always possible to suppress symptoms and signs of arthritis completely without risking drug toxicity. Drugs that modify the inflammatory response are employed in therapy. Of the available anti-inflammatory drugs, salicylates are the safest and best for most patients. Although in overdose they are commonly poisonous to children, salicylates can be given safely even to small children if physicians and parents are informed of possible side effects and careful follow-up is made. In adequate dosages for sufficient periods of time (blood salicylate levels of 20 to 30 mg* for a trial of at least several months' duration), salicylates will adequately control disease in most children with JRA. All other antirheumatic agents are fraught with more serious toxic effects for children. If salicylates alone do not work, however, other drugs should be tried. Injections of gold salts are effective in controlling arthritis in many patients, but must be given by a physician who is cognizant of their toxicity. Chloroquine, indomethacin and Butazolidin are toxic drugs with limited usefulness in children. Corticosteroids are dramatic in suppressing symptoms and signs of arthritis, but their long-term use is fraught with severe toxic hazards, and they have been a cause of considerable morbidity and even mortality in children. Corticosteroids do not cure JRA; joint destruction may proceed even while they are being given. Corticosteroids, once started in a chronic disease such as JRA, may be required for years, and their side effects are unavoidable. Corticosteroids should not be used to provide symptomatic relief for arthritis unless all other measures have failed; if they must be used, the lowest possible dosages should be employed.

Physical therapy is extremely important in preserving joint range of motion and muscle strength. All children should be started on a home program of daily exercises designed to retain normal joint function early in disease. Bed rest and prolonged immobilization of joints are generally contraindicated. Simple measures such as hot baths in the morning may be helpful in relieving joint stiffness. Exercises and judicious splinting may also be useful in correcting existing deformities.

---

*For children of less than 25 kg body weight, 100 mg/kg/day in four divided doses will generally give appropriate blood levels. For children of 25 to 50 kg body weight, doses between 40 grains (2.4 gm) and 70 grains (4.2 gm) are appropriate.

Occasionally, orthopedic surgical procedures are needed. Early prophylactic removal of inflamed synovium (synovectomy) may benefit certain patients. Joint replacement procedures may be helpful in severe cases after full growth is attained.

Salicylates are also usually effective in controlling the systemic manifestations of JRA. If high fever and other debilitating manifestations are uncontrolled after several weeks of adequate salicylate therapy, however, a short course of corticosteroids may be warranted. Since fever and other systemic manifestations usually remit spontaneously after several months, corticosteroids can generally be tapered and discontinued within a few months and the patient maintained on salicylates.

Therapy of iridocyclitis should be managed with help of an ophthalmologist. Early recognition of this complication by periodic slit lamp examinations is crucial for good results. The eye disease may be controlled with topical corticosteroids alone; occasionally systemic corticosteroids are needed.

The use of drugs such as cyclophosphamide and azathioprine in JRA is experimental and would seem rarely if ever warranted in a non-fatal disease with a generally good outlook.

RHEUMATIC FEVER

Rheumatic fever is a post-streptococcal disease characterized by non-suppurative inflammation of various organs, particularly the heart. It is the most common cause of acquired heart disease in children and young adults. The attack rate of rheumatic fever after group A streptococcal pharyngitis is about 3 per cent. Rheumatic fever does not follow skin infection with group A streptococci, although acute glomerulonephritis may result from such an infection; the reasons for this difference are unknown. Rheumatic fever rarely occurs before age five years, suggesting that repeated streptococcal exposures may be required prior to its development. The mechanisms by which streptococcal infections lead to rheumatic fever remain unknown despite much investigative work. No evidence has been found that rheumatic fever results from persistence of streptococci or their variants in the patient or from toxic effects of streptococcal components or products. Antibodies reactive with heart tissues have been found in sera of rheumatic fever patients; deposits of gamma globulin and complement have been identified in rheumatic heart tissues; and antigens cross-reactive between streptococci and heart muscle have been demonstrated. The significance of these observations is not known, however, and the role of "autoimmunity" in rheumatic fever remains uncertain.

Clinical manifestations. The clinical picture of rheumatic fever varies, depending on sites of involvement and severity of disease. The preceding streptococcal pharyngitis may be severe, mild or even subclinical. Following the streptococcal infection there is a latent asymptomatic period of one to several weeks before symptoms and signs of rheumatic fever become apparent. The major clinical manifestations of rheumatic fever are carditis, arthritis, chorea, subcutaneous nodules and erythema marginatum. Fever and arthritis are the most frequent presenting complaints.

The carditis of acute rheumatic fever is its most unique characteristic and the only disease manifestation that permanently damages the host. The incidence of carditis during initial attacks of rheumatic fever is 40 to 50 per cent. Endocardium, myocardium or pericardium may be affected. Carditis usually occurs during the first week or two of the attack if it is going to occur. It is usually unassociated with specific cardiac symptoms when the patient seeks medical attention. Signs of carditis include heart murmurs (mitral systolic, mitral or aortic diastolic), pericardial friction rubs, cardiac enlargement and cardiac decompensation. Special care must be taken to interpret heart murmurs accurately and to differentiate the benign functional murmurs commonly heard in children or the murmurs of congenital heart disease from the pathological murmurs of carditis. Non-specific findings such as prolongation of the PR interval on electrocardiogram, gallop rhythms and tachycardia with fever should not alone be accepted as evidence of rheumatic carditis.

Arthritis occurs in three fourths of patients with rheumatic fever and is the most common disease manifestation. The arthritis affects one or more large joints and rarely lasts more than one week in a given joint. It may involve several joints simultaneously or migrate from joint to joint. Affected joints are usually swollen, hot, painful and sometimes erythematous, but sometimes only arthralgia may be present.

Chorea is the strangest manifestation of rheumatic fever and often appears after a longer latent period than do other disease manifestations. Signs of chorea include purposeless motions, poor neuromuscular coordination and emotional lability. A significant number of children with chorea have associated mild carditis. Occasionally chorea occurs as the sole manifestation of acute rheumatic fever; such patients may lack fever or other signs of active inflammation. Attacks of chorea may last from weeks to months but eventually clear without neurological residue.

Erythema marginatum and subcutaneous nodules occur in 10 per cent or fewer of patients. Erythema marginatum begins as faint red macules, usually over the trunk and proximal limbs. Lesions enlarge peripherally, leading to a ring-like or serpiginous pattern. Subcutaneous nodules, resembling those of JRA, may occur over pressure points. Other less specific clinical manifestations of acute rheumatic fever include fever, malaise, epistaxis and abdominal pain. Rheumatic pneumonia may occur in a few patients.

Course and prognosis. Periods of active rheumatic fever (attacks) rarely exceed six months in duration but may recur unless group A streptococcal infections are prevented. During acute attacks of rheumatic fever death rarely occurs from fulminating carditis. The only potentially damaging sequela of acute rheumatic fever is residual cardiac damage. For the 50 to 60 per cent of patients without carditis during the initial attack of rheumatic fever the long-term prognosis is excellent, with complete recovery the rule; patients who do not initially have carditis rarely develop significant carditis on follow-up even though subsequent attacks of rheumatic fever occur. Of the 40 to 50 per cent of patients who do have carditis during initial attacks of rheumatic fever, about one third will also have no residual heart disease on follow-up. The incidence and severity of residual heart disease appear related to the severity of carditis when the patient is first seen. Patients with carditis during the initial attack of rheumatic fever may be expected to suffer further heart damage with subsequent disease attacks and may indeed be even more prone to develop recurrent rheumatic attacks. Much of the disability and death in rheumatic fever is related to recurrent attacks of disease with additive cardiac damage. The prognosis is therefore largely dependent on prevention of recurrent disease attacks by adequate antistreptococcal prophylaxis, particularly in those patients who have had carditis.

Laboratory tests. There are no diagnostic laboratory tests for acute rheumatic fever. Acute phase phenomena such as elevated sedimentation rates are usually demonstrable during active disease. Rheumatic fever is not associated with rheumatoid factors, antinuclear antibodies, LE cells or lowered serum complement levels.

Documentation of preceding streptococcal infection should be made in all patients. Streptococci may or may not be cultured from the pharynx when rheumatic fever has become manifest. Elevation of antibodies to streptococcal antigens provides evidence of preceding streptococcal infection. These antibodies begin to rise in titer about one week after the streptococcal infection and remain elevated for several months. Antibodies to streptolysin O (ASO titer) are most commonly measured; increased ASO titers are present in 80 per cent of patients with acute rheumatic fever. Patients without elevated ASO titers can be shown to have elevated antibody titers to other streptococcal antigens or enzymes. The streptozyme test measures antibodies to several streptococcal products simultaneously; a large percentage of patients with prior streptococcal infections have positive test results, but the ultimate usefulness of this procedure remains to be determined. It must be realized, however, that positive throat cultures for streptococci and elevated antibodies are diagnostic *only* of streptococcal disease and not of rheumatic fever.

Diagnosis. The diagnosis of rheumatic fever is clinical and should not be lightly made. There are no single diagnostic sign and no diagnostic laboratory tests. The modified Jones Criteria shown in Table 32–2 are diagnostic guides. Two major criteria or one major and two minor criteria are

TABLE 32-2 JONES CRITERIA FOR RHEUMATIC FEVER (REVISED)*

Major Manifestations	Minor Manifestations
Carditis	Fever
Polyarthritis	Arthralgia
Chorea	Previous rheumatic fever or rheumatic heart disease
Erythema marginatum	Elevated ESR or positive CRP
Subcutaneous nodules	Prolonged PR interval

Plus

Supporting evidence of preceding streptococcal infection
History of recent scarlet fever
Positive throat culture for group A streptococcus
Increased ASO titer or other streptococcal antibodies

*Circulation, 32:664, 1965.

suggestive of rheumatic fever; however, no combinations are entirely diagnostic of the disease. Carditis, the most important manifestation of rheumatic fever, is present in only 40 to 50 per cent of patients; heart murmurs and signs of carditis are not specific for rheumatic fever, occurring also in viral pericarditis, myocarditis, bacterial endocarditis and congenital heart disease. Arthritis is common in rheumatic fever (75 per cent of patients) but not very specific; the combination of arthritis and any two minor criteria could be consistent with any rheumatic disease and many infectious diseases as well. The nature and course of the arthritis (acute, self-limited) may be important in deciding whether the arthritis is due to rheumatic fever. Chorea, erythema marginatum and subcutaneous nodules occur in a minority of patients and thus are of less diagnostic usefulness. Other clinical findings such as fever, abdominal pain and epistaxis are so non-specific as to be of little diagnostic use. Before assigning a diagnosis of rheumatic fever to any patient, it behooves the physician to be sure that he is standing on firm ground. Many children have been damaged by needless long periods of bedrest and fear of heart disease because of over-enthusiastic diagnoses of rheumatic fever.

Therapy. Eradication of streptococci with adequate penicillin during the acute attack and subsequent adequate streptococcal prophylaxis to prevent further streptococcal infections and recurrences of rheumatic fever are of paramount importance. The monthly injection of 1.2 million units of benzathine penicillin is the most effective prophylaxis regimen for patients with rheumatic fever. If patients faithfully take oral medications, adequate prophylaxis can also be maintained with oral penicillin.

Therapy of attacks of rheumatic fever remains controversial. Treatment of the rheumatic manifestations entails the use of anti-inflammatory drugs. Both salicylates and steroids have been advocated for therapy, and both are effective in relieving symptoms of acute disease such as arthritis, fever and malaise. Although corticosteroids are more potent anti-inflammatory agents than salicylates, it has never been demonstrated that corticosteroids have any advantage over salicylates in affecting the incidence or severity of residual heart disease at follow-up. Carditis appears to be established early in the attack of rheumatic fever, and drugs thus rarely, if ever, prevent its occurrence. Furthermore, the incidence and severity of residual heart damage appear related to the extent of carditis when the patient is first seen, rather than to any specific therapy. Treatment with corticosteroids would seem indicated for patients with severe carditis where rapid control of inflammation will prevent mortality and morbidity during the acute attack. Opinions vary about the therapy of children with mild carditis; either salicylates or steroids are used. Most physicians would treat children having no carditis with salicylates alone. Bedrest may be indicated during periods of active carditis, but there appears to be little rationale for prolonged bedrest. Therapy for chorea is supportive; there are no specific drugs to control the neurological manifestations, and there is no evidence that anti-inflammatory drugs ameliorate the process.

SYSTEMIC LUPUS ERYTHEMATOSUS (SLE)

Systemic lupus erythematosus (SLE) is a much less common disease than juvenile rheumatoid arthritis or rheumatic fever, but it is of interest because of its known associations with immune mechanisms. SLE is characterized by typical cutaneous manifestations, multisystem disease and the formation of antibodies to a number of body constituents. The characteristic cutaneous manifestations may occur alone (discoid lupus erythematosus) unassociated with serological abnormalities.

Although the etiology of SLE remains unknown, much has recently been learned about the pathogenesis of some of its manifestations, particularly the nephritis and vasculitis that make SLE a severe disease in many patients. The discovery of the LE cell by Hargraves in the 1940's was fortuitous, and it opened the door to many immunological studies in SLE. Hargraves noted the presence of characteristic inclusion-containing cells in the bone marrows from several patients with SLE; he demonstrated that these cells resulted from a factor in lupus serum ("LE factor"), and that the inclusions in LE cells were composed of nuclear material that had been phagocytosed by leukocytes. The LE factor was subsequently shown to be an antibody that reacted with the deoxyribonucleoprotein of isolated cell nuclei, rendering them susceptible to phagocytosis. After the realization that LE cells resulted from an antibody directed against a nuclear protein, a number of additional antibodies reactive with nuclear constituents (antinuclear antibodies) were found. Other antibodies were also identified in the sera of lupus patients, including antibodies reactive with gamma globulin (rheumatoid factors), red blood cells (positive Coombs' test), platelets, antigens used in serological tests for syphilis and blood coagulation factors. The identification of these antibodies led to speculation that SLE was an "autoimmune disease." None of these antibodies could be shown to cause the disease SLE, however, and aside from antibodies directed against red cells and platelets, none could be implicated as causing direct tissue damage. Transfusion of lupus sera did not cause detectable disease in normal recipients. Recently, it has been recognized, however, that at least some of these antibodies cause tissue damage in SLE, not by direct "autoimmunity," but through the mechanism of immune complex disease. Immune complexes circulate in the blood, fix complement and localize in the walls of blood vessels and renal glomeruli, causing inflammation and tissue damage. DNA, antibodies to DNA, and complement can be identified in renal tissue from lupus nephritis patients and by immunofluorescent staining techniques or by elution and direct measurement. Levels of serum hemolytic complement and some of its components are regularly lowered in lupus patients with active immune complex disease, particularly nephritis.

Many questions remain to be answered about SLE, however. The basic cause of the disease remains unknown. Although it is well known that lupuslike illnesses can be set off by a variety of drugs, the role of foreign substances such as drugs or viruses in the disease remains uncertain. The predilection of SLE for females has never been explained (9 females to 1 male). Lupus appears to be familial in some instances, and serological abnormalities may sometimes be found in asymptomatic relatives of lupus patients.

About 20 per cent of cases of SLE begin in childhood, usually in girls over eight years of age.

Clinical manifestations. Systemic lupus erythematosus may be associated with a wide variety of clinical manifestations. The disease may begin insidiously, with vague symptoms dating back months or years prior to diagnosis, or explosively with sudden appearance of multisystem disease. Most frequently presenting manifestations in children are fever, malaise, arthritis or arthralgia, and rash.

Cutaneous manifestations affect most patients at some time during disease. The facial butterfly rash is characteristic of SLE, as are erythematous macules on the palms, soles, fingers or toes. Erythematous or ulcerative lesions appear frequently on oral and nasal mucous membranes or the hard palate. Alopecia secondary to involvement of hair follicles may occur. A rash similar to the butterfly rash may involve the extremities and trunk, and non-specific rashes resembling erythema multiforme may also appear. Arthritis and arthralgia are common; arthritis is usually transient and nondeforming. Myositis and aseptic necrosis of bones occur in some patients. Hepatosplenomegaly, generalized lymphadenopathy, pleuritis and pericarditis are frequent. Endocarditis may be present, as may interstitial pulmonary disease and gastrointestinal involvement. Involvement of the central nervous system may be severe and potentially fatal. Hematological problems including anemia, thrombocytopenia and leukopenia are common. Ocular involvement may also occur.

Nephritis occurs in the majority of children with SLE and is potentially the most serious disease manifestation. Signs of nephritis include abnormal urine sediment and proteinuria; the nephritis syndrome and signs of renal insufficiency occur in some patients.

Course and prognosis. The natural history of lupus is unpredictable. It is often considered a severe and progressive disorder that will terminate in death if untreated. However, spontaneous remissions or smoldering disease of many years' duration occur in some patients. The disease appears to be more acute and of greater severity in children than in adults. Most deaths in lupus now occur from infections, nephritis or central nervous system disease. Different types of nephritis occur in SLE; the ultimate prognosis of the nephritis may be related to the histological picture of the renal lesion. Not all lupus patients with nephritis have a dismal prognosis. Mild glomerular involvement (lupus glomerulitis) may never progress to severe renal disease and appears to have a relatively good prognosis. Widespread renal disease involving glomeruli and interstitial tissues (lupus glomerulonephritis), however, is usually progressive and appears to have a bad prognosis. Pure membranous glomerulonephritis occurs in a few lupus patients and has an unpredictable outcome.

The prognosis in earlier published series of children with lupus appeared gloomy with more than 50 per cent mortality, but it is now apparent that some children do have mild SLE and that vigorous therapy with early control of disease activity may improve the outlook for children with severe disease. The disease is potentially ever

present, however, and careful follow-up is mandatory.

Laboratory tests. Patients with active SLE invariably have positive tests for antinuclear antibodies; the antinuclear antibody test is the best screening test for SLE. Antinuclear antibodies are most frequently detected by immunofluorescent techniques. The LE cell is caused by the presence of sufficient antinuclear antibody to deoxyribonucleoprotein. Although LE cells are usually demonstrable at some time during the disease course, they may not always be present, and thus the LE cell is not a good screening test for the disease. Antibodies to deoxyribonucleic acid (DNA) are present in many lupus patients and are generally indicative of active immune complex disease. Other antibodies may also be found in lupus patients, including positive Coombs' test, false-positive serological test for syphilis, rheumatoid factors and circulating anticoagulants. Levels of serum immunoglobulins are generally elevated. Serum complement levels are regularly lowered in patients with active immune complex disease, particularly nephritis. Patients with nephritis have abnormal urine sediments and proteinuria and may have depressed renal function. Histology of renal tissue obtained by percutaneous kidney biopsy may be diagnostically helpful, although the histological picture is not entirely specific for SLE; examination of renal histology should be made in patients with clinical nephritis to assess the type and severity of renal involvement. The acute phase phenomena (ESR, C-reactive protein) are of no diagnostic usefulness but simply reflect active inflammatory disease. The histology of lupus rash is characteristic; occasionally dermal biopsies may be diagnostically useful, particularly in discoid lupus.

Diagnosis. The diagnosis of lupus is chiefly clinical, based on the presence of typical cutaneous or multisystem disease, and is confirmed by laboratory tests. It must be remembered that antinuclear antibodies are not diagnostic of SLE but occur also in a number of other conditions. The diagnosis of SLE should be considered in any child with arthritis. It is important to make the diagnosis early in the disease before irreversible damage has occurred.

Therapy. Therapy in lupus is designed

to combat inflammation and possibly to retard the production of immune complexes. Before undertaking therapy it is crucial to determine the extent and severity of systemic involvement, including nephritis. Therapy should be geared to the individual patient. For individuals with mild lupus without clinical nephritis and with normal levels of serum complement, symptomatic therapy with salicylates, chloroquine or small doses of corticosteroids may suffice. For individuals with more severe lupus, particularly with nephritis and low levels of serum complement, more vigorous therapy is indicated. The most valuable indices of disease control currently available are the return of levels of serum complement and antibodies to DNA to normal values. Rapid and effective control of disease is important to prevention of irreparable tissue damage, particularly to the kidneys. To this end, unpleasantly large doses of corticosteroids for prolonged periods of time may be required. The use of drugs such as azathioprine and cyclophosphamide has also been advocated; although these drugs have been termed "immunosuppressive," their mechanism of action in diseases such as lupus remains unknown, and there are as yet no controlled studies to show their efficacy. Their use may be warranted in severe lupus but should be made only under careful study conditions and with recognition of severe potential toxicities such as disseminated viral infections, possible induction of malignancies and possible damaging effects on reproductive cells in young individuals. The cutaneous manifestations of LE, particularly the facial rash, may be ameliorated by topical corticosteroid therapy or antimalarial drugs.

The treatment of lupus entails meticulous follow-up of patients for many years.

REFERENCES

Juvenile Rheumatoid Arthritis

Bywaters, E. G. L.: Categorization in medicine: A survey of Still's disease. Ann. Rheum. Dis., 26:185, 1967.

Calabro, J. J., and Marchesano, J. M.: The early natural history of juvenile rheumatoid arthritis. Med. Clin. North Am., 52:567, 1968.

Schaller, J., Kupfer, C., and Wedgwood, R. J.: Iridocyclitis in juvenile rheumatoid arthritis. Pediatrics, 44:92, 1969.

Schaller, J., Ochs, H. D., Thomas, E. D., Nisperos, B., Feigl, P., and Wedgwood, R. J.: Histocompatibility antigens in childhood-onset arthritis. J. Pediatr., 88:926, 1976.

Schaller, J., and Wedgwood, R. J.: Is Juvenile Rheumatoid Arthritis a Single Disease? A review. Pediatrics 50:940–953, 1972.

Still, G. F.: On a form of chronic joint disease in children. Med. Chir. Trans., 80:47, 1897.

Rheumatic Fever

Feinstein, A. R., and Spagnuolo, M.: The clinical patterns of acute rheumatic fever: A reappraisal. Medicine, 41:279, 1962.

Markowitz, M., and Gordis, L.: Rheumatic fever, 2nd ed. Philadelphia, W. B. Saunders Co., 1972, p. 309.

Wannamaker, L. W.: Differences between streptococcal infections of the throat and of the skin. N. Engl. J. Med., 282:23–31, 78–85, 1970.

Lupus Erythematosus

Christian, C. L.: Immune complex disease. N. Engl. J. Med., 280:878, 1969.

Dubois, E. L. (Ed.): Lupus erythematosus, 2nd ed. Los Angeles, University of Southern California Press, 1974, p. 798.

Koffler, D., and Kunkel, H. G.: Mechanisms of renal injury in systemic lupus erythematosus. Am. J. Med., 45:165, 1968.

Meislin, A. G., and Rothfield, N.: Systemic lupus erythematosus in childhood. Pediatrics, 42:37, 1968.

Schur, P. H., and Sandson, J.: Immunologic factors and clinical activity in systemic lupus erythematosus. N. Engl. J. Med., 278:533, 1968.

Hargraves, M. M.: Discovery of the LE cell and its morphology. Mayo Clin. Proc., 44:579, 1969.

Orthopedics

33

Lynn T. Staheli

INTRODUCTION

Children's orthopedics has changed dramatically during the past two decades. Medical centers were previously filled with children afflicted with poliomyelitis, tuberculosis or pyogenic infections. Today, congenital defects are the chief concern of the pediatric orthopedist. Cerebral palsy and myelodysplasia (meningomyelocele) rank first and second in this country as producers of crippling in children. Children with myelodysplasia now survive infancy because of the availability of antibiotics and improved neurosurgical techniques. Osteomyelitis and septic arthritis can be cured if treatment is initiated early. Congenital hip dislocation, if detected during the first few months of life, is treated simply and effectively with splints. The "Milwaukee" and "Boston" braces are revolutionizing the treatment of scoliosis and juvenile kyphosis. The deformity of clubfeet can usually be eliminated by serial casts applied in early infancy. Early recognition and institution of treatment are key factors in the proper management of the majority of these problems.

The term *orthopedic* is derived from two Greek words, *orthos*, or straight, and *paidios*, or child. Nicholas André, who coined the name of this specialty, recognized the need for proper care of orthopedic problems during childhood and emphasized the importance of early treatment in preventing deformity. The primary objective of the modern orthopedist is the preservation of function of the musculoskeletal system. Secondary objectives include eliminating pain, improving appearance and facilitating nursing care in the severely disabled.

Orthopedic problems are common. Injuries are frequent in children, who are also often seen for flat feet, intoeing gait or other limb growth variations. The clinical problems encountered number into the thousands, the majority of which may be classified under the following headings:

Etiology	*Example*
Congenital	Clubfeet; hip dysplasia
Developmental	Perthes' disease; scoliosis
Traumatic	Fractures; dislocations
Inflammatory	
Septic	Osteomyelitis
Aseptic	Osgood-Schlatter disease
Neoplastic	
Malignant	Osteogenic sarcoma
Non-malignant	Osteochondroma
Neuromuscular	
Central	Cerebral palsy
Peripheral	Poliomyelitis

EVALUATION OF PATIENT

Diagnosis of musculoskeletal system disorders is made by following the same approach used in other branches of medicine. A careful history is followed by a complete physical examination. Appropriate roentgenograms and laboratory studies complete the evaluation.

Medical History

Information regarding onset, course and previous treatment of the problem is obtained. A history of pain in the child is usually significant. Functional pain is less common in children than in adolescents or adults. A history of trauma is frequently obtained in children, especially boys. One should be cautious about attributing the

323

presenting problem to some injury. Patients with sepsis or tumors often give a history of injury. Assessing the child's developmental level and relating it to his age are helpful when evaluating the neurologically handicapped child.

Physical Examination

The examination is performed either as a screening evaluation or to explore a specific complaint. Ideally, screening should be performed at birth and periodically during infancy and childhood. Screening at birth should be aimed at detecting congenital hip instability.

Screening examination. In the newborn, hip instability is evaluated by Ortolani's test (see the section on congenital hip deformities later in this chapter). In the older child, the following screening examination is suggested:

General inspection: Assess posture, symmetry, deformity and presence of any masses (Fig. 33–1A).

Gait: Observe the general pattern; note asymmetry; evaluate each joint independently; note shoe wear; evaluate muscle strength and balance by heel-and-toe walking (Fig. 33–1B).

Back: While standing behind the patient, ask him to bend forward; look for truncal or thoracic asymmetry (scoliosis) (Fig. 33–1C). Note any pelvic tilt (leg length inequality) (Fig. 33–1D). Ask the patient to stand on one leg at a time and note any drop of the unweighted side (Trendelenburg test) (Fig. 33–1E). This is a sign of abductor weakness, which may be present in muscle diseases and congenital hip dysplasia.

Range of motion: The range of motion (ROM) of abnormal joints should be measured. The position of the joint is neutral (zero) when the patient is in the "anatomical position" (elbow and knee extended, ankle at right angle). The arc through which the patient can move the joint is the "active range of motion"; the arc through which the examiner can move the joint is the "passive range of motion."

Muscle strength: The collective strength of the muscles moving a joint in one direction is easily rated using the following scale:

0–No contraction
1–Trace
2–Poor (moves joint with gravity eliminated)
3–Fair (moves joint against gravity)
4–Good (moves against gravity and some resistance)
5–Normal

Deformity and terminology: Deformity may consist of a grotesque distortion or simply a slight joint stiffness. Deformities are often referred to in descriptive terms, e.g., "shepherd's crook deformity," indicating lateral bowing of the femur (fibrous dysplasia); "mallet finger"; "swan-neck deformity"; and "hammer toe." Most deformities are described by the direction of angulation of the part distal to the site of deformity. The terms *valgus* (turning out) and *varus* (turning in) are applied.

Pain and tenderness: Pain with joint motion and localized tenderness are extremely useful elements of the examination. The exact anatomic localization of the tenderness will frequently allow a presumptive diagnosis.

Radiology

The majority of children with musculoskeletal problems should be studied radiographically. With a few exceptions, films should be made in two planes—anteroposterior and lateral views. In roentgenographic interpretation in children, several suggestions may be useful:

1. Roentgenograms are of very little value in detecting hip dislocations and dysplasia in the newborn (Fig. 33–2). Later, they are indispensable.

2. Roentgenograms are normal (except for soft tissue swelling) in osteomyelitis and septic arthritis for the first 10 to 14 days.

3. Subtle fractures should be detected by accurate localization of the point of maximal tenderness during physical examination and confirmed by the demonstration of an interruption or abrupt change in contour of the bony cortex on the films. Various vague lines through the shaft are often misleading.

4. Accessory ossicles may be confused with fracture. Their location and especially the absence of tenderness allow the differentiation (Fig. 33–3).

5. When in doubt, take roentgenograms

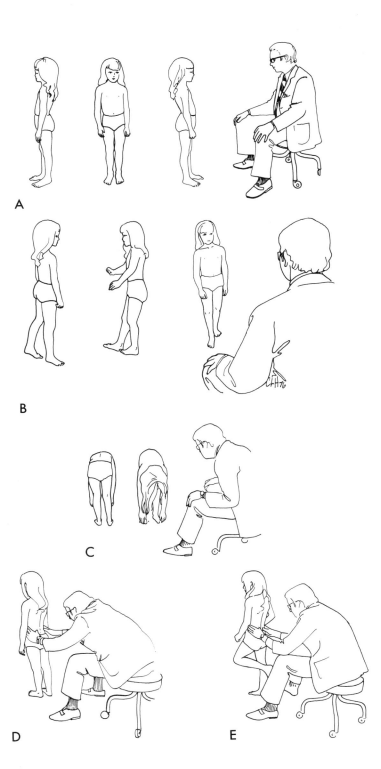

Figure 33–1 Orthopedic screening examination. *A*, General inspection. *B*, Assessment of gait, with heel and toe walking. *C*, Assessment for spinal curvature and for scoliosis. *D*, Leg length inequality check by noting pelvic position. *E*, Assessment of the Trendelenburg sign, indicating the presence of weakness of hip abductors present in conditions such as hip dysplasia.

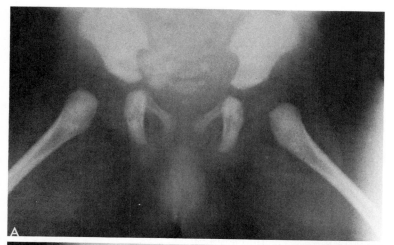

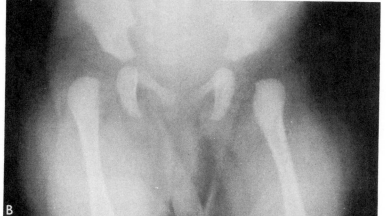

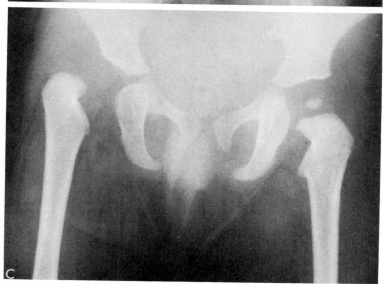

Figure 33–2 Congenital hip dysplasia. *A* and *B* show x-rays taken in the newborn period because of a positive Ortolani's sign on the right side. The radiographs were interpreted as normal, and therefore no treatment was instituted. The patient was next seen at the age of 13 months (*C*), just beginning to walk, with a limp, and showing an obvious dislocation. X-rays in the newborn period are not reliable in ruling out congenital hip dysplasia.

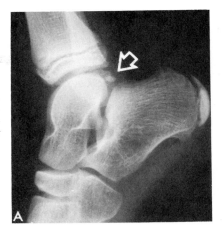
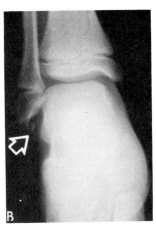

Figure 33–3 Accessory ossicles. The os trigonum (left) or the os fibulare (right) are relatively common accessory ossicles of the foot that may be confused with a fracture.

of the other extremity in the same position for comparison.

6. Some fractures are not visible on initial roentgenograms. Immobilize and restudy in 7 to 10 days. The fracture may be apparent later.

Bone scans. Bone scanning is becoming a useful tool in the early evaluation of certain disorders. It is particularly useful in localizing osteomyelitis, septic arthritis and discitis in the stage before radiographs show any abnormalities. Bone scanning is also useful for localization of tumors, particularly in the spine, early diagnosis of osteochondritis such as Perthes' disease, the determination of activity of bone lesions and verification of the preslip state of the proximal femoral epiphysis (Fig. 33–4).

Laboratory

The erythrocyte sedimentation rate (ESR) is very useful for separating pyogenic infections from other inflammatory states and traumatic lesions. The ESR is nearly always elevated in osteomyelitis and septic arthritis. The white blood count is often normal in these conditions. Laboratory studies are also useful in evaluating bacterial infections, muscular dystrophy, metabolic bone disease and collagen disorders. The importance of blood cultures in septic problems should not be overlooked.

TREATMENT PRINCIPLES

The primary objective of treatment is the restoration of function. In most instances complete restoration to a normal status is possible. In the more severely involved child (e.g., cerebral palsy, muscular dystrophy) one must assess the specific needs of the child first and then tailor the management to meet those objectives.

Shoe Corrections

Shoe manufacturers proclaim the value of corrective or "orthopedic" shoes. It has been clearly established that where climate and custom permit, bare feet are most healthy. The most important characteristic of a good shoe is that it is large enough to avoid cramping and distorting the growth of the foot. The relative values of common shoe corrections are given here:

Of Probable Value	*Of Doubtful Value*
Heel or sole lifts for leg length inequality	Thomas heels and arch supports for flat feet
Reverse last shoes for metatarsus adductus	Sole and heel patches for intoeing gait patterns
	Heel and sole wedges for bowlegs and knock-knees

Immobilization Moulding and Traction

Limiting motion often relieves pain, prevents deformity and may facilitate healing. Bedrest provides partial immobilization of the entire body. Children tolerate bedrest extremely well as compared with adults. A variety of methods of providing more complete immobilization is available.

Plaster casts are most commonly used to provide temporary immobilization following injury or surgery. They are also

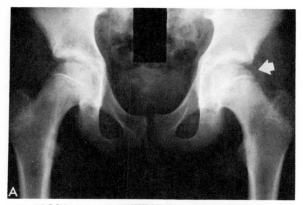

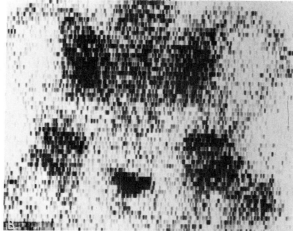

Figure 33–4 Bone scanning for slipped epiphysis. This 14-year-old boy had left hip pain, and radiographs were thought to show a preslipped state (*A*). This was verified by the presence of a hot bone scan (*B*). A good result followed pinning *in situ* to prevent further slip and initiate fusion of the epiphysis (*C*).

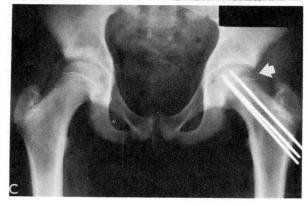

useful in correcting deformities in infants, such as clubfeet.

Braces are useful in providing stability or corrective force in the active patient. The most commonly used braces include the "Boston" and "Milwaukee" braces for scoliosis and the short leg brace to correct the drop foot gait in the neuromuscularly disabled child.

Splints, in contrast to braces, are usually used to maintain correction in the nonambulatory patient. Often, they are used in the ambulatory patient at night. They can be removed for bathing.

Traction is usually used in treating fractures (Fig. 33–5). It is occasionally useful in correcting deformity and relieving muscle spasm. Usually skin traction is satisfactory. Occasionally, skeletal traction (traction applied to pins extending through

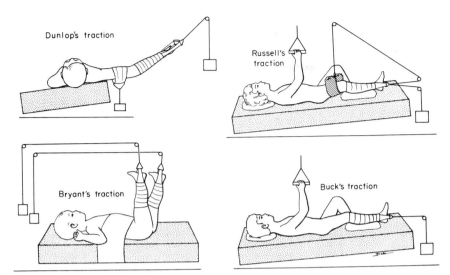

Figure 33–5 Common traction methods used for treating children with various injuries.

bone) is necessary when pull exceeds 5 to 10 pounds or when used for prolonged periods.

Physical and Occupational Therapy

The therapist strives to improve function by improving muscle strength, restoring joint motion and using special training programs.

Exercises. Exercise improves muscle strength and tone and may increase joint motion. *Isotonic* exercises are designed to move the joint against increasing resistance. In some situations motion of the joint may not be possible, e.g., the limb may be in a cast or injured, or it may be undesirable, as in an arthritic joint. *Isometric* exercises are then used. In this method, maximal contraction of the muscle is made with joint motion.

Range of motion. Joint motion may often be increased if the patient actively moves the joint throughout its range frequently and vigorously. Passive range of motion programs are valuable for patients unable to cooperate or those with neuromuscular disorders.

Gait training. The therapist may help the patient to establish efficient gait patterns with or without crutches. This is done through demonstration and repetition of the correct pattern.

Controlling spasticity. Spasticity can be reduced by proper positioning of the patient, inhibiting pathological reflexes and facilitating normal reactions.

Improving self-care. The handicapped child who is able to feed, toilet, entertain and propel himself is happier, better adjusted and much less demanding on the family and society. This is accomplished through training, special tools and modification of the environment when possible.

Drugs

The medications most commonly used in orthopedics are antibiotics and analgesics. The most useful antibiotics are penicillin and its derivatives. Parenteral antibiotics are indicated for osteomyelitis and septic arthritis. Preoperatively administered antibiotics are indicated for open fractures and for surgical procedures involving bones or joints in which the operative time is expected to exceed one and a half to two hours. Analgesics of greatest usefulness include aspirin, codeine and morphine. Aspirin should be avoided postoperatively, however, and in other situations in which one does not wish to mask body temperature elevations. Fever is a useful early sign of postoperative sepsis.

Surgery

Surgical treatment is an additional tool of the orthopedist for restoring, improving or maintaining function. Surgical treatment may be more "conservative" than non-operative methods of therapy. For example, early surgical correction of the resistant clubfoot by releasing restraining soft tissue structures is preferable to repeated forceful castings, which often produce permanent damage to the joints of the foot and ankle. The number of surgical procedures available runs into the thousands.

PRESENTING COMPLAINTS

The patient is usually seen by the physician for pain, deformity or altered function.

Pain

In children, pain is most commonly due to trauma or inflammatory lesions. Pain manifests itself in different ways at various ages. In the infant, pain may be manifested by increased irritability. The part involved is usually "splinted," and the loss of motion is sometimes referred to as *pseudoparalysis*. A painful condition such as a fracture of the clavicle may be misdiagnosed as a brachial plexus injury in the newborn. In the infant, septic arthritis may be first suggested when one extremity is not moved spontaneously. Pain in the back or lower limb usually produces a limp in the older child. The *antalgic* (painful) limp is characterized by a shortening of the *stance phase* (period of time the extremity is in contact with the ground) on the affected side.

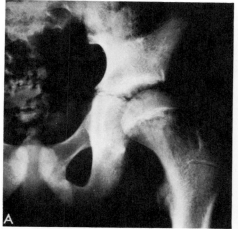
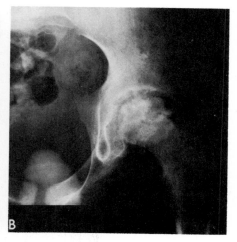
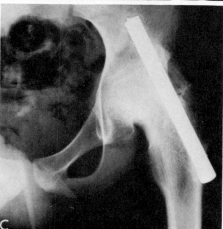

Figure 33–6 Septic arthritis. This 12-year-old boy developed pain in the left hip and fever, which was initially diagnosed as a "hip strain." Treatment was delayed, and when seen 14 days after the onset of symptoms, he was found to have a septic joint. The radiograph (A) shows deossification of the femoral neck with deossification of the head due to loss of blood supply. Subsequent x-rays show avascular necrosis and septic cartilage necrosis (B), necessitating fusion (C).

Septic arthritis. This is a most common urgent problem in pediatric orthopedics (Fig. 33–6). The synovium is usually seeded by a hematogenous route, although in the hip joint in which the metaphysis is intra-articular, direct extension from a focus of osteomyelitis in the femoral neck may occur. The most common organism in the child under two years is *Hemophilus influenzae*; later, *Staphylococcus* predominates. Untreated, the joint is destroyed by protolytic enzymes, and furthermore, the vascularity to the epiphysis may be jeopardized by increased intra-articular pressure and vascular obstruction. Diagnosis is established by aspiration of the joint and fluid examination. A Gram stain of the aspirate and appropriate cultures are made. In approximately 1 of 4 cases, the organism is not identified, and treatment with antibiotics is empirical. Drainage is essential. Open drainage of hip joint infections is necessary; other joints are at less risk and can frequently be managed by repeated needle aspiration.

The diagnostic problems of young infants are greater. The only consistent physical finding is reduced spontaneous mobility of the extremity. Bone scanning may be useful in localizing the site of involvement if it does not delay treatment, but the final diagnosis is made by aspiration. Avoiding delay is essential.

Osteomyelitis. Osteomyelitis usually occurs from hematogenous seeding of the metaphysis with bacteria. Untreated, the "cellulitic" phase progresses to suppuration. The abcess may then penetrate the cortex, elevate the periosteum and finally rupture into the soft tissue. Surgical drainage is indicated if suppuration has occurred. This may be apparent on physical examination and usually is present if treatment has been delayed or if significant clinical improvement fails to occur after 24 hours of antibiotic treatment. Bone scans may be useful in localizing occult infection, as conventional radiographs show no osseous changes for the first 10 to 14 days.

Leg aches (growing pains). Aching pain in the legs occurs in 10 to 20 per cent of children. The pain usually is present in the calves, frequently occurs in the evening at about bedtime and is most common after exposure to cold or damp weather. More serious causes can be excluded by careful

examination. A negative x-ray film, a normal sedimentation rate and the absence of tenderness, joint motion limitation, muscle atrophy or masses confirm the impression of "idiopathic myalgia of childhood." This is best managed by reassurance of the family, aspirin and local heat.

Osgood-Schlatter disease. This is a traction injury at the site of attachment of the patellar tendon to the tibial tubercle (Fig. 33–7). Inflammation occurs and heterotrophic bone forms within the tendon. The condition is usually self-limited, and healing occurs if stress is reduced. This may be achieved simply by restricting activity or, in more persistent forms, by four to six weeks of immobilization in a cylinder cast.

"Shin splints". Pain over the tibia is common and may occur from several different mechanisms. These include stress fractures, compartment syndromes, muscle hernias, periostitis and tenosynovitis. Differentiation is often difficult. Simple initial measures include avoiding running on hard surfaces, reducing the distance or speed of running and building up slowly at a rate below that which causes pain. If the pain persists, referral is appropriate.

Injury. Multiple injuries are suspected in the patient hurt in an automobile acci-

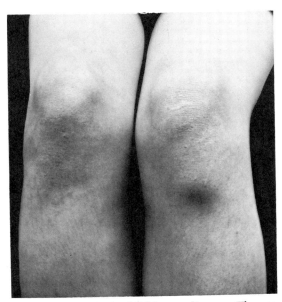

Figure 33–7 Osgood-Schlatter disease. The patient's left knee shows a typical swelling over the tibial tubercle, characteristic of Osgood-Schlatter disease. This is an attraction apophysitis that occurs commonly in the prepubescent child.

dent or by a fall from a height. The patient must be fully examined systematically. If the patient is conscious, fractures and other significant injuries can nearly always be ruled out by the absence of tenderness. Each bony part and joint should be palpated. If not tender, the joint is then moved. If this elicits no pain, the absence of significant injury is confirmed. If tenderness or pain is found, the site should be exactly localized to aid in establishing the nature of the injury and guide the examiner in ordering and interpreting the radiographs.

Open wounds require emergency treatment. In deep wounds, the integrity of the adjacent structures should be determined. Circulation is assessed by skin temperature, color, capillary filling, pulse and pain in the limb distal to the injury. Pain is an early sign of ischemia. Sensation and motor function should be carefully assessed and any deficit noted. In deep wounds, roentgenograms are required to rule out bony injury and may aid in detecting radiopaque foreign bodies. Optimal management includes: (1) cleansing of the adjacent skin with soap, (2) debridement of the wound as necessary and (3) irrigation with saline solution. Primary closure of a wound is justified if foreign matter and non-viable tissue have been completely removed by debridement. Tetanus prophylaxis should not be overlooked. Antibiotics, preferably methicillin and ampicillin, should be given as soon as possible after open bony injuries.

Fractures are common in childhood and are managed differently in children than in adults. Fortunately, the problems of post-fracture joint stiffness and non-union common in adults are extremely rare in children. Remodeling will correct deformity in the immature child, and judgment is required in deciding whether an angulated fracture requires reduction. In general, greater deformity can be accepted under the following circumstances:

1. Early childhood or infancy—more time is available for remodeling before growth ceases.

2. Deformity in the plane of motion of the adjacent joint—the joint can compensate for the deformity.

3. Deformity close to the end of a bone—greater deformity can be tolerated, for example, in a distal than in a midshaft forearm fracture.

Anatomic reduction is generally not necessary in children unless the fracture extends into the joint or through an epiphysis. In the older child, especially the female, remodeling may be limited because of advanced skeletal maturity, and caution should be exercised in leaving deformity, since complete remodeling may not occur before the epiphysis closes and remodeling ceases.

Side-to-side "bayonet" apposition in the child is acceptable if the alignment is satisfactory. In femoral shaft fractures, bayonet apposition is desirable, since the fracture stimulates growth and end-on apposition would result in excessive length of the fractured side. It is desirable to leave approximately 1 to 1.5 cm of shortening to compensate for subsequent overgrowth.

The time required for healing depends upon the age of the child and the size of the bone. The younger child heals more rapidly. As a general rule, the following guide is useful for children in midchildhood:

Immobilization for
4 weeks—Very small bones (phalange, metacarpal)
6 weeks—Small bones (radius, ulna)
8 weeks—Large bones (tibia, humerus)
10 weeks—Very large bones (femur)

When in doubt, it is preferable to err in extending the period of immobilization rather than in making it too short. During the period of immobilization it is very important to take serial x-ray films to assure maintenance of reduction of position. X-ray films should be taken only while the fracture can still be moved. In the usual forearm fracture it is wise to take films just after reduction and again at 3 and 10 days. The joints above and below the fracture should be immobilized. Following removal of the cast, some transient stiffness can be expected. Physical therapy is seldom necessary. Only active motion should be permitted, as passive stretching may result in a progressive loss of motion due to scar formation.

Epiphyseal injuries are a form of fracture that extends through all or part of the epiphyseal plate (Fig. 33–8). Epiphyseal injuries are handled somewhat differently from other fractures. As growth occurs at the epiphysis, certain types of epiphyseal injuries may result in a growth disturbance,

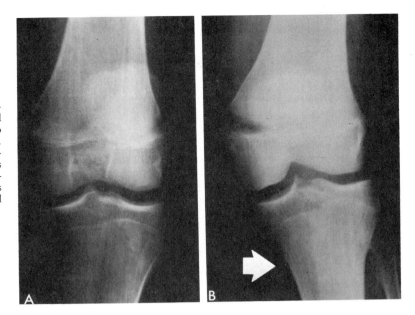

Figure 33–8 Occult epiphyseal injury. This is a 15-year-old boy who sustained an injury to his knee while playing football. The initial x-ray (A) shows no abnormality; however, on stress views (B) the fracture of the epiphysis becomes evident. This may be confused with a medial collateral ligament injury.

producing a progressively increasing deformity. Fractures through the epiphysis occur at the zone of provisional calcification or hypertrophied chondrocytes on the metaphyseal side of the epiphyseal plate (Fig. 33–9). This is the side opposite the germinal zone, and thus with the simple epiphyseal "slip" or fracture, growth abnormalities are uncommon. When the fracture line extends into the epiphysis itself and thus extends through the germinal zone, growth arrest may occur. In such fractures anatomic reduction is essential, and open operation may be necessary to

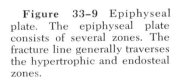

Figure 33–9 Epiphyseal plate. The epiphyseal plate consists of several zones. The fracture line generally traverses the hypertrophic and endosteal zones.

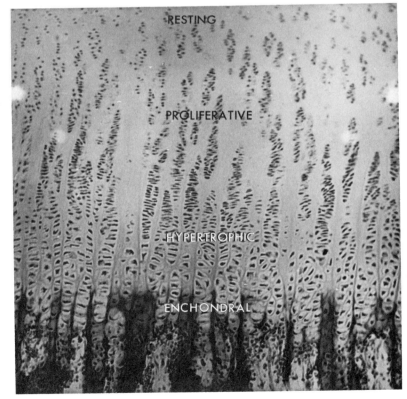

achieve this goal. In addition, the prognosis is guarded, and serial x-ray films and examinations are necessary to assess growth and determine whether deformity is developing. Such deformity is usually treated by performing an osteotomy of either an "opening wedge" or "closing wedge" type. Epiphyseal injuries heal somewhat more rapidly than simple bony fractures; thus the period of immobilization may be reduced by approximately one third.

Sprains are partial or complete ruptures of a ligament. A complete rupture is usually manifested by severe soft tissue swelling, and joint instability can be demonstrated by stress roentgenograms under appropriate local or general anesthesia. Sprains are most common about the ankle and knee. Frequent sites include the medial and lateral collateral ligament of the ankle, the calcanocuboid ligament and the medial and lateral collateral ligament of the knee. Sprains are usually best treated by cast immobilization for two to six weeks.

Slipped capital femoral epiphysis. This condition is most common in the pubescent male. Most slips are gradual, without significant injury. The patient complains of an aching pain, sometimes in the hip but frequently referred to the knee. Ideally, before the slip has become advanced the diagnosis is made by appropriate x-ray films of the hip (Fig. 33–10). The lateral x-ray is most important, as early slips may appear normal on the anteroposterior view. If the diagnosis is made early, the slippage can be arrested by placing pins across the

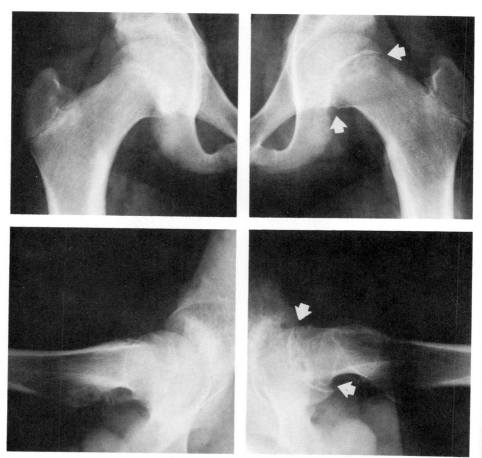

Figure 33–10 Slipped epiphysis (early). The two x-rays on the right show a very early slip of the left capital femoral epiphysis. Note that the irregularity of the metaphyseal side of the epiphyseal plate was the only significant finding in the anteroposterior x-ray. The lateral view, however, shows some posterior displacement of the head. This demonstrates the importance of the lateral view in picking up an early slip.

epiphyseal plate. If the diagnosis is delayed, treatment is much less satisfactory, and permanent disability may follow.

Deformity

Variations in the pattern of development are frequent in the growing child. Spontaneous correction occurs in the majority of children with flat feet, bowlegs and torsional deformities. Some deformities are more serious, however, and require treatment (see also Chapter 21).

Metatarsus adductus. This is generally a positional deformity in which the forefoot is adducted in relationship to the hind foot. The deformity is managed by manipulation and stretching exercises and if not resolved by five or six months is then treated by braces or casts.

Clubfoot. A *clubfoot* deformity with equinus, varus of the heel and adduction of the forefoot is more rigid and more serious than metatarsus adductus. Treatment with serial casts or strapping should begin immediately after birth because the deformity is most supple at that time. In about half the cases, the deformity is rigid and requires surgical correction in addition to casting.

Congenital hip dysplasia. Congenital hip dislocations can be diagnosed in the newborn and treated with complete correction by simple splinting. If the diagnosis is made after the child has begun to walk, treatment is complicated and prolonged, and the child is often committed to a lifelong disability. Every newborn should be examined to rule out hip instability. The infant is examined in the supine position. The hip and knee are flexed to a right angle. The thigh is then flexed, adducted and downward pressure is applied. This will posteriorly dislocate the unstable hip. The thigh is slowly brought into abduction, and the low-pitched "clunk" of relocation (Ortolani's sign) will be felt. High-pitched "clicks" are common, occurring in about 1 of 3 examinations, and are of no significance. Ortolani's sign may only be present during the first few days after birth. Later in infancy, hip abduction becomes limited and is the most reliable physical sign. Radiographs are of little value in diagnosing hip dysplasia in early infancy. In later in-

fancy and childhood, they may be the only certain way of diagnosing the condition.

Rotational abnormalities. "Toeing in," or "pigeon toed" gait, is very common in childhood. Occasionally, the deformity is dynamic (due only to muscle imbalance), but usually it is structural. This rotational malalignment may occur in the hip, tibia or foot. One should first observe the child's gait to determine the severity of the problem. The child is then examined in the prone position with the knees flexed to a right angle. If internal rotation of the hip is greater than 70 degrees, medial femoral torsion exists. If the axis of the foot turns in, in relation to the thigh axis as viewed from above, internal tibial torsion is present (Fig. 33–11). If the lateral margin of the sole is convex, metatarsus adductus or varus is present. These abnormalities may be single or multiple. In the infant or young child, tibial torsion is treated with night splints that hold the legs externally rotated. Metatarsus adductus is treated with corrective plaster casts. In the older child, significant deformities are treated surgically.

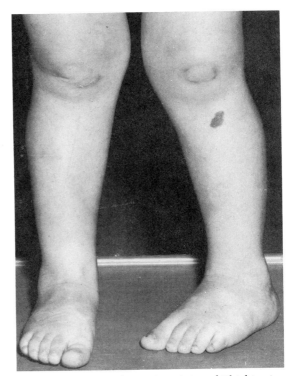

Figure 33–11 In this patient, internal tibial torsion has occurred on the left leg. Note that the patella is directed straight ahead.

"TOEING OUT". External rotation deformities are most common in infancy. The hips can be externally rotated to 90 degrees, and internal rotation may be restricted. This is due to capsular contracture, which will resolve spontaneously and requires only the reassurance of the mother. Excessive external tibial torsion often becomes worse with age and, if severe, may require operative correction.

BOWLEGS AND KNOCK-KNEES. Normally, infantile bowlegs are relatively mild and correct spontaneously by the second year. If the condition is more severe or persistent, active treatment is indicated. If the deformity is not great, it can be managed with a bar splint, which simply holds the feet widely separated (15 to 30 inches). In more severe cases, night bracing, corrective casts or, rarely, surgical correction is necessary.

Knock-knees occur in the preschool child. The normal range includes children with up to 2½ inches between the malleoli, with skin of the knees just touching. Figure 33–12 shows an unusual degree of knock-knee.

The pathological forms of these conditions usually result from rickets, rheuma-

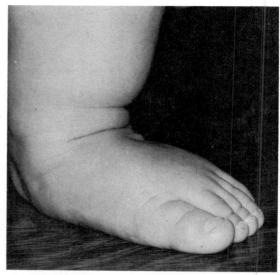

Figure 33–13 A typical (normal) infantile flat foot with a prominent fat pad obscuring the longitudinal arch.

toid arthritis, deformity secondary to injury or tibia vara (Blount's disease).

Flat feet. All infants, most young children and many older children have flat feet (Fig. 33–13). In infancy, a fat pad is present in the long arch. When the fat pad disappears, most children slowly develop a longitudinal arch. Failure of the longitudinal arch to develop is usually due to ligamentous laxity, which is often familial. Treatment of the familial or common "hypermobile" flat foot with shoe corrections, i.e., "orthopedic shoes" with Thomas heels (extended heel, or medial side and medial wedge, and arch supports) is of doubtful value. In addition, the adult with a hypermobile flat foot seldom has foot problems. Conversely, foot disability is common in adults who have high arches, varus (inverted) or stiff feet.

Other causes of flat feet are associated with disability and should be ruled out in each situation as shown on the opposite page.

Each of these conditions can be ruled out on physical examination. The vertical talus produces a prominent palpable mass (head of talus) in the longitudinal arch, and the accessory navicular can produce a prominence over the medial aspect of the foot. Dorsiflexion of the ankle will be limited if the Achilles tendon is contracted, and sub-

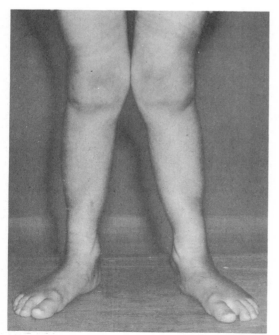

Figure 33–12 A child with moderately severe genu valgum (knock-knees).

Age Presenting	Deformity	X-ray	Treatment
Infancy	Congenital vertical talus (Fig. 33–14)	Talus vertical	Surgical correction
Late childhood and adolescence	Tarsal coalition (Fig. 33–15)	Oblique	Resection of coalition
	Tight Achilles tendon	None	Heel cord stretching or surgical lengthening
	Accessory navicular (Fig. 33–16)	Accessory ossicle, medial side of navicular	Excision of ossicle

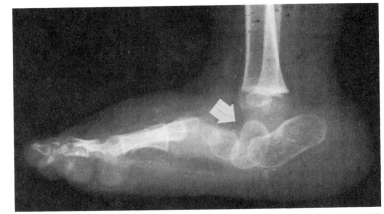

Figure 33–14 Congenital vertical talus (arrow). This produces a convexity on the plantar aspect of the hind foot.

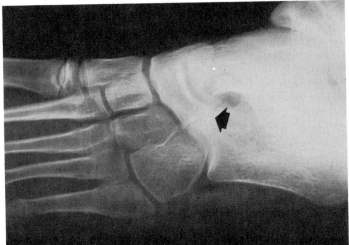

Figure 33–15 Roentgenogram of a foot with a tarsal coalition (arrow), between the calcaneus and the navicular bone. The secondary manifestation is peroneal spasm and foot pain. This results in reduction of the normal range of inversion and eversion of the hind foot.

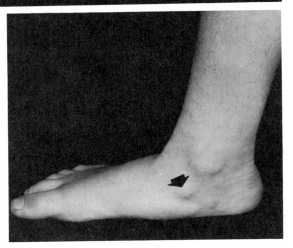

Figure 33–16 A foot with an accessory navicular bone (arrow) producing prominence over the medial aspect of the foot. Because of the associated anomalous insertion of the posterior tibial tendon, there is loss of the medial arch giving rise to a flat foot.

talar motion, i.e., inversion and eversion, will be restricted if a tarsal coalition is present. Absence of the talar and navicular prominences and a full range of motion of the ankle and subtalar joint therefore allow one to readily rule out the flat foot that requires treatment.

Baker's cysts. Baker's cysts are synovial cysts that occur in the popliteal fossa between the medial head of the gastrocnemius and semitendinosis tendons. The mass is firm, smooth, fixed, usually nontender and characteristic in location (Fig. 33–17). The majority of these cysts often resolve spontaneously over several years. In some instances the mass persists, and surgical removal may be necessary.

Scoliosis. Scoliosis is a lateral curvature of the spine that is accompanied by rotation, which accounts for most of the truncal asymmetry. Early diagnosis of scoliosis is important, as early curves can be effectively treated by bracing. Untreated, scoliosis may progress until skeletal maturity. If severe, it produces an ugly deformity and restriction of cardiopulmonary function. Early scoliosis can best be detected by truncal or thoracic asymmetry. Any asymmetry should be evaluated with radiographs of the spine. Nearly all patients with scoliosis should be evaluated by an orthopedist.

Altered Function

Conditions that produce pain in adults often produce only altered function or deformity in children. A painful condition such as Perthes' disease may result in a limp with no complaint of pain. Herniated disc in the adult is generally very painful; when the onset occurs in adolescence, however, stiffness and scoliosis may be the only findings.

Limping. The common causes of limping have definite age patterns. Other causes, such as osteomyelitis, septic arthritis and trauma, may occur at any age. The common age-related causes of limping include:

Early childhood	Congenital hip dysplasia
Midchildhood	Observation hip (synovitis)
	Perthes' disease
	Muscular dystrophy
	Cerebral palsy
Older child	Slipped capital femoral epiphysis
	Osteochondritis dissecans
	Osgood-Schlatter disease

"Nursemaid's elbow." This condition occurs when the child's arm is suddenly pulled, usually by the parent. Traction on the radial head results in a tear of the attachment of the annular ligament to the neck of the radius (Fig. 33–18). The ligament then becomes trapped between the radial head and capitellum and results in limitation of motion. The entrapment may be freed by rotation of the forearm into supination, generally accompanied by a "click." The child may not complain of pain but may simply refuse to move the elbow. Radiographs show no abnormality, and the condition generally does not recur.

ATHLETIC INJURIES

Participation in athletic activities is an important part of the social, emotional and

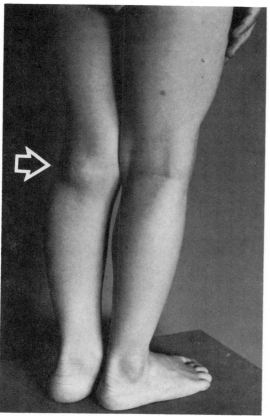

Figure 33–17 Baker's cysts. Swelling in the popliteal fossa in a child is usually due to a Baker's cyst. The cyst is identified by its characteristic location, smooth margins and positive translumination. The diagnosis may be confirmed by needle aspiration of a thick clear fluid content.

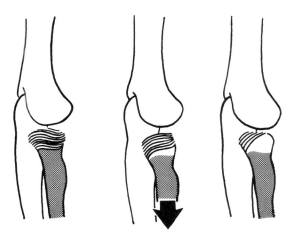

Figure 33–18 Nursemaid's elbow. Nursemaid's elbow results from a pull on the outstretched arm which tears the synovial lining of the annular ligament from part of the neck of the radius. This allows the annular ligament to slide into the joint when the traction is removed. With the rotation of the forearm the annular ligament slips back to its original location.

physical development of children and adolescents. Even children with physical handicaps find participation an enjoyable and valuable experience if properly structured. Injuries do occur but are less frequent than in adults, and healing and functional recovery are more rapid. The types of injuries in children are somewhat unique owing to the presence of an epiphyseal plate.

Epiphyseal fractures. Fractures often occur through the epiphyseal plate, as it is weaker than the adjacent bone or ligaments, particularly in torsional loading. Healing is more rapid than for fractures of adjacent bone. For fractures that extend through the epiphyseal plate or extend into the metaphysis, healing is more rapid, and the child may return to athletic activity after about four weeks if tenderness is absent. If the fracture extends through the epiphysis, immobilization should be con-

tinued for six weeks and contact sports avoided for one year.

"Little League Elbow." This condition results from repeated exposure to intense traction and compressive forces across the elbow during pitching. These forces are greater if a "curve ball" is thrown. The most common injury is partial or complete traction avulsion of the medial epicondyle. Compression on the radial side of the joint may produce avascular necrosis of the radial head or capitellum. The condition is best prevented by not throwing curve balls, limiting practice and allowing only two innings of pitching per game. Any shoulder or elbow pain should be reported immediately. Stress fractures of the humerus or epiphyseal separation of the proximal humeral epiphysis may also occur from pitching but are less frequent.

Management Principles

It is the role of the physician to assess the child's problem accurately, keep restrictions to a minimum and remove them as soon as possible. If activity restrictions are necessary, it is essential to explain them very carefully, specifically and often repeatedly to be certain that both child and parent understand. Frequently, the parent will impose greater restrictions than are medically justified, and the physician must often assume the role of the child's advocate. If restrictions are necessary, they can be graded. In grading the level of activity it should be noted that injury rates are many times higher during participation in competition than in practice. Participation in competitive playing is the last restriction to be lifted. A typical grading system is:

Mild	Walking, jogging, bicycle riding
Moderate	Tennis, roller and ice skating, baseball, basketball, swimming
Vigorous	Football, skiing, soccer, competition

Oral Disorders

M. Michael Cohen, Jr., and James R. Hooley

CONGENITAL MALFORMATIONS

Cleft lip and palate. These are common malformations, observed in approximately 1 of 750 births. Both the type and the extent of clefting vary (Fig. 34–1). Cleft lip with or without cleft palate is etiologically distinct from isolated cleft palate. Only one form ever recurs within the same family. In both forms, however, a polygenic recurrence risk of about 2 to 5 per cent can usually be given, provided clefting is the only malformation and no other family members are affected.

Clefting may also occur as part of a broader pattern of abnormalities, and more than 140 such conditions have been recog-

nized to date. The clinician should strive to make a specific diagnosis from the overall pattern of defects. Different diagnoses imply different recurrence risks, since various monogenic, chromosomal and teratogenic syndromes are known to occur.

Cleft lip should be surgically repaired as early as possible to encourage acceptance of the child by the parents. Cleft palate is usually closed at approximately 18 months of age to permit better growth in the width of the maxilla. Variation in the time of closure of the lip or palate may occur, depending upon the overall size of the infant, the presence of other abnormalities, the degree of development of the prolabium and lateral lip, the amount of protru-

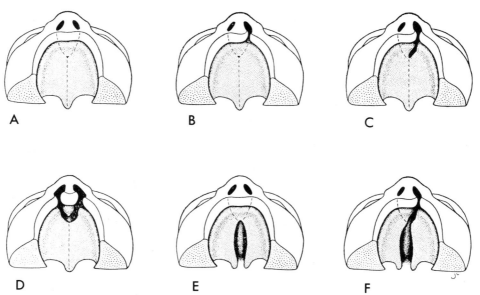

Figure 34–1 Ventral view of palate, gum, lip and nose. *A,* Normal. *B,* Unilateral cleft lip. *C,* Unilateral cleft involving lip and jaw, and extending to incisive foramen. *D,* Bilateral cleft involving lip and jaw. *E,* Isolated cleft palate. *F,* Cleft palate combined with unilateral anterior cleft. (*From* Langman, J.: *Medical Embryology.* Baltimore, Williams and Wilkins Co., 1963, p. 308.)

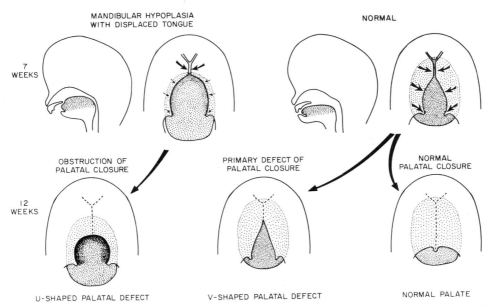

Figure 34–2 Diagram comparing the U-shaped cleft of the Robin anomalad with the more common V-shaped cleft palate. (*From* Hanson, J. W., Smith, D. W., J. Pediatr., 87:30, 1975.)

sion of the premaxilla and the degree of collapse of the palatal segments.

Management of the patient with cleft lip or palate is very complex and continues from birth through adulthood. A team approach typically includes a pediatrician, plastic surgeon, dentist, oral surgeon, orthodontist, speech pathologist and psychologist. Patients should be carefully followed for the development of otitis media and subsequent hearing deficit.

Robin anomalad. The Robin anomalad consists of cleft palate, micrognathia and glossoptosis. Pathogenesis is based on arrested development of the mandible, which prevents the normal descent of the tongue between the palatal shelves, obstructing closure. Thus, the palate in the Robin anomalad is U-shaped in contrast to the more frequently observed V-shaped cleft palate (Fig. 34–2). As with cleft lip with or without cleft palate and isolated cleft palate, the Robin anomalad may occur alone or as part of a broader pattern of abnormalities. Again, proper management and counseling depend upon proper overall diagnosis.

An important early problem in patients with the Robin anomalad is decent maintenance of the airway since the tongue interferes with respiration. In some cases, simply keeping the infant in a prone position serves to keep the tongue forward. In other cases, the tongue is temporarily sutured to the lower lip or a Kirshner wire is inserted from the angle of the mandible on one side through the posterior part of the tongue to the angle of the mandible on the other side. In severe cases with pronounced cyanosis, tracheostomy may be necessary.

Macroglossia. A large tongue (macroglossia) may occur as an isolated finding or may be a diagnostic clue in a broader pattern of abnormalities (Table 34–1). In some instances, partial glossectomy may be nec-

TABLE 34–1 SOME CONDITIONS WITH MACROGLOSSIA

Isolated Macroglossia Present at Birth
  Muscular macroglossia
  Hemangioma of tongue
  Lymphangioma of tongue

Generalized Disorders With Macroglossia Present at Birth
  Trisomy 21 syndrome
  Hypothyroidism
  Beckwith-Wiedemann syndrome

Generalized Disorders With Macroglossia of Postnatal Onset
  Hurler syndrome
  Pompé syndrome
  Neurofibromatosis

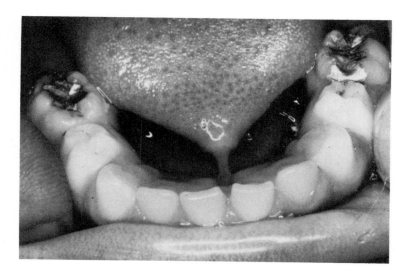

Figure 34–3 Ankyloglossia (tongue-tie).

essary to prevent anterior open bite and speech impediments.

Ankyloglossia. In tongue-tie (ankyloglossia) (Fig. 34–3), the lingual frenum is congenitally short, restricting tongue movement, especially extension. Treatment is not required in mild cases; in severe cases, the frenum should be clipped to avoid future speech defects.

Lingual thyroid tissue. This arises from incomplete embryological descent of the thyroid gland. It is more common in girls and is sometimes associated with hypothyroidism. The tissue is found most frequently at the base of the tongue. It may be raised, purple in color and occasionally associated with hemorrhage. In some cases, the condition may first become evident during puberty, with difficulties in speech and swallowing.

DISEASES OF THE ORAL MUCOSA

Primary herpes simplex. This infection usually occurs between the ages of one and five years. Systemic involvement includes fever, dehydration, irritability, malaise, headache, nausea, dysphagia and regional lymphadenitis. Less commonly, somnolence and convulsions may occur. Acute herpetic gingivostomatitis is characterized initially by swollen gums, increased salivation, pain and foul breath. Shortly thereafter, clear vesicles develop on the oral mucosa; they eventually rupture, forming shallow, painful erosions covered by a yellow pseudomembrane with an erythematous margin (Fig. 34–4). Uneventful spontaneous recovery ensues within 10 to 14 days. Recurrence of the primary form is extremely rare.

Secondary herpes infection. This may be precipitated by factors such as exposure to sunlight, trauma, stress and emotional strain. Initial symptoms include a burning sensation, swelling and soreness at the sites at which vesicular lesions will appear. Clear vesicles develop in small confluent groups, usually at the vermilion border of the lips; they soon rupture and become covered with a brownish-yellow crust. Pustules may also appear. The lesions heal without scarring within 4 to 10 days. Regional lymphadenitis is absent. Recurrent lesions may reappear in the same area; a cyclic pattern has been observed in some patients. Early application of topical corticosteroid preparations may lessen the severity of an attack.

Moniliasis. Moniliasis is a regional and, at times, chronic or systemic disease caused by the yeastlike fungus *Candida albicans*. It most frequently occurs in the mouth; in the newborn it may result from maternal vaginal moniliasis. It may also be associated with prematurity, debility, nutritional disorders, prolonged antibiotic and steroid therapy, diabetes mellitus and malignancy.

In the mouth, moniliasis is characterized by creamy plaques that leave a raw, painful, bleeding surface when removed (Fig. 34–5). Any area of the oral mucosa may be

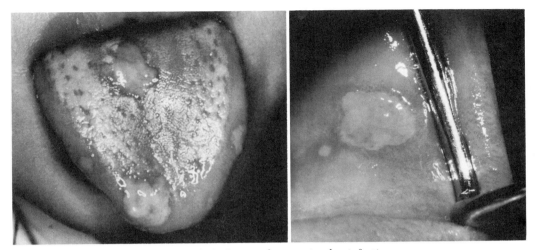

Figure 34-4 Primary herpes simplex infection.

involved. Monilial infection of the lips may cause erosion and cracks at the labial commissures known as perlèche.

Most frequently, the diagnosis is made clinically, especially in infants. Examination of scrapings treated with a 10 per cent potassium hydroxide solution reveals spore clusters and intertwining hyphae that confirm the diagnosis. Nystatin therapy is usually curative. Most cases of moniliasis induced by antibiotic therapy resolve after the drug in question is discontinued.

SALIVARY GLAND DISORDERS

Parotitis. *Mumps*, the most frequent disorder affecting the salivary glands, is discussed in Chapter 15 on infectious disease.

Another form of *acute parotitis* may occur occasionally following surgery or prolonged fever or conditions characterized by poor fluid balance. Hemolytic streptococci and staphylococci are responsible for most cases. Unilateral or bilateral swelling of the parotid gland occurs together with fever, elevated erythrocyte sedimentation rate and leukocytosis. Proper antibiotic treatment, drainage and rehydration resolve the infection.

Salivary flow. A great many conditions may be associated with excessive or diminished salivation. Some of the more common causes are listed in Table 34-2.

A mucocele is a firm, spherical, glistening mass that arises on the oral mucosa above an underlying mucus minor salivary gland (Fig. 34-6). Trauma to a salivary duct

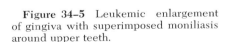

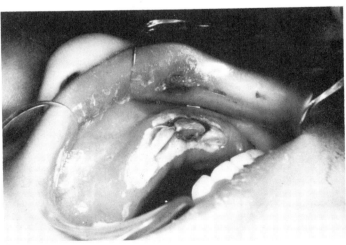

Figure 34-5 Leukemic enlargement of gingiva with superimposed moniliasis around upper teeth.

TABLE 34-2 SOME CONDITIONS AFFECTING SALIVARY FLOW

Excessive Salivation
 Teething
 Acute oral inflammation (e.g., herpes simplex)
 Neurological disturbance (e.g., epilepsy, chorea, mental deficiency)
 Cystic fibrosis
 Drugs (e.g., pilocarpine, mercury poisoning)

Seemingly Excessive Salivation
 Esophageal atresia
 Paralysis of tongue or pharyngeal muscles

Diminished Salivation
 Parotitis (e.g., mumps, post-surgical parotitis)
 Dehydration (fever, diarrhea, blood loss, renal disease)
 Drugs (e.g., atropine, belladonna, antihistamine)
 Anxiety states

Seemingly Diminished Salivation
 Mouth breathing

allows the secretion to escape into the supporting stroma. Mucoceles occur most commonly on the lower lip. Treatment consists of complete surgical excision, including the associated minor salivary gland. Recurrences are common with inadequate treatment such as incision and drainage or surgical "deroofing" of the lesion.

GINGIVAL DISORDERS

Gingival cysts of the newborn probably arise from remnants of the dental lamina. *Palatal cysts* of the newborn arise from epithelial rests incorporated during palatal fusion. Both types of cyst appear as small nodules on the mucosa, become superficial, rupture and resolve within the first few months of life. No treatment is necessary.

An *eruption cyst* is a dilated follicular space around the crown of an erupting tooth; it forms a dome-shaped swelling on the alveolar mucosa. Trauma may cause the cyst to become filled with blood. The lesion almost always occurs with eruption of a deciduous tooth. Although no treatment is usually required, incision may be necessary in rare instances.

Mild, transitory *eruption gingivitis* may accompany the emergence of teeth and should be considered normal. *Marginal gingivitis* in children usually results from poor oral hygiene and lack of abrasive foods. *Puberty gingivitis*, an exaggerated and temporary response to hormonal changes, is usually limited to the anterior part of the mouth, the interdental papillae becoming bulbous.

In *Dilantin hyperplasia*, painless overgrowth results from prolonged therapeutic use of diphenylhydantoin sodium; hyperplastic tissue may sometimes cover the teeth. Surgery is indicated in severe cases, and good oral hygiene aids in retarding growth.

DENTAL DISORDERS

Dental caries. Dental caries is the most prevalent chronic disorder of man. Although the etiology is extremely complex,

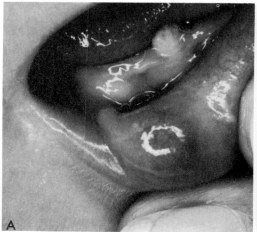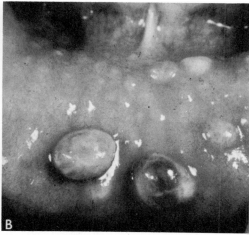

Figure 34-6 *A*, Large mucocele of lower lip. *B*, Multiple mucoceles of lower lip.

TABLE 34-3 NORMAL CHRONOLOGICAL DEVELOPMENT OF DECIDUOUS TEETH

Tooth	Initiation (week in utero)	Calcification Begins (week in utero)	Crown Completed (month)	Eruption (month)	Root Completed (year)	Root Resorption Begins (year)	Tooth Shed (year)
Central incisor	7	14 (13–16)	1–3	6–9	1½–2	5–6	7–8
Lateral incisor	7	16 (14½–16½)	2–3	7–10	1½–2	5–6	7–9
Canine	7½	17 (15–18)	9	16–20	2½–3¼	6–7	10–12
First molar	8	15½ (14½–17)	6	12–16	2–2½	4–5	9–11
Second molar	10	18½ (16–23½)	10–12	20–30	3	4–5	11–12

Sources: Logan, W. H. G., and Kronfeld, R.: Development of the human jaws and surrounding structures from birth to the age of 15 years. *J. Am. Dent. Assoc.*, 20:379, 1933; Lunt, R. C., and Law, D. B.: A review of the chronology of calcification of the deciduous teeth. *J. Am. Dent. Assoc.*, 89:599, 1974; Schour, I., and Massler, M.: Studies in tooth development. The growth pattern of human teeth. *J. Am. Dent. Assoc.*, 27:1918, 1940.

the problem is related to the consumption of refined carbohydrates. Untreated lesions may lead to pulpitis and periapical abscess. Methods of control include (1) good oral hygiene, (2) restoration of carious teeth, (3) dental examination every six months, (4) avoidance of sweets and fine sticky foods and (5) use of fluorides (fluoridation of community water supplies and topical applications). Children should begin regular dental examinations at age three years or as soon as all the primary teeth have erupted.

Natal and neonatal teeth. These are seen in approximately 1 of 3000 births in the general population, but are more frequently observed in association with cleft lip and palate and with several malformation syndromes, in which they may be a diagnostic clue. In most cases, the erupted teeth are deciduous incisors rather than supernumerary teeth. If such teeth are not firmly rooted, they should be extracted to prevent possible aspiration.

Tooth eruption. Normal chronological development of the deciduous and permanent dentition is presented in Tables 34–3 and 34–4. The timing of tooth eruption is quite variable. In general there is poor correlation between tooth age and bone age. Retarded dental development occurs in hypothyroidism, hypopituitarism and trisomy 21 syndrome. Accelerated eruption may be found in congenital adrenal hyperplasia and cerebral gigantism. Of all these conditions, however, only in *hypothyroidism* is deviation in the timing of erup-

TABLE 34-4 NORMAL CHRONOLOGICAL DEVELOPMENT OF PERMANENT TEETH

Tooth	Initiation (month)	Calcification Begins	Crown Completed (year)	Eruption (year)	Root Completed (year)
Maxilla:					
Central incisor	5–5¼ *in utero*	3–4 months	4–5	7–8	10
Lateral incisor	5–5¼ *in utero*	1 year	4–5	8–9	11
Canine	5½–6 *in utero*	4–5 months	6–7	11–12	13–15
First premolar	Birth	1½–1¾ years	5–6	10–11	12–13
Second premolar	7½–8	2–2½ years	6–7	10–12	12–14
First molar	3½–4 *in utero*	Birth	2½–3	6–7	9–10
Second molar	8½–9	2½–3 years	7–8	12–13	14–16
Third molar	3½–4 (yr)	7–9 years	12–16	17–25	18–25
Mandible:					
Central incisor	5–5¼ *in utero*	3–4 months	4–5	6–7	9
Lateral incisor	5–5¼ *in utero*	3–4 months	4–5	7–8	10
Canine	5½–6 *in utero*	4–5 months	6–7	9–11	12–14
First premolar	Birth	1¾–2 years	5–6	10–12	12–13
Second premolar	7½–8	2¼–2½ years	6–7	11–12	13–14
First molar	3½–4 *in utero*	Birth	2½–3	6–7	9–10
Second molar	8½–9	2½–3 years	7–8	11–13	14–15
Third molar	3½–4 (yr)	8–10 years	12–16	17–25	18–25

Sources: Logan, W. H. G., and Kronfeld, R.: Development of the human jaws and surrounding structures from birth to the age of 15 years. *J. Am. Dent. Assoc.*, 20:379, 1933; Schour, I., and Massler, M.: Studies in tooth development. The growth pattern of human teeth. *J. Am. Dent. Assoc.*, 27:1918, 1940.

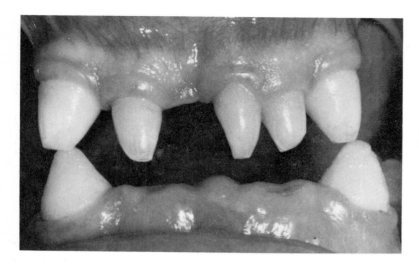

Figure 34–7 Missing teeth and conically shaped teeth in hypohidrotic ectodermal dysplasia.

tion sufficiently altered to be a clinically useful sign.

Missing teeth. These may occur alone or as part of a broader pattern of abnormalities. The most commonly missing teeth are the permanent maxillary lateral incisors, sometimes expressed as conically shaped teeth, frequently inherited as an autosomal dominant trait, occurring in approximately 2 per cent of the general population. Missing teeth and conically shaped teeth are features of hypohydrotic ectodermal dysplasia (Fig. 34–7), a genetic condition associated with sparse hair and limited ability to sweat.

Tooth loss. Premature tooth loss in children may result from a variety of causes, most commonly trauma. Avulsed permanent teeth may be replanted with splinting. Although not successful in many cases, replanting is still recommended since the

tooth is retained occasionally and serves as a space maintainer. Immediate dental consultation is indicated in all cases of avulsed teeth, fractured teeth and intrusion or displacement of teeth.

Enamel hypoplasia. This has a variety of causes, including exanthematous diseases, idiopathic hypoparathyroidism, vitamin D deficiency and localized infection or trauma. Hypoplasia results only when the insult occurs during the formative stage of enamel development, however. Thus, by knowing the chronology of tooth development, the clinician can determine from the location of the defects on various teeth the approximate time at which the insult occurred (Fig. 34–8).

Tooth discoloration. A number of conditions are associated with tooth discoloration. *Trauma* with internal bleeding of the dental pulp is the most common cause.

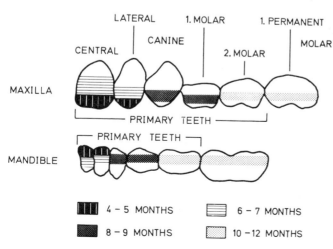

Figure 34–8 Chronology of onset of pre- and postnatal enamel hypoplasia. Time is indicated in months from the onset of gestation. (From Via, W. F., and Churchill, J. A.: J. Am. Dent. Assoc., 59:702, 1959.)

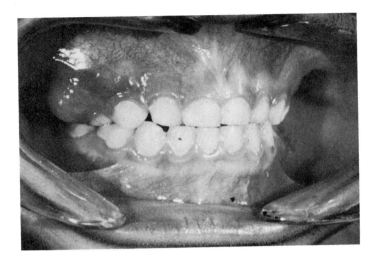

Figure 34–9 "Gum boil" from tooth infection.

Staining due to *tetracycline*, which was once a frequently used antibiotic in children, depends on dosage, time and length of administration and type of tetracycline employed. Staining varies from yellow to grayish brown. The condition may or may not be accompanied by enamel hypoplasia.

When the fluoride content of the drinking water exceeds 1 ppm, *mottled enamel* occurs. Staining varies from white spotting to yellow-brown wavy lines, and occasionally, ill-defined brownish black patches. Enamel hypoplasia is uncommon.

Yellow to green discoloration of the deciduous teeth with or without enamel hypoplasia may be observed in *erythroblastosis fetalis* and is due to indirect hyperbilirubinemia.

Abscess. Acute alveolar abscess is usually accompanied by excruciating, burrowing pain. The patient may also complain that the affected tooth throbs, becomes exquisitely sensitive during mastication and "feels long." Treatment consists of extraction or, in salvageable secondary teeth, opening and debriding the dental pulp chamber to establish drainage. Antibiotics are used in cases accompanied by swelling, facial cellulitis, dysphagia, trismus, hyperpyrexia and leukocytosis. Antibiotic therapy alone does not constitute adequate treatment. Without extraction or treatment of the root canal, a number of sequelae are possible, including recurrent acute abscess, chronic periapical abscess, "gum boil" (Fig. 34–9), periapical granuloma and facial cellulitis with extraoral fistula.

Malocclusion. Malocclusion occurs with such high frequency in the general population that the overwhelming majority of these conditions could more appropriately be called *occlusal dysharmony*. The term malocclusion seems to be a misnomer because it implies a pathological state. The etiology of occlusal dysharmony is extremely complex. Some of the more common causes include (1) discrepancy in the relationship between the maxilla and the mandible, (2) incompatibility of tooth size and jaw size, (3) prolonged retention of primary teeth and (4) premature tooth loss. Orthodontic consultation and treatment should be sought in cases in which occlusal dysharmony seems to be a problem. In most cases, the need for orthodontic treatment can be assessed by the degree of dissatisfaction the patient expresses about his dentition or facial appearance. In more severe handicapping oral-facial conditions such as micrognathia, prognathism or the severe midface deficiency of the Apert or Crouzon syndromes, orthognathic surgery is available.

REFERENCES

Cohen, M. M., Jr.: Pediatric Oral Pathology. *In* Kelley, V. C. (Ed.): *Brennemann's Practice of Pediatrics.* Hagerstown, Md., Harper and Row Publishers, Inc., Vol. 3, Ch. 1, pp. 1–19.

Cohen, M. M., Jr.: Syndromes with cleft lip and palate. J. Oral Surg., in press.

Cohen, M. M., Jr.: The Robin anomalad—its non-specificity and associated syndromes. J. Oral Surg., 34:587, 1976.

Gorlin, R. J., and Goldman, H. M., (Eds.): *Thoma's Oral Pathology*, 5th ed. St. Louis, The C. V. Mosby Co., 1970.

Gorlin, R. J., Pindborg, J. J., and Cohen, M. M., Jr.: *Syndromes of the Head and Neck*, 2nd ed. New York, McGraw-Hill Book Co., 1976.

Hooley, J. R.: The infant's mouth. J. Am. Dent. Assoc., 75:95, 1967.

35

Skin Disorders

Nancy B. Esterly

Skin disorders constitute a significant proportion of presenting complaints in pediatric practice, yet many physicians feel ill-equipped to diagnose and manage these problems. Perhaps it is because the proper interpretation of skin lesions depends on noticing subtle differences in structure, character and color, a skill developed only by persistence and experience. If the clinician recognizes the value of an accurate history, however, by asking appropriate questions he may obtain information that suggests certain diagnoses prior to inspection of the lesions. Pertinent historical data should include site and time of onset, duration, course (whether chronic or intermittent), response to medications, relationship to drug intake, contactants or environmental factors, the presence or absence of local symptoms such as pain and pruritus and systemic signs and symptoms such as fever and malaise. Information concerning household pets, recent travel experience, exposure to individuals with contagious diseases, exposure to insects or parasite vectors, systemic illnesses and family history or past history of skin disease is also often relevant.

EXAMINATION OF THE PATIENT

Thoughtful assessment of cutaneous signs in the pediatric patient can provide the clinician with valuable information regarding general health as well as specific disease processes. All too often, examination of the skin and its appendages is performed in a cursory and incomplete manner, with little attention directed to subtle or even obvious changes. It is important to undress the patient fully and examine the entire body surface as well as the hair, nails and mucous membranes. Good lighting is essential, and natural daylight without glare is the best source of illumination. Frequently, patients or parents have failed to notice minor cutaneous changes and emerging or asymptomatic skin lesions of diagnostic importance. If multiple lesions are present, it is wise to examine all of them before making a definitive diagnosis. A single lesion of one disorder may mimic those of another but, when viewed in the context of the total picture, may be correctly identified with confidence.

General examination of the skin includes assessment of color, texture, turgor, temperature, sweating, hair growth, nails and mucous membranes. Deviations in color may signify anemia (pallor), cardiorespiratory disease (cyanosis), shock (pallor), vasodilatation (erythema), endocrine disorders (hyperpigmentation) and liver disease or hemolytic states (icterus). Likewise, changes in texture may indicate the presence of a chronic skin disease such as ichthyosis or may be a sign of disease in other organs (e.g., thyroid disorders). In infants and small children, evaluation of skin turgor is critical in diseases that cause dehydration or edema.

Specific lesions should be described in terms of type, size, color, texture, firmness, configuration, location and distribution. Lesions must be felt as well as seen in order to characterize them completely. The resulting descriptive composite often suggests the appropriate diagnosis. Skin lesions in a patient may be uniform or diverse in appearance, depending on their stage of evolution. It is important to attempt to identify the primary lesion, since modifying factors such as excoriation or superimposed infection may alter an eruption significantly.

Primary lesions include macules, papules, nodules, tumors, vesicles, bullae, pustules, cysts and wheals. *Macules* are flat lesions of various sizes with distinct or indistinct, smooth or irregular borders. They represent alterations in skin color and cannot be felt. *Papules* are circumscribed, palpable, solid lesions of less than 1 cm that may be soft or firm and of any color. If they involve the pilosebaceous orifice, they are called follicular papules. *Nodules* are similar to papules but are deeper and larger. *Tumors* are even larger masses and may vary in consistency and mobility. *Vesicles* are discrete, elevated lesions containing clear or turbid fluid. *Bullae* differ from vesicles only in that they are larger. Superficial blisters (subcorneal or intraepidermal) are often flaccid and rupture easily, whereas deeper blisters (subepidermal) are usually tense and firm. Since the level of separation is typical for a given disease, an estimation of the location of the cleavage plane is often helpful in making a clinical diagnosis. When lesions contain purulent material, they are called *pustules*. Thick-walled lesions containing fluid or semisolid matter are called *cysts;* these lesions are usually located deep in the skin and are covered by relatively normal epidermis. *Wheals* are evanescent, flat-topped lesions with smooth or irregular borders that represent collections of edema fluid in the dermis. Aggregations of any of these lesions may be referred to as *plaques*.

Secondary lesions include scales, ulcers, excoriations, fissures, crusts and scars. *Scales* are compressed laminae of corneal cells that are retained on the surface of the epidermis. Their color may range from white to brown, and they may be thin, delicate and translucent or thick, opaque and odoriferous. *Ulcers* are excavations caused by loss of tissue by necrosis or trauma. *Excoriations* also represent loss of tissue but are more superficial and, because they are induced by scratching, are usually linear or angular in outline. *Fissures* are cracks or clefts in the skin due to injury or a disease process. *Crusts* or scabs are composed of dried serum, blood or pus mixed with dirt, bacteria and epithelial debris. They may be thin or thick, soft and friable or tough and adherent to the underlying tissue. *Scars* consist of fibrous connective tissue that has proliferated to replace skin that has been lost. Usually flat, pliable and hypopigmented, alternatively, scars may be hypertrophic, cordlike, erythematous, hyperpigmented, atrophic, wrinkled or telangiectatic.

In addition to classifying lesions morphologically, it is necessary to note their configuration or arrangement, which may provide clues to the identity of the eruption. Certain lesions are typically grouped. Some lesions are linear, others annular and ring-shaped and some serpiginous or geographic in outline. Individual lesions may remain discrete or merge and become confluent. Several skin diseases have a consistent and characteristic distribution that can be recognized readily. The particular distribution of an eruption can influence the final diagnosis when individual skin lesions of several diseases resemble each other morphologically.

LABORATORY PROCEDURES

Following completion of the history and physical examination, additional information may be gained from relatively simple laboratory procedures. Most of the following procedures can be carried out with ease in any pediatric outpatient facility.

Wood's lamp examination. The Wood's lamp is equipped with a filter that transmits long-wave ultraviolet light, mainly of a 3650 A wavelength. In certain superficial fungous infections of the scalp (tinea capitis due to organisms of the *Microsporum* species), a blue-green fluorescence can be detected when the patient is examined in a dark room. Debris, crusts and scales may give off a faint yellow glow, which should not be interpreted as a positive Wood's lamp examination. In tinea capitis, a discrete, fluorescent particle is visible at the base of each infected hair or in the follicular opening. Although it is common practice to perform a Wood's lamp examination in patients suspected of having tinea corporis (body ringworm), it is inappropriate to do so, since the lesions of tinea corporis do not fluoresce. Pale yellow fluorescence may be observed in lesions of tinea versicolor; however, this disease is more easily diagnosed with the aid of a KOH preparation.

A Wood's lamp is also useful in situations in which there is altered pigmentation, since examination in a dark room heightens the contrast between areas of skin that differ in color. This method of examination is particularly useful for the newborn infant, whose skin color is naturally pale owing to functional immaturity of the melanocytes. For example, white leaf macules, the hypopigmented lesions of tuberous sclerosis, may be barely perceptible in ordinary light but are readily demonstrated with a Wood's lamp and may provide a visual clue to the correct diagnosis in an infant with seizures. Likewise, the lesions of vitiligo in the older child will stand out more dramatically when viewed in this fashion.

Smears and cultures. The contents of vesicles and pustules may be smeared and stained with Gram stain or Wright stain for the purpose of identifying intralesional cells and bacteria. Cell morphology is best delineated by Wright stain, which, for example, will distinguish the neutrophils of a bacterial pyoderma from the monomorphous infiltrate of eosinophils found in pustules of erythema toxicum. Bacteria are demonstrable on Gram stain preparations and often can be classified with enough surety to initiate antibiotic therapy. When obtaining material for smears, it is important to cleanse the surface of intact lesions thoroughly with alcohol before rupturing them to avoid contamination with surface organisms. The pustules of an inflammatory skin disorder (e.g., miliaria, fungal kerion) may be confused clinically with a bacterial pyoderma, and properly prepared smears can be critical in distinguishing between lesions of different etiologies.

TZANCK SMEAR. This technique is rarely used in pediatrics, but is applicable in several situations. Tzanck smears are prepared by rupturing fresh, intact vesicles or pustules and draining away the fluid. Scrapings are then obtained from the base of the unroofed lesions. The smeared material may be treated with either Giemsa or Wright stain, but smears stained with Giemsa are the easiest to interpret. If the lesions are due to infection with a herpesvirus (*H. simplex* or *Varicella-zoster* virus), multinucleated giant cells and large, bizarre balloon cells can be identified in the smear. These cells represent altered infected epidermal cells; viral inclusions are not easily visualized with these stains. This technique can be used to confirm chicken pox, recurrent herpes simplex infection, herpes zoster and eczema herpeticum. Multinucleated giant cells are not present in vesicles produced by other viral agents.

KOH preparation. If fungous disease is suspected, a KOH preparation is indicated for confirmation of the diagnosis. This technique is particularly useful in dermatophyte infections, for, unlike yeasts, these organisms often take a few weeks to grow out on culture media. Scales obtained by scraping a lesion with a dull-edged instrument are placed on a slide with a few drops of 10 per cent potassium hydroxide and a cover slip. The preparation is heated gently and then viewed under the microscope. It is important to obtain scales from the active border of a skin lesion or, in tinea pedis, from the toe webs, since the yield of infected stratum corneum cells is likely to be greater from these areas. If vesicles are present, a blister top may be clipped off and treated in the same manner. False negative tests can result from improper choice of material or from inadequate clearing of the stratum corneum cells. In positive KOH preparations, the hyphae stand out as branched, slender, irregular filaments that cross cell borders. It is common for the inexperienced viewer to mistake intercellular spaces and cloth or cotton fibers for hyphae. In yeast infections such as candidiasis or tinea versicolor, both spores and hyphae may be visualized. In tinea capitis, fungal elements cannot be demonstrated in scales from the scalp; hairs must be plucked from the active border of the lesion and treated in the fashion described. Spores may be present either within the hair shaft (endothrix) or along its surface (ectothrix), depending on the type of infecting organism.

Scraping for mites. It is often possible to demonstrate the mite or its ova and feces in scrapings from patients with scabies. The most reliable technique is to apply a drop or two of mineral oil to a fresh papule, vesicle or burrow, and to scrape vigorously with a dull-edged instrument. The scrapings are collected in the oil droplet and can be transferred to a slide and viewed under the microscope without a cover slip. The mite remains alive in the oil and can be detected under low magnification. Ova and dark-colored feces will not dissolve in the oil as they do in KOH and may provide evidence for scabies infestation if the mite is not seen.

COMMON SKIN DISORDERS IN THE INFANT

Although many of the common dermatological disorders of childhood also occur in neonates and infants, there are a number of cutaneous abnormalities that are peculiar to this age group. Some of these lesions are benign and transient and require no therapy; others have a more prolonged course or are permanent defects. All are of concern to parents and should be explained fully, including prognosis. Some of the more common disorders are described here.

Milia.   These lesions are pearly white, 1 to 2 mm papules that, in newborn infants, are found most frequently on the face but occasionally occur in other areas. They represent epidermal inclusion cysts and usually rupture spontaneously during the first few weeks of life. Similar papules are present in the midline of the palate in about 80 per cent of newborns and are known as Epstein's pearls. Milia may also arise on the gingivae and, in older children, in sites of injury or scars. Persistent lesions may be gently shelled out with a sterile needle.

Mongolian spots.   These blue-gray macular lesions are exceedingly common in black and oriental infants, but also occur occasionally in white infants as well. They are most frequently seen in the lumbosacral area, but also may be found on the buttocks, legs, shoulders and, rarely, on the arms and face. The blue-gray hue is due to the presence of melanocytes in the dermis. Mongolian spots usually disappear during the first few years of life, but deeply pigmented lesions and those in less typical sites (e.g., the shoulders or face) may persist indefinitely.

Erythema toxicum.   This eruption occurs in approximately 50 per cent of term infants and has a peak incidence on the second day of life. The lesions are characteristically white papules or pustules on an erythematous base (Fig. 35–1). Splotchy erythema may be the only manifestation of the disorder, however. Lesions may be sparse or numerous and may affect all body

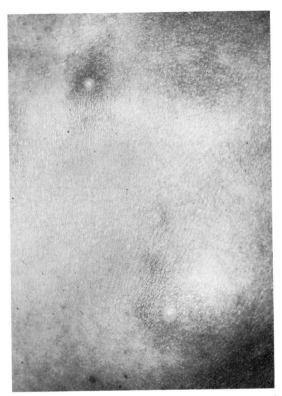

Figure 35–1   Raised papulopustules with surrounding erythema characteristic of erythema toxicum.

surfaces, although the palms and soles are virtually always spared. The infant is otherwise healthy, but may demonstrate mild peripheral eosinophilia. Smears of intralesional contents disclose a monomorphous infiltrate of eosinophils. Bacteria are never present on Gram stain, thus permitting differentiation of erythema toxicum from staphylococcal pyoderma. Individual lesions are transient, and the course of the eruption rarely exceeds two to three days. The cause is unknown, and treatment is unnecessary.

Miliaria.   Miliaria results from obstruction of the eccrine sweat gland duct and is colloquially known as prickly heat. In the newborn, a form known as miliaria crystallina is more frequent and consists of very superficial, easily ruptured, non-inflamed vesicles. Deeper lesions known as miliaria rubra are more usual in older infants. These lesions are erythematous papules or pustules that are often confined to intertriginous areas. The absence of bacteria and yeasts on Gram stain of the pustule contents distinguishes these lesions from a cutaneous infection. Since excessive warmth and humidity cause the eruption, simple measures to keep the infant cool usually suffice. Application of topical agents may be harmful rather than helpful.

Diaper dermatitis. Dermatitis in the diaper area can have a variety of causes but most frequently can be attributed to irritation from prolonged contact with urine and feces and the friction of diapers on macerated skin. Proprietary preparations and soaps and detergents may contribute to the problem. Primary irritant contact dermatitis is most often erythematous and scaly and involves the lower abdomen, perineum and proximal thighs, but often spares the depths of the inguinal folds (Fig. 35–2), a helpful point in differential diagnosis. If the eruption is permitted to persist, it may become erosive and secondarily infected or hypertrophic and papular. This type of diaper dermatitis responds to frequent diaper changes and protection of the skin with a bland ointment such as petrolatum or zinc oxide. If intense inflammation is present, application of a mild corticosteroid preparation (1 per cent hydrocortisone) with each diaper change may be required for a few days.

Candidal infection in the diaper area may supervene, since a proportion of infants, like adults, are intestinal carriers of yeast. When the organism is spilled onto the perineal skin it flourishes in the warm, moist environment. Candidal infection presents as a brilliant red, scaly, confluent plaque of dermatitis, with discrete borders

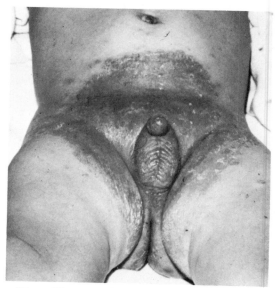

Figure 35–3 Candidal diaper dermatitis. Confluent, deeply erythematous, scaly eruption with sharp borders involving folds, genitalia and perianal skin. Satellite pustules are present.

and satellite vesicopustules on the skin adjacent to the main plaque of dermatitis (Fig. 35–3). Characteristically, the inguinal folds and perianal skin are involved. A KOH preparation is helpful since hyphae and budding yeasts usually can be demonstrated. Cultures should be performed if the diagnosis is unclear. The dermatitis responds to topical applications of nystatin, amphotericin B or miconazole. Although creams are often used, ointments tend to be more soothing and do not contain preservatives that may be irritating to inflamed skin.

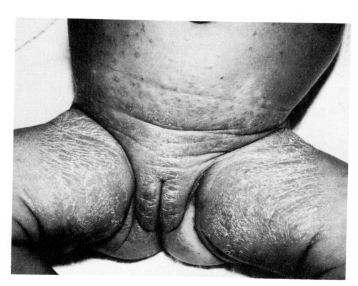

Figure 35–2 Primary irritant diaper dermatitis. Scaly, erythematous eruption with indistinct borders and relative sparing of the inguinal folds.

Dermatitis in the diaper area may also be a manifestation of atopic dermatitis, seborrheic dermatitis, bacterial pyoderma or, less commonly, allergic contact dermatitis, viral infections or syphilis. Additional historical data and identification of lesions elsewhere on the skin may provide clues to the correct diagnosis. A Gram stain of material from pustular lesions, a Tzanck smear and a VDRL test may be indicated in some instances.

Vascular lesions. Macular hemangiomas *(salmon patch)* are present in 30 to 50 per cent of normal newborns. These pale pink lesions are usually relatively small, have diffuse borders and occur most frequently on the upper eyelids, glabella and upper lip. They are inconsequential and fade completely during the first year or two of life. *Nuchal hemangiomas,* which commonly appear on the occiput in newborn infants, may be darker in color and more discrete; a considerable proportion of these lesions persist indefinitely, but since they become covered by hair, they are rarely of concern to parents. True *nevus flammeus* (port wine stain) is a macular hemangioma that may be small or large, pink to deep purple in color, and may occur on any body surface. These lesions represent proliferations of mature blood vessels and are permanent defects. Lesions in the trigeminal area should alert the physician to the possibility of Sturge-Weber syndrome (vascular lesions in the brain manifested by seizures, ipsilateral intracranial calcification, contralateral hemiparesis). Infants with a facial nevus flammeus should have a thorough ophthalmological examination periodically to detect glaucoma, which also may be a manifestation of Sturge-Weber syndrome. Although the nevus flammeus cannot be removed easily, in the older child, applications of Covermark, a cosmetic preparation blended to match the normal skin color, will mask the defect very effectively.

Capillary hemangiomas (strawberry mark) are soft, compressible, bright red protuberances that may be present at birth but more often appear during the first two months of life. Initially pallor, telangiectasia or a bruiselike mark may be the only indication that a hemangioma will develop in that site. Once these lesions appear, it is usual for them to increase in size over a period of weeks to months. Gray, fibrotic

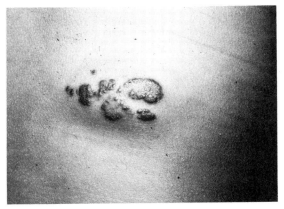

Figure 35–4 Mixed hemangioma with capillary and cavernous components.

areas on the surface of the hemangioma herald involution, which occurs spontaneously in the majority of patients. Since these nevi are self-limited, it is common practice to reassure parents and follow a course of non-intervention. Total regression may require several years. Deeper bluish lesions are called *cavernous hemangiomas.* These tumors also exhibit an active growth phase, but usually regress spontaneously, like capillary hemangiomas (Fig. 35–4).

Occasionally, the physician may be required to intervene, if vascular lesions impinge on vital structures, become so large as to be grotesque, cause thrombocytopenia and bleeding (Kasabach-Merritt syndrome) or are associated with multiple vascular lesions in the viscera. Treatment by surgery, irradiation or prednisone therapy may be indicated in those instances.

COMMON CHILDHOOD DERMATOLOGICAL PROBLEMS

Many of the diseases included in this section can and do occur in all age groups, but are most common during childhood.

Molluscum contagiosum. Molluscum lesions are discrete, pearly white, firm, often umbilicated papules that vary in size from 1 to several millimeters (Fig. 35–5). Because they are caused by a virus, they are disseminated by autoinoculation and hence occur in clusters. They are most often mistaken for warts and, occasionally, obscured by an eczematous eruption that

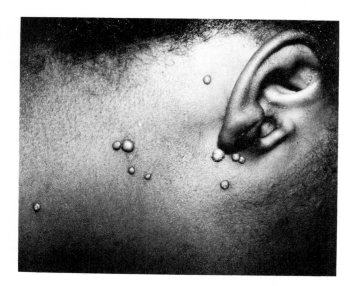

Figure 35–5 Grouped papular lesions of molluscum contagiosum. Note umbilication of several of the papules.

occurs in the surrounding skin. Destruction can be accomplished by applications of liquid nitrogen, Cantharone without occlusion, curettage or expression of the contents of the papules by a sterile needle.

Verrucae. All verrucae are of viral etiology and may be classified as follows: (1) common warts, which are hyperkeratotic and conical or filiform (Fig. 35–6), (2) flat warts, which are minimally hyperkeratotic and may occur in profusion, particularly on the face and dorsum of the hands (Fig. 35–7), (3) plantar or palmar warts, which are flat and round with depressed central cores, (4) mucous membrane warts called condylomata acuminata, which are soft and moist and occur mainly on the genitalia and perianal skin.

Treatment is always destructive and aimed at removing the infected epidermal cells. Therapeutic measures for warts are legion and include application of blistering agents such as liquid nitrogen or Cantharone or peeling agents such as 40 per cent salicylic acid plaster (especially useful for plantar warts), 10 per cent salicylic acid and 10 per cent lactic acid in flexible collodion applied daily or vitamin A acid preparations. Condylomata can be treated with liquid nitrogen or weekly applications of 20 per cent podophyllin in tincture of benzoin. All topical agents should be applied only to warty tissue, as surrounding normal skin can be easily damaged. Spontaneous resolution of warts is common but not invariable.

Scabies. The incidence of this infestation has reached epidemic proportions in recent years, and this disorder should be considered in all patients, even infants, with a severely pruritic, chronic eruption. The dermatitis is caused by the mite *Sarcoptes scabiei*, which burrows in the stratum corneum, causing papules, vesicles, nodules, pustules and burrows. The characteristic burrows in intertriginous areas and interdigital spaces present in older children and adults are often absent in infants. Likewise, the face, scalp, palms and soles,

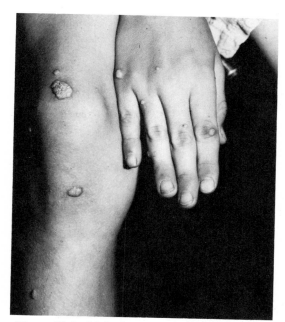

Figure 35–6 Multiple common warts on the hand and knee.

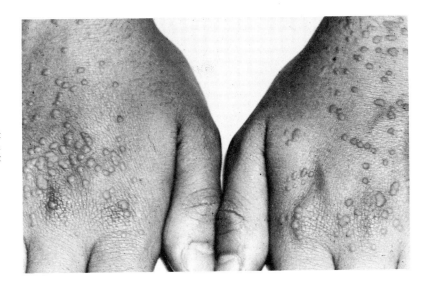

Figure 35-7 Numerous flat warts on the dorsum of both hands. Linear streaks suggest spread by autoinoculation.

which are rarely involved in children and adults, are often affected in infants. A secondary eczematous eruption due to scratching may mask the underlying primary lesions (Fig. 35-8).

The offending mite and its ova and feces may be identified in scrapings from fresh lesions (see Laboratory Procedures). Treatment with lindane lotion or cream is usually effective. The hazards of intoxication must be considered in infants, and a brief treatment (up to four hours) to the total body surface may suffice. An alternative therapy is 4 to 6 per cent sulfur ointment applied for 24 hours and repeated in one week. Control of the intense pruritus and eczema may require application of a

topical corticosteroid cream for a few days. Since scabies is usually acquired by skin contact with infected humans, the entire family should be carefully examined and treated as needed.

Tinea versicolor. This superficial fungous infection most often affects older children or teenagers. The lesions are scaly, mildly pruritic macules that may be hypopigmented or hyperpigmented in contrast to the surrounding skin. Typical areas of involvement are the chest, back and shoulders, although the neck and face may be affected. The causative organism, *Malassezia furfur*, probably represents the filamentous form of the normal skin resident *Pityrosporum orbiculare*. Recurrence

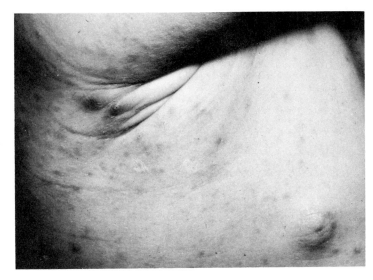

Figure 35-8 Scabies in an infant. Erythematous nodules in the axilla with eczematous dermatitis of surrounding skin.

in individuals with this infection is likely, particularly during warm weather. Affected areas of skin do not tan. Diagnosis is confirmed by yellow fluorescence under a Wood's lamp and a positive KOH preparation showing grouped, thick-walled, round spores and short, thick hyphae. Although certain topical antifungal agents are effective, treatment with these agents can be expensive. Also efficacious are applications of 25 per cent sodium hyposulfite solution twice a day for two to three weeks, selenium sulfide suspension (Selsun) applied nightly for five days and repeated one week later or acne lotions containing salicylic acid or resorcinol.

Dermatophytosis (ringworm). Dermatophyte infections are named according to the part of the body affected. Three groups of fungi cause this disease: *Microsporum, Trichophyton* and *Epidermophyton.* Some are indigenous to man, others to animals and some are natural inhabitants of the soil.

Tinea corporis. Body ringworm occurs at any age and is characterized by pruritic, sharply demarcated, erythematous, scaly lesions with raised inflammatory borders composed of tiny papules or papulovesicles (Fig. 35–9). Central clearing, which results

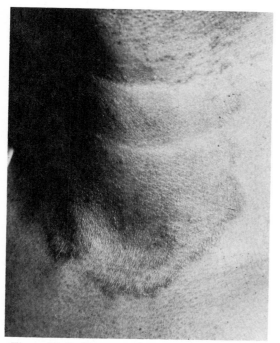

Figure 35–9 Tinea corporis on the neck. Note the sharp, elevated erythematous border.

in an annular configuration, is not always present. A positive KOH preparation is diagnostic, but scales should be cultured on Sabouraud or Mycosel media if the diagnosis is in doubt. Patients with papular eczema often develop round, scaly lesions that can be mistaken for tinea corporis. Granuloma annulare is another condition also frequently confused with ringworm. Treatment with topical antifungal agents such as tolnaftate, haloprogin or miconazole twice daily for two to four weeks will clear limited infections. Widespread lesions may require treatment with oral griseofulvin for a similar period of time.

Tinea pedis. Although frequently diagnosed in children, athlete's foot is more commonly found in adolescent and adult males. It is manifested by scaling, erythema, fissuring and vesicular lesions of the soles. Toe web involvement is virtually always present. Pruritus and burning may be troublesome for some patients. A KOH preparation test is mandatory, since eczema (contact dermatitis, irritant dermatitis, dyshidrotic eczema, atopic dermatitis) is frequently misdiagnosed as tinea pedis and aggravated by inappropriate treatment. Toenail involvement occurs in some patients, but dystrophic nails can also result from long-standing eczema, and KOH preparations and cultures should be obtained to verify a diagnosis of dermatophytosis. Specific treatment is the same as for tinea corporis. Nail involvement necessitates treatment with griseofulvin for many months. Non-specific measures should include meticulous drying of feet, particularly toe webs, and avoidance of occlusive shoes and heavy socks.

Tinea capitis. Scalp lesions may be caused by organisms of either the *Microsporum* or *Trichophyton* species. The lesions may appear as slightly red, scaly areas with hair loss and broken off hairs or as circumscribed, boggy granulomas surmounted by pustules (kerion) (Fig. 35–10). Differential diagnosis includes alopecia areata, pyoderma, seborrhea and psoriasis. Lesions due to *Microsporum* infections will show the characteristic blue-green fluorescence with a Wood's lamp. KOH preparation of infected hairs will demonstrate spores on the outside of the shaft (*Microsporum* sp.) or within the hair shaft (*Trichophyton* sp.). Tinea capitis does not respond

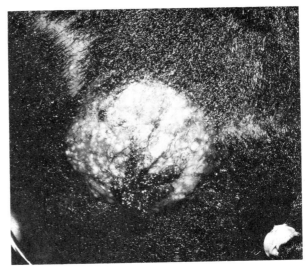

Figure 35-10 Raised, circumscribed, boggy mass with hair loss and superficial pustules typical of a fungal kerion (tinea capitis).

to topical therapy and must be treated with oral griseofulvin for approximately four weeks. It is helpful to scrub the scalp with an antiseborrheic shampoo to decrease scaling and to eradicate infected hairs. It is not necessary to shave the hair. Regrowth of hair, disappearance of fluorescence and a negative KOH preparation provide reassurance that the infection has been adequately treated.

Impetigo. Impetigo may be caused by the β-hemolytic streptococcus or *Staphylococcus aureus*; in mixed infections the staphylococcus is considered a secondary invader. Streptococcal lesions are transient, superficial pustules that, when ruptured, become covered with thick, moist, honey-colored crusts (Fig. 35-11). Gram positive cocci in chains can be demonstrated on Gram stain of the exudate. Certain strains of streptococci have a predilection for the skin; some of these strains are nephritogenic and may cause subsequent acute glomerulonephritis. Staphylococcal lesions are typically bullous and, when ruptured, become covered with thin, varnish-like crusts (Fig. 35-12). Both types of impetigo are spread by autoinoculation and are quite contagious. Impetigo is frequently secondary to underlying eczema, scabies, viral infections and insect bites.

Impetigo should be treated with compresses of tap water, Burow's solution or normal saline to remove adherent crusts

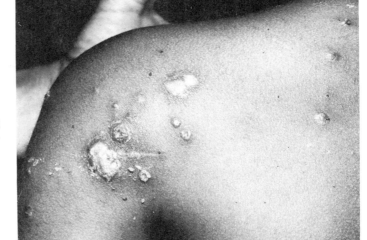

Figure 35-11 Superficial oozing and crusting lesions of streptococcal impetigo.

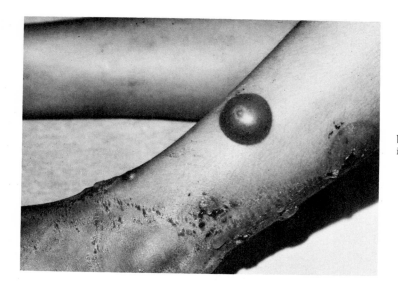

Figure 35–12 Intact and ruptured bullae characteristic of staphylococcal impetigo.

and debris. Scrubbing with antibacterial soap and germicidal agents is probably not necessary. Systemically administered penicillin or erythromycin for 10 days is indicated for streptococcal lesions. Staphylococcal lesions will respond to a topical antibiotic ointment such as Polysporin, but extensive lesions may require systemic administration of a semisynthetic penicillin.

Alopecia areata. Most often confused with tinea capitis, this disorder consists of solitary or multiple, sharply defined areas of alopecia. The scalp is always normal in appearance. The etiology is unknown but the disorder is self-limited and rarely requires treatment. High-potency topical corticosteroid ointments under occlusion may sometimes encourage regrowth of hair. Rarely, this condition is recurrent, involves the entire scalp (alopecia totalis) and body hair (alopecia universalis) and results in permanent hair loss.

Pigmented lesions. *Café au lait spots* may be present in newborns or develop in early childhood. They are tan to brown macules of varying sizes and represent an increased number of melanocytes in the epidermis. Six or more lesions larger than 1.5 cm are characteristic of patients with neurofibromatosis, a neurocutaneous multisystem disease inherited as an autosomal dominant trait. Large, unilateral café au lait spots with irregular borders are typical of McCune-Albright syndrome.

Pigmented nevi are ubiquitous lesions that occur occasionally in newborn infants, but more often arise during childhood.

Early lesions, known as junctional nevi, are flat and brown and may occur on any body surface. Lesions on palms, soles and genitalia usually remain junctional (nevus cells in epidermis above the basement membrane), but elsewhere they may evolve into compound or dermal moles. Small lesions are benign and need be removed only for cosmetic reasons. Congenital junctional nevi and giant hairy nevi should be removed because of an increased risk of malignancy.

Pityriasis rosea. This common, minimally symptomatic eruption is often limited to the trunk and proximal extremities, although all body surfaces may be involved. The initial lesion, called the herald patch, precedes the generalized eruption by five to seven days and is usually the largest lesion. Typically, the lesions are round to ovoid, erythematous, scaly maculopapules that follow the natural skin lines. In some patients, the lesions are papular or annular and may become quite profuse. Total duration is four to six weeks. The etiological agent is presumed to be viral but has never been identified. Differential diagnosis includes secondary syphilis (patients should have a VDRL test), drug and viral eruptions. Treatment is usually unnecessary; if itching is present it can be controlled with oral antihistamines and a lubricant containing 0.25 per cent menthol.

Papular urticaria. This disease occurs most often during the summer months in children between the ages of 2 and 10 years. Lesions occur predominantly on exposed areas and consist of very pruritic, inflamed wheals and papules. They are thought to represent a delayed hypersensitivity reaction to insect bites. The eruption is difficult to control, as the etiological agent is often obscure. Treatment of the patient should include an oral antihistamine preparation and topical antipruritic agents (a lubricant with menthol or a corticosteroid cream). Thorough spraying and dusting of the house, furniture and pets with insecticides are mandatory. Despite such measures, the disorder may persist for several months.

Erythema multiforme. This generalized eruption is a hypersensitivity reaction that can often be attributed to antecedent drug therapy or an infection, particularly with viral agents. The cutaneous manifestations are polymorphous and include urticaria, erythematous macules, papules, nodules, bullae and target or iris lesions, which are pathognomonic. Lesions are most often present on the extensor surfaces of the limbs, face, palms, soles and oral mucous membranes. Associated systemic symptoms such as fever, malaise, anorexia and arthralgia are frequent. When the cutaneous lesions are localized mainly to the mucous membranes and affect at least two sites (eyes, mouth, nasal mucosa, genitalia) the disorder may be designated Stevens-Johnson syndrome. Mucosal lesions may become erosive, pseudomembranous and secondarily infected, causing severe and permanent damage, particularly to the eyes. Ophthalmological consultation should be obtained if there is eye involvement. The cutaneous eruption rarely requires treatment. Pruritus can be managed effectively with oral antihistamines. Systemic corticosteroids have been recommended when the disease is severe, but their effectiveness is questionable. Therapy should be supportive and directed to the underlying problem.

Erythema nodosum. This eruption is also regarded as a hypersensitivity reaction and may be associated with streptococcal infections, tuberculosis, deep fungal infections, inflammatory bowel disease, drug ingestion and sarcoidosis. Individual lesions are discrete, deeply erythematous, tender, warm nodules up to several centimeters in diameter that are seen in the pretibial areas but also may appear on the thighs and upper arms. As the lesions subside, they develop a bruiselike appearance and a scaly surface; total duration is usually one to two weeks. Prodromes of fever, malaise, chills, migratory arthralgia and pharyngitis are common. The erythrocyte sedimentation rate is usually elevated. Laboratory studies should be directed toward elucidation of the underlying disorder. Bedrest and analgesics are all that is necessary for the cutaneous eruption.

Eczema. The term eczema describes a cutaneous reaction pattern characterized by a weeping, erythematous, microvesicular dermatitis in the acute phase and a dry, scaly, lichenified (accentuated skin markings), hyper- or hypopigmented eruption in the chronic phase. The histological hallmark is edema in the epidermis (spongiosis). The eczemas of childhood include atopic dermatitis, seborrheic dermatitis, allergic and primary irritant contact dermatitis, dyshidrotic and nummular eczema as well as several other less common entities. Certain morphological features facilitate recognition of several of these disorders.

Atopic dermatitis is the most common type of eczema in infancy and childhood. This disorder is frequently associated with asthma and hay fever and is probably inherited. The cause is unknown, although it is grouped with the allergic diseases. Onset is usually after two to three months of life. In infants, the distribution of the eruption is generalized, localization to extensor extremities is characteristic in the toddler age group and flexural predilection is noted in the older child (Fig. 35–13). Dry skin and pruritus are virtually always present.

The success of a treatment regimen in atopic dermatitis depends on alleviation of dryness and pruritus. It is essential to control aggravating environmental factors and minimize friction, sweating, exposure to extremes of temperature and irritation by topical preparations, perfumes and scratchy fabrics. Bathing need not be curtailed if lubrication is provided by a bath oil or superfatted soap and, immediately following the bath, by application of a simple unscented emollient. Moist, weeping lesions will benefit from compressing with cool tap water or Burow's solution. Topical corticosteroids are the mainstay of treat-

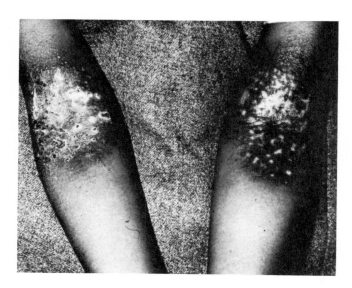

Figure 35–13 Hyperpigmentation, lichen-ification and secondary infection in the ante-cubital fossae of a patient with atopic derma-titis.

ment because of their antipruritic and in-flammatory effect. They should be applied four times per day in the acute phase of the disease. Generally, ointments are more lu-bricating and less irritating than creams. One of the fluorinated steroids may be required to initiate treatment and bring the dermatitis under control. Hydrocortisone preparations are useful for maintenance therapy. Systemic corticosteroids are rarely, if ever, indicated. Additional meas-ures include tars (e.g., 5 per cent liquor car-bonis detergens in an appropriate base) for chronic lichenified dermatitis, oral antihis-tamines for sedation and antibiotics for sec-ondary infection. It is more effective to be aggressive for the first few days than to alleviate symptoms completely.

Seborrheic dermatitis in infants may re-semble atopic dermatitis but is drier, more scaly and rarely itches (Fig. 35–14). Scaling of the scalp and retroauricular, axillary and diaper area involvement are all usual. In the older child, the dermatitis may be con-fined to the scalp or may involve the eye-brows, eyelids, nasolabial folds and ret-roauricular areas and, less commonly, other intertriginous areas. Scalp lesions can be controlled by shampooing two to three times per week with a shampoo containing sulfur, salicylic acid, tars and antiseptic agents. When an inflammatory dermatitis is present, a topical corticosteroid cream, lo-tion or gel may be applied two to three times per day. A sulfur ointment (3 to 5 per cent) is also moderately effective. Response

is prompt, but recurrences are common in some patients.

Contact dermatitis may be of the pri-mary irritant type (e.g., diaper dermatitis) or may be due to a true allergic reaction.

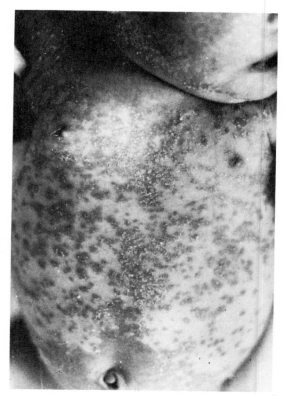

Figure 35–14 Infant with severe seborrheic derma-titis. Multiple dry, erythematous, scaly lesions, which are confluent in the diaper area and neck folds.

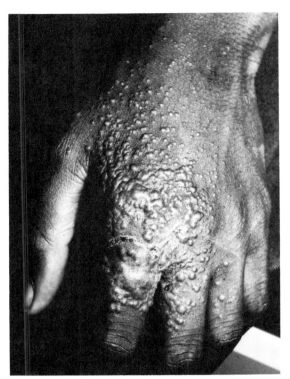

Figure 35-15 Bullous contact dermatitis on the dorsum of the hand surrounding an abrasion treated with tincture of Merthiolate. Patch test to thimerosal was positive.

The most common allergens in children are Rhus antigen (poison ivy or oak), cosmetics and deodorants, topical medications (Fig. 35-15), substances used in tanning leather, metals (nickel) and fabric finishers. The dermatitis may be acute in onset and vesiculobullous in character. The distribution and morphology of the lesions are often a clue to etiology. For example, linear streaks of vesicles are seen in plant dermatitis where the leaves have brushed against the skin. Nickel dermatitis occurs at sites of contact with jewelry, zippers and other metal closures on clothing.

Treatment for acute contact dermatitis consists of compresses with tap water or Burow's solution four to six times per day. Large bullae may be decompressed but should not be unroofed, as they provide protection for damaged skin. Oral antihistamines will alleviate pruritus. A topical corticosteroid preparation is also indicated. The offending allergen must be avoided or the dermatitis will not clear. If the reaction is severe and widespread, a brief course of an oral corticosteroid may be of great benefit.

DISEASES OF THE ADOLESCENT

Acne vulgaris. Acne is so prevalent in the adolescent population that it can almost be regarded as a physiological process. Clinically, acne is characterized by open and closed comedones (blackheads and whiteheads), erythematous papules, pustules, nodules and cysts that occur on the face, upper chest and back. Patients with severe acne frequently produce increased amounts of sebum and have oily skin. Plugging of the pilosebaceous canals with keratotic debris and sebum results in comedones and papules. When the follicular pore is dilated, the oxidized keratinous mass is perceived as a blackhead. Extravasation of follicular contents into the surrounding dermis incites an inflammatory response producing pustules, nodules and cysts. Free fatty acids, produced by the action of bacterial lipases of normal cutaneous flora (*Staphylococcus epidermidis, Corynebacterium acnes*) on serum triglycerides, are thought to be the irritating substances.

Therapy can be very effective in controlling acne and should be instituted to prevent scarring. Simple topical measures may be all that is required in mild disease. Acne scrubs, gels and lotions that contain sulfur and salicylic acid cause drying and peeling, a desirable result if it is not excessive. Acne gels and lotions containing benzoyl peroxide are extremely effective when used on a daily basis. Benzoyl peroxide is keratolytic and promotes drying and peeling, which help open the plugged pileosebaceous unit. Vitamin A acid used once daily or alternated with a benzoyl peroxide preparation is indicated for comedone and pustular acne. The strength of the preparations chosen and frequency of use should be titered for each patient to achieve an optimal effect, depending on the individual's tolerance. Certain antimicrobial agents, particularly tetracycline and erythromycin, may be used for severe pustular and cystic acne. The initial dose of 1 gm daily (in divided doses) may be gradually decreased after two to three weeks of therapy to a maintenance dose of 250 or 500 mg daily.

Alternatively, these antibiotics can be used topically. Sun exposure with tanning and peeling is an effective ancillary measure in some patients. Staphylococcal vaccines and oral vitamin A are not indicated in patients with acne.

The psychological effects of acne should be appreciated by the physician. The patient should be educated about the pathogenesis of acne lesions and should appreciate that acne therapy rarely results in abrupt improvement but requires several weeks to effect a change. Occlusive cosmetics, such as moisturizing cream and greasy make-up, and oily hair preparations should be avoided. Dietary manipulations are unnecessary, since ingestion of greasy foods does not alter the type or amount of lipid secreted by the sebaceous gland. If acne persists despite adequate therapy, the patient should be referred to a dermatologist. Some patients may require acne surgery (extraction of comedones, intralesional corticosteroids, drainage of cysts and cryosurgery). Causes of refractory acne include ingestion of acnegenic drugs (iodides, corticosteroids, antiepileptics, certain oral contraceptives), exposure to topical acnegenic preparations such as heavy oils and greases, and certain systemic diseases.

REFERENCES

Arndt, K.: *A Manual of Dermatologic Therapeutics.* Boston, Little, Brown and Co., 1974.

Domonkos, A. M.: *Andrews' Diseases of the Skin,* 6th ed. Philadelphia, W. B. Saunders Co., 1971.

Jacobs, A. H. (Ed.): *Symposium on pediatric dermatology.* Pediatr. Clin. North Am., *18*:3, 1971.

Korting, G. W., Curth, W., and Curth, H. O.: *Diseases of the Skin in Children and Adolescents.* Philadelphia, W. B. Saunders Co., 1970.

Rajka, G.: *Atopic Dermatitis.* Philadelphia, W. B. Saunders Co., 1975.

Solomon, L. M., and Esterly, N. B.: *Neonatal Dermatology.* Philadelphia, W. B. Saunders Co., 1973.

Weinberg, S., Leider, M., and Shapiro, L.: *Color Atlas of Pediatric Dermatology.* New York, McGraw-Hill, 1975.

Pediatric Gastroenterology

36

Marvin E. Ament

MAJOR CONGENITAL ABNORMALITIES OF THE GASTROINTESTINAL TRACT

Tracheoesophageal fistula. Tracheoesophageal fistula is the most common anomaly of the esophagus. Its incidence is about 1 per 3000 births, and it occurs equally in both males and females. The condition results from faulty separation of the embryonic foregut into trachea and esophagus during the fourth to sixth week of gestation.

The condition is associated with polyhydramnios and with low birth weight in one third of cases. Half of these infants have other congenital anomalies; 50 per cent have multiple anomalies and 25 per cent have life-threatening anomalies. The cardiovascular and gastrointestinal systems are principally involved. Cardiovascular anomalies most often seen are atrial septal defect, ventricular septal defect and patent ductus. Imperforate anus is the most common associated gastrointestinal anomaly. In 85 to 90 per cent of these cases, the proximal esophagus ends in a blind pouch, with the distal esophagus connected to the trachea.

Symptoms are present from birth. Because these infants are unable to swallow, there is a constant drooling of frothy saliva. Episodes of regurgitation, choking, coughing and cyanosis with evidence of respiratory distress occur from aspiration of accumulated saliva in the nasopharynx. Pulmonary symptoms result from either aspiration of saliva or reflux of acid gastric contents through a distal segment fistula.

In an infant with esophageal atresia, a catheter will be felt to stick at 10 to 12 cm from the nares, as the tip becomes lodged in the blind proximal esophagus. Treatment of tracheoesophageal fistula is by surgical correction. In the predominant form, the fistula is ligated and the blind proximal pouch is anastomosed to the distal portion.

Hypertrophic pyloric stenosis. Hypertrophic pyloric stenosis (HPS) is the gastrointestinal disorder that most often requires surgery among Caucasians, and it occurs in 3 out of 1000 live births. Its etiology and pathogenesis remain unknown. Males are affected three or four times as frequently as females. HPS may be one feature in a pattern of malformation such as trisomy 18, XO Turner syndrome, Smith-Lemli-Opitz syndrome or de Lange syndrome.

Gross hypertrophy of the circular muscle of the pylorus produces a marked swelling, which may be 2 or 3 cm long. The distal end of the tumor is externally distinct and ends abruptly at the duodenum, but the proximal end merges into the gastric antrum.

Typically, the child is well until the third or fourth week and then starts to vomit. The vomiting is non-bilious and initially starts as regurgitation but gradually becomes projectile. Bowel movements become constipated and irregular.

Signs at physical examination that are diagnostic include visible gastric peristalsis and a palpable pyloric tumor. Jaundice occurs in 2 to 3 per cent of patients with pyloric stenosis. If physical examination does not clearly establish the diagnosis, an upper gastrointestinal series should be done. Prior to surgery these patients should have abnormalities in electrolytes and water corrected.

The standard treatment for HPS is the Ramstedt pyloromyotomy, in which the pyloric muscle is split longitudinally down to the mucosa.

Small Intestinal Obstruction

Small intestinal obstruction may be complete or partial. In the duodenum, it is most commonly due to extrinsic bands or atresia, in the midgut and jejunum to volvulus and atresia and in the ileum to meconium ileus, atresia, duplication and volvulus.

Meckel's diverticulum. This anomaly is often an asymptomatic disorder. It may present clinically with massive rectal bleeding secondary to peptic ulceration of ectopic gastric mucosa and less commonly to intestinal obstruction. Radiological diagnosis is usually confined to demonstrating intestinal obstruction in children when this occurs, usually without demonstrating its cause. Most bleeding Meckel's diverticula can be detected by technetium scan. It is treated by surgical resection.

Congenital Abnormalities of the Large Intestine

Imperforate anus and Hirschprung's disease are common causes of large bowel neonatal obstruction.

Hirschprung's disease. This is characterized by congenital absence of the intrinsic ganglionic plexus of Auerbach and Meissner, as well as hypertrophy of the intrinsic nerve bundles. The anomaly extends from the sphincter area of the anal canal proximally for a variable level. It may involve a short rectal segment, rectosigmoid, whole colon or colon plus small intestine.

Symptoms may be present at birth, with failure to pass meconium or with meconium peritonitis after intrauterine perforation. Partial or complete intestinal obstruction with bile-stained vomitus and abdominal distension may be the initial manifestation in the first week of life. In rare cases, diagnosis is delayed until after early infancy. The clinical course is usually one of gradually increasing constipation and abdominal distension, fecal masses palpable in the abdomen and a characteristically empty rectum, except in the very short segment type. There may be bouts of diarrhea between periods of constipation, and enterocolitis may develop at any time.

The incidence in the general population is 1 in 5000. Diagnosis is established by rectal suction or full thickness biopsies, looking for absence of submucosal ganglion cells and hypertrophy of extramural parasympathetic nerves. Anal manometry is a new diagnostic technique used to diagnose Hirschprung's disease, but it is not universally accepted. Barium enema may be diagnostic and typically shows a spastic rectum or rectosigmoid and a dilated proximal colon. If the entire colon is involved, it will look like a microcolon. Barium enema is often not diagnostic in the first month of life.

Surgery is the only preferable form of treatment and is done in two stages. A sigmoid or left transverse colostomy is placed in most infants at the time of diagnosis. Completion of the correction is done by one of three surgical procedures — the Swenson, Duhamel or Soave method when the patient weighs 10 kg or is a year old.

Imperforate anus. Imperforate anus is found in 1 in 3000 to 1 in 5000 live births and is more common in males. These infants have normal birth weights. Associated developmental anomalies may include esophageal and duodenal atresia.

Obstructions above the puborectalis muscle in the pelvic floor form the high group and require immediate initial treatment by colostomy. Obstructions below the puborectalis constitute the low group and are treatable by direct surgical approach from the perineum.

Plain radiography in the true lateral inverted position, with the thighs flexed and centering over the pelvis, is the conventional method of separating high from low defects. An associated developmental anomaly of the sacrum and evidence of a fistula by the detection of air in the bladder or, rarely, the vagina, favors a high lesion as opposed to a low one.

Gastroesophageal Reflux

Gastroesophageal reflux or chalasia is a common occurrence during early infancy.

In most instances it is more of a nuisance for the parents than a major problem. The primary symptom of reflux is vomiting or "spitting up." Physicians should be concerned with the problem only if the infant is failing to gain weight or grow at a normal rate. Other symptoms are cough and chronic bronchitis or aspiration pneumonia. The diagnosis is established through several studies. A barium swallow is a very poor way to demonstrate reflux, showing it in only 25 per cent of cases; a cinéesophagram is a better study and shows it in the majority of cases. Measurement of lower esophageal sphincter pressure and monitoring pH in the lower esophagus after the stomach is filled with .1N hydrochloric acid are the best means to establish the presence of significant reflux.

If these tests and the upper gastrointestinal series are normal, the physician should suspect vomiting due to functional causes. In older school-age children, the symptoms of gastroesophageal reflux may be similar to those of infants, but other complaints may include dysphagia, retrosternal burning and hematemesis.

Diagnostic studies are similar to those in infants, but in addition, the acid drip or Bernstein test is used.

Treatment in early infancy is initially medical and consists of keeping the infant in an upright position between feedings and giving him equal volume feedings around the clock. If the infant gains weight and grows normally with treatment, surgery is unnecessary. Fundoplication of the stomach around the lower esophagus is the surgical treatment of choice in patients who do not respond to medical management. Peptic esophagitis and stricture are immediate indications for surgery.

Achalasia

This is the rarest motility disorder of the esophagus and may present at any time during infancy or childhood. It presents with symptoms of vomiting solids but not liquids, unless the liquids must pass around an impacted piece of solid food in the distal esophagus. Diagnosis is established by an esophagogram that shows a nonperistaltic esophagus that tapers to a fine point. It differs from a stricture because the narrowed portion dilates with passage of fluid. Esophageal motility studies show that the lower esophageal sphincter fails to relax with initiation of swallowing, and there is no propagation of a primary peristaltic wave.

Achalasia must be treated either surgically or with pneumatic dilation.

Peptic Ulcer Disease

The true incidence of duodenal and gastric ulcers in children is unknown. The condition is relatively rare and is more prevalent in males, occurring in a ratio of 3 or 4 to 1. Peptic ulcers occur in families, and a near majority of affected children will have fathers who have the condition.

Unless the patient presents with hematemesis and melena, the diagnosis may be difficult. Abdominal pain is the most frequently noted symptom of peptic ulcer, but it does not have a typical pattern in the preadolescent individual. Its location is midepigastric or periumbilical and can occur during the day as well as at night. Peptic ulcer disease must be differentiated from functional abdominal pain. Children with peptic ulcers, like adults on the average, hypersecrete gastric acid.

An upper gastrointestinal series should be the initial diagnostic study. Upper intestinal endoscopy is the diagnostic procedure of choice in individuals with hematemesis or melena or occult blood positive gastric aspirate. This procedure should be done for abdominal pain if the radiographic study is equivocal or if the pain persists and becomes incapacitating.

Upper Gastrointestinal Hemorrhage

The four usual causes of upper gastrointestinal hemorrhage in children are: peptic ulcers in the stomach and duodenum, duodenal and gastric ulcers secondary to stress or aspirin, gastritis and esophageal varices.

The diagnostic procedure of choice is flexible fiberoptic upper intestinal endoscopy.

SMALL INTESTINE

The most frequent causes of chronic diarrhea and malabsorption of infancy in childhood include cystic fibrosis, celiac sprue, congenital sucrase–isomaltase deficiency, giardiasis and injury to intestinal mucosa by invasive microorganisms and cow's milk and soy proteins.

Cystic fibrosis. Cystic fibrosis is a hereditary disease characterized by generalized dysfunction of exocrine glands (see also Chapter 40). The three customary features of the disease are chronic pulmonary disease, intestinal malabsorption from pancreatic insufficiency and elevated concentrations of sodium and chloride in the sweat.

Cystic fibrosis is primarily a disease of Caucasians, but it has been described in Negroes and those of the Mongolian race. The incidence in the Caucasian population is 1 per 2500 live births, and it has an autosomal recessive inheritance. Until adolescence, the sex incidence is equal; however, after adolescence, males predominate significantly.

The earliest manifestation of cystic fibrosis can be neonatal intestinal obstruction due to blockage of the small bowel lumen by thick and tenacious meconium. Vomiting and abdominal distension develop within a few hours of life. Vomiting is first bile-stained and then feculent. Meconium peritonitis may complicate meconium ileus. If the complications of perforation, volvulus, gangrene, peritonitis or small bowel atresia are suspected, immediate operation is indicated. In uncomplicated cases non-operative management may be preferred.

Eighty to 90 per cent of patients with cystic fibrosis have no pancreatic exocrine secretion of either enzymes or bicarbonate. This results in pale, bulky, unpleasant-smelling stools. Infants have voracious appetites but fail to gain weight at a normal rate. Because of the maldigestion and malabsorption they may develop hypoproteinemia, edema and bleeding diatheses secondary to prothrombin deficiency.

Patients who do not have malabsorption usually are not diagnosed during infancy. Chronic pulmonary infection alone will usually be the presenting feature.

Abdominal pain is common in older patients. The pain is usually colicky and often severe. It migrates from the midabdomen to localize in the right hypochondrium or right iliac fossa. A mass is usually palpable in the right lower quadrant and is called the meconium ileus equivalent.

Multinodular biliary cirrhosis occurs, and

is being seen more often with prolonged survival. The clinical features of liver disease are non-specific. Enlargement of the liver occurs first, jaundice second and splenomegaly with portal hypertension and varices last. Death from liver disease is rare.

Elevated sweat electrolyte concentration is the most constant feature of cystic fibrosis, and the sweat test is the main diagnostic test. In children, the normal sweat sodium and chloride are less than 60 mEq/l.

Pancreatic insufficiency is managed with pancreatic replacement therapy.

Celiac sprue. Celiac sprue is a permanent inability to tolerate dietary gluten found in wheat, barley, rye and oats. The condition is characterized by non-specific flat mucosal lesion at the duodenal jejunal junction and clinical response to a gluten-free diet. The latter is characterized by disappearance of signs of malabsorption and return to normal weight gain and growth.

The mechanism by which gluten causes the morphological and functional changes to the mucosa is unknown. The damage induced by gluten is most severe in the proximal small intestine. Malabsorption results from a decreased area for absorption and impaired intestinal mucosal enzyme activity.

The incidence of the disease varies from 1 in 300 in Ireland to 1 in 6500 in Sweden. The disease is familial, but its mode of inheritance is still unclear.

The typical child presents at 9 to 12 months of age with impaired growth, finger clubbing, vomiting, abnormal stools, abdominal distension, poor appetite, muscle wasting and slowing in development. In the majority of cases, symptoms develop three to six months after the first gluten is ingested. Stools usually are pale, soft, bulky and rancid. Rarely, they may be firm and pale and passed every three days if the patient has anorexia.

Older children have less obvious features and abnormal stools may not be readily recognized. Growth failure, anemia and rickets are more typical of cases recognized later in childhood.

Fat balance study is the best way to establish steatorrhea and its severity. Small intestine biopsy is the next test to perform if sweat chloride is normal and the patient has evidence of malabsorption.

Other tests that should be done are

prothrombin time and partial thromboplastin time, serum proteins, electrolytes, calcium, magnesium, serum iron and total iron binding capacity.

Treatment consists of a gluten-free diet for life. Weight returns to normal within six months and height within one year. Mucosa may return to normal within three months, but it may take a year.

Congenital sucrase-isomaltase deficiency. This is the predominant primary disaccharidase deficiency. It has autosomal recessive inheritance and has an increased incidence in the Eskimo.

The condition presents anytime after the introduction of sucrose-containing formulas or foods into the diet. It is characterized by abdominal distension, rarely vomiting, and watery acid diarrhea.

Diagnosis is established by testing stools for the presence of acid and increased amounts of sucrose. Since sucrose is not a reducing sugar, stools must be acid hydrolyzed and boiled prior to Clinitest. Sucrose tolerance test results in a flat curve and appearance of abnormal amounts of acid and sugar in the stool.

Treatment consists of eliminating sucrose from the diet. The condition is life-long.

Giardiasis. Giardiasis is a protozoan infection caused by the parasite *G. lamblia*. It is endemic in some areas of the United States and is the most common cause of parasite-induced diarrhea and malabsorption. The infection rarely occurs before six months of age. It is characterized by a 7 to 10 day incubation period and a variety of gastrointestinal symptoms. Fever is rarely seen. Initial symptoms are anorexia, nausea and borborygmi. These are followed by diarrhea, abdominal distension and steatorrhea.

The undiagnosed and untreated case can last for two to three months.

Diagnosis by examining stools is a relatively poor way to establish the diagnosis. If parasites are not found in the stools, then a duodenal aspirate or small intestinal biopsies must be obtained to look for trophozoites.

Giardiasis can result in a generalized malabsorption syndrome. Treatment with Atabrine or metronidazole results in complete reversal of malabsorption and mucosal lesions.

Gastrointestinal injury induced by cow's milk and soy proteins. Gastrointestinal mucosal damage induced by cow's milk and soy proteins is a diagnosis difficult to establish because it requires withdrawal of the offending formula and rechallenge with that agent at another time.

The spectrum of the condition is quite broad. It may present on the first day of life or as late as six months of age. Typically, it is characterized by gradual onset of diarrhea associated with generalized malabsorption and vomiting. In some, there is associated colitis, with bright red blood in the stool. Some patients may present with only the latter symptoms. There is no screening test for milk and soy protein intolerance.

Some patients may have severe damage and require total parenteral nutrition for weeks before feeding can be reinstituted. Elemental formulas should be fed to such infants. Intolerance to them persists until they are one to two years old.

Invasive *E. coli* duoviruses may penetrate the enterocytes and severely damage them, resulting in a malabsorption syndrome similar to and not separable from the one induced by formulas.

DISEASES OF THE COLON

Rectal bleeding in infancy and childhood. Colitis induced by milk and soy proteins, not anal fissures, is the most frequent cause of rectal bleeding in the neonatal period. Stools in these infants are usually loose or seedy and are streaked with blood.

Juvenile polyps do not occur before the end of the first year of life. The peak incidence for juvenile polyps is between four and six years of age. Bleeding and rectal prolapse of the polyp are the usual presenting signs. Bleeding is usually not severe, and patients rarely become anemic. Most polyps are within reach of the proctosigmoidoscope and should be removed to stop bleeding.

Ulcerative colitis and Crohn's disease. These may occur at any age but they are most often seen in adolescents.

Ulcerative colitis may be mild or moderate to severe. The majority of affected infants and children have moderate to severe disease. It may present with blood streaking of formed stool or profuse bloody diarrhea. Associated symptoms may include fever, arthralgia, arthritis, erythema nodosum and pyoderma gangrenosum. These features may occur independently of the bowel disease. Diagnosis is established by proctosigmoidoscopy, rectal biopsy, barium enema and negative cultures for *Shigella* and *Salmonella* and examination for trophozoites of *E. histolytica*.

Crohn's disease of the colon has many features in common with ulcerative colitis but more typically has perianal fistula, fissures and rectal ulcers. Changes in the mucosa are patchy at proctosigmoidoscopy. Medical treatment for both conditions depends primarily on the use of adrenocorticosteroids and salicylazosulfapyridene.

The majority of pediatric patients with ulcerative colitis require colectomy within five years because of intractable disease and growth failure.

Surgery for Crohn's colitis is performed less frequently, because of the high recurrence rate.

REFERENCES

Ament, M. E.: Inflammatory bowel disease of the colon. J. Pediatr., 86:322, 1975.

Anderson, C. M., and Burke, V. (Eds.): *Pediatric Gastroenterology*. Oxford, Blackwell Scientific Publications, 1975.

Battersby, J. S., Tolly, W. W., and Fess, S. W.: Esophageal atresia: A comprehensive study of 210 patients. Bull. Soc. Int. Chir., 230:415, 1971.

Cloud, D. T., White, R. F., Linker, L. M., and Taylor, L. C.: Surgical treatment of esophageal achalasia in children. J. Pediatr. Surg., 1:137, 1966.

Euler, A. R., and Ament, M. E.: Effect of Nissen fundoplication on the lower esophageal sphincter (LES) pressure of children with gastroesophageal reflux. Gastroenterology (accepted for publication).

Nissan, S., and Bar-Maor, J. A.: Changing trends in presentation and management of Hirschprung's disease. J. Pediatr. Surg., 6:10, 1971.

Noblett, H. R.: A rectal suction biopsy tube for use in the diagnosis of Hirschprung's disease. J. Pediatr. Surg., 4:406, 1969.

Prosser, R.: Infantile hypertrophic pyloric stenosis. Surgery, 58:881, 1965.

Santulli, T. V., Schullinger, T. N., Kiesewetter, W. B., and Bill, A. H.: Imperforate anus: A survey from the members of the surgical section of the American Academy of Pediatrics. J. Pediatr. Surg., 6:484, 1971.

Renal Disorders In Children

37

Fred G. Smith, Jr.

Introduction

In general, the spectrum of renal disorders in children does not differ greatly from that in the adult; however, many disorders that do not become apparent until adulthood have their origin in childhood. It is therefore important, from a preventive standpoint, to know that renal disease may be present throughout childhood without obvious symptoms or signs and then become clinically apparent in late adolescence or adulthood.

This chapter emphasizes some of the more frequently encountered renal disorders and provides information regarding the detection, evaluation and management of these disorders. Urinary tract infections are covered in Chapter 15.

EVALUATION OF THE CHILD WITH HEMATURIA OR PROTEINURIA

Hematuria

Because of the multitude of clinical conditions that can be associated with hematuria, it is important to have a systematic approach to hematuria in mind (Table 37–1). How then does one approach the diagnostic problem of the child with blood in his urine? Following a medical history and a physical examination, one should have a reasonable idea of whether the hematuria is associated with other organ systems or is localized to the urinary tract. The history should also distinguish whether it has resulted from trauma, is a familial problem, is recurrent and whether there is an associated abdominal mass or evidence of bleeding elsewhere.

Diagnosis of hematuria cannot be made unless a routine urinalysis is part of the evaluation of every child coming to the physician. Urinalysis should be performed on a fresh and, when possible, a concentrated sample, since the formed elements are best preserved in a concentrated and acid urine. The exact nature of the lesion causing hematuria may be difficult to determine by urinalysis alone, but the urinalysis may be helpful in differentiating a renal lesion from an extrarenal cause of hematuria. Red urine with or without blood clots suggests trauma or lower urinary tract bleeding. Blood at the initiation of voiding suggests urethritis or meatal stenosis in young boys. Terminal hematuria usually arises from the posterior urethra, bladder neck or trigone. Urine of patients with glomerulonephritis is often dark brown or smokey in color. Microscopic hematuria is usually painless; however, acute gross hemorrhage is often accompanied by suprapubic tenderness, frequency and dysuria. With the introduction of chemically impregnated "dip stix," the detection of hematuria and certain other urine abnormalities has become easy and efficient, requiring very little physician or technician time. The "dip stix" analysis of the urine should be coupled with careful examination of the sediment and measurement of

TABLE 37–1 ETIOLOGIC CLASSIFICATION OF HEMATURIA

Glomerulonephritides
Infectious disease of the urinary tract
Familial and congenital renal disease
Bleeding and vascular disorders
Neoplastic disease
Renal trauma
Drug or chemically induced
Recurrent asymptomatic

the specific gravity when urine volume is adequate. Before proceeding with detailed evaluation of the patient with suspected hematuria it is important to repeat the urinalysis to determine whether the hematuria is persistent or not. In young adolescent girls who are menstruating, it is obviously important to determine the time of the last menstrual period in order to evaluate the significance of red cells in the urine.

The remaining work-up suggested for hematuria is described in Table 37–1. The blood chemical studies of particular value include either blood urea nitrogen or serum creatinine, total serum protein, serum albumin and serum cholesterol. This general scheme for the evaluation of patients with hematuria is often obscure. If the history and physical examination and a few selected laboratory studies indicate that the patient has acute glomerulonephritis, many of the recommended studies in this scheme need not be done. For example, if the diagnosis is acute glomerulonephritis, it is obviously not necessary to carry out a urological evaluation. Diagnostic work-up is complete when the physician has enough information to make a specific diagnosis.

The intravenous pyelogram should be done on all patients who have traumatic hematuria. A cystourethrogram should be obtained from all patients having hematuria associated with bacteriuria or in whom lower urinary tract disease is suspected. There are occasions when a retrograde pyelogram may be indicated, but this should not be considered as routine in the evaluation of hematuria. Cystoscopy is warranted when the pyelogram and voiding cystourethrogram are normal, there is no evidence of renal impairment and the only remaining question is whether the hematuria is unilateral or bilateral. The decision to perform a renal biopsy, either percutaneous or open, should be made on an individual basis. In general, renal biopsy should be performed when the diagnosis is not established and the hematuria is believed to be intrarenal. For example, when a form of chronic glomerulonephritis is being considered, a biopsy may be very helpful in evaluating structural damage and the severity of the lesion, in addition to providing some basis for prognosis. Percutaneous renal biopsy should not be at-

tempted on any patient having an unidentified renal mass, a solitary kidney or severe uncontrolled hypertension. In addition, it is extremely important to evaluate the patient's coagulation status before the biopsy is performed.

The last clinical entity in the etiological classification of hematuria (Table 37–1) defines a select, but not uncommon, group of patients with hematuria. These patients may have recurring episodes of gross, along with microscopic, hematuria, and this symptom alone may be very puzzling to the patient and the physician because the cause is seldom apparent. This has been referred to as benign hematuria of childhood, recurrent monosymptomatic hematuria and also as idiopathic hematuria. The etiology of the hematuria is unknown in this group of patients, and onset may occur anywhere from one year to adulthood. The episodes of gross hematuria appear most commonly in association with an upper respiratory tract infection but can also occur after strenuous exercise and other stressful experiences. This diagnosis can only be made when all of the recommended studies have been completed and are normal. Renal function studies are always normal, as are the intravenous pyelogram, voiding cystourethrogram, cystoscopy and retrograde pyelogram. In addition, serum complement levels are normal.

The diagnostic approach to patients with this entity should include all the tests listed in Table 37–2 except for renal biopsy. If the hematuria is the only evidence of renal malfunction, the biopsy is not necessary. The patient should be ob-

TABLE 37–2 DIAGNOSTIC APPROACH TO HEMATURIA

   I. Medical History
  II. Physical Examination
 III. Laboratory
    A. Urinalysis
    B. Complete blood count, erythrocyte sedimentation rate
    C. Blood Chemistries
    D. Other: Antinuclear antibody, Complement (B_{1C}), ASO
    E. Clotting Studies (PTT, PT, Platelet)
  IV. Urological Evaluation
    A. Intravenous pyelogram
    B. Voiding cystourethrogram
    C. Cystoscopy
   V. Renal Biopsy

---

served with periodic urinalysis, however, and simple tests of renal function and evaluation for proteinuria should be repeated at regular intervals over a three- to four-year period. If the patient develops persistent proteinuria or any other symptom of renal disease along with the hematuria, a renal biopsy should be performed.

Proteinuria

Proteinuria in an asymptomatic patient requires careful differentiation. If it is transient or postural, which can be determined by a relatively simple approach, the prognosis is good, especially in young patients. The older child in whom no primary cause is apparent, presents a much more difficult problem. In this case, a renal biopsy is essential to establish a diagnosis and to provide optimal management. Proteinuria is one of the most common clinical expressions of renal dysfunction, but its exact pathophysiology has not yet been carefully delineated. A general outline of the causes of proteinuria are depicted in Table 37–3. This cannot be considered a conclusive list of the causes of proteinuria because this discussion does not deal with all of the causes.

When proteinuria is encountered, the first priority is to determine whether it is transient, orthostatic or persistent (Table 37–4). As with hematuria, there may be many clues to the diagnosis in the history, physical examination and complete urinalysis. In order to classify the proteinuria, two 12-hour quantitative urine protein determinations should be performed, the first in the supine position and the second in the erect position. This urine collection can be used also to measure the endogenous creatinine clearance, which will serve as an estimate of renal function. If the 24-hour protein is less than 250 mg, the creatinine

TABLE 37–4 CLINICAL CLASSIFICATION OF PROTEINURIA

I. Intermittent proteinuria
II. Persistent proteinuria
III. Orthostatic proteinuria
A. Intermittent
B. Persistent
IV. Exercise proteinuria

clearance is normal. If this is coupled with urines that are negative for protein, the patient may be classified as having transient proteinuria, and further evaluation is not necessary. If children, adolescents and young adults have fixed and reproducible orthostatic proteinuria, the prognosis is considered to be generally good, and no further studies need be done except for an intravenous pyelogram. When the 24-hour urine protein excretion exceeds 250 mg and is persistent, further evaluation is necessary (Table 37–5). These studies are designed to determine the nature and severity of the renal parenchymal disease that underlies the proteinuria. A renal biopsy should be performed in the apparently healthy child with significant proteinuria who does not have hypertension or other systemic illnesses, such as lupus erythematosis or diabetes, or who shows no other evidence of renal disease, such as abnormal urine sediment or excretory pyelogram. It is our practice to perform renal biopsies on all patients whose 24-hour protein excretion is in excess of 500 mg/24 hours. In patients excreting less than 500 mg of protein per 24 hours, 24-hour urine protein determinations, as well as creatinine clearances, should be repeated at regular intervals. It should again be emphasized that in patients who have both persistent hematuria

TABLE 37–5 LABORATORY EVALUATION OF THE PATIENT WITH SIGNIFICANT PERSISTENT PROTEINURIA

Complete blood count, sedimentation rate, urinalysis
Quantitative urine protein
Endogenous creatinine clearance
Antinuclear antibody titer
Complement level ($C3\ B_{1C}$)
Total serum protein and protein electrophoresis or total albumin
Serum cholesterol
Intravenous pyelogram
Renal biopsy

TABLE 37–3 ETIOLOGY OF PROTEINURIA

Exercise, cold, orthostasis
Disorders not primarily renal: fever, drug, cardiac
Systemic disorders producing renal lesions
Pregnancy (eclampsia)
Primary renal disease
Urological problems
Asymptomatic

and proteinuria, renal biopsies should be performed because of the high incidence of renal parenchymal disease.

NEPHROTIC SYNDROME IN CHILDREN

The nephrotic syndrome is characterized by edema, proteinuria, hypoalbuminemia and hypercholesterolemia that may extend over many months or years. The frequency of nephrosis is not precisely known; however, an incidence of approximately 7 per 100,000 population under the age of five years has been estimated. It is primarily a disease of childhood, with the average age of onset being approximately two and one half years. It is uncommon in those under one year of age and is more common in boys than in girls.

Nephrotic syndrome may be due to intrinsic renal disease or it may result from systemic abnormalities that damage the glomeruli (Table 37–6). The age of the patient is quite important in this regard. Nephrotic syndrome in a preadolescent child has about a 90 per cent chance of being caused by intrinsic renal abnormality and not a systemic disorder, while this is true of approximately 80 per cent of adults. A careful history and physical examination may reveal whether any systemic abnormality exists.

Certain laboratory studies are also essential in delineating the cause of the nephrotic syndrome. Urinalysis will reveal the degree of proteinuria, and it will also detect the presence of hematuria, which if persistent is a poor prognostic sign. A complete blood count and erythrocyte sedimentation rate may give clues to the chronicity and severity of the illness. Urine should be collected for 12 or 24 hours and analyzed for quantitative loss of protein. The same urine specimen may be used for assessment of the creatinine clearance. An antinuclear antibody (ANA) determination should be done to exclude systemic lupus erythematosus, and beta 1_c globulin, which is equivalent to complement component 3 (C3), should also be determined. The latter is usually diminished in systemic lupus erythematosus, post-streptococcal acute glomerulonephritis and hypocomplementemic membranoproliferative

TABLE 37–6 PRINCIPAL CAUSES OF NEPHROTIC SYNDROME

Systemic Infections	Syphilis
	Malaria
Toxins	Mercurials
	Bismuth
	Gold
	Trimethadione (Tridione) and Paramethadione (Paradione)
	Probenecid
	Meglumine diatrizoate (Renografin)
	Heroin
Allergens	Poison oak
	Bee sting
	Serum sickness
	Inhaled pollens
Mechanical causes	Renal vein thrombosis
	IVC thrombosis of obstruction
	Constrictive pericarditis
	Tricuspid valve disease
Generalized disease processes	Amyloidosis
	Multiple myeloma
	Diabetic glomerulopathy
	Juvenile diabetes mellitus
	Mucopolysaccharidoses
	Malignancies
	Systemic lupus erythematosus
	Henoch-Schonlein purpura
Intrinsic renal Congenital Familial Minimal change — Nil disease glomerulonephritis	Focal sclerosis
	Proliferative, including post-streptococcus acute glomerulonephritis
	Membranous nephropathy
	Membranoproliferative

glomerulonephritis. Further specialized studies may be needed to determine whether or not there is systemic cause in nephrotic syndrome.

The Pathophysiology in Nephrotic Syndrome

In nephrotic syndrome, the glomerular capillary, which is normally impermeable to albumin and other larger proteins, becomes permeable to these proteins, thus circulating blood proteins can leak into the urine. If protein synthesis is unable to compensate for this loss of protein, hypoproteinuria (primarily hypoalbuminemia)

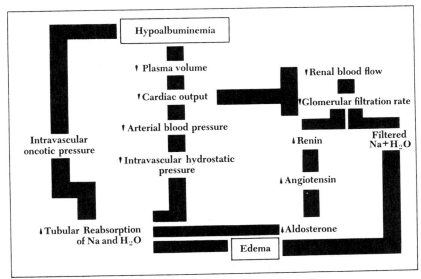

Figure 37–1 Pathophysiology of nephrotic syndrome.

ensues (Fig. 37–1). As a result, intravascular oncotic pressure decreases, and fluid shifts from the blood vessels into the extracellular space. Consequently, edema develops and intravascular volume decreases. Hypovolemia then induces protective homeostatic responses such as release of renin-angiotensin and aldosterone to promote retention of sodium and water.

Management

In the patient with edema, sodium and water enter the extracellular space, while the intravascular space is depleted. This signals the renin-angiotensin-aldosterone system and prevents sodium loss in the urine. Consequently, any sodium that is ingested cannot be excreted and instead increases the edema fluid. To prevent increased build-up of edema, dietary sodium must be limited. A diet containing 1 to 2 gm/day of sodium is usually tolerable for a brief time while other measures have a chance to take effect. There is no need for rigid water restriction; in fact, this may be dangerous. The nephrotic syndrome patient is hypovolemic, thus a significant rapid decrease in intake or an increase in fluid output could lead to a further decrease in intravascular volume. A generous protein diet is beneficial in a child without azotemia and is especially important in a growing child. The presence of azotemia

and renal failure is, of course, a contraindication to a high protein diet.

Diuretic therapy, while not curative, can give prompt relief to the unhappy edematous child with nephrotic syndrome while he is waiting the 14 to 28 days for steroids to take effect. They can also alleviate the symptoms of the partially improved adult patient who is already receiving steroids or immunosuppressive agents. In the child, however, diuretics should be given cautiously, for the reasons mentioned here. The child should be under hospital observation during the initial diuresis, and his blood pressure and peripheral circulation should be regularly assessed. Generally, the use of hydrochlorothiazide and spironolactone (initially 2 mg/kg/day of each in divided doses) promotes a safe, effective diuresis. In less responsive children, more potent diuretics such as furosemide may be required. Initially 1 mg/kg/day of furosemide is usually effective, but up to 250 mg or more may be required, especially in the face of renal impairment. Whether hyponatremia or hypokalemia are present should be determined by serial serum measurements and corrected by appropriate drug and dietary adjustment.

Adrenocortical steroids have been used in therapy of nephrotic syndrome since 1950. Based on their therapeutic response to steroids, nephrotic patients may be classified in three groups: (1) the steroid-sensitive group, which responds to a single short course of steroids with no relapse after cessation of therapy (40 per cent of the children with nephrotic syndrome are in this category); (2) those who respond to steroids but have relapses when steroids are withdrawn and require repeated courses of prednisone (50 per cent); and (3) steroid resistant patients (7 to 10 per cent of children and 70 to 80 per cent of adult patients). Response to steroids can often be predicted by the results of the patient's renal biopsy. In children with nephrotic syndrome, most of whom show minimal changes, steroids are remarkably successful in clearing the urine of protein. A dose of 60 mg/m²/day of prednisone (up to a maximum of 60 mg/day) produces diuresis, ends proteinuria and clears edema generally within 14 to 21 days. Patients with other histological types appear to respond rather poorly, if at all, to adrenocortical steroids. In general, patients with evidence of chronic glomerulonephritis do not respond favorably to steroids, and in many instances, steroids may be contraindicated.

In light of these facts, a rational approach to the treatment of nephrotic syndrome has emerged (Table 37–7). In children under 10 years of age who do not have hematuria or hypertension, a biopsy is usually not performed initially. The patient is given a 28-day trial of prednisone therapy. Response to prednisone generally indicates that the child has minimal change disease. Lack of complete response within 28 days implies that the child is in another category, and renal biopsy should be performed. A patient who is under 10 years of age and has no evidence of persistent hypertension or hematuria should be started on 60 mg/m²/day (maximum 60 mg/day); this dose is given until the urine becomes free of protein, and at that point, the same amount is given to the patient every other day. Patients in our clinic are generally treated in this manner for two to four months, and then the steroids are withdrawn over another month-long period.

The absence of proteinuria for two to three years after therapy usually indicates successful treatment. More than half the patients have relapse, however, at which time they are given another course of prednisone. The steroid-dependent patients, that is, those that relapse frequently, can be maintained free of nephrotic syndrome but are highly susceptible to complications of

TABLE 37–7 TREATMENT OF NEPHROTIC SYNDROME

Child under 10 years old	With no hematuria and no hypertension—prednisone, 60 mg/m²/day (maximum 60 mg) daily, until protein free; then 60 mg/m² every other day for 2 to 4 months; then taper to 0 mg over 1 month
	If relapse occurs, restart prednisone, 60 mg/m²/day (maximum 60 mg) daily until protein free; then 60 mg/m² every other day for 1 month; then taper to 0 mg over 1 month
	If no response to prednisone within 28 days, perform renal biopsy to ascertain underlying lesion; symptomatic therapy with diuretics, high-protein diet; consider cyclophosphamide, 2.5 to 3 mg/kg/day for 8 weeks, with informed consent
Adult or child over 10 years old	Exclude systemic disease process; renal biopsy to ascertain underlying lesion; trial of prednisone for 28 days, especially if there is minimal change lesion
	Prednisone, 60 to 80 mg/day until protein free; then 60 to 80 mg every other day for 2 to 4 months; then taper to 0 mg over 1 month
	If no response to prednisone within 28 days, consider cyclophosphamide therapy; symptomatic therapy with diuretics

steroids such as growth failure, hypertension, gastrointestinal bleeding, Cushing syndrome, osteoporosis, infections and diabetes mellitus.

For patients who demonstrate various steroid side effects and for the steroid-resistent patient, consideration of cytoxan (Cyclophosphamide), a nitrogen mustard derivative, is indicated. This drug has been shown to be a very effective agent in steroid-sensitive relapsing nephrotic children. It is our feeling, however, that this drug should only be used in patients in whom serious steroid side effects have arisen or who are resistant or moderately resistant to steroids. Side effects from cyclophosphamide are numerous, including leukopenia, alopecia, nausea and vomiting, hemorrhagic cystitis and more importantly, damage the gonads.

It is difficult to assess the overall prognosis for children with nephrotic syndrome; however, several retrospective studies indicate a five-year survival rate of approximately 75 per cent. Since most of the survival studies have not included renal biopsy studies, it is difficult to know the types of renal lesions that were included in the groupings.

ACUTE POSTSTREPTOCOCCAL GLOMERULONEPHRITIS

Post-streptococcal glomerulonephritis is one of the most frequent glomerulonephritidies observed in children. Infections of the skin and soft tissue, as well as the pharynx, due to the group A streptococcus have long been recognized as important causes of acute glomerulonephritis, especially in children. The signs and symptoms of acute glomerulonephritis are characteristically preceded by a latent period of 7 to 14 days, following infection with group A nephritogenic streptococcus. Acute rheumatic fever or acute glomerulonephritis may occur after streptococcal infections of either the throat or skin. Historically, streptococcal pyoderma has played an important role in the epidemiology of acute glomerulonephritis in several sections of the United States. In the past two decades, a large number of specific serotypes of group A beta hemolytic streptococcus have been shown to be nephritogenic. It is clear now that pyoderma-nephritis serotypes are clearly different from major nephritogenic strains found in the throat; therefore, definitive serological classification of strains of group A streptococcus is of fundamental importance in streptococcal epidemiology. Nephritis may occur sporadically or may be associated with epidemics of streptococcal pharyngitis or pyoderma.

Clinical Manifestations

Diagnosis of acute post-streptococcal glomerulonephritis is not difficult. Findings such as history of a recent beta hemolytic streptococcal infection in either skin or pharynx, elevation of blood pressure, impairment of renal function, hematuria and proteinuria associated with hypertension

TABLE 37–8 CLINICAL MANIFESTATIONS OF ACUTE GLOMERULONEPHRITIS

Hematuria
Oliguria
Edema
Hypertension
Anemia
Heart failure
Elevated ASO or anti-Dnase B titer
Decreased serum complement (B_{1C})

suggest acute glomerulonephritis (Table 37–8).

Selected serological studies should be performed in order to document an antecedent streptococcal infection. Streptococcal antibodies can be detected in the serum by a number of serological determinations. The antistreptolysin-O test, in the past, was the most commonly used; however, it has been recognized that it will detect only 60 to 70 per cent of previous group A beta hemolytic streptococcal infections. More recently, it has been shown that the antideoxyribonuclease B (anti-DNase B) titer is a much more sensitive test to document streptococcal infection, especially in patients with streptococcal pyoderma; however, it is not universally available. The latter test will identify approximately 90 per cent of previous streptococcal infection. The measurement of serum complement as either total hemolytic complement or as B_{1c} (C3) should also be measured because of its value in following the resolution phase of the nephritis. Measurements of the blood chemistries, including blood urea nitrogen, creatinine and serum potassium, should also be measured, especially if oliguria is a prominent feature of the clinical course.

The differential diagnosis of glomerulonephritis includes anaphylactoid purpura, viral nephritides (ECHO, Coxsackie), hemolytic uremic syndrome, lupus erythematosus, polyarteritis, toxic nephropathy and other forms of chronic glomerulonephritis. If the presenting clinical manifestations are equivocal or the glomerulonephritis could represent a manifestation of a systemic disease or other entity, renal biopsy may be indicated. Renal biopsy may also be helpful when there is persistence of abnormal urinary findings for an extended period of time.

Management

Until we have a complete understanding of the pathogenic mechanisms involved in acute streptococcal glomerulonephritis, no specific therapy can be developed. Therapy is therefore directed at management of those pathophysiological problems that arise as consequences of disturbances in renal function caused by the primary disease process. The overall aim of therapy is to carry the patient through the acute period into a period of convalescence, avoiding serious iatrogenic complications. The most important complications of acute glomerulonephritis are listed in Table 37–9. The cause of hypertension in acute glomerulonephritis is unknown, but the frequent correlation with salt and water balance suggests that the expansion of extracellular or intravascular volume may have an important role. Hypertension is often found in the edematous patient and typically subsides as the spontaneous diuresis ensues.

Antihypertensive therapy in acute nephritis involves three components: control of sodium balance, avoidance or reduction of hypervolemia and the use of specific antihypertensive drugs. If the hypertension is of mild to moderate degree, dietary restriction may be all that is necessary in the therapy. Usually, sodium intake should be limited to 1 gm/m²/day as long as hypertension is present. In more severe hypertension, with diastolic pressures in excess of 100 mm Hg, especially when there is associated hypervolemia, specific therapeutic measures should be instituted. Presence of hypervolemia attributes to the development of cardiac failure; therefore, when hypervolemia exists, diuretics should be considered. The less potent diuretics such as chlorthiazides are usually not effective, and therefore, more potent "loop" diuretics such as furosemide should be used. Furosemide may be given

TABLE 37–9 COMPLICATIONS OF ACUTE GLOMERULONEPHRITIS

Hypertension
Encephalopathy
Circulatory congestion and edema
Renal failure
Infection

intravenously in doses of 1 to 2 mg/kg or may be given orally in doses of 2 to 4 mg/kg.

Other antihypertensive drugs should also be considered when the diastolic pressure is greater than 100 mm Hg. Reserpine in doses of 0.07 mg/kg (maximum 2.5 mg) may be administered intramuscularly and is usually effective. If the diastolic pressure is 100 mm Hg or greater, hydralazine should be added to the regimen in doses of 0.1 to 0.15 mg/kg. Most episodes of hypertension associated with acute streptococcal nephritis may be controlled with either one or both of these agents. In a severe hypertensive crisis associated with encephalopathy, the use of diazoxide, 5 mg/kg, as a single rapid intravenous infusion should be considered. Nitroprusside may also be given as a slow intravenous drip (100 mg nitroprusside in 500 ml of 5 per cent dextrose and water). The nitroprusside should be administered via a constant infusion pump and the blood pressure monitored continuously as therapy is induced. The blood pressure must be monitored carefully when nitroprusside is used.

Moderate edema may also complicate acute glomerulonephritis, and when it exists in mild to moderate degree, salt intake should be restricted to 1 gm/m²/day. If the edema is severe or progressive in spite of restriction of salt intake, diuretic therapy as outlined should be utilized. If renal failure is present, as evidenced by mild or moderate oliguria or anuria, careful intake and output records should be maintained for all patients with acute glomerulonephritis in order to detect renal failure and avoid serious fluid overload and electrolyte imbalance. Disturbances such as hyperkalemia, hyponatremia and metabolic acidosis occur almost exclusively in patients with severe oliguria or anuria. In the severely oliguric patient, water restriction is necessary. Fluid intake should equal the calculated insensible loss plus urine output. Measures to prevent and treat hyperkalemia are also vital; therefore, curtailment of protein intake and maintenance of a high carbohydrate intake should be attempted. Dietary protein restriction need not be continued, however, once the azotemia has subsided.

When the serum potassium is rising rapidly or is above 6.5 mEq/l or more, measures for reducing potassium levels must be instituted. The administration of a cation-exchange resin such as sodium polystyrene sulfonate (kayexalate) is effective in lowering the serum potassium if used soon enough. The desired amount of resin can be administered rectally or orally as a 20 to 30 per cent suspension. When more severe hyperkalemia is evident, e.g., a serum potassium of 6.5 mEq/l or greater or electrocardiographic evidence of potassium intoxication, dialysis is indicated.

In glomerulonephritis, cardiac failure with pulmonary edema is usually associated with hypervolemia and hypertension. Therefore, cardiac failure can usually be avoided if hypertension is controlled and hypervolemia avoided. Bedrest is desirable in the early stage of the nephritis when hypertension is present; however, it is not indicated after gross hematuria, hypertension and edema are no longer present. The convalescent patient may be reambulated slowly, provided these signs do not recur, and may return to normal physical activity usually within one to two months after acute onset of nephritis.

ACUTE RENAL FAILURE

Acute renal failure is an abrupt, frequently reversible, impairment or cessation of renal function, expressed clinically by oliguria or anuria. The patient with acute renal failure usually has "oliguria" with daily urine volume less than 300 ml/m².

A summary of the main causes of acute renal failure in children is shown in Table 37–10. Despite the diversity of clinical situations, the main causes of true acute renal failure fall into two major categories, each of which results in distinctive pathological lesions. The first of these is nephrotoxic substances, and in this category are drugs, solvents, heavy metals and certain products of hemolysis that are directly toxic to the renal tubular cells. In most instances, these foreign substances are filtered to the glomeruli and are reabsorbed by cells of the proximal tubules. Subsequently, high local concentration of these substances may produce necrosis of tubular cells. The other major category is that of renal ischemia. Many clinical situations causing acute renal failure in children are associated with

TABLE 37–10 CAUSES OF ACUTE RENAL FAILURE

I. *Prerenal Failure* (circulatory insufficiency)
1. Severe dehydration
2. Hemorrhage
3. Severe burns
II. *Renal Failure* (intrinsic)
1. Parenchymatous disease
  Acute glomerulonephritis
  Renal cortical necrosis
  Acute pyelonephritis
2. Nephrotoxins
  Heavy metals
  Chemical (C Cl₄, DDT)
3. Vascular disease
4. Intravascular hemolysis
III. *Postrenal Failure* (obstructive uropathy)
1. Ureteral obstruction
2. Obstruction at bladder neck

the loss of effective blood volume, hypotension or severe dehydration. All these situations set off a train of hemodynamic changes, which if prolonged or extensive, can result in renal tubular damage. These mechanisms, shown in Figure 37–1, are frequently seen in severe dehydration, hemorrhage or severe burns.

Intrinsic renal diseases that are frequently associated with acute renal failure are acute glomerulonephritis, renal cortical necrosis and hemolytic uremic syndrome. In any instance in which there is an abrupt cessation of renal flow, one must also consider post-renal failure that may be due to renal obstruction, which may be bilateral or unilateral, in the case of a solitary kidney. Acute obstruction at the bladder neck, although a rare cause, should also be considered.

In order to distinguish between acute renal sufficiency and other reversible causes of oliguria and azotemia, the initial examination should include blood pressure, pulse rate, assessment of the state of dehydration by examination of the skin turgor, serum sodium, hematocrit, examination for evidence of congestive heart failure, including the measurement of central venous pressure if necessary, and evaluation for possible occult causes, of blood loss such as gastrointestinal hemorrhage or enclosed space hemorrhage, such as extremity fractures. Initial evaluation will detect those cases of oliguria and azotemia due to hypovolemia, hypotension or congestive heart failure and will not identify those instances due to bilateral, artery or venous obstruction or urinary tract obstruction. Renal artery or venous obstruction occurs rarely, however, and diagnostic evaluation for these entities is needed only when the clinical setting is suggestive of them. On the other hand, in any patient except one in whom the clinical findings clearly indicate an alternative diagnosis, urinary tract obstruction must be suspected initially. Under these circumstances, a unilateral retrograde pyelogram will be necessary to exclude urinary tract obstruction.

In some cases, it may be difficult to differentiate between oliguria due to fluid and electrolyte depletion and renal insufficiency due to various parenchymatous kidney diseases. Renal function tests may permit some preliminary conclusions. For example, a urine-urea to plasma-urea nitrogen concentration ratio of less than 10:1 suggests parenchymal renal disease. A ratio greater than 10:1 virtually excludes true acute renal insufficiency.

Management

The major components of management of acute renal failure are shown in Table 37–11. Hypovolemia is probably the largest contributing factor to prerenal failure and is usually reversible if recognized early and treated promptly. If severe, hypovolemia should be treated by intravenous infusion of a volume expander, preferably whole blood or plasma, if the patient is bleeding. A variety of electrolyte solutions

TABLE 37–11 MANAGEMENT OF ACUTE RENAL FAILURE

1. Restoration of extracellular fluid volume
   a. Mannitol
2. Treatment of hyperkalemia
3. Restoration of fluid and electrolyte balance
   a. Edema
   b. Hyponatremia-hypernatremia
   c. Phosphate
   d. Acidosis-alkalosis
4. Minimize protein catabolism
   a. Glucose (50%)
5. Restore blood volume
   a. Anemia
   b. Hypertension
6. Infection
   a. Sepsis
   b. Pyelonephritis (Catheter problem)

may also be used in correcting the hypovolemic state. Solutions containing 115 to 154 mEq/l of sodium and 70 to 154 mEq/l of chloride should be given as the initial expander at the rate of 20 ml/kg or 400 ml/m² over a 40- to 60-minute period. This maneuver usually stimulates urine flow in most patients except those with severe dehydration; this may be repeated within one or two hours after the initial infusion. It is extremely important, however, to avoid overloading the patient, because he cannot excrete fluid and electrolytes.

In the absence of an increase in urine output after volume depletion is corrected, a test dose of 20 per cent mannitol, 0.2 to 0.5 gm/kg intravenously over a 10- to 20-minute period with or without furosemide (1 to 2 mg/kg intravenously) can be given. Mannitol should not be given to a patient in cardiac failure; nor should furosemide if the patient is hypovolemic. Mannitol and furosemide may induce diuresis in reversible intrinsic renal failure. In the initial volume expansion, bicarbonate may be substituted for chloride in the solution when the patient is symptomatically acidotic.

After reversible causes of acute renal failure have been eliminated, hypertension has been corrected, and gross water and electrolyte losses have been restored, therapy should be designed to maintain as normal a state as possible until spontaneous diuresis takes place. This is accomplished largely by meticulous fluid balance and a provision of enough calories to slow down protein catabolism and prevent ketosis. Fluid intake should be based on insensible loss, especially in children; therefore, it is important to weigh the patient daily as accurately as possible. Ideally, there should be a small daily weight loss of 150 to 300 gm/day.

Most of the serious metabolic derangements of acute renal failure stem from the products of protein breakdown. Therefore, any protein intake should be effectively eliminated and foods containing sodium should also be withheld. One should attempt to give 50 to 75 gm/m²/day of glucose in order to maintain a relatively antiketogenic, anticatabolic state. The patient should therefore receive all the fluid requirements as 10 per cent dextrose and water either orally or intravenously depending upon the patient's condition. "Christmas candy," butterballs and so on may be added to increase total caloric intake, if the patient is not vomiting. If more concentrated glucose solutions are given intravenously, catheters should be inserted into larger veins to minimize chances of venous thrombosis secondary to hypertonic glucose.

The next major concern in the treatment of acute renal failure is that of hyperkalemia, which may require immediate therapy. Hyperkalemia is one of the most common sources of catastrophe in the management of patients with acute renal failure. Hyperkalemia, particularly with cardiotoxic manifestations, is all too often not recognized as an acute medical emergency. In any patient with oliguria or anuria, the serum potassium should be monitored frequently. Hyperkalemia should be treated expectantly, and one should not wait for the development of serious toxicity. In our practice, we utilize the exchange resin sodium polystyrene sulfonate (Kayexalate) when there are T wave changes on the electrocardiogram or serum potassium levels greater than 6.5 mEq/l. It must be used early in the development of hypokalemia. Kayexalate may be given in a dose of 15 to 25 gm every four to eight hours by mouth or by retention enema. Approximately 1 mEq/l of potassium is exchanged for each gram of resin. The resin also exchanges for calcium and magnesium; therefore, if it is used for more than 12 to 24 hours, serum calcium and magnesium should be monitored.

When there is acute onset of severe hypokalemia with electrocardiogram changes such as markedly peaked waves or prolongation of the QT interval, glucose and insulin may be given intravenously to lower the serum potassium (one unit of insulin per 3 to 4 gm carbohydrate). Calcium gluconate may also be given at a rate of 100 to 200 mg/min with continuous electrocardiogram monitoring. Sodium bicarbonate may also be administered intravenously, in order to lower serum potassium concentration. These modes of therapy should only be considered in instances in which the potassium levels have to be lowered immediately. There is frequently a rapid rise of serum potassium following the cessation of insulin-glucose transfusions; therefore, the patient should be prepared for peritoneal dialysis when the potassium level is controlled by the insulin-glucose infusion.

With severe hyperkalemia or a rapidly rising serum potassium, therapy by peritoneal dialysis or hemodialysis should be considered. Other indications for peritoneal dialysis in acute renal failure are severe congestive heart failure associated with the hypervolemia, intractable acidosis or hypertension.

The prognosis for acute renal failure is directly related to the etiology and severity of the underlying cause of the renal failure; however, acute renal failure is usually a reversible disorder of renal function in which the patient generally achieves near normal renal function if he survives the initial course and complications that may occur. Meticulous attention to the complications associated with acute renal failure and to the metabolic derangements that occur will undoubtedly reduce the morbidity and mortality of this disorder.

REFERENCES

Hematuria and Proteinuria

McConville, J. M., West, C. D., and McAdams, A. J.: Familial and non-familial benign hematuria. J. Pediatr., 69:207, 1966.

Northway, J. D.: Hematuria in Children. J. Pediatr., 78:381, 1971.

Thompson, A. L., Durrett, R. R., and Robinson, R. R.: Fixed and reproducible orthostatic proteinuria VI. Results of a 10 year follow-up evaluation. Ann. Intern. Med., 73:235, 1970.

Wagner, M. C., Smith, F. G., Jr., Tinglof, B. O., Jr., and Cornberg, E.: Epidemiology of proteinuria. J. Pediatr., 73:825, 1968.

Nephrotic Syndrome

Smith, F. G., Jr., Gonick, H., Stanley, T. M., and McIntosh, R. M.: The nephrotic syndrome: Current concepts. Ann. Intern. Med., 76:463, 1972.

Acute Glomerulonephritis

Dillon, H. C., and Reeves, M. S.: Streptococcal immune responses in nephritis after skin infection. Am. J. Med., 56:333, 1974.

Perlman, L. V., Herdman, R. C., Kleinman, H., and Vernier, R. L.: Post-streptococcal glomerulonephritis: A ten year follow-up of an epidemic. J.A.M.A., 194:63, 1965.

38

Parenteral Fluid Therapy in Children

William E. Segar and Russell W. Chesney

Parenteral fluids are used whenever a child is unable to ingest the amount of water and electrolytes needed to (1) meet the ongoing daily physiological losses of water and electrolytes, (2) restore pre-existing body fluid deficits and (3) replace abnormal continuing losses of water and electrolytes. The intravenous route is the only safe means by which this can be provided. The volume of parenteral fluid should always be calculated as the amount needed by the child per 24 hours, and the fluid usually should be administered at a constant rate during the entire 24-hour period unless abnormal continuing losses of fluids occur at an inconstant rate.

MAINTENANCE THERAPY

Every patient normally loses reasonably predictable quantities of water, electrolytes and calories each day. Fluid therapy aimed at replacing these losses is termed maintenance therapy. If the patient is in an adequate state of hydration when therapy is started and is not undergoing large concurrent losses of fluid or electrolytes, maintenance therapy will meet the entire requirement.

Many systems are recommended for the calculation of maintenance water requirement. It has been shown that daily physiological water losses are directly proportionate to caloric expenditure. It follows, therefore, that maintenance water requirements are also proportionate to caloric expenditure. Under most circumstances, water requirement is constant from one pa-

tient to the next, when expressed as water needed per unit of reference. The usual reference unit in calculating maintenance fluid requirements is per 100 kcal. For the average hospitalized child, the approximate caloric expenditure in kilocalories can be estimated from one of the following formulas: (1) For the child who weighs up to 10 kg, caloric expenditure is 100 times the weight in kilograms. (2) For the child who weighs 10 to 20 kg, caloric expenditure is 1000 plus (kg − 10) times 50. (3) For the child who weighs more than 20 kg, caloric expenditure is 1500 plus (kg − 20) times 20. The caloric expenditure per day of three children weighing 5 kg, 15 kg and 25 kg would be estimated as 500 kcal, 1250 kcal and 1600 kcal, respectively.

The maintenance water requirement is the sum of insensible and urinary water losses. Water lost from the lungs, skin and in the stool represent the main sources of insensible loss. When environmental temperature and humidity are normal, approximately 50 ml/100 kcal/day of water are lost via these routes. Renal water loss varies with the amount of solute that must be excreted and with the solute concentration of the urine. If we assume that a normal solute load will vary from 10 to 40 mOsm/100 kcal, then 67 ml/100 kcal of water will permit this solute load to be excreted at a urinary solute concentration of 150 to 600 mOsm/l. This concentration range can easily be achieved by any child without severe renal disease. The total maintenance water requirement is the sum of the insensible losses plus renal requirement or 50 ml + 67 ml = 117 ml/100 kcal/day. Approximately 15 to 20 ml/100 kcal of water is produced, however, as a result of oxidative metabolism each day. Thus, the amount to be given by parenteral administration is 117 ml − 17 ml = 100 ml/100 kcal/day of water.

Maintenance water requirements must be augmented when either insensible or renal water losses are increased. Insensible losses may increase if the child is in a hot environment, has a persistent fever or has significant hyperventilation. The newborn infant under bilirubin lights or a child with hyperventilation, as in salicylism or asthma, will have increased water losses. Extra water, usually 25 to 50 ml/100 kcal/day, should be provided in these circumstances. Renal water requirement will be increased if the child is undergoing an osmotic diuresis, as in the diabetic with hyperglycemia, or if he is unable to concentrate urine normally owing to the fixed urine osmolality caused by renal disease or nephrogenic diabetes insipidus. In these patients, the renal water allotment must be increased from 50 to 250 per cent, and this can be done properly only by monitoring the serum sodium concentration and the weight of the patient. If the level of serum sodium decreases and the body weight increases, less water should be given; if the sodium concentration increases and body weight decreases, more water is needed.

Insensible losses may be decreased if the patient is in a cool environment, is hypothermic or is breathing air saturated or supersaturated with water vapor. In these instances, less water should be given to meet insensible needs. This is particularly important if the patient cannot excrete dilute urine owing to renal disease or to the presence of appreciable concentrations of circulating antidiuretic hormone (ADH).

Less water is needed to meet renal water requirement if the patient can produce only a concentrated urine (caused by high blood levels of antidiuretic hormone acting on the renal medulla) or if the patient is oliguric. Stress, shock, meningitis, pneumonia and recovery from surgery often produce high blood levels of ADH, and since patients having such high levels are unable to excrete excess water, they often cannot tolerate a total water intake of more than 60 to 75 ml/100 kcal/day. Overhydration and hyponatremia frequently occur in these circumstances, and patients should be weighed daily and their serum sodium concentrations determined frequently. The anuric patient needs no water except that necessary to replace insensible loss. Thus his water intake is 50 ml − 17 ml = 33 ml/100 kcal/day. Even this amount is frequently excessive, and a total water requirement of 20 ml/100 kcal/day is usually more appropriate. Overhydration is a real danger, and the anuric child should be weighed at least once daily. Ideally, his weight should decrease about 0.5 per cent per day if overhydration is to be avoided.

Maintenance electrolyte therapy is always necessary to replace the normal urinary, fecal and skin losses of sodium, potassium and chloride. The appropriate requirements can also be determined on the basis of caloric expenditure. One can assume that the child usually needs 3 mEq of sodium, 2 mEq of chloride, and 2 mEq of potassium per 100 kcal per day to meet his electrolyte maintenance requirements. These electrolyte requirements usually do not need to be altered when the maintenance water requirement is varied. This quantity of sodium should not be given to patients with heart failure or liver disease, however, or in other circumstances in which a low sodium intake is necessary. Potassium is omitted if the child is oliguric, in shock, suspected of having adrenal insufficiency or in the immediate post-operative period, since the surgical procedure may cause excess tissue loss of K+.

Glucose must also be included to prevent acidosis and ketosis and to lessen protein catabolism. At least 5 gm/100 kcal/day of glucose should be given, and if less than 100 ml/100 kcal/day of water is ordered, the glucose concentration in the infusate should be increased to more than 5 per cent.

To summarize, the typical patient needs 100 ml of water, 3 mEq of sodium, 2 mEq of chloride, 2 mEq of potassium, and 5 gm of carbohydrate per 100 kcal of energy expenditure per day. In addition to the several exceptions noted, 60 to 80 per cent of the usual maintenance therapy should be given to premature infants and to full-term newborns during the first few days of life. The glucose concentration in these solutions should usually be greater than 5 gm/100 ml of infusate.

DEFICIT THERAPY

Many children have extensive losses of body fluids from pre-existing illnesses, with deficits of both water and the electrolyte contained in that water. If the amount of sodium lost with water is proportionate to the concentration of sodium in body fluids, no change in body fluid tonicity occurs, and the child has isotonic dehydration. If proportionately more water than sodium is lost, the concentration of serum sodium and the serum osmolality are increased, producing hypertonic dehydration. If sodium losses are proportionately greater, the serum sodium level and the serum osmolality are less than normal, resulting in hypotonic dehydration. Experience has shown that of 100 children with dehydration, about 80 will have normal serum tonicity.

Isotonic Dehydration

When body fluids are lost, a portion of that loss originates in the extracellular compartment (approximately 60 per cent); the remainder represents a loss of intracellular fluid (40 per cent). By definition, the loss of 1 liter of extracellular fluid (ECF) in these patients will include 140 mEq of sodium and 100 mEq of chloride, whereas approximately 150 mEq of potassium is lost in association with the loss of 1 liter of intracellular fluid (ICF). Deficit therapy consists of replacing the estimated amount of ECF and ICF lost. If a child has lost 1 liter of ECF and 500 ml of ICF, then replacement therapy would consist of 1000 ml of 5 per cent glucose in water containing 140 mEq of sodium and 100 mEq of chloride, plus 500 ml of 5 per cent glucose in water containing 75 mEq of potassium.

Laboratory tests are of little help in estimating the magnitude of body fluid deficit. Only the history and physical examination are useful. Certain physical findings correlate in a general way with the degree of fluid deficit. A mild deficit represents the loss of 20 to 40 ml/kg of body fluid, or a quantity of fluid equal to 2 to 4 per cent of the body weight. A patient with such a deficit may demonstrate thirst and dry mucous membranes but little else. A child with a moderate deficit (5 to 7 per cent) has, in ad-

dition, obvious fluid loss around the eyes and, occasionally, slight changes in tissue turgor. The skin may "tent" after being picked up, owing to loss of elasticity. A depressed fontanelle will be found in infants. A patient with a severe deficit (8 to 12 per cent) demonstrates marked changes in skin turgor, depression of the fontanelle, a dry tongue, tachycardia and oliguria. As the deficit approaches 120 ml/kg (12 per cent), marked oliguria, acidosis and evidence of shock will be observed.

Under most circumstances, about 60 per cent of body fluid deficit represents loss of extracellular fluid and 40 per cent loss of intracellular fluid. If the illness has lasted less than 48 hours, proportionally less intracellular fluid has probably been lost, and the total fluid loss is somewhat less than might be estimated from the physical findings. If, however, the illness is protracted (more than seven days), the physician should assume a proportionately greater loss of intracellular fluid and understand that he may underestimate the magnitude of dehydration if he relies on physical findings alone. One should estimate the deficit as accurately as possible and return that amount of fluid to the patient, along with his maintenance fluid requirement.

Three examples may clarify the manner in which this is done.

Example 1. A 5-kg infant has been vomiting all feedings for 72 hours and displays the physical findings of severe (10 per cent) dehydration. Two assumptions are made: (1) normal maintenance therapy for a child with a caloric expenditure of 500 kcal will be needed and (2) the child's total body fluid deficit of 500 ml (5 kg × 10 per cent) represents the loss of 300 ml of ECF (60 per cent of 500 ml) and 200 ml of ICF (40 per cent of 500 ml). The 300 ml of ECF

TABLE 38–1   DEFICIT THERAPY
REQUIREMENTS FOR 5-KG INFANT
WITH SEVERE ISOTONIC DEHYDRATION

| | Water (ml) | Electrolyte, mEq | | |
		Na	K	Cl
Maintenance	500	15	10	10
ECF deficit	300	42		30
ICF deficit	200		30	
Total	1000	57	40	40

should contain $300 \div 1000 \times 140 = 42$ mEq of sodium and $300 \div 1000 \times 100 = 30$ mEq of chloride, whereas the 200 ml of ICF should contain $200 \div 1000 \times 150 = 30$ mEq of potassium. These requirements are shown in Table 38–1. Thus, this infant requires 1000 ml of 5 per cent glucose in water to which 40 mEq of potassium chloride and 57 mEq of sodium have been added. Since the patient's chloride requirement has been met by the administration of KCl, the sodium can be provided as sodium bicarbonate or sodium lactate.

Example 2. A 20-kg girl has had diarrhea for 48 hours and demonstrates the physical findings of mild dehydration. We assume that: (1) maintenance therapy should be based on a caloric expenditure of 1500 kcal/day, (2) total-body fluid deficits are 600 ml (20 kg × 3 per cent), of which approximately 400 ml represents the loss of ECF and 200 ml the loss of ICF and (3) electrolyte losses are proportionate. The requirements are shown in Table 38–2. Since our assumptions involve errors of greater than 5 per cent, we would probably give this child 2000 ml of 5 per cent glucose, to which 70 mEq of potassium chloride and 100 mEq of sodium bicarbonate had been added.

Example 3. A 10-kg boy has been ill overnight. He has dry mucous membranes, sunken eyes and barely perceptible changes in tissue turgor. We assume that: (1) the maintenance requirements are normal, (2) since the child has suffered rapid dehydration, the total deficit is only 5 per cent, or less than that indicated by examination and (3) of the fluid lost (500 ml), more than 60 per cent, perhaps 80 per cent (400 ml), was extracellular and only 20 per cent (100 ml) was intracellular. The

TABLE 38–2 DEFICIT THERAPY REQUIREMENTS FOR 20-KG CHILD WITH MILD ISOTONIC DEHYDRATION

	Water (ml)	Electrolyte, mEq		
		Na	K	Cl
Maintenance	1500	45	30	30
ECF deficit	400	56		40
ICF deficit	200		30	
Total	2100	101	60	70

TABLE 38–3 DEFICIT THERAPY REQUIREMENTS FOR 10-KG CHILD WITH RAPID ISOTONIC DEHYDRATION

	Water (ml)	Electrolyte, mEq		
		Na	K	Cl
Maintenance	1000	30	20	20
ECF deficit	400	56		40
ICF deficit	100		15	
Total	1500	86	35	60

requirements are shown in Table 38–3. We would give the patient 1500 ml of 5 per cent glucose in water, to which 35 mEq of potassium chloride, 25 mEq of sodium chloride and 60 mEq of sodium bicarbonate had been added.

Hypertonic Dehydration

Hypernatremia (a serum sodium concentration greater than 155 mEq/l) is a serious complication of dehydration because it is associated with a significant increase in mortality rate; of those children who survive an episode of hypernatremic dehydration, many are left with permanent central nervous system damage. Hypernatremia may be the result of the excessive parenteral or oral administration of sodium to children with diarrheal dehydration and, as such, is often the result of mismanagement of a relatively benign illness. Hypernatremia also occurs as a result of the unwitting or conscious denial of water to a child, and in the latter situation, represents another form of child abuse. In order to prevent cerebral edema during therapy, care must be taken to reduce the serum sodium concentration slowly. The usual requirement for maintenance therapy is first determined. The fluid deficit in hypernatremia dehydration is always great, and deficit therapy of at least 100 ml/kg (10 per cent) is usually required. One third to one half of the deficit is replaced by 5 per cent glucose in water, and the remainder is provided by isotonic deficit therapy as described previously. Such therapy should gradually lower the serum sodium concentration by 10 to 12.5 mEq/day.

Example 4. A 5-kg infant girl with severe

TABLE 38-4 FLUID THERAPY REQUIREMENTS FOR 5-KG INFANT WITH SEVERE HYPERTONIC DEHYDRATION

	Water (ml)	Electrolyte, mEq		
		Na	K	Cl
Maintenance	500	15	10	10
Deficit (water only)	200			
ECF deficit	200	28		20
ICF deficit	100		15	
Total	1000	43	25	30

dehydration is seen, whose mother has fed her only boiled skim milk for four days. The serum sodium concentration is 170 mEq/liter. The therapeutic assumptions are that: (1) normal maintenance therapy is indicated, (2) total body fluid deficit is 500 ml, of which 40 per cent (200 ml) will be given as 5 per cent glucose in water (this portion of the deficit therapy should not contain electrolyte), and (3) 60 per cent (approximately 200 ml) of the remaining deficit should be replaced with ECF and 40 per cent (approximately 100 ml) with ICF. The requirements are shown in Table 38-4.

Hypotonic Dehydration

Hyponatremia (serum sodium concentration of less than 130 mEq/l) is occasionally present in dehydration and is treated by providing the patient with additional salt. Extra salt must be given cautiously, and water restriction may be more appropriate in treatment of the child who has dilutional hyponatremia and overhydration. Treatment of children with hyptonic dehydration consists of maintenance therapy, plus the usual deficit therapy, plus additional NaCl in an amount sufficient to bring the serum sodium concentration to normal (135 mEq/l). Since 0.6 mEq/kg of sodium will increase the sodium concentration by approximately 1 mEq/l, the use of the formula, (135 − the observed sodium) × 0.6 × weight in kilograms, permits an estimate of the extra NaCl required. Three per cent sodium chloride provides 0.5 mEq/ml of sodium and can be used in the

treatment of the profoundly hyponatremic patient.

Example 5. A 10-kg infant has 5 per cent dehydration due to vomiting and diarrhea. The serum sodium concentration is 120 mEq/l. The assumptions are that: (1) the child needs normal maintenance and deficit therapy, (2) the sodium concentration should be increased 15 mEq (135 − 120), so 15 × 0.6 × 10 = 90 additional mEq of NaCl are required and (3) if the child has convulsions or stupor, this added salt may be given rapidly (15 to 60 minutes) as a hypertonic solution; otherwise it should be added to the parenteral fluids. The requirements are shown in Table 38-5.

Shock

Shock caused by dehydration, as may occur with severe diarrhea, is due to the loss of large quantities of extracellular fluid. Shock caused by burns, by crushing injuries or by retroperitoneal or abdominal surgery is related to the transudation of ECF into the injured tissue. The treatment for shock is the rapid infusion of Ringer's lactate solution, 20 to 40 ml/kg/hr, until a stable clinical state is obtained. As the injury heals, gradual resorption of this solution will occur, leading to saline diuresis. If plasma or blood is used, hypervolemia, congestive failure and pulmonary edema may occur, since these substances cannot easily be removed from the vascular system.

REPLACEMENT OF ABNORMAL LOSSES

Maintenance therapy replaces normal water and electrolyte losses, and deficit

TABLE 38-5 FLUID THERAPY REQUIREMENTS FOR 10-KG INFANT WITH HYPOTONIC DEHYDRATION

	Water (ml)	Electrolyte, mEq		
		Na	K	Cl
Maintenance	1000	30	20	20
ECF deficit	300	42		30
ICF deficit	200		30	
Additional NaCl		90		90
Total	1500	162	50	140

therapy restores pre-existing body fluid deficiencies. Occasionally, a patient will have exceptionally large unremitting body fluid losses. These losses may include upper or lower gastrointestinal fluids, as would occur with continuous gastric or duodenal aspiration or with persistent vomiting or diarrhea; drainage from a fistula or from colostomy; severe polyuria; persistent sweating; or prolonged hyperventilation. Both the quantity and composition of the fluid should be measured (or estimated) and replaced (volume for volume) by a parenteral solution having a comparable electrolyte composition. Commercial solutions with the electrolyte composition of "average" upper and lower gastrointestinal secretions are available and should be used. Large sweat losses can be replaced by additional maintenance fluids, whereas respiratory losses should be replaced with 5 per cent glucose in water. The electrolyte composition of the urine should govern the appropriate replacement therapy for patients with persistent polyuria.

Fluids designed to replace abnormal losses must be given in addition to the usual maintenance therapy and, should a deficit exist, to deficit therapy as well. When replacement fluids are added to a running intravenous infusion, the flow rate must be increased so that all necessary fluids are given in 24 hours.

Example 6. A 10-kg infant undergoing chronic gastric suction appears to have 5 per cent dehydration. During the past 12 hours, 500 ml of gastric juice has been removed. The assumptions are that: (1) the child needs normal maintenance and deficit therapy, and (2) during the next 24 hours he will need an additional 1000 ml of

TABLE 38–6 FLUID THERAPY REPLACEMENT FOR ABNORMAL WATER AND ELECTROLYTE LOSSES IN 10-KG CHILD

| | Water (ml) | Electrolyte, mEq | | |
		Na	K	Cl
Maintenance	1000	30	20	20
ECF deficit	300	42		30
ICF deficit	200		30	
Replacement	1000	63	15	150
Total	2500	135	65	200

fluid that has the electrolyte composition of gastric juice. These requirements are shown in Table 38–6. The patient requires 2500 ml of 5 per cent glucose in water plus 135 mEq of NaCl and 65 mEq of KCl during the subsequent 24 hours.

Many patients requiring parenteral fluid therapy will have metabolic acidosis because of dehydration and caloric deprivation. If glucose is provided, however, and body fluid deficits are corrected, the acidosis will be corrected by homeostatic mechanisms. "Titration" of the serum CO_2 with $NaHCO_2$ or Na lactate is then unnecessary, and indeed, can be potentially dangerous.

In conclusion, the total water and electrolyte requirements of the child should be calculated, and the necessary amounts of Na, K and Cl, which are commercially available as concentrated solutions, should be added to the appropriate volume of 5 per cent glucose in water, thereby providing each child with fluid therapy designed specifically for him.

Inborn Enzymatic Errors

C. Ronald Scott

Over 120 inborn errors of metabolism have now been recognized, many of which are associated with mental retardation or neurological degeneration. Individually the disorders are rare, but collectively they constitute a significant number of patients. Many of these conditions lend themselves to easy recognition and the possibility of treatment. Because of the high emotional and monetary costs to individual families and society for care of the physically and mentally retarded, early recognition, diagnosis and therapy of treatable disorders have become mandatory. In an attempt to blunt the impact of these diseases on society, many countries and states have initiated newborn screening programs to identify infants at risk for treatable metabolic abnormalities.

Screening programs have been initiated throughout the world, and detection of three disorders has been found practical during the newborn period: phenylketonuria, galactosemia and hypothyroidism. Detection of these three disorders relies on the discovery of an elevated level of phenylalanine, an absence of galactose-1-PO_4 uridyl transferase or a decreased level of T_4 in the blood of a newly born infant. Interpretation of these screening tests places a heavy burden on the physician responsible for the care of infants. The following disorders need to be considered in interpreting reports for the screening of phenylketonuria and galactosemia.

Phenylketonuria

Phenylketonuria (PKU) is one of the "common" inborn errors of metabolism. It is an autosomal recessive condition and occurs with a frequency of 1:10,000 to 1:15,000 in most northern European populations. This incidence gives an estimated gene frequency of 1:100, or approximately 1 person in 50 is a heterozygote for PKU. The allele for PKU exists in greater frequency in the Irish population, with 1 in 5000 to 8000 infants born with PKU. It is rare in the black population, with only 1 child in 1,000,000 births affected. This low frequency of the allele for PKU in blacks precludes the necessity of screening for PKU in a population that is predominantly black.

The deficient enzyme in phenylketonuria is phenylalanine hydroxylase (Fig. 39-1). This enzyme exists primarily in the liver and catalyses the conversion of phenylalanine to tyrosine. In PKU, the complete absence of phenylalanine hydroxylase activity has been documented in liver tissue obtained by biopsy. This absence of activity prevents the conversion of phenylalanine to tyrosine; consequently, phenylalanine accumulates in bodily fluids. The accumulation of phenylalanine allows it to be converted to other aromatic products, namely phenylpyruvic acid, phenyllactic acid, phenylacetic acid, phenylacetyl glutamine and O-OH-phenylacetic acid. Phenylpyruvic acid excreted in the urine of untreated children with PKU reacts with ferric chloride to give a characteristic dark green color.

Children born with phenylketonuria appear normal at birth and usually do not exhibit evidence of mental retardation until six months to one year of age. They typically will have delayed maturational landmarks and delayed speech. It is between the ages of two and four years that parents

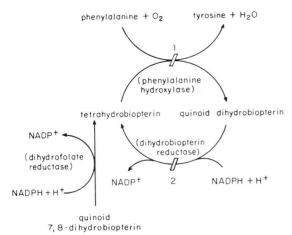

phenylalanine + O_2 tyrosine + H_2O

1

(phenylalanine hydroxylase)

tetrahydrobiopterin   quinoid dihydrobiopterin

$NADP^+$

(dihydrofolate reductase)

(dihydrobiopterin reductase)

$NADPH + H^+$ $NADP^+$ 2 $NADPH + H^+$

quinoid 7, 8-dihydrobiopterin

Figure 39–1 Two different enzyme defects may cause phenylketonuria. In classic phenylketonuria a deficiency of phenylalanine hydroxylase (site 1) prevents the oxidation of phenylalanine to tyrosine. A rare mutation, dehydrobiopterin reductase deficiency (site 2) prevents the reduction of quinoid dehydrobiopterin to tetrahydrobiopterin. The latter compound is necessary for phenylalanine hydroxylase activity.

seek medical counsel for their "slow" child. It is thought that most children with phenylketonuria, if untreated, will have an eventual IQ between 10 and 50. Many will never walk, talk or develop voluntary sphincter control. Only a small percentage will have IQs above 50, and a relatively rare person with PKU will have normal intelligence.

Table 39–1 describes the major clinical findings in the older child or adult with phenylketonuria who has not been treated.

Most infants born today are tested for an elevated plasma phenylalanine level prior to leaving the hospital. For the testing procedure to be reliable, the specimen should be obtained after the infant is 72 hours (three days) of age. If a blood specimen is collected prior to 72 hours, a second specimen should be obtained for phenylalanine before the infant is six weeks of age.

A blood phenylalanine concentration greater than 4 mg/100 ml of plasma in an infant is considered "elevated." The test should be repeated immediately, and if the level is still elevated, further studies are required to establish the proper diagnosis. The most frequent causes of an elevated phenylalanine level are listed in Table 39–2. A child with a persistent elevation of his blood phenylalanine concentration, however, should be carefully evaluated at a medical center with the laboratory expertise to establish a precise diagnosis.

The initiation of a low phenylalanine diet has been shown to be effective in the prevention of mental retardation in patients with phenylketonuria. The diet is aimed at lowering the serum phenylalanine concentration to near normal levels and supplying extra tyrosine for metabolic needs. Dietary control is considered adequate if the serum phenylalanine is maintained between 2 and 10 mg/100 ml and the serum tyrosine is between 1 and 3 mg/100 ml. In the United States, a low phenylalanine milk substitute called Lofenalac is available commerically. This dietary preparation is used as a replacement for milk products and high protein foods that contribute the majority of

TABLE 39–1   CLINICAL FINDINGS IN PHENYLKETONURIA

Finding	Incidence, per cent	Finding	Incidence, per cent
Agitated behavior	32–90	Inability to talk	63
EEG abnormalities	80	Hyperkinesis	50
Muscular hypertonicity	75	Inability to walk (and usually incontinence)	35
Hyperactive reflexes	66	Tremors	30
Blond hair, blue eyes	62	Eczema	19–34
		Seizures	26

From: Phenylketonuria by W. Eugene Knox in *The Metabolic Basis of Inherited Disease.* 2nd ed. Edited by Stanbury, Wyngaarden and Fredrickson. New York, used with permission of McGraw-Hill Book Company, 1966.

TABLE 39–2 CHEMICAL CRITERIA IN DIAGNOSIS OF ELEVATED SERUM PHENYLALANINE

Condition	Diagnostic Aids	Treatment
Normal infant	Serum phenylalanine < 4 mg/100 ml Serum tyrosine < 4 mg/100 ml No excess excretion of urinary phenolic acids	Normal diet

Phenylketonuria	Serum phenylalanine >15 mg/100 ml
	Serum tyrosine < 3 mg/100 ml
	Excess urinary excretion of:
	  Phenylalanine
	  Phenylpyruvic acid (PPA)
	  O-Hydroxyphenylacetic
	   acid (O-HPAA)
		Low phenylalanine
		  diet

Benign hyperphenyl-
alaninemia
	Serum phenylalanine 5–15 mg/100 ml
	Serum tyrosine < 3 mg/100 ml
	Excess urinary excretion of
	  phenylalanine, but usually not
	  PPA or O-HPAA
		None necessary

Dihydropteridine reductase deficiency	Serum phenylalanine >15 mg/100 ml Serum tyrosine < 4 mg/100 ml Excess excretion of urinary phenolic acids: ?	? Biopterin
Hereditary tyrosinemia	Serum phenylalanine 3–10 mg/100 ml Serum tyrosine > 5 mg/100 ml Serum methionine—elevated Excess tyrosyl products in urine	Diet low in phenylalanine and tyrosine

Tyrosinemia of
prematurity
	Premature infant
	Serum phenylalanine—variable
	Serum tyrosine > 5 mg/100 ml
	Excess excretion of tyrosine
	  in urine
		None indicated (ascorbic
		  acid may rapidly reverse
		  the elevated tyrosine)

? Phenylalanine transaminase deficiency	Serum phenylalanine—elevated Serum tyrosine—normal No excess excretion of urinary phenolic acids (PPA or O-HPAA)	?
Laboratory error in serum phenylalanine determination	—	—

dietary phenylalanine. The level of phenylalanine in the infant's blood is regulated by the amount of milk and low-protein fruits and vegetables required to keep his serum phenylalanine in a satisfactory range. This must be adjusted for each child on an individual basis.

Three major problems exist in the management of phenylketonuric children. The first is placing a non-phenylketonuric child on a low phenylalanine diet. In such cases, the serum phenylalanine falls to very low values (less than 1 mg/100 ml) and can result in growth failure, permanent mental retardation and even death. This is usually the fault of an improper diagnosis, based on a single elevated phenylalanine value, with no confirming laboratory studies.

The second problem is too severe a diet for a child with phenylketonuria. In such cases, the child will have poor growth, long bone changes at the metaphyses, neutropenia with a megaloblastic marrow, frequent infections and occasionally a scurvy-like clinical appearance. These signs are related to phenylalanine deficiency and are reversed by allowing a more generous protein intake.

The third problem is the most common: poor dietary control with high serum phenylalanine values. This may occur because of poor communication or poor nutritional counseling by the physician, poor dietary regulation at home, a social situation that precludes careful dietary control, rebellion to the diet by older children or psychological problems in the family that mitigate against a carefully controlled diet.

Long-term, successful management can best be obtained by having the children managed in centers in which nutritionists, psychologists, parent groups and medical personnel with special expertise interact in the care of children with metabolic disorders.

Hyperphenylalaninemia

There exists a group of infants with high serum phenylalanine values who do not have PKU and who usually do not require treatment. Disorders of this group have been designated "hyperphenylalaninemia of the newborn" or "benign hyperphenylalaninemia."

Infants with hyperphenylalaninemia have been detected by the newborn screening programs for PKU. They exhibit serum phenylalanine values greater than 4 mg/100 ml but usually less than 15 mg/100 ml on two or more examinations. Their serum tyrosine values are normal, and urinary values for phenylpyruvic acid and O-hydroxyphenylacetic acid are usually not elevated. Thus, the infants share the elevated serum phenylalanine but not the secondary metabolic findings characteristic of phenylketonuria.

The precise metabolic defect in these children is unclear. Several infants have had liver biopsies, and decreased activity for the phenylalanine hydroxylase complex has been reported. The vast majority of children classified as having "hyperphenylalaninemia," however, have not been enzymatically evaluated. There undoubtedly exist several biochemical mechanisms for hyperphenylalaninemia.

There is no confirming evidence that untreated cases of benign hyperphenylalaninemia progress to develop mental retardation or signs of chronic neurological damage. If infants with hyperphenylalaninemia are placed on a strict low phenylalanine diet, however, their serum phenylalanine levels promptly decrease below normal values, and they develop symptoms of phenylalanine deficiency. Several infants with apparent benign hyperphenylalaninemia have died from being treated for phenylketonuria.

This disorder may be as common as phenylketonuria. The gene for hyperphenylalaninemia appears to be more common in the Mediterranean population than in other Caucasian groups, but adequate genetic information is not yet available.

Dihydrobiopterin Reductase Deficiency

A rare cause of elevated phenylalanine in the blood may be from a deficiency of dihydrobiopterin reductase (see Fig. 39–1). This enzyme is necessary to maintain adequate concentrations of tetrahydrobiopterin, an essential cofactor for the phenylalanine hydroxylase complex. Several infants have been detected through newborn screening programs because they possessed high levels of phenylalanine, but have subsequently been shown to have a deficiency of dihydrobiopterin reductase. They were not distinguishable from infants with classic phenylketonuria by phenylalanine or tyrosine values in the blood. Dietary restriction of phenylalanine was successful in lowering their serum phenylalanine levels, but the children had developed significant neurological damage by one year of age. The proper diagnosis in children suspected of having this disorder can only be achieved by assaying the enzyme activity in cultured skin fibroblasts or a liver biopsy. A satisfactory therapy for these children has not yet been found. This condition is quite rare and probably accounts for no more than 5 per cent of children who have previously been diagnosed as having PKU.

Neonatal Tyrosinemia

The most common cause of elevated serum phenylalanine in a newborn is from neonatal tyrosinemia. Infants with this condition will be detected because of phenylalanine concentrations between 4 and 10 mg/100 ml. If a serum tyrosine level is requested, it often is above 10 mg/100 ml and may be as high as 60 mg/100 ml. A normal serum tyrosine concentration should not exceed 3 mg/100 ml. Depending upon the criteria for establishing the diagnosis of neonatal tyrosinemia, it may occur as frequently as 30 per cent in premature infants and 10 per cent in full-term infants.

This phenomenon of an elevated tyrosine level in clinically healthy newborns may exist for the first week or two of life and then spontaneously recede. It has been established that these newborns have a delay in the developmental expression of their p-hydroxyphenylpyruvic acid oxidase system. This enzyme is responsible for the conversion of p-hydroxyphenylpyruvic acid (p-HPPA) to homogentisic acid. The accumulation of p-HPPA interferes with the normal metabolism of tyrosine and allows tyrosine to accumulate to greater than normal physiological concentrations. As the tyrosine accumulates, it acts as a competitive inhibitor of phenylalanine hydroxylase, allowing phenylalanine to increase above normal concentrations.

Ascorbic acid, 100 mg/day, should be administered to infants with suspected neonatal tyrosinemia. Ascorbic acid will prevent the inhibition of p-HPPA oxidase by its substrate, p-HPPA, and allow the enzyme to perform more efficiently. The administration of ascorbic acid will normally lower the serum tyrosine concentration within three days in newborns with neonatal tyrosinemia.

It is beneficial to limit the amount of protein the infant is receiving to 2 to 3 gms/kg/day. Protein in excess of this amount supplies extra phenylalanine and tyrosine that the infant must metabolize through his compromised pathway.

Neonatal tyrosinemia is thought to be a benign condition that does not cause long-term sequelae for intellectual development. This is probably true for most infants with this condition. Some concern, however, has been raised about premature infants with birthweights greater than 2000 gm who have had persistent tyrosinemia. Several of these infants have been reported to have detectable intellectual impairment in later childhood.

Hereditary Tyrosinemia

A rare cause of an elevated phenylalanine in the newborn is hereditary tyrosinemia. This condition is associated with a persistent deficiency of p-hydroxyphenylpyruvic acid oxidase, the same enzyme that is transiently depressed in neonatal tyrosinemia.

Infants with hereditary tyrosinemia usually have a severe clinical course, typified by cirrhosis of the liver, vitamin D resistant rickets, vomiting, diarrhea and failure to thrive. Hypoglycemia may be a prominent finding. Laboratory studies have shown a tyrosinemia, methioninemia, anemia, hypoproteinemia, hypophosphatemia and hyperphosphatemia. Urinary excretion of tyrosine products is prominent. Serum phenylalanine levels are characteristically between 5 and 10 mg/100 ml, and serum tyrosine values are in the range of 3 to 10 mg/ml. The tyrosine concentration in the serum is usually not as elevated as that in neonatal tyrosinemia. Plasma nethionine is often markedly elevated and may be the most prominent amino acid abnormality.

Infants with hereditary tyrosinemia, if untreated, usually die of liver failure. The pathological mechanism responsible for the liver damage is not understood. A dietary program similar to that of phenylketonuria, but with low tyrosine as well as low phenylalanine, has been tried with some success. Some infants have responded dramatically to this dietary manipulation, but the same pitfalls exist in the management of patients with hereditary tyrosinemia as in the dietary treatment of phenylketonuria.

Hereditary tyrosinemia is genetically determined and inherited as an autosomal recessive condition. It is less common than phenylketonuria and has a distinctive geographic distribution—it has been most commonly observed in the Swedish and French-Canadian populations.

Galactosemia

In some areas of the world, newborn infants are screened for galactosemia during the newborn period. This test is done in conjunction with screening for phenylketonuria. Most screening systems use a small portion of the infant's blood sample that has been impregnated on a piece of filter paper. A small disc of filter paper is incubated in the presence of an *E. coli* mutant that is lacking galactose-1-phosphate uridyltransferase. If the infant's blood has an increased concentration of galactase or a zone of inhibited growth is observed around the disc, a positive bacterial inhibition test is confirmed by the direct measurement of the infant's blood sample for galactose-1-PO_4 uridyl transferase, the enzyme deficient in "classical" galactosemia (Fig. 39–2).

Infants with galatosemia have an intolerance to milk and develop severe clinical symptoms in the first weeks of life. The triad of hepatosplenomegaly, cataracts and mental retardation has characterized older

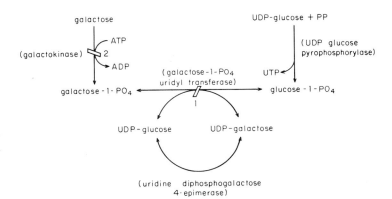

Figure 39–2 Two enzyme deficiencies exist that may cause the accumulation of galactose in body tissues. The absence of galactose-1-PO$_4$ uridyl transferase (site 1) is responsible for classic galactosemia. An absence of galactokinase (site 2) may cause elevated levels of galactose and lead to the formation of cataracts.

children with galactosemia, while failure to thrive, jaundice, vomiting and diarrhea are more characteristic of affected infants. Many cases of galactosemia are quite fulminating during the first few weeks of life, and death occurs from acute liver failure or sepsis from *E. coli*. Documented hypoglycemia associated with seizures may occur following milk ingestion, even when the serum galactose is significantly elevated.

The major source of galactose is from the lactose (glucose-galactose disaccharide) content of human or cow's milk. Infants with galactosemia who have not been detected through a screening program will often show a "milk intolerance." Such infants are often placed on a milk substitute, usually meat-base or a soybean milk product, with clinical improvement. This is done prior to the actual knowledge that galactosemia exists. In such cases, clinical symptoms may not be typical, and the identification of galactose in body fluids may be difficult.

The earliest clue to the diagnosis of galactosemia in a sick infant may be the finding of a strong reducing substance in the urine that is not glucose. When analyzed, this reducing substance is identified as galactose. The detection of a non-glucose reducing substance is easily performed by the combined use of Benedict's reagent (Clinitest) and the glucose oxidase paper strips (Tes-tape or Clinistix). Benedict's reagent is a non-specific agent for reducing substances and will be positive with most monosaccharides and disaccharides except sucrose. The glucose oxidase strips are specific for glucose. This, a positive Benedict's test and a negative glucose oxidase test indicate a non-glucose reducing substance.

Confirmational tests for galactosemia are

dependent upon the assay for galactose-1-phosphate uridyl transferase. A galactose tolerance test should not be performed because of serious reactions associated with elevations of the blood galactose. If galactosemia is suspected, the enzyme should be measured directly in the infant's red blood cells.

The clinical features observed in galactosemia are probably due to the elevated concentration of galactose and galactose-1-PO$_4$ in body tissues. The development of cataracts in the lens of the eye results from the formation of galactitol, a galactose alcohol. The galactitol concentration increases in the lens of the eye and is not further metabolized. Its accumulation causes overhydration of the lens, with resultant cataract formation.

The hepatomegaly, jaundice, brain damage, clotting difficulties, vomiting and failure to thrive are believed to be secondary to the accumulation of galactose-1-PO$_4$. This compound is thought to be a potent inhibitor of enzyme reactions in the carbohydrate pathway that are dependent upon phosphorylated intermediate.

Dietary treatment of galactosemia is rewarding if the child is started on therapy before irreversible damage has occurred. The cornerstone of therapy rests on the replacement of human or cow's milk with a non-lactose containing milk substitute. This is usually Nutramigen or a soybean milk formula.

With removal of galactose from the diet, the vomiting, diarrhea, hepatomegaly and jaundice promptly reverse, and weight gain begins. The child is immediately less irritable and easier to care for. Long-term therapy is accomplished best with the aid of a nutritionist to aid the parents selecting food free of galactose - containing products.

Classical galactosemia occurs in 1 of 30,000 to 70,000 live births in various populations. It is inherited as an autosomal recessive condition. Heterozygosity for the gene occurs in 1 in 100 to 1 in 130 persons. Heterozygotes may be detected by the quantitative measurement of galactose-1-PO_4 uridyl transferase in red blood cells combined with electrophoresis.

Allelic variants exist for the galactose-1-PO_4 uridyl transferase enzyme. A common variant is the "Duarte" protein. This enzyme has a different electrophoretic migration and lower enzyme activity than the normal enzyme. A person homozygous for the Duarte variant has 50 per cent of normal activity for galactose-1-PO_4 uridyl transferase. This does not cause galactose accumulation or clinical symptoms. Approximately 10 per cent of the population is heterozygous for the Duarte allele.

Some infants are heterozygous for both the classical and the Duarte alleles and have only 25 per cent of normal enzyme activity. These infants may be detected in screening programs and may be diagnosed as having classical galactosemia. The 25 per cent residual activity is apparently adequate for normal growth and development. They do not develop symptoms of galactosemia and should not be removed from galactose-containing products.

Newborn screening tests for galactosemia that use *E. coli* bacterial inhibition assay may also detect cases of galactokinase deficiency. This is a rare autosomal recessive condition in which galactose is unable to be converted to galactose-1-PO_4 and galactose accumulates in body tissues. The clinical consequences are the development of cataracts from the formation of galactitol in the lens. Brain and liver damage do not occur, apparently because galactose-1-PO_4 cannot be synthesized.

Detection and proper classification of infants with galactokinase deficiency are important. Removal of galactose from the diet of children with galactokinase deficiency should help in the prevention of cataract formation and the preservation of their sight.

The exact incidence of galactokinase deficiency is unknown, but it is probably no more frequent than galactosemia.

REFERENCES

Phenylalanine and Tyrosine

Avery, M. E., Clow, C. L., Menkes, J. H., *et al.*: Transient tyrosinemia of the newborn: Dietary and clinical aspects. Pediatrics, 39:378, 1967.

Dobson, J. C., Kushida, E., Williamson, M., and Friedman, E. G.: Intellectual performance of 36 phenylketonuria patients and their nonaffected siblings. Pediatrics, 58:53, 1976.

Dontanville, V. K., and Cunningham, G. C.: Effect of feeding on screening for PKU in infants. Pediatrics, 51:531, 1973.

Friedman, P. A., Fisher, D. B., Kang, E. S., and Kaufman, S.: Detection of hepatic phenylalanine 4-hydroxylase in classical phenylketonuria. Proc. Natl. Acad. Sci. USA, 70:552, 1973.

Friedman, P. A., Kaufman, S., and Kang, E. S.: Nature of the molecular defect in phenylketonuria and hyperphenylalaninaemia. Nature, 240:157, 1972.

Hansen, H.: Risk of fetal damage in maternal phenylketonuria. J. Pediatr., 83:506, 1973.

Holtzman, N. A., Meek, A. G., and Mellits, E. D.: Neonatal screening for phenylketonuria. I. Effectiveness. J.A.M.A., 229:667, 1974.

Holtzman, N. A., Mellits, E. D., and Kallman, C. H.: Neonatal screening for phenylketonuria. II. Age dependence of initial phenylalanine in infants with PKU. Pediatrics, 53:353, 1974.

Holtzman, N. A., Welcher, D. W., and Mellits, E. D.: Termination of restricted diet in children with phenylketonuria: A randomized controlled study. N. Engl. J. Med., 293:1121, 1975.

Howell, R. R., and Stevenson, R. E.: The offspring of phenylketonuric women. Soc. Biol., 18:S19, 1971.

Kaufman, S., Holtzman, N. A., Milstien, S., *et al.*: Phenylketonuria due to a deficiency of dihydropteridine reductase. N. Engl. J. Med., 293:785, 1975.

Knox, W. E.: Phenylketonuria., *In* Stanbury, J. B., Wyngaarden, J. B., and Fredrickson, D. S. (Eds.): *The Metabolic Basis of Inherited Disease*, 3rd ed. New York, McGraw-Hill Book Company, 1972.

Levy, H. L.: Genetic screening. Adv. Hum. Genet., 4:1, 1973.

Levy, H. L.: Neonatal screening for inborn errors of amino acid metabolism. Clin. Endocrinol. Metabol., 3:153, 1974.

Levy, H. L., Karolkewicz, V., Houghton, S. A., and MacCready, R. A.: Screening the "normal" population in Massachusetts for phenylketonuria. N. Engl. J. Med., 282:1455, 1970.

Levy, H. L., Shih, V. E., Madigan, P. M., and MacCready, R. A.: Transient tyrosinemia in full-term infants. J.A.M.A., 209:249, 1969.

MacCready, R. A., and Levy, H. L.: The problem of maternal phenylketonuria. Am. J. Obstet. Gynecol., 113:121, 1972.

Perry, T. L., Hansen, S., Tischler, B., Richards, F. M., and Sokol, M.: Unrecognized adult phenylketonuria. Implications for obstetrics and psychiatry. N. Engl. J. Med., 289:395, 1973.

Rosenberg, L. E.: Diagnosis and management of inherited aminoacidopathies in the newborn and the unborn. Clin. Endocrinol. Metabol., 3:145, 1974.

Scriver, C. R., Larochelle, J., and Silberberg, M.: Hereditary tyrosinemia and tyrosyluria in a French Canandian geographic isolate. Am. J. Dis. Child., *113*:41, 1967.

Smith, I., and Wolff, O. H.: Natural history of phenylketonuria and influence of early treatment. Lancet, *2*:540, 1974.

Starfield, B., and Holtzman, N. A.: A comparison of effectiveness of screening for phenylketonuria in the United States, United Kingdom and Ireland. N. Engl. J. Med., *293*:118, 1975.

Galactose

Beutler, E., Baluda, M. C., Sturgeon, P., *et al.*: A new genetic abnormality resulting in galactose-1-phosphate uridyltransferase deficiency. Lancet, *1*:353, 1965.

Beutler, E., Matsumoto, F., Kuhl, W., *et al.*: Galactokinase deficiency as a cause of cataracts. N. Engl. J. Med., *288*:1203, 1973.

Cogan, D. G.: The lens, cataracts and galactosemia. N. Engl. J. Med., *288*:1239, 1973.

Cohn, R. M., and Segal, S.: Galactose metabolism and its regulation. Metabolism, *22*:627, 1973.

Donnell, G. N.: Pitfalls in the diagnosis of galactosemia. J. Pediatr., *83*:515, 1973.

Donnell, G. N., Bergren, W. R., and Ng, W. G.: Galactosemia. Biochem. Med., *1*:29, 1967.

Fishler, K., Donnell, G. N., Bergren, W. R., and Koch, R.: Intellectual and personality development in children with galactosemia. Pediatrics, *50*:412, 1972.

Levy, N. S., Krill, A. E., and Beutler, E.: Galactokinase deficiency and cataracts. Am. J. Ophthalmol., *74*:41, 1972.

Segal, S.: Disorders of galactose metabolism. *In* Stanbury, J. B., Wyngaarden, J. B., and Fredrickson, D. S. (Eds.): *The Metabolic Basis of Inherited Disease*, 3rd ed. New York, McGraw-Hill Book Company, 1972.

Shih, V. E., Levy, H. L., Karolkewicz, V., *et al.*: Galactosemia screening of newborns in Massachusetts. N. Engl. J. Med., *284*:753, 1971.

Tedesco, T. A.: Human galactose-1-phosphate uridyltransferase. Purification, antibody production, and comparison of the wild type, Duarte variant, and galactosemic gene products. J. Biol. Chem., *247*:6631, 1972.

Tedesco, T. A., Wu, J. W., Boches, F. S., and Mellman, W. J.: The genetic defect in galactosemia. N. Engl. J. Med., *292*:737, 1975.

40

Cystic Fibrosis

Jack M. Docter

Description and Incidence

Cystic fibrosis is a generalized autosomal recessively inherited disorder of children, adolescents and young adults in which there is widespread dysfunction of the mucus-secreting glands. In fully manifested cases, chronic pulmonary disease, growth deficiency and abnormally high sweat electrolyte levels are present. The disorder is characterized by differing degrees of involvement of affected organs, resulting in marked variation in clinical severity. It ranges from very mildly involved, non-handicapped patients to very severely involved, completely incapacitated patients who are dying.

Cystic fibrosis is one of the more common serious chronic diseases of childhood and adolescence and is the most frequent lethal genetic disease among white children. In the United States at the present time, cystic fibrosis accounts for virtually all cases of pancreatic enzyme deficiency in children, for the majority of young patients with chronic obstructive pulmonary disease and for many children with biliary cirrhosis and portal hypertension. In the past, the disorder was confined to children because of the high mortality in infancy and early childhood. Cystic fibrosis is now seen with increasing frequency among adolescents and young adults.

Cystic fibrosis has been recognized throughout the world. It is a disease primarily of the Caucasian race, although proven cases have been found in black Americans. The incidence is believed to be 1 in 2000 live births, with the carrier incidence estimated at 3 to 6 per cent of the population. As of 1976, there is no generally reproducible laboratory means to identify the heterozygote. Because cystic fibrosis is carried as an autosomal recessive trait, a mating of two heterozygotes has a 25 per cent chance of producing an affected child in each pregnancy.

Pathophysiology

The non-mucous glands (the exocrine sweat glands and parotid glands) exhibit no pathological or histological changes, although the chemical composition of their secretion is abnormal. Mucus-producing glands throughout the body produce thick, viscid secretions, leading to ductal obstruction and dilatation of the secretory organ itself. The most striking changes are found in the pancreas. These consist of obstruction of the pancreatic ducts by abnormal secretions, dilatation of the secretory acini and, as the process progresses, fibrosis and fatty replacement of the acinar tissue. The islands of Langerhans usually remain structurally normal. As a result of the pancreatic involvement, trypsin, lipase and amylase may be decreased or completely absent in pancreatic secretions. Duodenal aspirate is more acidic than normal and has increased viscosity. These enzyme deficiencies impair alimentary digestion and absorption. Stools are foul smelling and bulky and contain an excess of both fat and protein. Variable but relatively large amounts of liposoluble vitamins (A, D, E and K) are lost as part of the malabsorption. Attempts at maintaining a positive nitrogen balance are made through a markedly increased dietary intake.

Increased viscosity of the secretions of the tracheobronchial tree results in obstruction of the smaller bronchioles, with retention

394

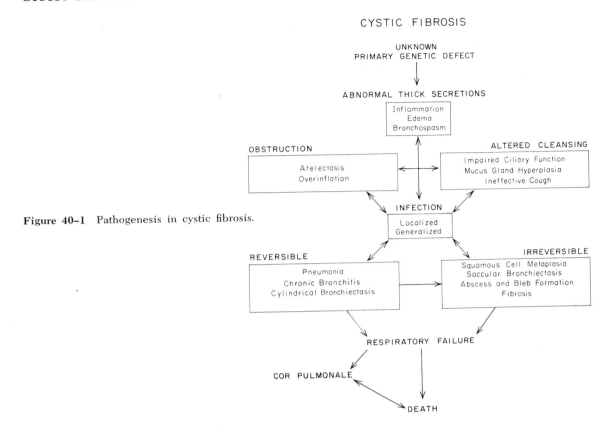

CYSTIC FIBROSIS

UNKNOWN
PRIMARY GENETIC DEFECT

ABNORMAL THICK SECRETIONS

Inflammation
Edema
Bronchospasm

OBSTRUCTION

Atelectasis
Overinflation

ALTERED CLEANSING

Impaired Ciliary Function
Mucus Gland Hyperplasia
Ineffective Cough

INFECTION
Localized
Generalized

REVERSIBLE

Pneumonia
Chronic Bronchitis
Cylindrical Bronchiectasis

IRREVERSIBLE

Squamous Cell Metaplasia
Saccular Bronchiectasis
Abscess and Bleb Formation
Fibrosis

RESPIRATORY FAILURE

COR PULMONALE

DEATH

Figure 40-1 Pathogenesis in cystic fibrosis.

and stagnation of the fluid distal to the obstruction. This results in stagnation of secretions, with infection, inflammation and suppuration causing a markedly diminished air exchange. The impairment of air flow results in a progressive increase in residual volume and a decreased vital capacity. The ratio of residual volume to total lung capacity increases. Regional difference in ventilation-perfusion results in hypoxemia and carbon dioxide retention. A gradual, continuing increase in number of obstructive lesions produces chronic bronchitis and impairment of mucociliary function, with eventual onset of irreversible changes with multiple abscesses and bronchiectasis. The bronchial arteries become dilated around the areas of chronic suppuration, and there is shunting of pulmonary capillary blood away from the obstructed alveolar areas. These changes, plus the limitation or loss of gas exchange surface area, lead to pulmonary insufficiency, respiratory failure, cor pulmonale and right heart failure. The usual cause of death in cystic fibrosis is heart failure secondary to cor pulmonale (Fig. 40-1).

Manifestations

Clinically, patients present in a variety of ways. The earliest manifestation of cystic fibrosis is small bowel obstruction in the newborn period, i.e., meconium ileus. The obstruction is produced by inspissated bowel contents in the distal jejunum or ileum. Complications associated with meconium ileus are volvulus, atresia, perforation of the bowel, and chemical peritonitis. Meconium ileus occurs in 5 to 15 per cent of cystic fibrosis patients and usually requires surgery, although occasionally the obstruction may be relieved medically. Another gastrointestinal complication is prolapse of the rectum. Cystic fibrosis is the most common cause of rectal prolapse in infants and children in the United States. It usually occurs in mildly involved patients and may be the presenting symptom anywhere from six months to four years of age, and if present in an otherwise healthy child, should always suggest the possibility of cystic fibrosis. Delayed bowel obstruction may occur at any time in a patient with cystic fibrosis and results from the thickened intestinal contents obstructing the small bowel. It may be associated with intussusception or volvulus and has been mistaken for tumor and appendicitis. Other gastrointestinal complications include edema and anasarca, usually occurring in the first six months of life and associated with hypoproteinemia resulting from poor absorption. Biliary cirrhosis may occur, rarely manifested by esophageal varices and gastrointestinal hemorrhage with a nodular, palpable liver, enlarged spleen and clubbed digits. Most adult males with cystic fibrosis are sterile as a result of congenital malformation or absence of the vas deferens.

The respiratory tract may be involved from the nose to the alveoli, and usually in the mildly involved patient paranasal sinus opacification and nasal polyps may be presenting symptoms. These result in obstruction of the eustachian tube, with chronic serous otitis media and hearing difficulty. Nasal polyposis is probably as commonly caused by cystic fibrosis as by allergic rhinitis in the childhood and adolescent period. Chronic pulmonary disease dominates the clinical picture and determines the fate of the majority of patients. The earliest symptoms referable to the bronchial system are cough and increased respiratory rate. Initially, the cough may be dry and nonproductive, but as time progresses, it becomes more moist, eventually producing varied amounts of purulent sputum that usually harbors *Staphylococcus aureus* or *Pseudomonas aeruginosa*. The changes, as measured by pulmonary function, accompany a number of physical findings: (1) enlargement of the thoracic cage (barrel chest); (2) limited respiratory movement; (3) use of accessory muscles of respiration; (4) clubbing of the digits (pulmonary osteoarthropathy); and (5) cyanosis. As the pulmonary disease progresses, varied and serious complications may ensue, such as lobar atelectasis, bronchiectasis, abscess and cyst formation, pneumothorax, hemoptysis, respiratory failure and asphyxia. The eventual outcome is usually cor pulmonale, heart failure and death.

Diagnosis

Diagnosis of cystic fibrosis is established by an awareness of the disease and its many symptoms and ramifications, with confirmation by a positive quantitative sweat test confirmed by a second, or perhaps third, sweat test. No other disease that could be confused with cystic fibrosis on a clinical basis has a constant elevation of sweat electrolyte level. The reliability of the sweat test, when properly performed, is greater than 99 per cent in children. A child with any of the symptoms or signs described and a family history of cystic fibrosis, coupled with a positive sweat test (properly performed), has cystic fibrosis. Stimulation of the sweat glands by pilocarpine iontophoresis and chemical analysis of the electrolytes is currently the most reliable sweat test available.

Treatment and Prognosis

As a disease of unknown etiology with widespread manifestations, treatment must be non-specific, non-curative and primarily symptomatic and prophylactic. Treatment modes in current vogue are largely symptomatic, empirical, subjective and the result of a trial and error program.

A prophylactic approach to treatment lies in the attempted prevention and treatment of: (1) bronchial and bronchiolar obstruction, (2) pulmonary infection and (3) pancreatic exocrine and nutritional deficiencies. It is generally believed that improvement of life expectancy in cystic fibrosis has resulted at least partially from advances in treatment that have occurred over the years. These include: (1) dietary regulation with vitamin and pancreatin replacement therapy; (2) antibiotic therapy; (3) inhalation therapy and physical therapy; and (4) a continuing home pulmonary-care program. Over the past 35 years, concurrent with the development of these therapy programs, the life expectancy of patients with cystic fibrosis has increased from 5 to 20 years. This increased life expectancy has led to a continually changing spectrum of patients with cystic fibrosis and has added consideration of the problems of educational and occupational preparation, marriage, childbearing and family responsibility to the burdens, as well as to the joys and pleasures of the patient with cystic fibrosis.

REFERENCE

Special Education Committee of the National Cystic Fibrosis Research Foundation: A Guide to Diagnosis and Management of Cystic Fibrosis, revised ed. Atlanta, Georgia, 1971.

Hematology

41

W. Archie Bleyer and James H. Feusner

This chapter offers practical, logical approaches to the differential diagnosis of anemia and bleeding in infancy and childhood. History, physical examination and simple laboratory tests are emphasized. Treatment is not discussed.

ANEMIA

Interpretation of a low hematocrit or hemoglobin in an infant or child requires a different approach from that used in adult medicine. First, one must determine whether the observed value is definitely abnormal for the age of the child. Second, one must know what causes of anemia are likely to occur at various ages. Third, one should be able to investigate and treat the anemia in an effective, logical and safe manner, avoiding excessive and overly traumatic procedures.

Normal Values

Hematocrit. Figure 41–1 shows the normal hematocrit and reticulocyte count, each expressed as the mean and two standard deviations above and below the mean. Note first that at birth the hematocrit is higher and more variable than later in life. The higher levels reflect the increased red cell mass resulting from the relative hypoxia of the intrauterine environment. The variability is due to the infant's gestational age (the more premature the infant, the lower the hematocrit), the time of clamping of the umbilical cord (the later the clamping, the more blood allowed to flow from the placenta into the neonate) and vagaries in blood sampling (capillary hematocrits average 2 to 10 percentage

points higher than venous hematocrits). As the oxygen content of the blood increases immediately after birth, erythropoietin stimulation promptly ceases, and the hematocrit then decreases rapidly, dropping to an initial nadir between 27 and 37 per cent at about two months of age. This dip is referred to as a "physiological anemia," in that it represents a switch from the cessation of red blood cell production shortly after birth to a delayed resumption of red blood cell production by the bone marrow. It is not caused by iron deficiency. A few months thereafter, however, the rapidly regenerating erythroid marrow depletes iron stores, and the ability of the bone marrow to supply red blood cells becomes limited by the amount of iron available. A relative "iron-limiting anemia" ensues, with a slight second dip in the hematocrit at approximately one year of age. The hematocrit

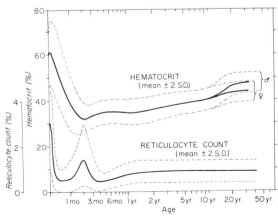

Figure 41–1 Normal hematocrit and reticulocyte count, expressed as mean ± two standard deviations. Note that the reticulocyte count is given as percentage × 10⁻¹. These normal curves were derived from the data of Matoth et. al., Schulman, Maurer, and Gorten and Cross.

rises slowly, thereafter, until adult levels are achieved, except during adolescence in males, when there is a relative acceleration (see Fig. 41–1).

Reticulocyte count. At birth, the reticulocyte count is four to eight times higher than in adults. This reticulocytosis disappears by one week of age. When the hematocrit falls below 35 per cent at approximately one month of age, erythropoietin production resumes, and the reticulocyte count increases to a peak of 2 to 4 per cent at two months of age. A second dip in the reticulocyte count occurs between four and six months of age.

Red cell indices. Normal red cell indices are given in Table 41–1. Note again the dynamic changes during the first year of life. Initially, the cells are relatively macrocytic, with mean cell volumes ranging between 100 to 140 femtoliters. A nadir is observed at one year of age, when the red cell volume ranges between 70 to 84 femtoliters (Koerper et. al.). The mean cell hemoglobin content follows a similar pattern, but the mean cell hemoglobin concentration is relatively constant throughout childhood.

Peripheral blood smear. In general, red cell morphology in infants and children is identical to that found in adults. The immediate neonatal period is an exception, during which the cells appear macrocytic, polychromasia is prominent and nucleated red cells may be found.

Premature infants. The sequence of events in premature infants apparently differs only quantitatively from that de-scribed for full-term infants. The basic adjustments and their mechanisms are the same. In the premature infant, the hematocrit declines to a lower value than that seen in the full-term infant, with the initial nadir between 21 and 35 per cent. The reticulocyte count peaks between 4 and 15 per cent. The initial nadir and peak also tend to occur at an earlier post-natal age. If notice is taken of growth, however, it can be seen that during this time the infant is growing rapidly, his blood volume is expanding and his red cell volume and hemoglobin mass are increasing. There has been much discussion and speculation about why the premature exhibits the more exaggerated fall and seemingly slower response, but as yet there is no clear understanding of these phenomena.

A Practical Approach

Documentation of a significantly reduced hematocrit or hemoglobin must be followed by correct diagnosis and treatment. The approach described here provides the user with a simple, practical and efficient method to establish etiology in the majority of instances. It is based on three simple laboratory determinations that can be obtained in an office setting: peripheral blood smear, reticulocyte index and red cell indices. Another advantage is that it is also based on the most common causes of anemia in children that are, in the order of frequency, iron deficiency, hemolysis, hypoproliferative states and maturation abnormalities. A somewhat different approach is suggested for anemia during the neonatal period, since the differential diagnosis in newborn infants differs greatly from that later in life, and the most common causes, in the order of incidence, are hemolysis, hemorrhage and hypoproliferative states. Because fetal hemoglobin predominates during the first three months of life, abnormalities in the synthesis of the beta chains of hemoglobin such as sickle cell disease and β-thalassemia are not clinically detectable during this period.

The authors' approach to anemia in childhood is diagrammed in Figure 41–2. The first step is to examine the peripheral blood smear. If it discloses microcytosis and hypochromia, *iron deficiency* is by far the most likely cause. Confirmation can

TABLE 41–1 NORMAL RED CELL INDICES

Age	Mean Cell Volume Mean	Mean Cell Volume SD	Mean Cell Hemoglobin Mean	Mean Cell Hemoglobin SD	Mean Cell Hgb Concentration Mean	Mean Cell Hgb Concentration SD
Birth	120	±10	38		34	±2
Months						
1	100	±8	35		35	±2
2	95	±13	31		33	±2
4	87	±4	29		33	±2
8	80	±3	27		33	±2
Years						
1	77	±4	26	±2	32	±2
2	78	±3	27	±2	32	±2
5	82	±3	27		33	±2
10	85		28		33	±2
20	90	±8	31	±2	33	±2

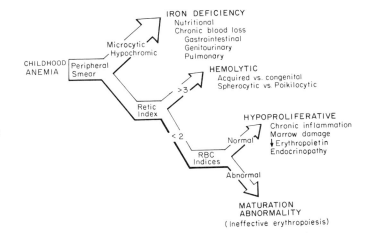

Figure 41–2 Approach to anemia in children over three months of age.

come from documentation of a low serum iron level and a high total iron binding capacity (per cent saturation <15) or by demonstrating a significant rise in the hematocrit within one week after starting adequate iron replacement therapy. If the smear does not demonstrate small, poorly hemoglobinized red cells, the reticulocyte count should be obtained and the reticulocyte index calculated (Hillman and Finch). If the index is greater than 3, the child has a *hemolytic anemia*. If the index is less than 2, the red cell indices should then be examined. If they are normal, the child has a hypoproliferative anemia; that is, red cell production in the bone marrow is suppressed. If the red cell indices are abnormal, the child has an anemia of ineffective erythropoiesis, otherwise known as a *maturation abnormality*.

Iron deficiency anemia may be either nutritional or due to chronic hemorrhage, with enhanced iron losses from the body. It is usually caused by a deficiency in dietary iron that fails to meet the demands of rapid growth and the concomitant expanding blood volumes. It is seen most frequently in those between six months and three years of age, when the demand is greatest, prenatally-acquired iron stores have been depleted and the diet may be largely milk, which is a poor source of iron. In children, the gastrointestinal tract is the most common site of chronic blood loss. Iron deficiency itself may lead to low-grade blood loss by altering the integrity of the intestinal mucosa. Bleeding gastrointestinal lesions may also be diagnosed in children, with aspirin-induced mucositis, peptic

ulcer and Meckel's diverticulum being the most common causes. Other sites of blood loss include the urinary tract (hemosiderinuria or chronic intravascular hemolysis) and the pulmonary tract (idiopathic pulmonary hemosiderosis and Goodpasture syndrome). The adolescent female is particularly prone to iron deficiency anemia, because of monthly menstrual blood losses of 40 to 50 ml and certain dietary indiscretions. Additional diagnostic tests for this group of anemias include the stool guaiac, urine hemosiderin and radiographs of the chest and gastrointestinal tracts. Because technetium is secreted by gastric mucosa, a technetium abdominal scan may reveal the ectopic gastric mucosa contained in a Meckel's diverticulum.

Hemolytic anemia may be due to acquired and inherited causes. Among the congenital causes are hereditary spherocytosis, sickle cell anemia, glucose-6-phosphate dehydrogenase deficiency and the congenital Heinz-body anemias. Acquired causes include autoimmune hemolytic anemia, disseminated intravascular coagulation, hypersplenism, vascular disease, the presence of a prosthetic cardiac valve and either hepatic or renal failure. Which test will confirm the suspected etiology depends on clinical factors. For example, in a black child, a sickle cell test or hemoglobin electrophoresis would be most likely to disclose the cause. In a child of Mediterranean heritage, a glucose-6-phosphate dehydrogenase analysis and a Heinz-body stain would probably provide the correct diagnosis. In the sick child suspected of having disseminated intravascular coagulation, a coagulation screen and platelet count would suggest the diagnosis. The presence of a large spleen on physical examination should prompt the clinician to obtain osmotic fragility and autohemolysis tests (congenital spherocytosis, pyruvate kinase deficiency), a Coombs' test (autoimmune hemolytic anemia) or determination of the white cell and platelet counts (hypersplenism).

For **hypoproliferative anemia** the following causes should be suspected: red cell aplasia, either congenital (Blackfan-Diamond syndrome) or acquired (pure red cell anemia, thymoma-related anemia), marrow damage (acute leukemia, aplastic anemia, drug-induced myelosuppression), erythropoietin suppression (chronic renal disease), endocrinopathy (hypothyroidism) or the anemia of chronic inflammation. Often, the appropriate tests in this category are bone marrow aspiration, renal function tests, thyroid tests, total iron-binding capacity and transferrin saturation.

Maturation abnormality will raise or lower the mean cell volume. If the mean cell volume is too large, a nuclear maturation arrest is indicated: folic acid deficiency, vitamin B_{12} deficiency, a defect in DNA synthesis (formiminotransferase deficiency, transcobalamin II deficiency, orotic aciduria) or DiGuglielmo syndrome. Serum folate and vitamin B_{12} levels should be obtained. If the mean cell volume is too small, a cytoplasmic maturation arrest is probable. Such an arrest is due to a defect either in globin synthesis, such as thalassemia, or in heme synthesis. The latter constitutes the so-called "sideroblastic" anemias associated with lead intoxication, porphyria, vitamin B_6 deficiency or depen-

dency or unknown factors. Appropriate studies are quantitative analysis of hemoglobins F And A_2, red cell protoporphyrin determination, serum lead level and iron stains of bone marrow aspirates.

Anemia in the neonate poses a different differential diagnosis from that for older children. The recommended test scheme is modified as depicted in Figure 41–3. The first step is to obtain a reticulocyte count. If it is subnormal, a hypoproliferative anemia such as congenital hypoplastic anemia of Blackfan and Diamond should be considered and a bone marrow examination performed. If the reticulocyte count is normal or elevated, a peripheral blood smear should then be examined. A hemolytic anemia may be suggested by poikilocytosis, red cell fragments or by specific morphological abnormalities such as spherocytes, elliptocytes, stomatocytes or pyknocytes. If these findings are present, a Coombs' test should be obtained. If the Coombs' test is positive, an isoimmune anemia such as Rh or ABO incompatibility should be considered, the mother and infant should be typed for red cell antigens and the neonate's serum should be examined for maternal antibodies. If the smear discloses hypochromic, microcytic red cells, chronic fetomaternal transfusion is likely. If no abnormalities are noted on the peripheral blood smear, one should then determine whether or not the neonate has hepatosplenomegaly or hyperbilirubinemia. If these findings are not present, then acute perinatal blood loss is likely; for example, fetomaternal hemorrhage, placenta previa, abruptio placentae, vasa previa or cesarean section. If the infant is jaundiced but does not have hepatosplenomegaly, a congenital

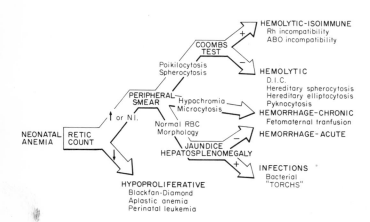

Figure 41–3 Approach to anemia in newborn infants.

enzymatic defect of the red cell, such as glucose-6-phosphate dehydrogenase or pyruvate kinase deficiencies, is likely. If the infant has both hepatosplenomegaly and jaundice, an infection is likely. This includes bacterial infection or any of the components of the TORCHS complex: *toxo*plasmosis, *rubella*, *cytomegalovirus*, *herpes* simplex, *syphilis*.

HEMOSTASIS

This section presents the distinctive features of abnormal hemostasis in the infant and neonate. Normal and abnormal hemostasis in older children and adolescents are similar to those of adults and are not discussed. The approach presented is not inclusive and should, in fact, also illustrate the need for a better understanding of the normal mechanisms, both qualitative and quantitative, of hemostasis in neonates and infants.

Normal Values

In approaching the problem of a bleeding infant, one should consider the state of three critical factors: (1) platelets (quantity and function), (2) blood vessels and (3) coagulation factors (quantity, function and presence of inhibitors). Table 41–2 shows the normal values, according to gestational age, for these determinants. Most investigators agree that platelet counts less than 100,000/μl should be considered abnormal in neonates, even in premature infants. Platelet function is less well defined, although there is evidence that platelet aggregation to collagen, epinephrine and ADP is impaired in the neonate, compared to adult standards. The bleeding time is reported to be the same as in adults, although this observation should be confirmed. The role of vascular factors in hemostasis is even less well defined. Fibrinogen and factors V, VIII and XIII are

TABLE 41–2 NORMAL HEMOSTATIC VALUES

	Normal Adult/Child	Premature, 27–31 weeks	Premature, 32–36 weeks	Full-term	Adult Level Attained
Platelet count (μl^{-1})	300,000 ± 50,000	275,000 ± 60,000	290,000 ± 70,000	310,000 ± 68,000	–
Bleeding time (min)	4 ± 1.5	–	4 ± 1.5	4 ± 1.5	–
Platelet aggregation	Normal	↓ to ADP, collagen	↓ to ADP, collagen	↓ to ADP, collagen epinephrine	?
PTT (sec)	35–45	–	70–145	55 (45–65)	2–9 months
PT (sec)	12–14	23	17 (12–21)	16 (13–20)	3–4 days
TT (sec)	10–12	–	14 (11–17)	12 (10–16)	few days
Fibrinogen (mg/100 ml)	200–400	270 ± 140	226 ± 70	246 ± 55	prenatal
II (%)	100	30 ± 10	35 ± 12	45 ± 15	2–12 months
V (%)	100	72 ± 25	91 ± 23	98 ± 40	prenatal
VII–X (%)	100	32 ± 15	39 ± 14	56 ± 16	2–12 months
VIII (%)	50–200	70 ± 30	98 ± 40	105 ± 35	prenatal
IX (%)	75–125	27 ± 10	?	28 ± 8	3–9 months
XI (%)	100	5–20(?)	?	30	1–2 months
XII (%)	100	?	30	51	9–14 days
XIII (%)	100	100	100	100	prenatal
FSP (μg/ml)	0–7	0–10	0–7	0–7	

Data for term and preterm infants represent either smoothed means ± 1 standard deviation, or ranges from cord blood samples or venous samples obtained in first 24 hours of life.

Data for adults represent either the normal range or percent of normal where 1μ/ml activity is taken as normal.

Bleeding time data are unconfirmed.

equivalent to adult levels. The remaining factors are normally low at birth and attain adult values at varying times during the first postnatal year (Table 41–2).

Disorders of Hemostasis

Blood vessels. A vascular defect is rarely a primary factor in the bleeding infant. Disorders most likely to be encountered include endotoxemia, hemolytic-uremic syndrome and the vascular side effects of steroid therapy. Entities presenting later in childhood include Henoch-Schönlein purpura and homocystinuria, but these are rare. Vascular integrity is assessed by the bleeding time and tissue biopsy. The tourniquet test is no longer employed.

Platelets. The pathogenetic classification of thrombocytopenia is quite similar to that in older children and adults. Some distinctly neonatal entities (Table 41–3) include passively acquired forms (isoimmune neonatal thrombocytopenia and either idiopathic thrombocytopenic purpura or systemic lupus erythematosus in the mother), giant hemangiomata, those associated with congenital anomalies (e.g., radial aplasia syndrome, trisomy 13, trisomy 18) and that occasionally found with metabolic aberrations (methylmalonic acidemia, isovaleric acidemia, glycinemia). The most common causes of platelet dysfunction in children are von Willebrand syndrome and aspirin exposure. Congenital forms, such as Glanzmann's thrombasthenia, Bernard-Soulier syndrome and storage-pool disease, are rare. Maternal aspirin ingestion has been shown to cause bleeding in some newborn infants. Promethazine and a large number of other drugs may also be associated with platelet dysfunction. Other conditions that may interfere with platelet function include hyperbilirubinemia, uremia and disseminated intravascular coagulation.

An optimal approach to the thrombocytopenic infant consists of a thorough history, a directed physical examination and laboratory tests obtained in a logical sequence. The physician should determine what illnesses (especially bleeding dyscrasias), or drugs the mother may have had, as well as any previously affected infants the mother may have had. Jaundice, hepatosplenomegaly and congenital anomalies are important clues on physical examination of the infant. Laboratory tests follow, beginning with a complete blood count and a peripheral blood smear. Helpful findings include leukocytosis (infection,

TABLE 41–3 NEONATAL THROMBOCYTOPENIA

I. Impaired Production
  A. Hypoplasia
    1. Congenital amegakaryocytic
    2. Congenital infections
    3. Maternal drugs
  B. Marrow replacement
    1. Congenital leukemia
    2. Neuroblastoma
    3. Reticuloendotheliosis
II. Increased Destruction
  A. Immune mediated
    1. Isoimmune neonatal thrombocytopenia
    2. Maternal drugs – thiazides, digitoxin, quinidine
    3. Maternal idiopathic thrombocytopenic purpura or lupus erythematosus
    4. Erythroblastosis(?)
  B. Consumptive
    1. Disseminated intravascular coagulation
    2. Microangiopathic process (e.g., hemolytic-uremic syndrome)
    3. Giant hemangioma
  C. Other
    1. Wiskott-Aldrich syndrome
    2. May-Hegglin anomaly
III. Abnormal Distribution (hypersplenism)
  A. Cirrhosis
  B. Portal or splenic vein thrombosis
  C. Storage disease
  D. Myeloproliferative syndrome
  E. Congenital hemolytic anemia with splenomegaly
IV. Other
  A. Congenital thyrotoxicosis
  B. Metabolic (e.g., methylmalonic acidemia, isovaleric acidemia, hyperglycinemia)

TABLE 41–4 DISORDERS OF COAGULATION – NEONATAL

I. Isolated Genetic Defects
  A. ↓ Synthesis
    1. Fibrinogen
    °2. von Willebrand syndrome
    3. II, V, VII, XIII
  B. Defective Synthesis
    °1. VIII (Hemophilia A)
    °2. IX (Hemophilia B, Christmas disease)
    3. Dysfibrinogenemia
    4. II, V, VII, XI, XIII
II. Multiple Acquired
  A. ↓ Synthesis
    1. Liver disease
  B. Defective Synthesis
    °1. Vitamin K deficiency
  C. ↑ Destruction
    °1. Disseminated intravascular coagulation
    2. Enzymatic (e.g., acute pancreatitis)

°Indicates more common causes.

TABLE 41–5   ABNORMALITIES OF CLOTTING SCREEN

Smear	PT	PTT	TT	Abnormality
Normal	Normal	↑	Normal	↓ VIII, ↓ IX, ↓ XI, ↓ XII, and von Willebrand syndrome
Normal	↑	↑	Normal	Vitamin K deficiency, ↓ V, ↓ X, ↓ II, and fibrinogen, liver dysfunction
Normal	↑	Normal	Normal	↓ VII
Normal	Normal	Normal	↑	Presence of heparin, ↓ fibrinogen, ↑↑ bilirubin, ↑↑ BUN
Normal	Normal	Normal	Normal	↓ XIII, platelet dysfunction, occasionally von Willebrand syndrome
RBC fragmentation	↑	↑	↑	Disseminated intravascular coagulation

leukemia), Döhle bodies (bacteremia), red cell fragments (disseminated intravascular coagulation) and increased platelet size (consumptive coagulopathy, bacteremia). A platelet count should be done on the mother to evaluate whether or not she is thrombocytopenic. Further studies, if needed, can be performed in the following order: coagulation screen (disseminated intravascular coagulation; see next section), bone marrow aspiration (neoplasia, congenital amegakaryocytic thrombocytopenia), prolonged survival of platelets transfused from mother versus a random donor (isoimmune thrombocytopenia), amino acid screen and chromosomal karyotyping if indicated.

Coagulation factors. Table 41–4 presents a classification of coagulopathies in infancy. The more common causes are designated by an asterisk. Now that vitamin K is routinely administered to newborn infants, disseminated intravascular coagulation is by far the most common cause. Precise diagnosis of this condition requires a careful comparison of the clotting tests with the known normal values for newborn infants (Table 41–2). The genetic defects of hemophilia (factor VIII or IX deficiency) and von Willebrand syndrome are rare except in infants with an affected sibling or parent. The most informative laboratory tests are the partial thromboplastin time, prothrombin time, thrombin time and peripheral blood smear. This battery of tests will usually reveal the diagnosis (Table 41–5). The battery will not detect factor XIII deficiency, however, which often presents in the neonatal period as umbilical cord hemorrhage. This diagnosis requires demonstration of increased clot solubility in a 5 M urea solution. Additional studies may be indicated but are beyond the scope of this discussion.

In summary, normal hemostasis in early childhood needs further definition. However, a logical approach with the data currently available will uncover the etiology in most instances.

REFERENCES

Bleyer, W. A., Hakami, N., and Shepard, T. H.: Development of hemostasis in the human fetus and newborn infant, J. Pediatr., 79:838, 1971.

Chessels, J. M., and Hardisty, R. M.: Bleeding problems in the newborn infant. Progr. Hemost. Thromb., 2:333, 1974.

Gorten, M. K., and Cross, E. R.: Iron metabolism in premature infants, J. Pediatr., 64:509, 1964.

Harker, L. A.: *Hemostasis Manual*, 2nd ed. Philadelphia, F. A. Davis Co., 1974.

Hathaway, W. E.: The bleeding newborn. Seminars Hemat., 12:175, 1975.

Hillman, R. S., and Finch, C. A.: *Red Cell Manual*, 4th ed., Philadelphia, F. A. Davis Co., 1974, pp. 59–60.

Koerper, M. A., Mentzer, W. C., Brecker, G., and Dallman, P. R.: Developmental change in red blood cell volume: Implication in screening infants and children for iron deficiency and thalassemia trait. J. Pediatr., 89:580, 1976.

Matoth, Y., Zaizov, R. and Versano, I.: Postnatal changes in some red cell parameters. Acta Paediatr. Scand., 60:317, 1971.

Maurer, A. M.: *Pediatric Hematology*. New York, McGraw-Hill Co., 1972, pp. 3–6.

Oski, F. A., and Naiman, J. L.: *Hematologic Problems in the Newborn*, 2nd ed. Philadelphia, W. B. Saunders Co., 1972, pp. 11–17, 54–77, 236–311.

Schulman, I.: Fetal and neonatal erythropoiesis. *In* Barnett, H. L., and Einhorn, A. H. (Eds.): *Pediatrics*, 15th ed. New York, Meredith Corp., 1972, pp. 1155–1160.

42 Malignant Diseases

Ronald L. Chard, Jr. and Irwin D. Bernstein

Malignancy is now the second most frequent cause of death in those between the ages of 1 and 14 years. Tumors in children are properly considered apart from tumors in adults. The two groups of neoplasms differ not only with respect to the obvious age brackets, but also in respect to basic tumor types, sites of origin and clinical manifestations. In children, carcinomas are exceedingly uncommon. Most childhood malignancies are embryonal or mesenchymal in origin, and teratomas and sarcomas make up the bulk of the neoplasms. These tumors are largely concentrated in the first five years of life, in all probability a natural corollary of their origin.

A satisfactory classification of malignant neoplasms in childhood, based solely on anatomic area or organ system, is as follows: (1) leukemia and lymphoma; (2) tumors of the kidney, adrenals and sympathetic nerves; (3) tumors of the central nervous system and eye; (4) bone tumors; and (5) soft tissue tumors. According to this classification, the experience over a 26-year period, 1949–1975, in Seattle, shows the incidence pattern. See table opposite.

This experience compares well with the experience in other areas of the United States.

Considering those tumors that occur in children from the neonatal period through two years of age, neuroblastoma and Wilms' tumor predominate. Neuroblastoma is the more common in the first year, with Wilms' tumor more frequent during the next one to two years. For both these tumors there is an expected 50 per cent or more cure rate in patients diagnosed and treated adequately before two years of age.

Leukemia is seen during all ages of childhood, but most commonly occurs between the ages of two and five years. Above the age of five years, tumors of the central nervous system and eye occur almost with the same frequency as leukemia. There is no particular incidence difference, however, at any age from 2 to 12 years in tumors of the central nervous system.

Bone tumors show a predilection for the ages between 5 and 25 years, with the peak incidence toward age 15.

Early detection of malignant disease in children, as in adults, is one of the most important aspects of successful management of the disease. During the first two years of life a thorough physical examination, especially of the abdomen by palpation, is perhaps the most important single test, since both neuroblastoma and Wilms' tumor most frequently present as an abdominal mass. Over two years of age it is important to

	Number of Cases	Percentage
1. Leukemia	675	40.0
Lymphomas (including Hodgkin's disease)	124	7.3
	799	47%
2. Sympathetic nervous system (neuroblastoma)	140	8.3
Wilms' tumor	98	5.8
	238	14%
3. CNS and eye	273	16%
4. Bone tumors	78	5%
5. Miscellaneous		
Soft tissue sarcoma	89	5.3
Carcinoma	56	3.3
Teratoma	44	2.6
Other	111	6.6
	300	18%
	1688	

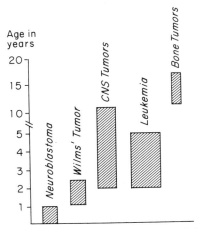

Figure 42–1 Peak ages of occurrence of the more common malignant diseases in children. The width of each bar reflects the relative frequency among tumors of childhood.

GENERAL CONSIDERATIONS OF MANAGEMENT

In treating children with malignant disease, one must use certain philosophical principles peculiar to the age group being considered. Since a child has a lifetime ahead of him, five-year survival rates, commonly used in dealing with adult malignancies, in most cases need to be modified in evaluating therapy. Since a great many recurrences occur within 12 to 24 months after the original diagnosis, aggressive "total therapy" is mandatory at the onset of therapy.

There have been rather marked improvements in disease-free survival and total survival in six of the major solid tumor types that occur in childhood, as illustrated in Figure 42–2. These advances have come about by clinical and scientific use of multimodal therapy involving surgery, radiotherapy, chemotherapy and pathogenesis. Two rather common solid tumors in childhood, brain tumor and neuroblastoma, continue to be clinical and scientific enigmas. Specifics for therapy are discussed in a later section. Leukemia therapy has become much improved through the combination of radiotherapy and chemotherapy.

recall that iron deficiency is a less common cause of anemia than in the age group between one and two. Therefore, a complete blood cell count, including platelets or at least a platelet estimate, as well as a physical examination for lymphadenopathy and organomegaly, is important in any child with anemia above the age of two. Children over two years of age with any sudden or persistent neurological abnormalities should have a central nervous system tumor evaluation in the differential diagnosis. Persistent lymphadenopathy or soft tissue masses should be biopsied at any age, and persistent bone pain deserves a radiological evaluation at any time, but probably earlier in the high-risk group for bone tumors.

SPECIFIC CONSIDERATIONS OF DIAGNOSIS AND MANAGEMENT

Leukemia

As stated, the most common age at onset is between two and five years. The specific

Figure 42–2 Progress in survival with multimodal therapy.

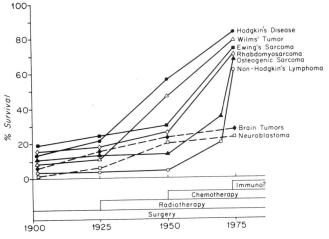

diagnostic test is bone marrow examination. Any child with anemia, thrombocytopenia, leukocytosis or pancytopenia with or without lymphadenopathy or organomegaly should have a bone marrow evaluation.

Eighty per cent of leukemia in childhood is acute lymphocytic (also called stem cell or undifferentiated). The cause is unknown, and there is no definite cure to date, but research test results at present are very encouraging. Untreated leukemia has a median survival rate of eight weeks. Before 1970, median survival with chemotherapy had been increased to between 24 and 36 months.

In acute lymphocytic leukemia, combining radiotherapy with chemotherapy was first shown to be beneficial in a study done at St. Jude's Hospital. In this program, children with acute lymphocytic leukemia were treated with multiple drugs, prednisone and vincristine induction and placed into remission; at that time they had central nervous system prophylactic therapy. This was done because as marrow remissions were improved, more and more children had central nervous system relapses and this became more life-threatening and difficult to handle than the bone marrow disease. The children at St. Jude's, after bone marrow remission, were treated with cranial-spinal irradiation of 2400 rads vs. cranial irradiation, 2400 rads, plus intrathecal methotrexate given biweekly for three weeks in six doses. At 28 months from the start of therapy, 70 per cent of the children showed no evidence of disease. In that program, all therapy was then stopped in all patients, and during the first year, 15 per cent had relapsed; thus approximately 55 per cent at three and one-half years were still well.

In 1972, the Children's Cancer Study group began its study with the use of prophylactic central nervous system therapy. It has become apparent that there may be more than one type of disease in childhood acute lymphocytic leukemia, as children with high counts did not do as well as those with low counts. In this study the patients were stratified by white count; that is, children with a white count of less than 20,000 received the same randomization as children with white counts greater than 20,000, but they were randomized as separate groups to prevent result bias from having more unfavorable patients in one group than the other. This program involved multiple drug induction consisting of prednisone and vincristine and L-asparaginase. Approximately 700 children were enrolled, and the induction rate was 93 per cent. This was significantly better than prednisone or vincristine alone, which previously had shown a remission rate of 86 per cent in approximately 500 children. After achieving remission, the patients received central nervous system prophylaxis consisting of radiation therapy and intrathecal methotrexate. Remission was then maintained, with daily 6-mercaptopurine, weekly oral methotrexate and monthly pulses of a single dose of vincristine and five days of prednisone. This study showed that, regardless of the central nervous system prophylaxis, children with low counts did significantly better than children with high counts. This study was further broken down to see if white counts in smaller categories and patient age at diagnosis were of significant prognostic importance. Results have been most gratifying. Of the approximately 700 children enrolled in this study, 175 were between the ages of three and seven with initial white counts of less than 10,000. Of these, 93 per cent are relapse-free three years after diagnosis. Children with initial white counts of over 50,000, regardless of age, are having the poorest disease-free remission and survival time. This is exceedingly important for future studies, as it further emphasizes that children who have a pathological diagnosis of acute lymphocytic leukemia do not necessarily have the same disease, since with the same treatments, the results are markedly different. Because of this, future studies will have at least three different treatment programs for these children.

To summarize briefly, treatment in a child with acute lymphocytic leukemia in the good risk group is becoming more standardized, involving multiple drug induction therapy, central nervous system prophylaxis and multiple drug maintenance therapy of at least three years' duration. In children with less favorable prognostic factors, we still need a great deal of improvement.

Twenty per cent of children with leukemia have acute non-lymphocytic leukemia or acute granulocytic leukemia, acute myelomonocytic leukemia, acute monocytic leukemia or acute erythrocytic leukemia.

This disease, although treatment results have improved, still shows rather poor results compared with acute lymphocytic leukemia. The best results, so far, are in a program using multiple drug induction and multiple drug maintenance therapy that shows a 60 per cent survival at one year, 33 per cent at two years and at three to four years, only 20 per cent. Another treatment mode that is evolving for children with acute leukemia is bone marrow transplantation. This can be an exceedingly successful program, and approximately 30 per cent of children so far transplanted have achieved a graft and have had significant maintenance durations of good quality. It has been well shown in children who have an HL-A–matched sibling that transplantation is more successful if done when they are relatively well rather than when they are relatively ill. As children with acute myelocytic leukemia have relatively short remission durations, it may well be that such a child who has an HL-A–matched sibling should receive a transplantation while in the initial remission. Also, children with acute lymphocytic leukemia who suffer bone marrow relapse, to this time, have had distressingly short second remission durations of only four months. This remission duration was the same in 1975 as in 1970 with different treatment programs. Therefore, children with an HL-A–matched sibling with acute lymphocytic leukemia who suffer bone marrow relapse perhaps should be transplanted after they achieve a second remission.

Lymphomas

Lymphomas are presently three types: Hodgkin's disease, nodular lymphomas or diffuse lymphomas. These can present with involvement of a single lymph node group or be widely disseminated at the time of diagnosis. Diagnosis is by tissue biopsy or excision. Bone marrow is not always diagnostic but it may be used to show the degree of involvement at the time of diagnosis.

Staging is extremely important in dealing with Hodgkin's disease. In Stage 1, involvement is localized to one lymph node group without involvement in any other area. In Stage II, involvement is in two or more continuous lymph node groups, but is limited to above or below the diaphragm. In Stage III, involvement is both above and below the diaphragm. In Stage IV, generalized involvement is of the reticuloendothelial system, with bone marrow invasion as well. Treatment and prognosis of this disease have depended on the degree of involvement at the time of diagnosis.

Recently, laparotomy and splenectomy, multiple open liver biopsies and periaorta and iliac node biopsies have been found more reliable than liver function tests and lymphangiograms alone in ruling out or identifying Stage III or IV disease.

Basically, Stage I disease in most centers receives only radiotherapy, which is felt to be curative. In many centers, the Stage IIa disease is also treated with only radiotherapy, but in some centers protocols are now being established to determine whether extended field radiotherapy alone should be used or if one can use involved field radiotherapy plus chemotherapy to give even better results. In Stage III and IV disease, chemotherapy plays a more important role. In Stage IV disease, chemotherapy using multiple drug programs is the primary treatment. The one used most often involves nitrogen mustard, vincristine, prednisone and Matulane or procarbazine. This is given in two-week cycles once a month. In adults, this gives very satisfying results in Stage IV disease if stopped after only six months of treatment; however, children have not remained disease-free as long. Therefore, they are usually treated for one to two years but using different drug combinations, because the nitrogen mustard is severely toxic, and many teenage patients will refuse to take this drug after several injections.

Nodular lymphoma in adults has a good treatment result, but unfortunately, this is rarely seen in children. The most common type of lymphoma in childhood is diffuse lymphoma, which has very poor treatment results with programs used to treat the nodular form of the disease.

Very recently, a nine-drug protocol was developed at the Sloan Kettering Memorial Hospital in New York with radiation therapy used as an adjuvant. That is, radiotherapy is given to bulk disease greater than 5 cm but is limited usually to 2000 to 2500 rads. The multiple drug program involves induction with high dose Cytoxan, followed by vincristine and prednisone with intrathecal methotrexate and two doses of dauno-mycin during the first month. Following this, consolidation therapy is done with cy-tosine arabinoside daily for two weeks, followed by twelve days of L-asparaginase on a daily basis. This is then followed by a maintenance program that consists of giv-ing two drugs for five days with a nine-day rest and then coming in with a different two drugs every two weeks. This is a very toxic program to the bone marrow, but at this time, 15 patients have been treated at this center, and only two have developed recurrent disease. The follow-up at present is anywhere from 6 to 18 months.

Wilms' Tumor (Nephroblastoma)

Wilms' tumor is a form of teratoma, in that there may be more than one type of cell that has become malignant in the tumor. It starts in the kidney tissue and may grow to tremendous size. It metasta-sizes characteristically to the lungs and sometimes to the local lymph nodes by direct extension. Five to ten per cent of Wilms' tumors have bilateral involvement at the time of presentation.

An abdominal mass with gross or micro-scopic hematuria is an indication of the presence of this tumor and demands imme-diate intravenous pyelography and chest x-ray. Characteristically, the intravenous pye-logram will show the kidney to be in nor-mal position, though there is typically dis-tortion of the renal calyces that is not present in neuroblastoma. Calcification in the tumor is also rare.

Treatment includes nephrectomy of the involved kidney where possible, radiation therapy to the abdomen on the side of ex-cision and chemotherapy, which has signif-icantly increased survival rates.

It has now been shown that there are two very successful drugs to treat Wilms' tumor, actinomycin-D and vincristine or Oncovin. A third drug, adriamycin, has shown response in patients with metastatic disease. Age also appears to be quite im-portant—children under two years of age who have disease localized to the kidney have now been shown to respond as well to chemotherapy alone as to chemotherapy and radiotherapy to the tumor bed. At the present time, the recommendation for a child less than two years of age with a tumor localized to the kidney is that he re-ceive post-operatively only chemotherapy consisting of actinomycin and vincristine. The present national study is designed to determine how long chemotherapy should be given, and a randomized trial is under way, in which patients receive three courses, or three months of therapy, *vs.* seven courses, or fifteen months of therapy, which had been the previous standard. For children with localized disease to the kid-ney over the age of two years, the answer to whether radiotherapy is needed or not post-operatively is equivocal. At the Chil-dren's Orthopedic Hospital and Medical Center of Seattle, children over two years of age who have a tumor localized to the kid-ney receive radiation therapy to the tumor bed in addition to the chemotherapy de-scribed. Patients with more widespread dis-ease all receive post-operative radiotherapy plus a randomized trial of actinomycin-D and vincristine *vs.* actinomycin-D and vin-cristine and adriamycin. This tumor in childhood has a very good response (80 to 90 per cent) in a good risk patient.

Soft Tissue Sarcomas

A variety of soft tissue sarcomas are seen in the early age group. One of the more frequent is rhabdomyosarcoma, or malig-nancy of striated muscle. This originates most frequently in the female generative tract or in the region of the prostate in the male, and then frequently in the face, be-neath the orbit of the pterygoid or the zygomatic region. It may also originate in the orbit itself. This tumor is highly malig-nant, but it may be removed by early and complete excision. Metastases are most fre-quently found in the lungs.

Because of the increased survival with cyclic, maintenance chemotherapy added to complete surgical removal of the tumor or radiation therapy in Wilms' tumor, com-bination, cyclic chemotherapy programs for 12 to 18 months post-operatively are being added to other solid tumor treatment pro-grams. Specifically, in rhabdomyosarcoma, the use of actinomycin, vincristine and cy-clophosphamide has shown two years of disease-free survival in 80 to 90 per cent of patients with rhabdomyosarcoma. The duration of cyclic chemotherapy in solid tumors is based on the natural history of these tumors, which indicates that metastases occur 50 per cent within 6 months of diagnosis, 80 per cent within 12 months and 95 per cent within 24 months. Therefore, if patients are two years from diagnosis and free of evidence of tumor, it is felt that they have a 95 per cent chance for cure.

Bone Tumors

Tumors of bone are some of the more serious malignancies seen in childhood. The types seen are chondrosarcoma and osteogenic sarcoma, 80 per cent of which are osteogenic; Ewing's sarcoma, 15 per cent; and other rare types 5 per cent. Malignant degeneration of benign osteochondromas or giant cell tumor does not occur in children.

The sarcomas usually appear in the metaphyses or shafts of long bones. There will be both proliferation and destruction of bone in the same area. The sarcomas are new growths from the periosteum.

The symptom leading to the diagnosis of a bone tumor is, as a rule, pain in the bone. This is frequently traced to trauma, probably without foundation. After the early pain, there is usually swelling of the soft parts over the bone. The x-ray appearance is that of elevation and lamellation of the periosteum, sometimes with cortical destruction.

Differential diagnosis of bone lesions producing lytic destruction includes metastatic neuroblastoma and also lesions of reticuloendotheliosis. Lesions producing new bone include osteomyelitis, osteocytic osteoma, benign osteochondroma and osteoma. Diagnosis must be made by tissue biopsy.

Significant improvements have been made in the last five years in osteogenic sarcoma and Ewing's sarcoma.

It has been long recognized that the primary tumor site in Ewing's sarcoma could be sterilized or cured by high dose radiotherapy. Approximately 90 per cent of patients were dying rapidly, however, from metastatic disease that was not evident at the time of initial diagnosis. Because of the rapid development of these lesions, primarily in the lung, the disease had to be present microscopically at the time of diagnosis. Therefore, in Ewing's sarcoma, heavy reliance was made on chemotherapy, and several drugs have shown marked benefit, including cyclophosphamide, vincristine, actinomycin-D and adriamycin. In a current national study, children with Ewing's sarcoma receive biopsy only of the lesion without amputation. They then receive radiotherapy to the primary tumor, and on a random basis, some children additionally receive prophylactic radiotherapy to both lungs. In addition, all patients receive cyclophosphamide, actinomycin and vincristine, and on a random basis, some children in addition receive adriamycin. At this time, the radiotherapy to the lungs in a prophylactic manner does not appear to improve disease-free survival, but either drug is showing approximately 60 to 70 per cent of children free of disease at two years from diagnosis.

Results in osteogenic sarcoma are perhaps even more dramatic, with the use of large doses of methotrexate and adriamycin as the two primary effective agents. Methotrexate for leukemia is commonly given in a dose of 20 mg/m² or about 1 mg/kg orally once a week. Large doses of methotrexate for osteogenic sarcoma are 100 to 300 mg/kg given intravenously over six hours, followed by citrovorum or folinic acid rescue or 960 mg/m² of methotrexate, given over a 42-hour infusion, again with citrovorum or folinic acid rescue. Remarkably, the folinic acid rescue prevents bone marrow and gastrointestinal toxicity but does not prevent the therapeutic effect. At this time, amputation of the primary lesion is the initial therapy, followed by chemotherapy. If results of chemotherapy continue to show this marked improvement of 50 to 70 per cent of children well after two years, it is possible that in the future, children with osteogenic sarcoma may be able to receive local resection surgery without amputation. This is still speculative, though, and today amputation of the primary lesion is still recommended in most centers.

Retinoblastoma

Retinoblastoma is said to be derived from the embryonic nerve elements of the eye. These tumors have a hereditary predisposition. Inheritance appears to be due to a single dominant gene that either is inherited or arises as a mutation in the patient. Once it exists, the abnormal gene is transmitted to the patient's children as an autosomal dominant with incomplete penetrance, and has been estimated to range between 80 and 90 per cent. Healthy parents who have one affected child without prior family history of the disease have only a 4 per cent chance of having another affected child. Cured patients have been shown to transmit the disease to 20 to 50 per cent of their children.

Retinoblastoma is the most common intraocular tumor of childhood. It occurs bilaterally in about one fourth to one third of cases reported. Onset in the second eye occurs several months, occasionally a year or two, after the disorder has been diagnosed in the first eye.

The care of these patients demands continued follow-up by an ophthalmologist. Treatment consists of enucleation, if a single eye is involved. If the disease is bilateral, radiation therapy and chemotherapy must be considered. Recently, the development of the laser beam has shown promising results in the treatment of this tumor.

Neuroblastoma

Neuroblastoma is said to arise from the ganglia of the sympathetic nervous system, which are located primarily along the vertebral column. The largest single collection of cells is the adrenal medulla. The disease may present as an abdominal mass. Neuroblastoma originating in the adrenal medulla will displace the kidney but not distort the kidney pelvis on intravenous pyelography. In the chest it presents as a posterior mediastinal mass. Neuroblastoma commonly metastasizes to the skull and long bones, and therefore, skeletal survey is part of the diagnostic work-up. Metastases also commonly go to the bone marrow, so that bone marrow examination is a valuable procedure to determine the full extent of the disease.

A 24-hour urine collection for vanillyl mandelic acid (VMA) may also be helpful, since it is often elevated in this disease. The only other tumor that shows this elevation of VMA is the rare pheochromocytoma.

Neuroblastoma, as can be seen in Figure 42–2, is one of the two pediatric solid tumors that remain a treatment enigma. For children who are over two years of age with metastatic disease including bone lesions, we have made no inroads into improving survival rate. Survival time has been increased through combination of cyclophosphamide, given on day 1, with imidiozol carboximide, given on days 1 through 5, and viscristine, given on day 5. This drug combination is repeated every three to four weeks. With this combination, we recently have seen a response rate of 70 per cent in approximately 90 children in the Children's Cancer Study Group, with approximately 50 per cent of the respondants, or 35 per cent of the total, still living at two years. However, most of the children still living at two years have had some recurrence of their disease already. In children with neuroblastoma under two years of age, those who present with an identifiable primary mass in the adrenal or along the perispinal region have a better prognosis, with or without bone marrow involvement, liver involvement or subcutaneous skin nodules. Children who have localized disease with any one of these three metastatic areas are classified as in Stage IV. These children seem to do very well despite whatever therapy they receive, and some children have done well with no therapy. For localized disease that is felt to be totally excised, a recent study has shown that radiotherapy or chemotherapy did not improve survival and a probable cure rate was 95 per cent. In children with a Stage II disease, that is, with gross tumor remaining after surgery, chemotherapy does add some improvement, but for those with Stage III or IV, as mentioned, although survival time has been improved, there has been no improvement in survival rate. Research into this disease continues to be very intensive, and particular immunological parameters are being looked at as possibilities for further therapeutic manipulations.

Central Nervous System Tumors

The common tumors of the first two decades of life are gliomas of the brain stem, optic nerve and cerebellum, pinealomas, craniopharyngiomas and teratomas. Meningiomas, neurofibromas, gliomas of the cerebral hemisphere and pituitary tumors occur most frequently in adults.

Unfortunately, about 50 per cent of all brain tumors are gliomas, which have a very rapid course, with death expected in 6 to 12 months. About 10 per cent of all gliomas are medulloblastomas, which are most frequently seen in infants or young children and are rare after the age of 20.

Brain tumors can present with many diversified symptoms. Therapy, in general, is limited to surgical procedures, although medulloblastomas are said to be moderately influenced by radiation therapy. To date, chemotherapy, both by local arterial perfusion and intravenous administration, has shown no definite additive benefits, but is still early in its inception.

IMMUNOLOGICAL CONSIDERATIONS

Immunotherapy

There is considerable clinical and laboratory evidence suggesting that patients respond immunologically to their tumor. It is intriguing to speculate that the observed spontaneous regression of certain tumors, most notably neuroblastoma in children, and the variation in the duration of maintenance in patients with leukemia may in fact be due to host immune responses. It is known for acute lymphocytic leukemia that patients in remission have cells detectable by biopsy, but not detectable by usual clinical parameters, e.g., in the kidney, and inhibition of progressive disease may be immunologically mediated. This possibility was suggested by Mathé and coworkers in the late 1960's, when they reported that treatment of patients with acute lymphocytic leukemia with an immunostimulant, BCG, or allogeneic leukemic cells or a combination of the two allowed for prolonged remission duration, as compared to untreated controls. Larger studies evaluating the effects of BCG given in addition to chemotherapy for the maintenance of remission in childhood acute lymphocytic leukemia, however, failed to show an effect. Unfortunately, different preparations of BCG were given in different ways, and the patients were induced with differing chemotherapies. Because of the success

with current therapeutic approaches to acute lymphocytic leukemia of childhood, it is unlikely that the earlier approach of Mathé will be directly tested. There is much interest in the immunotherapy of acute myelogenous leukemia. A variety of studies, primarily with adults, suggested that BCG or an extract of tubercle bacilli (MER) with or without leukemic cells from other patients, given in combination with chemotherapy, may prolong remission, as compared to the same chemotherapy alone. To date, some of these studies have not included control groups, while others are too new to draw any conclusions. These approaches are further reviewed by Bernstein and Wright. A number of investigators are also currently evaluating the use of immunostimulants such as BCG or MER given in addition to chemotherapy in the treatment of neuroblastoma. In the next five to ten years, the efficacy of immunological approaches to the treatment of neoplasia in childhood should be determined.

Immunodiagnosis. Immunological approaches are also allowing improved diagnosis of neoplasia. Of most interest to pediatricians is the immunoclassification of acute lymphocytic leukemia. Lymphocytes can be defined as either T cells (which form rosettes with sheep red cells), B cells (which can be identified by having immunoglobulin and complement receptors on their surface) or null cells (which have no surface markers as for T cells or B cells). Leukemia cells from most children with the acute lymphocytic type are null cells. Ten to 25 per cent of children have lymphoblasts that can be shown to be T cells. These tend to occur in older children, who often have mediastinal and other nodal masses and a high peripheral white blood count (20,000). These patients have a poor prognosis and require more aggressive therapy.

REFERENCES

Bernstein, I. D., and Wright, P. W.: Immunology and immunotherapy of childhood neoplasia. Pediatr. Clin. N. Am., 23:93, 1976.

Boles, E. T., Jr.: Tumors of the abdomen in children. Pediatr. Clin. N. Am., 9:467, 1962.

Department of Ophthalmology, Hospital for Sick Children, Toronto: *The Eye in Childhood*. Chicago, Year Book Medical Publishers, 1967.

Mathé, G., Amiel, J. L., Schwarzenbergh, L. *et al.*: Active immunotherapy for acute lymphoblastic leukemia. Lancet *1*:697, 1969.

Owens, G.: Brain tumors. Am. Acad. Gen. Pract., *34*:93, 1966.

Rosewall Park Memorial Institute Symposium: Conflicts in Childhood Cancer, Sept. 19–20, 1974, Buffalo, New York.

Simone, J.: Acute lymphocytic leukemia in childhood. Semin. Hematol., *11*:25, 1974.

Simone, J., Aur, R. S. A., Hustu, H. O., and Pinkel, D.: "Total therapy" studies of acute lymphocytic leukemia in children. Cancer, *30*:1488, 1972.

Sutow, W. W., Vietti, T. J., and Fernback, D. J.: *Clinical Pediatric Oncology*. St. Louis, C. V. Mosby, 1973.

Thomas, E. D., *et al.*: Bone-marrow transplantation. N. Engl. J. Med., *292*(16, 17):832, 895, 1975.

Sudden Infant Death Syndrome

43

Nora E. A. Davis

Few human events have the tragic impact of sudden infant death syndrome (SIDS), commonly known as crib death. It is estimated that approximately 8000 such deaths occur each year in the United States. SIDS kills more infants between the ages of 1 week and 12 months than any other disease and ranks second only to accidents in causes of death in children between 1 week and 15 years of age. The cause is still unknown; it has not been prevented.

A typical pattern emerges surrounding SIDS death. An apparently thriving infant is bedded down for the evening. The next morning, without warning or any intervening outcry, the infant is found dead. Death has come quickly and silently. This is only the beginning of the horror story the parents must endure. The tragedy of SIDS does not end with the death of the baby, but will continue to have a profound impact upon family members.

Pervasive guilt reactions occur among family members, and the psychiatric morbidity is enormous. Parents are overwhelmed with grief; they blame themselves for having done (or not done) something to cause the infant's death. SIDS has occurred only a few hours after a physician has examined the infant and pronounced him in excellent health.

While the health professional cannot aid the deceased infant, another role must be assumed. He must be a compassionate counselor and assist the family to confront this tragedy so they may cope more effectively during their grieving process. A compassionate counselor must assure the family that the death was in no way their responsibility and that SIDS, though still not fully explained, is nevertheless a definite disease entity.

Epidemiology

The epidemiology of SIDS is amazingly constant throughout the world, wherever the disease has been studied. It is estimated that a SIDS death will occur once in every 350 live births. It is more frequently seen in males, low birth weight babies and low socioeconomic class families and during the season of upper respiratory illness, i.e., fall-winter. About half the infants have a history of upper respiratory infection within two weeks before death. Genetic factors do not appear to play a significant role. The unique age distribution of SIDS (Fig. 43–1) has led to much speculation concerning its possible or probable causes.

Clinical Findings

There are two features of the disease that seem to be important. First, death seems to occur during a period of sleep. In our Seattle series of over 550 cases, all infants who were *observed* to die turned out to have some lethal cause demonstrated at autopsy, and thus did not have SIDS. All of our cases of SIDS died during sleep. Second is the apparent silent nature of death. In over one third of our proven cases, adults were sleeping in the same room as the infant but heard no noise during the night. Occasionally, a "crowing noise" from the child's

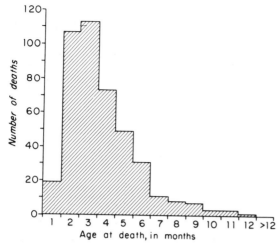

Figure 43–1 Age distribution of 425 sudden infant death syndrome cases from the Seattle study.

crib is heard shortly before finding his lifeless body, but this is rare.

When the infant is discovered, the death scene is often one of disarray. The infant is often discovered with his head covered by the blankets, giving rise to the invidious thought of possible suffocation. It was shown long ago that normal infants cannot suffocate in their usual bed clothing. In many cases, a blood-tinged froth, due to pulmonary edema, exudes from the nostrils and may stain the infant's clothing and sheets.

Pathological Findings

Diagnosis of SIDS can be readily made on the basis of an autopsy, which shows no obvious lethal cause. In about 15 per cent of cases of sudden, unexpected infant deaths a definite cause of death other than SIDS is determined; for example, meningococcemia, subdural hemorrhage or myocarditis. On internal examination, the lungs are filled with hemorrhagic edema fluid, and minor microscopic evidence of respiratory inflammation is often found. Intrathoracic petechiae dot the surfaces of lungs, pericardium and thymus in about 85 per cent of cases and are an important landmark of SIDS. It is believed that increased negative pressure in the thorax against an obstructed airway causes the petechiae. Respiratory viruses are discovered in about a third of cases; they are the same viruses that cause common colds.

Gastric contents appear in the trachea as a post-mortem phenomenon. Diagnosis of aspiration should be made only when bronchial obstruction and distal atelectasis are noted.

Etiology

The cause is unknown. Our Seattle research team feels that the terminal event (or final common pathway) of SIDS is respiratory obstruction of the larynx, mediated through the autonomic nervous system and "triggered" by some contingency factors. Viral inflammatory disease of the upper respiratory tract may be one factor. Death occurs as the result of complete upper airway obstruction, which comes on suddenly during sleep and evokes a brief, noiseless, sometimes agonal struggle. Steinschneider's studies have shown a relationship between sleep apnea, viral infections and SIDS. Naeye has found that SIDS victims have thickened pulmonary arteries characteristic of chronic hypoxia, suggesting that babies are not "normal" before death. Research in developmental neurophysiology should provide more conclusive answers. There is at present no evidence that monitors can prevent SIDS.

Emotional Reactions of Parents

SIDS has been cloaked in mystery and superstition, and guilt is pervasive and universal. Because the cause is unknown, parents feel responsible and often are blamed for their infant's death. There are three aspects of a SIDS death that cause a profound impact on families—the loss of a child, the sudden and unexpected nature of the death and the fact that the cause is unknown. Because the death is a sudden and unexpected happening at home, and not while the child is under medical supervision, SIDS becomes a matter for coroners, police and other legal authorities. They are concerned with establishing whether the death could be attributed to foul play. The grief-stricken parents may be callously questioned at the scene of the death about their "care" of the dead child. Terminology such as pneumonitis, aspiration or suffocation on the death certificate compounds the implication of parental neglect or blame. The fact that the cause of death is unknown again compounds the guilt and self-blame these parents experience. The "if onlys" plague parents' minds as they search for the things they feel they should have done to prevent the death. This feeling of guilt tends to persist with intensity for a considerable period of time, indeed if ever resolved, and can cause great discomfort to the parents.

Immediate and sustained grief reactions are inevitable. Feelings of shock and disbelief may last for several weeks. Common reactions include anger, helplessness and loss of meaning in life. Parents may fear they are losing their minds. There may be major disruptions of routine behavior, i.e., inability to care for family. Over the following weeks, parents often continue to deny the death of their infant, dreams of the dead child are common and there may be expressions of hostile feelings toward close friends and relatives. Reports of alcoholism, depression, suicide, drug abuse and divorce are not uncommon and illustrate the need for immediate supportive intervention. An understanding coroner, physician, nurse or other health professional should be ready to counsel and comfort a stricken family immediately after a SIDS tragedy and for some time thereafter.

Community Support Systems

Many communities have established SIDS management programs in which the health professional will come in contact with the family. The management program consists of four elements:

1. Autopsies should be available on all infants who die suddenly and unexpectedly and should be performed by qualified pathologists.

2. The term "Sudden Infant Death Syndrome" should be noted on the death certificates, when appropriate.

3. Families should be notified, either by telephone or letter, of the autopsy results within 24 hours.

4. Follow-up counseling and information about SIDS should be provided by a knowledgeable health consultant as the need arises.

Some parents who lose a child to SIDS may have long term counseling needs that require ongoing therapeutic psychotherapy. Understandably, this function is best *not* handled by the family's pediatrician or public health worker. Proper management of the SIDS family would then revert to those professionals with a specialization in mental health. Each community SIDS management program should have a mental health back-up system in which referrals of problem families can be made to qualified mental health professionals.

REFERENCES

Beckwith, J. B.: The Sudden Infant Death Syndrome. Curr. Probl. Pediatr., 3:8, 1973.

Bergman, A. B., Pomeroy, M. A., and Beckwith, J. B.: Psychiatric toll of the sudden infant death syndrome. GP, 60:6, 1969.

Canadian Foundation for the Study of Infant Deaths: Sudden Infant Death Syndrome—1974.

National Sudden Infant Death Syndrome Foundation: Facts About Sudden Infant Death Syndrome.

Proceedings of the Second International Conference on Causes of Sudden Death in Infants. Seattle, University of Washington Press, 1970.

Szybist, C.: The Subsequent Child. National Sudden Infant Death Syndrome Foundation, New York.

PART XII

APPENDIX

Growth Charts

NATIONAL CENTER FOR HEALTH STATISTICS PERCENTILE GROWTH CHARTS
FOR BOYS: BIRTH TO 36 MONTHS: LENGTH

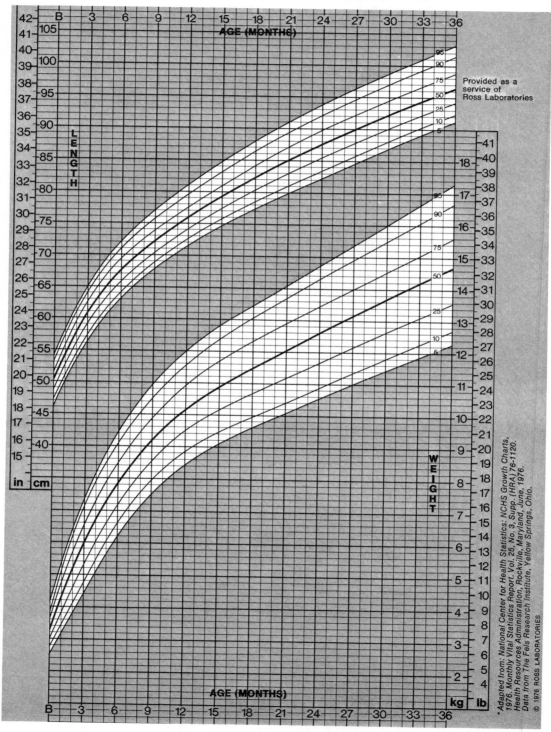

Provided as a
service of
Ross Laboratories

*Adapted from: National Center for Health Statistics: NCHS Growth Charts,
1976. Monthly Vital Statistics Report. Vol. 25, No. 3, Supp. (HRA) 76-1120.
Health Resources Administration, Rockville, Maryland, June, 1976.
Data from The Fels Research Institute, Yellow Springs, Ohio.

© 1976 ROSS LABORATORIES

APPENDIX

The recent National Center for Health Statistics growth charts for birth to 36 months were derived from the data of the Fels Research Institute in Yellow Springs, Ohio, and the growth charts for 2 to 18 years of age were derived from several large recent studies. These charts provide standards for comparing weight growth versus linear growth. The head circumference data only extend to age three years, and therefore, the more complete Nellhaus charts for head circumference are included. The Tanner-Whitehouse growth grids, based on British populations, are the best to use in Britain. The outdated Boston Stuart growth grids, which were developed 30 to 40 years ago, are included because they were the predominant growth charts used during the past 20 years, will be the ones most commonly found in past patient charts, and may still be the ones available to the student in some clinical settings.

NATIONAL CENTER FOR HEALTH STATISTICS PERCENTILE GROWTH CHARTS FOR BOYS: BIRTH TO 36 MONTHS: HEAD CIRCUMFERENCE

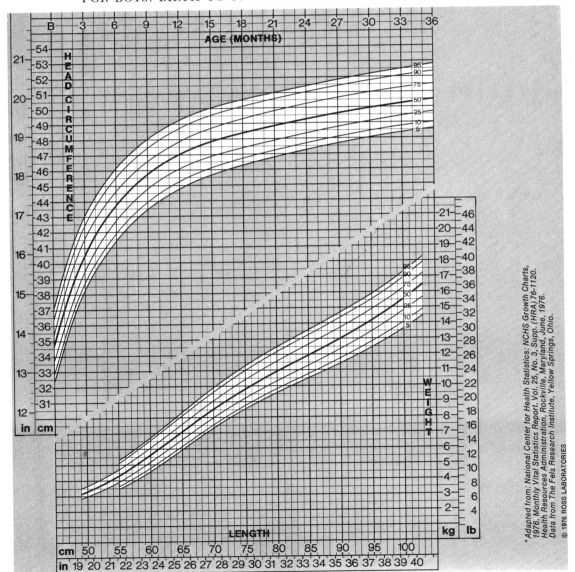

*Adapted from: National Center for Health Statistics: NCHS Growth Charts, 1976. Monthly Vital Statistics Report. Vol. 25, No. 3, Supp. (HRA) 76-1120. Health Resources Administration, Rockville, Maryland, June, 1976. Data from The Fels Research Institute, Yellow Springs, Ohio.

© 1976 ROSS LABORATORIES

NATIONAL CENTER FOR HEALTH STATISTICS PERCENTILE GROWTH CHART
FOR BOYS: 2 TO 18 YEARS

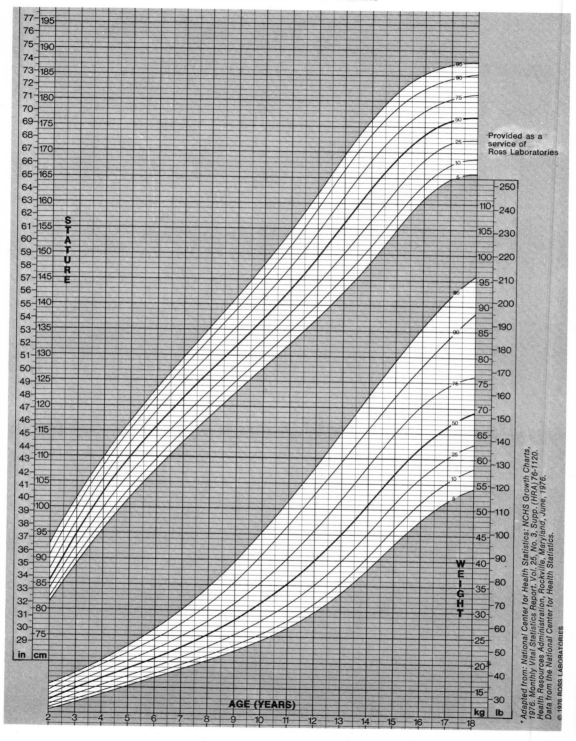

Provided as a service of Ross Laboratories

* Adapted from: National Center for Health Statistics: NCHS Growth Charts, 1976. Monthly Vital Statistics Report. Vol. 25, No. 3, Supp. (HRA) 76-1120. Health Resources Administration, Rockville, Maryland, June, 1976. Data from the National Center for Health Statistics.

© 1976 ROSS LABORATORIES

NATIONAL CENTER FOR HEALTH STATISTICS PERCENTILE GROWTH CHART FOR PREPUBESCENT BOYS

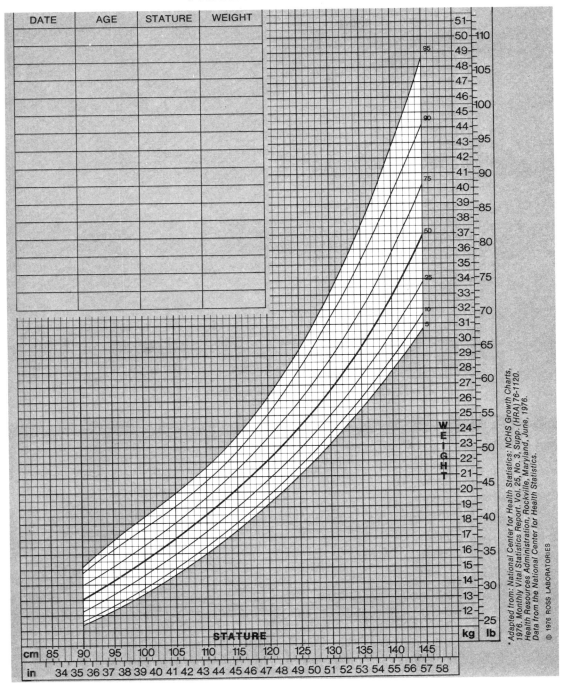

NATIONAL CENTER FOR HEALTH STATISTICS PERCENTILE GROWTH CHARTS
FOR GIRLS: BIRTH TO 36 MONTHS: LENGTH

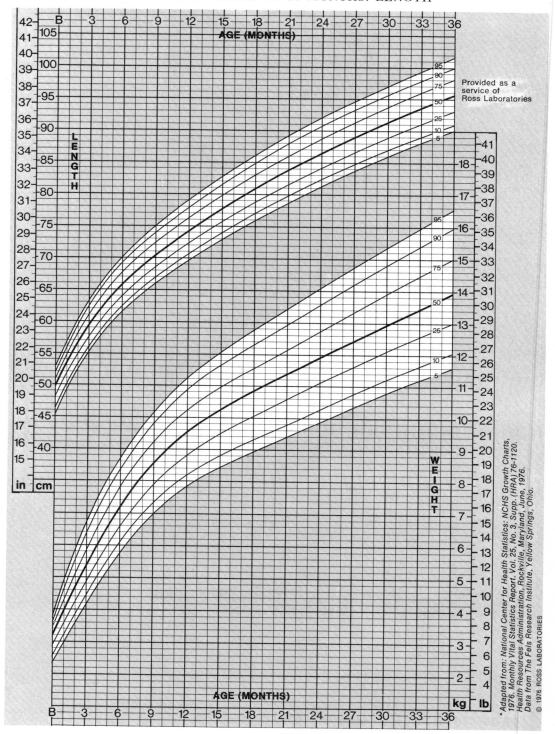

Provided as a
service of
Ross Laboratories

* Adapted from: National Center for Health Statistics: NCHS Growth Charts,
1976. Monthly Vital Statistics Report. Vol. 25, No. 3, Supp. (HRA) 76-1120.
Health Resources Administration, Rockville, Maryland, June, 1976.
Data from The Fels Research Institute, Yellow Springs, Ohio.

© 1976 ROSS LABORATORIES

NATIONAL CENTER FOR HEALTH STATISTICS PERCENTILE GROWTH CHARTS FOR GIRLS: BIRTH TO 36 MONTHS: HEAD CIRCUMFERENCE

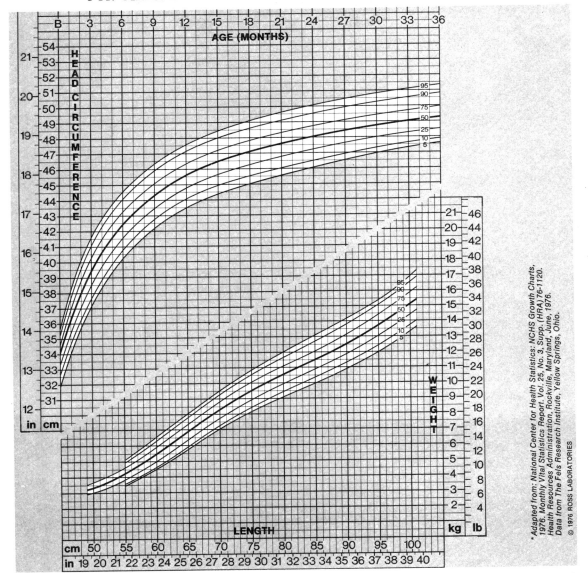

*Adapted from: National Center for Health Statistics: NCHS Growth Charts, 1976. Monthly Vital Statistics Report. Vol. 25, No. 3, Supp. (HRA) 76-1120. Health Resources Administration, Rockville, Maryland, June, 1976. Data from The Fels Research Institute, Yellow Springs, Ohio.

© 1976 ROSS LABORATORIES

NATIONAL CENTER FOR HEALTH STATISTICS PERCENTILE GROWTH CHART
FOR GIRLS: 2 TO 18 YEARS

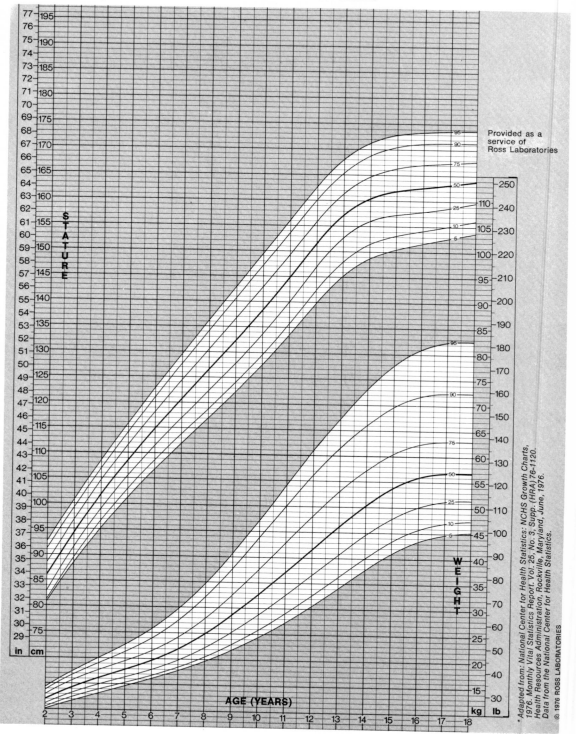

Provided as a
service of
Ross Laboratories

* Adapted from: National Center for Health Statistics: NCHS Growth Charts, 1976. Monthly Vital Statistics Report. Vol. 25, No. 3, Supp. (HRA) 76-1120. Health Resources Administration, Rockville, Maryland, June, 1976. Data from the National Center for Health Statistics.

NATIONAL CENTER FOR HEALTH STATISTICS PERCENTILE GROWTH CHART
FOR PREPUBESCENT GIRLS

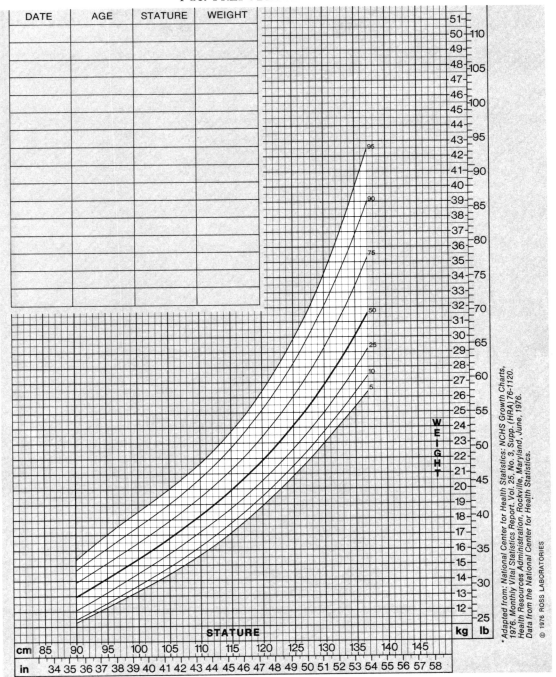

DATE	AGE	STATURE	WEIGHT

*Adapted from: National Center for Health Statistics: NCHS Growth Charts, 1976. Monthly Vital Statistics Report. Vol. 25, No. 3, Supp. (HRA) 76-1120. Health Resources Administration, Rockville, Maryland, June, 1976. Data from the National Center for Health Statistics.

© 1976 ROSS LABORATORIES

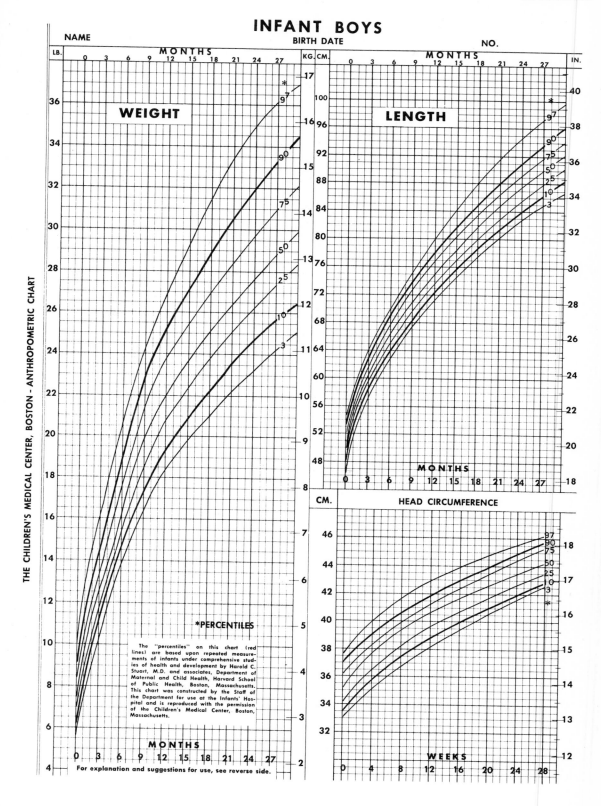

INFANT BOYS

NAME   **BIRTH DATE**   **NO.**

WEIGHT

LENGTH

HEAD CIRCUMFERENCE

THE CHILDREN'S MEDICAL CENTER, BOSTON - ANTHROPOMETRIC CHART

*PERCENTILES

The "percentiles" on this chart (red lines) are based upon repeated measurements of infants under comprehensive studies of health and development by Harold C. Stuart, M.D. and associates, Department of Maternal and Child Health, Harvard School of Public Health, Boston, Massachusetts. This chart was constructed by the Staff of the Department for use at the Infants' Hospital and is reproduced with the permission of the Children's Medical Center, Boston, Massachusetts.

For explanation and suggestions for use, see reverse side.

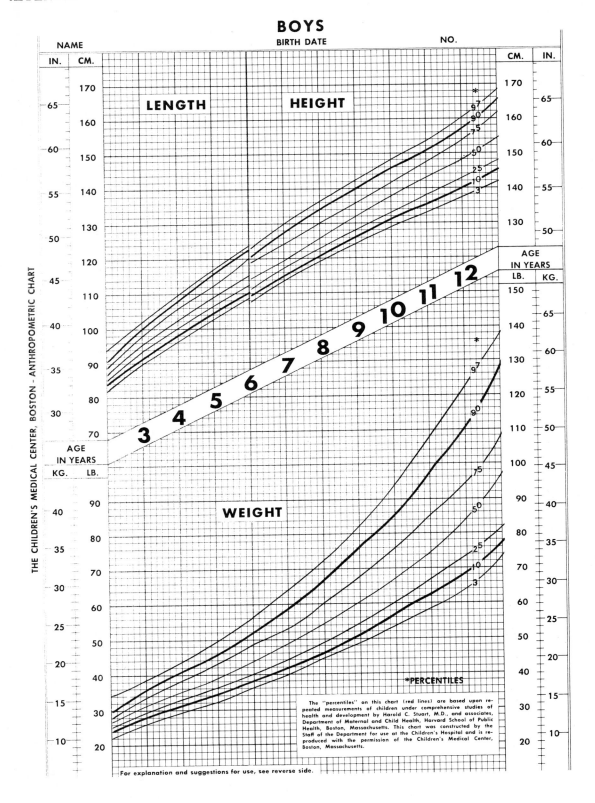

BOYS

NAME   BIRTH DATE   NO.

LENGTH   HEIGHT

WEIGHT

AGE IN YEARS

3 4 5 6 7 8 9 10 11 12

*PERCENTILES

The "percentiles" on this chart (red lines) are based upon repeated measurements of children under comprehensive studies of health and development by Harold C. Stuart, M.D., and associates, Department of Maternal and Child Health, Harvard School of Public Health, Boston, Massachusetts. This chart was constructed by the Staff of the Department for use at the Children's Hospital and is reproduced with the permission of the Children's Medical Center, Boston, Massachusetts.

For explanation and suggestions for use, see reverse side.

THE CHILDREN'S MEDICAL CENTER, BOSTON - ANTHROPOMETRIC CHART

INFANT GIRLS

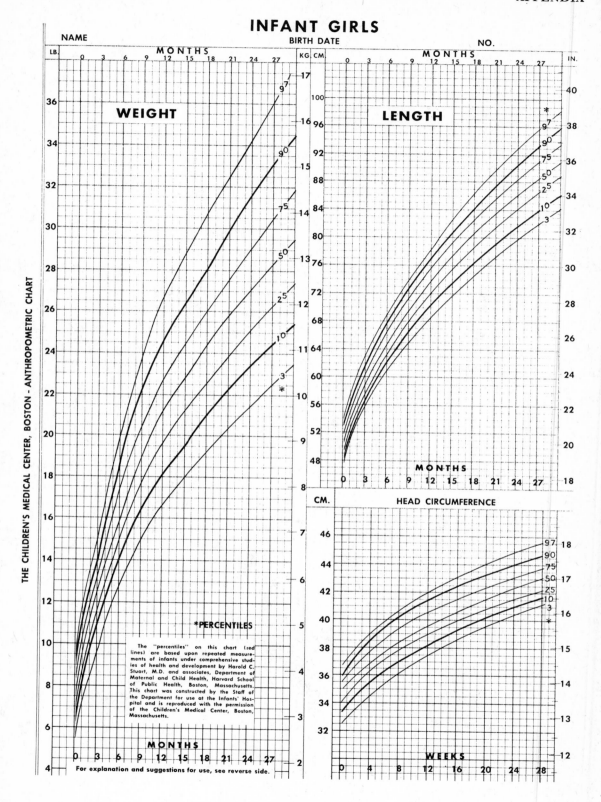

NAME   BIRTH DATE   NO.

WEIGHT

LENGTH

THE CHILDREN'S MEDICAL CENTER, BOSTON - ANTHROPOMETRIC CHART

*PERCENTILES

The "percentiles" on this chart (red lines) are based upon repeated measurements of infants under comprehensive studies of health and development by Harold C. Stuart, M.D. and associates, Department of Maternal and Child Health, Harvard School of Public Health, Boston, Massachusetts. This chart was constructed by the Staff of the Department for use at the Infants' Hospital and is reproduced with the permission of the Children's Medical Center, Boston, Massachusetts.

MONTHS

For explanation and suggestions for use, see reverse side.

HEAD CIRCUMFERENCE

MONTHS

WEEKS

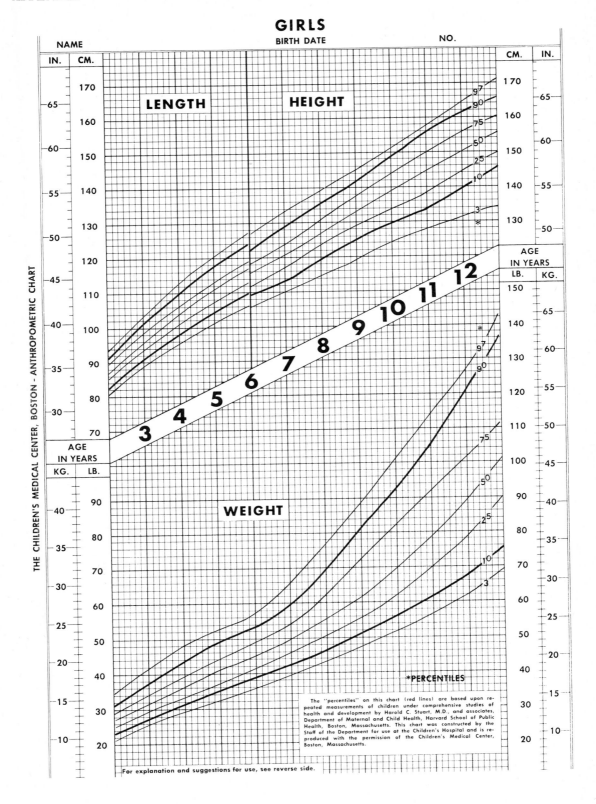

GIRLS

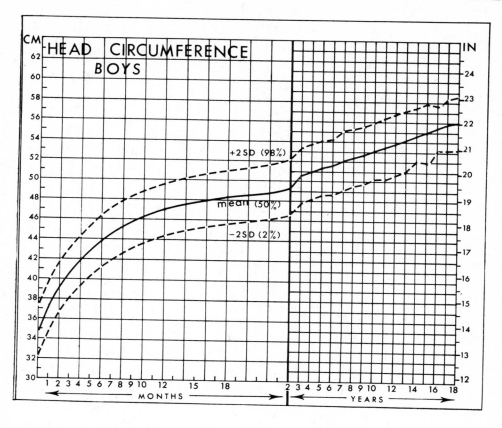

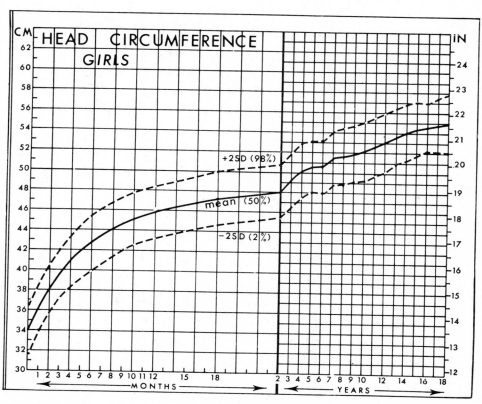

APPENDIX

THICKNESS OF TRICEPS AND SUBSCAPULAR SKINFOLDS AT VARIOUS AGES[*]

Age (months)	Percentiles	S.D.	Triceps (mm) Males	Triceps (mm) Females	Subscapular (mm) Males	Subscapular (mm) Females
1		−2	2.9	3.5	3.1	3.8
	10		4.0	4.5	4.2	4.9
	25		4.7	5.2	4.8	5.4
	50		5.3	5.8	5.6	6.2
	75		6.2	6.7	6.5	7.0
	90		7.0	7.6	7.5	7.9
		+2	8.1	8.3	8.3	9.0
3		−2	4.5	5.0	3.5	4.7
	10		6.0	6.2	4.9	5.9
	25		6.8	7.2	5.8	6.9
	50		8.1	8.2	6.9	8.0
	75		9.2	9.2	8.1	8.6
	90		10.3	10.5	9.0	9.4
		+2	11.7	11.8	10.7	11.1
6		−2	6.3	6.7	3.8	4.0
	10		7.8	8.2	5.5	5.9
	25		8.6	9.0	6.2	6.9
	50		9.7	10.4	7.1	8.1
	75		11.1	11.3	8.4	8.9
	90		11.8	12.7	10.1	10.3
		+2	13.5	13.9	11.0	12.4
9		−2	6.0	6.7	3.4	4.7
	10		7.5	7.9	5.3	6.0
	25		8.7	8.8	6.0	6.7
	50		9.9	10.1	7.1	7.6
	75		11.2	11.3	8.5	8.8
	90		12.5	12.5	9.7	10.1
		+2	14.0	13.5	11.4	11.1
12		−2	6.2	6.4	3.8	4.5
	10		7.8	7.6	5.3	6.0
	25		8.6	8.7	6.0	6.5
	50		9.8	9.8	7.2	7.5
	75		11.1	11.2	8.6	8.7
	90		12.2	12.2	9.6	9.8
		+2	13.8	13.6	11.0	10.9
18		−2	6.4	6.8	3.9	4.2
	10		7.7	7.9	5.3	5.7
	25		8.6	8.9	6.0	6.2
	50		9.9	10.3	6.8	7.1
	75		11.4	11.3	7.9	8.0
	90		12.2	12.3	9.3	9.0
		+2	13.6	13.6	10.3	10.2
24		−2	5.8	6.5	3.0	3.9
	10		7.4	8.3	4.6	5.3
	25		8.5	8.9	5.4	5.6
	50		9.8	10.1	6.5	6.5
	75		11.6	11.6	7.4	7.3
	90		13.1	12.8	8.3	8.4
		+3	14.2	14.1	10.2	9.5
36		−2	6.6	6.4	2.9	2.6
	10		7.8	8.2	4.5	4.7
	25		9.0	9.4	5.0	5.2
	50		9.8	10.3	5.5	6.1
	75		11.0	11.5	6.4	7.2
	90		12.2	12.5	7.1	8.6
		+2	13.4	14.4	8.9	10.6

[*] Based on data of Karlberg *et al.*: Acta Pediatr. Scand. (Suppl. 187): 48, 1968.

The Denver Developmental Screening Test: Clinical Utility

The Denver Developmental Screening Test (DDST) is a reliable and easily administered tool for assessing the developmental progress of children from birth to six years of age. Standardized on a large, mixed-racial sample of Denver, Colorado, infants and children in 1967, it is presently the most widely used and accepted developmental screening test. It can be used by physicians and a wide variety of health care professionals, once they are familiar with its administration.

It consists of 105 selected items divided into four major developmental sectors, i.e., gross motor (large muscle), fine motor (small muscle), language and personal-social (self-help skills). Each item is represented by a bar indicating the range between when 25 per cent of children pass it and when 90 per cent of children have mastered it. Many of the items, particularly those during the first year of life, are well-known developmental milestones that should be very familiar to professionals caring for infants and children.

The DDST, as its name indicates, is a screening instrument. It is not an intelligence test and does not yield an IQ score. Within the broad range of normal development this test does not predict subsequent school performance. Its purpose is to identify the child who is developing at an unusually slow rate so that appropriate investigative and intervention measures can be undertaken. By validation comparisons with the Stanford-Binet Intelligence Scale, it has been shown to be quite accurate at recognizing the developmentally abnormal child. Thus it is a particularly valuable tool for the practitioner during the first two years of life before the time when traditional psychological tests are given.

As with any instrument, the DDST must be appropriately administered and carefully scored in order to be interpreted meaningfully. Administration usually requires 15 to 30 minutes, and a prepared kit with blocks, rattle, bell and ball is needed. On the illustrated test form, a straight line is drawn from top to bottom at the child's chronological age. Items passed are so marked. Any item entirely to the left of the age line that is not passed is considered to be a failure or delay. Some items, as indicated, may be passed by parent's report, while others must be observed by the examiner.

Over-all test interpretation is divided into three categories: normal, abnormal or questionable. Development is considered abnormal if (1) two or more sectors each have two or more delays or (2) one sector has two or more delays *and* one other sector has one delay and in the same sector the age line does not intersect an item that is passed. Development is considered questionable if (1) any one sector has two or more delays or (2) one or more sectors have one delay *and* in the same sector the age line does not intersect an item that is passed. Children with abnormal or questionable tests are possibly developmentally retarded and deserve follow-up investigation.

Forrest C. Bennett, M.D.
Fellow in Child Development
University of Washington
Department of Pediatrics

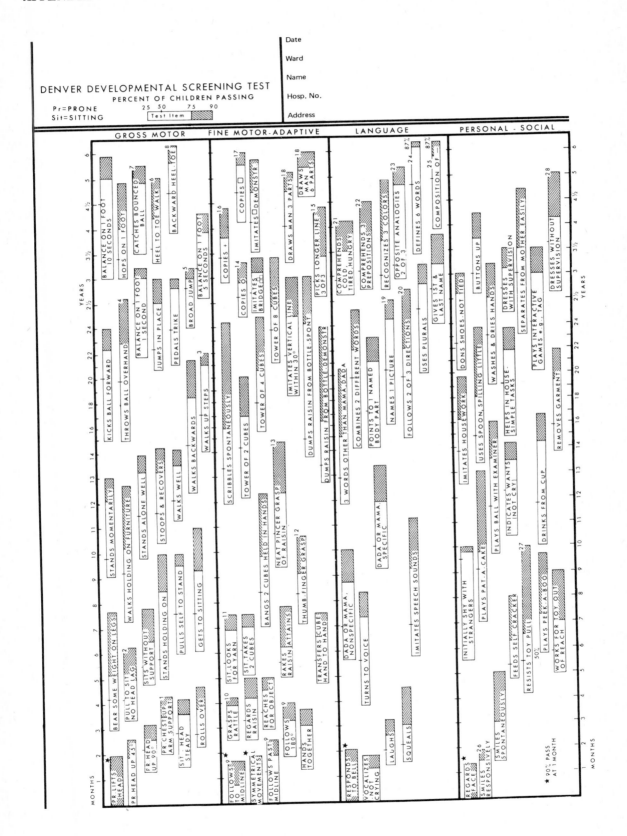

DENVER DEVELOPMENTAL SCREENING TEST

Date

Ward

Name

Hosp. No.

Address

DIRECTIONS

1. Infant, when prone, lifts chest off table with support of forearms and/or hands.
2. Examiner grasps child's hands, pulls him from supine to sitting, child has no head lag.
3. Child may use wall or rail only, not person, may not crawl.
4. Child throws ball overhand 3 feet to within examiner's reach.
5. Child performs standing broad jump over width of test sheet.
6. Ask child to walk forward, ⬤⬤⬤⬤⬤→ heel within 1 inch of toe.
7. Examiner bounces ball to child, child must catch with hands (2 of 3 trials).
8. Ask child to walk backwards, ←⬤⬤⬤⬤⬤ toe within 1 inch of heel.
9. Examiner moves yarn in arc from side to side 1 foot above baby's head. Note if eyes follow 90° to midline (past midline; 180°).
10. Infant grasps rattle when touched to his finger tips.
11. Child looks after yarn dropped from sight over table's edge.
12. Child grasps raisin between thumb and index finger.
13. Child performs overhand grasp of raisin with tips of thumb and index finger.

14. Copy: Pass any enclosed form. Do not demonstrate. Do not name form.

15. "Which line is longer?" (Not bigger.) Turn paper upside down, repeat (Pass 3 of 3).

16. Pass crossing lines, any angle.

17. Have child copy first. If fail, demonstrate. Pass figure with 4 square corners.

18. When scoring, symmetrical parts count as one (2 arms or 2 eyes count as one part only).
19. Point to picture and have child name it.

20. Examiner asks child to: "Give block to Mommie, put block on table, put block on floor" (2 of 3). Caution: Examiner not to gesture with head or eyes.
21. Child answers 2 of 3 questions: "What do you do when you are cold? hungry? tired?"
22. Examiner asks child to: "Put block on table, under table, in front of chair, behind chair." Caution: Examiner not to gesture with head or eyes.
23. Examiner asks child: "Fire is hot, ice is____. Mother is a woman, dad is a____. A horse is big, a mouse is____." (Pass if 2 of 3 are correct.)
24. Ask child to define 6: ball; lake; desk; house; banana; curtain; hedge; pavement. Pass if defined in terms of use, structure, composition or classification.
25. Examiner asks: "What is a spoon made of? a shoe made of? a door made of?" (No other objects may be substituted.) Must pass all 3.
26. Examiner attempts to elicit a smile by: smiling, talking or waving to infant, do not touch, baby smiles responsively in 2 or 3 attempts.
27. When child is playing with toy, pull it away from him. Pass if he resists.
28. Child need not be able to tie shoes or button in the back.

W. K. Frankenburg, M.D. and J. B. Dodds, Ph.D., Univ. of Colo. Medical Center, Denver, Colo.

DATE AND BEHAVIORAL OBSERVATIONS

(how child feels at time of the evaluation, relation to examiner, attention span, verbal behavior, self-confidence, etc.):

FOOD AND NUTRITION BOARD, NATIONAL ACADEMY OF SCIENCES–NATIONAL RESEARCH COUNCIL
RECOMMENDED DAILY DIETARY ALLOWANCES,ᵃ Revised 1974

Designed for the maintenance of good nutrition of practically all healthy people in the U.S.A.

	Age (years)	Weight (kg)	Weight (lbs)	Height (cm)	Height (in)	Energy (kcal)ᵇ	Protein (g)	Vita-min A Activity (RE)ᶜ	Vita-min A Activity (IU)	Vita-min D (IU)	Vita-min E Activityᵉ (IU)	Ascor-bic Acid (mg)	Fola-cinᶠ (µg)	Nia-cinᵍ (mg)	Ribo-flavin (mg)	Thia-min (mg)	Vita-min B₆ (mg)	Vita-min B₁₂ (µg)	Cal-cium (mg)	Phos-phorus (mg)	Iodine (µg)	Iron (mg)	Mag-nesium (mg)	Zinc (mg)
Infants	0.0–0.5	6	14	60	24	kg × 117	kg × 2.2	420ᵈ	1,400	400	4	35	50	5	0.4	0.3	0.3	0.3	360	240	35	10	60	3
	0.5–1.0	9	20	71	28	kg × 108	kg × 2.0	400	2,000	400	5	35	50	8	0.6	0.5	0.4	0.3	540	400	45	15	70	5
Children	1–3	13	28	86	34	1,300	23	400	2,000	400	7	40	100	9	0.8	0.7	0.6	1.0	800	800	60	15	150	10
	4–6	20	44	110	44	1,800	30	500	2,500	400	9	40	200	12	1.1	0.9	0.9	1.5	800	800	80	10	200	10
	7–10	30	66	135	54	2,400	36	700	3,300	400	10	40	300	16	1.2	1.2	1.2	2.0	800	800	110	10	250	10
Males	11–14	44	97	158	63	2,800	44	1,000	5,000	400	12	45	400	18	1.5	1.4	1.6	3.0	1,200	1,200	130	18	350	15
	15–18	61	134	172	69	3,000	54	1,000	5,000	400	15	45	400	20	1.8	1.5	2.0	3.0	1,200	1,200	150	18	400	15
	19–22	67	147	172	69	3,000	54	1,000	5,000	400	15	45	400	20	1.8	1.5	2.0	3.0	800	800	140	10	350	15
	23–50	70	154	172	69	2,700	56	1,000	5,000		15	45	400	18	1.6	1.4	2.0	3.0	800	800	130	10	350	15
	51+	70	154	172	69	2,400	56	1,000	5,000		15	45	400	16	1.5	1.2	2.0	3.0	800	800	110	10	350	15
Females	11–14	44	97	155	62	2,400	44	800	4,000	400	12	45	400	16	1.3	1.2	1.6	3.0	1,200	1,200	115	18	300	15
	15–18	54	119	162	65	2,100	48	800	4,000	400	12	45	400	14	1.4	1.1	2.0	3.0	1,200	1,200	115	18	300	15
	19–22	58	128	162	65	2,100	46	800	4,000	400	12	45	400	14	1.4	1.1	2.0	3.0	800	800	100	18	300	15
	23–50	58	128	162	65	2,000	46	800	4,000		12	45	400	13	1.2	1.0	2.0	3.0	800	800	100	18	300	15
	51+	58	128	162	65	1,800	46	800	4,000		12	45	400	12	1.1	1.0	2.0	3.0	800	800	80	10	300	15
Pregnant						+300	+30	1,000	5,000	400	15	60	800	+2	+0.3	+0.3	2.5	4.0	1,200	1,200	125	18+ʰ	450	20
Lactating						+500	+20	1,200	6,000	400	15	80	600	+4	+0.5	+0.3	2.5	4.0	1,200	1,200	150	18	450	25

ᵃ The allowances are intended to provide for individual variations among most normal persons as they live in the United States under usual environmental stresses. Diets should be based on a variety of common foods in order to provide other nutrients for which human requirements have been less well defined. See text for more detailed discussion of allowances and of nutrients not tabulated. See Table I (p. 6) for weights and heights by individual year of age.

ᵇ Kilojoules (kJ) = 4.2 × kcal.

ᶜ Retinol equivalents.

ᵈ Assumed to be all as retinol in milk during the first six months of life. All subsequent intakes are assumed to be half as retinol and half as β-carotene when calculated from international units. As retinol equivalents, three fourths are as retinol and one fourth as β-carotene.

ᵉ Total vitamin E activity, estimated to be 80 percent as α-tocopherol and 20 percent other tocopherols. See text for variation in allowances.

ᶠ The folacin allowances refer to dietary sources as determined by *Lactobacillus casei* assay. Pure forms of folacin may be effective in doses less than one fourth of the recommended dietary allowance.

ᵍ Although allowances are expressed as niacin, it is recognized that on the average 1 mg of niacin is derived from each 60 mg of dietary tryptophan.

ʰ This increased requirement cannot be met by ordinary diets; therefore, the use of supplemental iron is recommended.

CHEMISTRY LABORATORY REFERENCE STANDARDS FOR CHILDREN'S ORTHOPEDIC HOSPITAL

Test	Age	Source	Value
Albumin	NB and infant	P, S	2.9–5.5 g/dl
	Child and adult		
Aldolase	NB–1 yr	P, S	0.5–16 IU/l @ 37°C
	Child		1–8
	Adult		1–6
Ammonia	Adult	B1: Art.	up to 70 ⎫
		Ven.	up to 140 ⎬ μg/dl
Alanine Amino transferase (ALT) (SGPT)°	Infant	P, S	up to 54 IU/l @ 30°C
	Child–adult		1–25
	may be higher in premature and jaundiced infants		
Amylase	NB to 2 mo	P, S	may be undetectable
	2 mo–1 yr		incr. to adult level
	Adult		60–160 U/dl @ 37°C
Aspartate Amino transferase (AST) (SGOT)°	NB	P, S	2–55 IU/l @ 30°C
	over 2 yr		10–30
	Child-adult		5–20
Bilirubin, Total	up to 24 hr	P, S	up to 6 mg/dl
	up to 48 hr		up to 7.0
	3–5 days		up to 12
	1 mo–adult		0.2–0.8
(conjugated) Direct			0–0.3
Blood Gases			
pH	Child and adult	B1: Art.	7.35–7.45
		Ven.	7.32–7.42
PCO_2	NB–2 yr	Art.	26–40 mm Hg
	Child and adult	Art.	35–45
	All ages	Ven.	41–51
PO_2	NB	Art.	60–70 mm Hg
	Child and adult	Art.	80–90
	All ages	Ven.	25–40
BUN		P, S	6–20 mg/dl
Calcium, total	Premature first wk	S	6.0–10.0 mg/dl
	Full term first wk		7.0–13.0
	Child and adult		9.0–11.0
Cholesterol	NB	P, S	50–120 mg/dl
	Up to 1 yr		70–170
	2–16 yr		95–195
	Adult		120–255
Creatinine	NB–6 mo	P, S	0.1–1.0 mg/dl
	6 mo–2 yr		0.2–0.8
	Child		0.2–1.0
	Adult		0.2–1.2
Creatine kinase	NB, Prem.	P, S	0–170 @ 30°C
	NB, 3 mo		25–110
	Child and adult		4–75
CSF			
Glucose			45–55% of Plasma glucose
Protein, total	NB		up to 120 mg/dl
	Child and adult		up to 40
Electrolytes		P, S	
Na	NB		132–142 mEq/l
	Child and adult		135–145
K	NB		5.0–7.5 mEq/l
	2 days–3 mo		4.0–6.2
	Child and adult		3.5–5.5
Cl	NB		96–106 mEq/l
	Child and adult		97–104
CO_2 content			18–27

CHEMISTRY LABORATORY REFERENCE STANDARDS FOR CHILDREN'S ORTHOPEDIC HOSPITAL (*Continued*)

Test	Age	Source	Value
Glucose	0–24 hr 24–48 hr Child and adult	P	50–75 mg/dl 40–90 60–105
Iron, total	NB 4–10 mo 3–10 yr Adult	P, S	110–270 µg/dl 30–70 53–119 72–186
Iron Binding Capacity	NB Adult	P, S	59–175 µg/dl 250–400
Lactic Dehydrogenase (LDH)	NB Child Adult	S	up to 1000 IU/l @ 30°C gradual decrease to adult values 30–120
Magnesium	NB Child Adult	P, S	1.5–2.3 mEq/l 1.4–1.9 1.3–2.5
Osmolality		P, S	275–295 mOsm/kg
Phenylalanine	NB Child	S	up to 4.0 mg/dl 0.7–3.0
Phosphatase, Alk.	NB Child Adolescent Adult	P, S	70–260 IU/l at 30°C up to 275 up to 180 (higher in males) 20–80
Phosphorus, inorganic	NB Child Adult	P, S	4.2–9.0 mg/dl 4.0–6.0 3.0–4.5
Protein, total	NB up to 4 yr 4 yr–adult	S	4.6–7.0 gm/dl 5.5–7.5 6.0–8.2
Total Thyroxine, T_4	1–3 day 1 wk–1 mo 1–4 mo 4 mo–6 yr 6–10 yr Adult	S	11–23 µg/dl 9–18 7.5–16.5 5.5–14.5 5.0–12.5 4.0–12.0
Uric Acid	Child or Adult, F Adult, M	P, S	2.0–6.0 mg/dl 3.0–7.0
Miscellaneous Sweat Chloride Fecal Fat Urine osmolality	 72 hr collection Early infancy Child and adult		 up to 50 mEq/l up to 10% of total fat intake 50–600 mOsm/kg 50–1400

Definition of symbols: P = plasma   F = female
                        S = serum   M = male
                        NB = newborn   °Alternate designation
                        dl = 100 ml

These reference data represent a combination of laboratory experience at Children's Orthopedic Hospital and Medical Center and literature references.

Recommended References: Meites, S. (Ed.): *Pediatric Clinical Chemistry: A Survey of Normals, Methods and Instrumentation, with Commentary.* In press, September 1976.

Elizabeth K. Smith, Ph.D.
Director of Chemistry Laboratory
Children's Orthopedic Hospital and Medical Center
Seattle, Washington

REFERENCES

Frankenburg, W. K., and Dodds, J. B.: The Denver Developmental Screening Test. J. Pediatr., 71:181, 1967.

Frankenburg, W. K., Goldstein, A. D., and Camp, B. W.: The revised Denver Developmental Screening Test: Its accuracy as a screening instrument. J. Pediatr., 79:988, 1971.

INDEX

Note: *Italicized* page numbers indicate illustrations; numbers followed by (t) indicate tables.